THE EPIDEMIOLOGY OF CHILDHOOD DISORDERS

THE EPIDEMIOLOGY OF CHILDHOOD DISORDERS

Edited by

Ivan Barry Pless

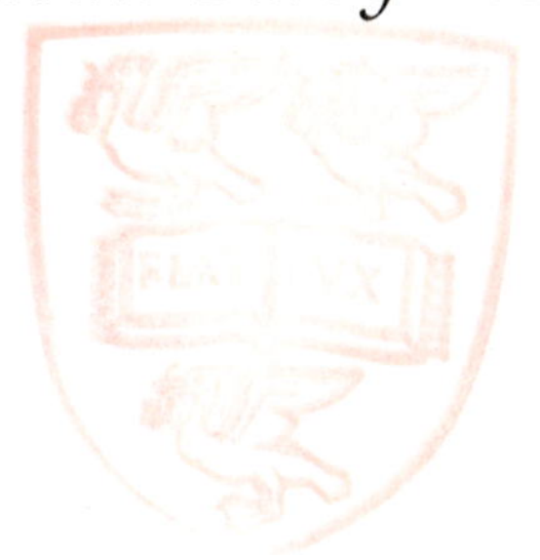

New York Oxford

OXFORD UNIVERSITY PRESS

1994

Oxford University Press

Oxford New York Toronto
Delhi Bombay Calcutta Madras Karachi
Kuala Lumpur Singapore Hong Kong Tokyo
Nairobi Dar es Salaam Cape Town
Melbourne Auckland Madrid

and associated companies in
Berlin Ibadan

Published by Oxford University Press, Inc.
200 Madison Avenue, New York, New York 10016

Library of Congress Cataloging-in-Publication Data
The Epidemiology of childhood disorders /
[edited by] Ivan Barry Pless.
p. cm. Includes bibliographical references and index.
ISBN 0-19-507516-1
1. Pediatric epidemiology.
I. Pless, Ivan B. (Ivan Barry).
[DNLM: 1. Child Development Disorders—epidemiology.
2. Child Behavior Disorders—epidemiology.
3. Pediatrics.
WS 16 E64 1993] RJ106.E65 1993
614.5′992—dc20
DNLM/DLC for Library of Congress 93-9760

1 3 5 7 9 8 6 4 2

Printed in the United States of America
on acid-free paper

Foreword

Epidemiologic thinking can be traced to the Hippocrateian days and epidemiology has been considered a basic science for the prevention of infectious diseases for more than a century. During the last fifty years epidemiology has become a distinct discipline with its own principles and methods and a broad spectrum of applications. These include investigations of outbreaks, identification of component causes of chronic, frequently non-infectious diseases, study of perinatal, developmental, and behavioral disorders, and the evaluation of diagnostic and therapeutic procedures, as well as macro-systems of health care.

A correlate of this expansion of epidemiology has been the publication of over fifty textbooks presenting, in variable depth and different emphasis, the principles and methods of the new discipline. By contrast, there have been relatively few books presenting the considerable substantive epidemiologic knowledge that has accumulated concerning specific categories of diseases or medical specialties. This is particularly striking with respect to childhood disorders, for which there is a wealth of epidemiologic information that has transformed the way we understand, prevent, treat and care for these disorders. "The Epidemiology of Childhood Disorders", superbly contributed to by a group of distinguished authors and masterly edited by Professor I.B. Pless, will successfully fill this gap.

The book is most valuable because it combines breadth and depth, highlights what is important and reasonably established, discusses what is controversial, avoids dogmatism and respects modern epidemiology's principles, rigor and, not least, terminology. The introductory part offers an outline of epidemiologic concepts and methods that should be useful to those less familiar with the theory and practice of epidemiology. The second chapter of this part discusses longitudinal studies with quantitative or qualitative outcome variables critical in growth and development. Parts I to V represent the main body of the book and cover the whole range of pediatric epidemiology, from perinatal disorders and infectious diseases to chronic disease, injuries, and behavioral problems.

The Epidemiology of Childhood Disorders is an important book. It summarizes the successes and outlines the problems in pediatric epidemiology. It represents a comprehensive and clearly written review of what is currently known about the epidemiology of childhood disorders. Readers of the book, whether medical students, physicians, pediatricians, epidemiologists or other health professionals, will come to appreciate the elegance and enormous potential of epidemiology, as applied to childhood disorders.

Boston
January 1993

Dimitrios Trichopoulos, M.D.
Vincent L. Gregory Professor of
Cancer Prevention and Epidemiology
Chairman, Department of Epidemiology
Harvard School of Public Health

Preface

It is perhaps not too great an exaggeration to claim that much of the most useful knowledge about the diseases of children has come from epidemiologic studies of one kind or another. The truth of this speaks not only to the vast improvements in the techniques employed by epidemiologists, especially over the last 30 years, but also to the increasing breadth of the territory over which the discipline lays claim.

Epidemiology has helped define the magnitude and patterns of occurrence of pediatric problems with ever greater precision and has done so in a manner that has yielded powerful clues to etiology. Studies of risk factors have increased our understanding of why and how children become ill. This, in turn, has led to proven or promising forms of intervention, from vaccines to seatbelts. Moreover, modern epidemiology has been applied with growing success to evaluate the outcomes of various forms of therapy, as well as other strategies intended to improve the health of children, such as screening. The results of these evaluation studies have often been sobering, forcing clinicians or public health officers to reign in unwarranted enthusiasms.

Concomitant with the growth of pediatric epidemiology has been a dramatic improvement in the health of children. Although all scientists know better than to attribute causality to such an association of events, the temptation is great. Whatever the true relationship, the benefits of the expansion of epidemiologic knowledge about child health have been manifold.

Until now the emphasis in textbooks has been on the methods of epidemiologic inquiry or on the facts needed by clinicians to help diagnose and treat children. This concentration has spawned many excellent texts, but few have attempted to summarize the substantive epidemiologic knowledge that has accumulated with amazing rapidity. If the distinction between "methods" and "substantive" books is a useful one, this text belongs almost entirely in the latter domain. With the exception of the first two chapters, all the authors have addressed a topic with a body of knowledge that is sufficiently rich to merit a comprehensive review. This book makes no pretense that all important areas have been addressed. What it does do, however, is to range widely enough to include not only the "old morbidity," but many elements of the "new morbidity" as well.

Thus, the contributors to this volume have succeeded in covering the large body of knowledge that has accumulated about the epidemiology of many of the important diseases of childhood. For most of these conditions, that knowledge includes detailed information about the patterns of occurrence, along with important data about risk factors. In addition, the effectiveness of various preventive or therapeutic interventions is highlighted in most chapters.

Until now, this knowledge has been scattered widely. It is found in a large number of sources, ranging from texts on specialized topics to a bewildering array of journals. The latter include mainstream, general pediatric publications, and specialist journals (i.e., organ or system-specific), as well as the epidemiologic, public health, and maternal and child health literature. Yet, no single text has addressed this topic as a whole. Hence, the task for any student, teacher, or investigator wishing to have these data at her or his fingertips has been a daunting one. This book seeks to fill this gap, drawing on the wisdom, experience, and skill of acknowledged experts.

The intention is to be comprehensive while avoiding excessive detail. It is assumed that most readers will make full use of the extensive references provided by each author to obtain whatever additional, more specific information they require. The contributors have each reviewed their topic in a consistent and lucid fashion. All but the introductory and concluding chapters have a similar structure. A brief overview is followed by a summary that describes, for the nonmedical reader, the salient biologic points about the disorder(s) under consideration. For example, the chapter on asthma reviews the main features of the pathophysiology, along with the evidence for genetic and allergic etiologic factors.

The main emphasis in each chapter, however, is on the patterns or frequency of occurrence. This section summarizes the most recent and accurate estimates of the incidence or prevalence of each disorder and provides basic descriptive data not readily available from other sources. Where appropriate, it also reviews what is known about major differences in rates of occurrence by age, sex, social class, and temporal trends. For example, in many instances the incidence and prevalence of the main disorders of childhood have changed markedly over the period during which reasonably accurate data have been available. The reader is reminded that some of these apparent changes may be due to altered definitions, classification, diagnostic criteria, or methods of data collection. Yet, to the extent that rates are comparable and show interesting trends, they are reviewed. In the case of malignancies, for example, although there may have been few changes over the last several decades with respect to the rate of occurrence, there has been a dramatic improvement in survival, which, of course, affects prevalence figures. National or international variations are considered as well. For example, there are striking national differences in suicide and in mortality resulting from unintentional and intentional injuries (violence) in childhood and adolescence. Frequently, these differences shed light on etiologic factors or on the relative success of various approaches to prevention or control.

Each chapter also includes a section on risk factors. For many readers this may prove to be the most interesting and useful section. Certainly for clinicians this discussion will be of great value, as will the section on interventions. The choice of this broad term enables the contributors to deal with the issue generically. Accordingly, equal attention is devoted (as justified by the available data) to interventions that have prevented the occurrence of some diseases (and thereby modified their incidence) and to the influence of effective therapies on survival.

The introductory chapters remind readers of the basic terms, concepts and methods used, with a special emphasis on longitudinal studies. The intention is to ensure that readers unfamiliar with epidemiologic language and methods will not be intimidated by the subsequent contributions. This introductory section is followed by three chapters dealing with perinatal disorders: prematurity, birth defects, and genetic disorders. Part II addresses infectious diseases: congenital, respiratory, gastrointestinal, and communicable. In Part III the mental and behavioral disorders are reviewed: mental retardation, emotional, and suicide. Part IV covers both intentional and unintentional injuries, which together account for as many deaths in childhood as all other causes combined. The next section, Part V, addresses several prototypical chronic disorders: asthma, malignancies, and cerebral palsy. The concluding chapter examines the rapidly growing body of data linking childhood disorders to those of adults.

The contributors are those whose work in specific disorders is recognized internationally. Some have been leaders in their field of interest for decades. Their goal, in brief, has been to review pediatric epidemiology both from the perspective of knowledge about etiology (traditional, or population epidemiology) and knowledge about outcomes (clinical epidemiology). It is hoped that this text will become the main resource for those requiring an expert, comprehensive overview of this field. It is intended to provide the epidemiologic information needed to complement the rapidly expanding body of clinical knowledge and thereby help maintain an appropriate perspective on the health problems of children.

Montreal, Canada
September 1993

I. B. P.

Acknowledgments

As editor, I wish to express my enormous gratitude to all the contributors to this volume. Each was motivated by the conviction that the very substantial effort required would benefit other scientists and the children they serve.

Spectrum Holobyte generously provided copies of their award-winning computer game "Tetris" for all the authors. This no doubt helped break the tedium of manuscript preparation and may explain some of the delays!

The support of Canada's National Health Research and Development Program, Health and Welfare, through my National Health Scientist Award, made it possible for me to devote the time needed to bring this book together, as did the hospitality of the Child Accident Prevention Trust during a sabbatical year in London. Charles Pless provided invaluable assistance in the preparation of the index, as did Diane Léger in the coordination of the entire undertaking.

I also wish to acknowledge the inspiration and guidance of Carol Buck, Bob Oseasohn and Bob Haggerty, each of whom prompted so many young investigators to look to epidemiology for answers to socially important questions that affect the health of children. Thanks too, to other mentors, now deceased, whose influence on me and other would-be pediatric epidemiologists, was pivotal: Donald Reid, Abe Adelstein, Ronnie MacKeith, Jack Connelly, and John Cassel.

My greatest debt is to my family for their forbearance, and especially to my always patient and loving wife, Ann, to whom this book is dedicated.

Contents

Part III Mental and Behavioral Disorders

Part IV Injuries and Violence

Part V Chronic Disorders

Contributors

Eva Alberman MD, FFCM, FRCP, FRCOG
Professor Emeritus
The Department of Preventive and Environmental Medicine
The Wolfson Institute of Preventive Medicine
London, England

Jessie Anderson MD, PhD, FRANZCP
Senior Lecturer
Department of Psychological Medicine
University of Otago
Dunedin, New Zealand

Caryn Bern, MD, MPH
Medical Epidemiologist
Viral Gastroenteritis Unit
Maternal and Child Nutrition Branch
Division of Nutrition
National Center for Chronic Disease Prevention and Health Promotion
Centers for Disease Control and Prevention
Atlanta, Georgia USA

Eve Blair, PhD
Research Officer
The Western Australian Research Institute for Child Health
Australia

Katherine Kaufer Christoffel MD, MPH
Professor, Pediatrics, Community Health & Preventive Medicine
Northwestern University Medical School
Attending Physician
Division of General & Emergency Pediatrics
Children's Memorial Hospital
Chicago, Illinois USA

Joseph T.R. Clarke, MD, PhD, FRCP(C), FCCMG
Professor, Department of Pediatrics
University of Toronto
Director, Division of Clinical Genetics
Departments of Pediatrics and Genetics
Hospital for Sick Children
Toronto, Canada

Roger I. Glass, MD
Chief
Viral Gastroenteritis Unit
Centers for Disease Control
Altanta, Georgia USA

Neil M.H. Graham, MBBS, MD, MPH, FAFPHM
Associate Professor
Departments of Epidemiology and Medicine
The Johns Hopkins University School of Medicine
School of Hygiene and Public Health
The Johns Hopkins University
Baltimore, Maryland USA

Roger Hicks, BA
Research Associate
Columbia University, College of Physicians & Surgeons
New York State Psychiatric Institute
New York, New York USA

Helene Koller, MS
Senior Associate
Department of Pediatrics
Albert Einstein College of Medicine
Bronx, New York USA

Ian Leck, MB, PhD, DSc, FRCP, FFPHM
Professor Emeritus
formerly, Professor of Epidemiology
University of Manchester
Manchester, England

Stuart Logan, MD
Senior Lecturer
Department of Paediatric Epidemiology
Institute of Child Health
London, England

Edward A. Mortimer, Jr., MD
Elisebeth Severance Prentiss Professor and Vice Chairman
Professor of Pediatrics
Department of Epidemiology and Biostatistics
School of Medicine Case Western Reserve University
Cleveland, Ohio USA

Terry Nolan, BMedSc, MBBS, PhD, FRACP
Senior Lecturer
Department of Paediatric Epidemiology
Head, Clinical Epidemiology and Biostatistics Unit
Royal Children's Hospital
Melbourne, Australia

Catherine S. Peckham, MD, FRCP
Professor
Department of Paediatric Epidemiology
Institute of Child Health
London, England

I.B. Pless, CM, MD, FRCP(C)
National Health Scientist
Professor of Pediatrics, and Epidemiology and Biostatistics
McGill University
Montreal, Qeubec, Canada

Christopher Power, PhD
Senior Lecturer
Department of Paediatric Epidemiology
Wolfson Child Health Monitoring Unit
Division of Public Health
Institute of Child Health
London, England

Fred P. Rivara, MD, MPH
Professor of Pediatrics
Director
Harborview Injury Prevention and Research Center
Seattle, Washington USA

Stephen A. Richardson, PhD
Professor Emeritus
Departments of Pediatrics and Epidemiology/Social Medicine
Albert Einstein College of Medicine
Bronx, New York USA

David Shaffer MB, BS, FRCP, FRCPsych.
Iriving Philips Professor of Child Psychiatry
Columbia University, College of Physicians & Surgeons
New York State Psychiatric Institute
New York, New York USA

Fiona J. Stanley, MD, FFPHM
Director, WA Research Institute for Child Health
Professor, Department of Paediatrics
University of Western Australia
Australia

Charles A. Stiller, MA, MSc
Research Statistician
Department of Paediatrics
University of Oxford
Childhood Cancer Research Group
Oxford, England

Michael E.J. Wadsworth, PhD
Director
Medical Research Council National Survey of Health and Development
Visiting Professor
Department of Epidemiology and Public Health
University College London
London, England

John Scott Werry, MD
Formerly, Professor and Head Chairman
Department of Psychiatry & Behavioural Science
School of Medicine, University of Auckland
Auckland, New Zealand

THE EPIDEMIOLOGY OF CHILDHOOD DISORDERS

1

Concepts, Terms, and Methods

I.B. PLESS

This chapter is intended to help readers who may be unfamiliar with some of the concepts, terms or methods used in epidemiology. The goal is to walk a thin line between providing sufficient knowledge to understand the subsequent chapters while avoiding the appearance of a mini-, how-to-do-it text. In short, this introduction is not meant to be a crash course in epidemiology and biostatistics.

The word "epidemiology" comes from the greek **epi** (upon), **demos** (people) and **logos** (the study of) and describes "the study of the distribution and determinants of diseases and injuries in human populations" (Mausner et al., 1985). It is also used in a broader sense to include the application of epidemiologic methods to the control of health problems. It follows that an epidemiologist is one who either studies patterns of disease or seeks to control them.

When defined in this manner, epidemiology can be viewed as a science in its own right or as an arm of public health. As a science, it is used to study the causes of disease or the outcomes of treatments or other interventions. In this context it is closely allied with biostatistics, and distinctions between the two are increasingly blurred. As a branch of public health, epidemiology helps define the magnitude and distribution of health problems and their risk factors. In both its research and applied manifestations, there are descriptive and inferential divisions.

Epidemiology's role in policy and program formulation in public health is complex, and in child health it often appears under the rubric of "Maternal and Child Health." Such programs encompass a variety of traditional as well as novel approaches to the care of children, as does pediatrics itself. The key distinction arises from the target or focus. For clinical pediatrics, the main concern is individual children or their families. When, however, the focus is on groups or populations of children, the clinical issues become epidemiologic.

Pediatric Epidemiology

Pediatric epidemiology deserves special attention for several reasons. First and foremost, but often overlooked, most childhood diseases are not simply variants of conditions with the same name found among adults. For example, the pediatric heart diseases are most often congenital, and therefore their etiology and prognosis are entirely different from the common, acquired cardiac diseases of adults. Furthermore, many conditions are found **only** among infants and children. Birth defects and illnesses in the perinatal period are obvious examples.

Second, because growth and development are so critically important in pediatrics, epidemiologic studies of children must take special account of changes over time. Doing so is often far from simple.

Third, pediatric epidemiology often includes parents (usually mothers), as well as children; hence, the pervasive combination of Maternal and Child Health. Child health problems have maternal origins (genetic, intrauterine, or obstetric events). Parents are central to communication in child health, both as proxy respondents and as intermediaries between physician and child. They transmit information (e.g., physician's orders) and are often responsible for administering treatment (and thus compliance). Accordingly, special techniques are needed to address this unusual duality.

Finally, pediatric epidemiology now requires a special place because the body of knowledge about childhood disorders has mushroomed in the last several decades. Although much of this information is found in standard textbooks, the epidemiologic aspects are often neglected, and even the most recent texts do little to remedy this failing.

This book attempts to provide much of what is missing, not only for clinicians and those responsible for child health programs but also for epidemiologists. The chapters describe substantive divisions of pediatric epidemiology, chosen because each contains a significant body of knowledge, and together they cover many of the important disorders of children. Yet, because the growth of epidemiologic knowledge has been so rapid, this book does not (and could not) pretend to be comprehensive. Many disorders are omitted: some because they are too rare or too technical and others because not enough is known to warrant a full chapter. In the end, difficult choices had to be made, and many of the exclusions are certain to appear arbitrary.

Other Branches of Epidemiology

Historically, epidemiology's roots grew out of the burden of infectious diseases that dominated health concerns until the early part of the 20th century. In the years following World War II, as noninfectious diseases came to displace infectious diseases as major sources of morbidity and mortality, interest in the former led to the development of chronic disease epidemiology. Subsequent divisions of epidemiology then emerged along disease lines (cancer, heart disease), particular forms of investigation (pharmacoepidemiology), or age groups (perinatal, pediatric, geriatric). It is important to stress, however, that despite their seeming diversity, the methods of inquiry remain constant: they form a core set of tools applicable to any health problem.

Terms and Concepts: An Evolutionary Process

As the discipline of epidemiology has advanced, many of the terms and concepts used have been subjected to increasing scrutiny. Inevitably, suggestions have been made for better, more apt, or seemingly more "correct" terms. To minimize confusion, whenever possible the definitions used in this chapter are those provided in *A Dictionary of Epidemiology* (Last, 1988). This dictionary reflects more than John Last's personal preferences: it is a handbook sponsored by the International Epidemiological Association and represents a consensus of the views of more than 60 contributing editors and an even larger number of corresponding editors. Although disagreement still surrounds many of these definitions, the nature of this disagreement is often esoteric and hair-splitting and need not concern most readers. Most terms are, of necessity, only reviewed briefly, and quotations without further attribution originate from *A Dictionary of Epidemiology* (Last, 1988).

The terms introduced in this chapter underlie the discipline of epidemiology and thus require careful consideration. A **hypothesis** is simply "a supposition or conjecture." Those of interest to researchers are formulated to be tested and then either accepted or refuted. They may arise from previous work, reflection, or imagination and even from folklore. **Pathogenesis** describes the mechanisms by which an etiologic agent produces disease and subsumes **etiology**, which is defined as "the cause or causes that initiate pathogenesis." A broader definition of etiology is "all factors that contribute to the occurrence of disease." It is therefore a matter of proximity to the initial cause that distinguishes these terms.

An **association** is the "statistical dependence between two or more events, characteristics, or other variables." However, the extensive discussion in Last makes it clear that this concept is not a straightforward one. In part, this is because it is usually laden with words and phrases tinged with hints of causality, despite the fact that we are reminded that "an association may be fortuitous or may be produced by various other circumstances; the presence of an association does not necessarily imply a causal relationship." When considering causal pathways, however, a useful distinction arises between "direct" and "indirect" association. The former represents an association that is *not* via a known third variable. An indirect association arises when a factor is associated with a disorder because both are related to a common underlying factor or when the two are associated with an intermediate or intervening factor. In this sense, then, a direct association is closer to the outcome in a causal pathway.

A **determinant** is "any factor (event, characteristic, etc.) that brings about change in a health condition." Accordingly, a **dependent** (or outcome) variable is one that depends on the effect of other variables in the relationship under study. For example, in linear regression, the dependent variable is predicted by the regression equation. An **independent** (or predictor) variable is "the characteristic being observed or measured that is hypothesized to influence an event."

The concept of risk carries with it a quantitative element. Strictly used, it is "the probability that an event will occur." It follows that a **risk factor** is virtually any variable that "on the basis of epidemiological evidence is known to be associated with ill health." An important distinction should be made when referring to a risk marker. This term should be reserved for an exposure associated with an adverse outcome, but one that is not viewed as causal.

Exposure defines those who "have been exposed to, or subjected to, a supposed cause of a disease or health state, or who have a characteristic that determines the health outcome under examination." For example, children who have not been immunized and who have not already experienced measles are "exposed" or at risk for contracting measles. In the context of infectious disease epidemiology, exposure is "proximity to a source of a disease agent such that transmission is possible." For other epidemiologists, it is the "*amount* of a factor to which a person at risk is exposed"; this definition gives rise to several surprisingly complex considerations.

Consider attempting to define exposure for the risk of an injury to a child bicyclist. Are those exposed all who are of bike-riding age, say 5 to 14 years; all who own or have access to bicycles; only those who use them often or regularly; or only those times when bicycles are actually in use?

To complicate matters further, "exposed" can also be used to denote protective effects (e.g., of a vaccine or the use of a bike helmet) and thus may be viewed as "positive risk factors." If one group of children who receive a vaccine are defined as those who are exposed and they experience the target disease significantly less often than others who do not receive the vaccine, exposure would in this case lower the risk, i.e., be protective.

To summarize, previously the shorthand phrase "at risk" was used. It should now be evident that a complete specification of this concept must include the notion of exposure, as well as consideration of time intervals and the presumption that no competing cause or event (such as death) acts during the time period in question. The fundamental point is that groups at risk cannot include those not exposed, whether it is because they have died, moved away, are the wrong sex, already have the disease, or are immune to it.

The broadening of epidemiology has led to the view that any factor may be an "exposure" or "outcome." To illustrate, bike helmet use may be the exposure of interest in a study assessing the protective effects of helmets following motor vehicle accidents, whereas for a health education initiative, bike helmet use following school visits may be the outcome of interest.

Measures of Risk

As has been stated, the related ideas of risk and exposure are essential to a proper understanding of **effect measures**—those that assess the effect of a factor on the frequency or risk of a health outcome. The critical issue is that those in the denominator must only include those who are able to experience the disease. Although this concept is elementary, it is frequently overlooked. It would be foolish, for example, to include all children under 18 years in a study of risk factors for teenage pregnancies, because neither boys, nor pre-pubertal girls, nor those who are already pregnant are "at risk."

Relative Effects

Relative risk (RR) or risk ratio may be viewed as a descriptive statistic, but it is most often found in analytic studies. It is one of the two main ways that rates can be compared. The term describes the ratio of the risk of a disease among those exposed to a risk factor, compared to the risk among those not exposed

(RR = Ie/Io). As with incidence and prevalence, all its variants are less confusing when the underlying idea is clearly understood.

There is, however, a confusing (and somewhat contentious) side to this term. RR is sometimes used as a synonym for the **odds ratio** (OR), although that is incorrect. Arithmetically, they are different because OR is the ratio of two odds (the probability of an event occurrence to the probability of its nonoccurrence). In betting, the odds of a win is the ratio of the chance or probability of winning to the chance or probability of losing. Risks range from 0 to 1, whereas odds may take any value from 0 to infinity. The OR is used in case-control studies (see later section) where the direct estimation of the probability or risk of an event is not possible because sampling is by outcome (or disease status). In epidemiology, odds ratios are the ratios of the odds of exposure in cases relative to exposure in controls. Thus, if Pe is the probability of exposure among cases and Po the probability of exposure for controls, the formula is as follows:

$$\mathrm{OR} = \mathrm{Pe}(1 - \mathrm{Po}) \,/\, \mathrm{Po}(1 - \mathrm{Pe})$$

It can be shown that when the outcome is rare, the RR and OR estimates are equivalent. (Unfortunately, statisticians are often reluctant to say how rare is rare).

Absolute Effects

Attributable risk (AR) is the *difference* between two risks and describes the extent to which disease can be attributed to a risk factor. It can be estimated for a population (**Population Attributable Risk** or PAR) or as an attributable fraction among the exposed (AFe). Either way, it is important to distinguish this risk difference measure from the relative risk (RR). The latter—which is a ratio of risks—serves as an estimate of the strength of the association between exposure and outcome. Accordingly, it is used in making inferences about causality (see previous). In contrast, the PAR is the risk in the exposed *minus* the risk in the nonexposed and thus indicates the frequency that the outcome in question may be attributed to the exposure in the population being sampled. Its main application is, therefore, in public health studies where it helps the investigator to determine what the effect of a preventive or therapeutic intervention is likely to be in a particular setting.

The PAR is similar to the **etiologic fraction** (EF) which measures "the *proportion* of all cases of outcome in the target population that are attributable to the exposure. Alternatively, the EF can be interpreted as the proportion of cases of the outcome that would disappear if exposure were eliminated in the target population" (Kramer, 1988). EF and RR are closely related, as can be seen from the formula: $\mathrm{EF} = \mathrm{Pe}(\mathrm{RR}-1)/\mathrm{Pe}(\mathrm{RR}-1)+1$, where Pe is the prevalence of exposure in the target population. When RR and other risk factors are constant, the EF can be used to compare populations with different prevalences of exposure.

Consider the example of hypercholesterolemia and assume that its prevalence in a population of children is 0.001. Even with an RR of 20, the PAR is only 1.9%. Conversely, a risk factor with a much lower RR—for example, 2.0 for maternal smoking and otitis media among preschoolers—could have a much larger PAR because so many mothers smoke. For example, if the prevalence of maternal smokers is estimated to be 20%, the PAR would be 16.7%. Therefore, if all pregnant women were to stop smoking, 16.7% of all otitis media among their children would be eliminated.

An analogous measure for preventive exposures (e.g., immunization) is the **preventable fraction** (PF). It measures the proportion of disease in the target population that would be prevented if the population was exposed to the preventive (or protective) factor (e.g., immunization) and is estimated as PF = 1 − RR. To illustrate, assume that chicken pox affects 80% of those exposed and that with complete immunization the rate would fall to 20%. The immunization PF in this example is then 75%. Expressed differently, if the RR for chicken pox following immunization is 0.25, then PF = 0.75 (for other examples, see Chapter 9).

Validity and Bias

Validity, or truth, for epidemiologists is most easily understood if we accept that its antonym is "error," which can be either systematic or nonsystematic, e.g., random. The distinction between the two concepts is critical. Systematic error is a potential source of bias and must always be considered as a possible explanation for associations that seem to be statistically significant. Nonsystematic error is "noise," which is usually assumed to be distributed randomly.

Random error is most easily thought of as "sampling" error. That is, any observed association depends on the particular sample drawn from the universe or population of all subjects comprising the target population. Different random samples from this population will necessarily provide different estimates of association. However, if the study was repeated on different samples, the differences in estimates due to random error would cancel out, i.e., the estimates would converge toward the true association. Statistical testing, which considers this theoretical notion of repeat sampling, quantifies the (un)certainty due to random error of any observed association.

Systematic error, or bias, would not cancel out with repeat studies. A biased study therefore provides a distorted estimate of the true association. Systematic error may occur during any stage of the research process. For such error to distort an estimate of association, however, the bias must occur differentially across the study groups. A bias occurring with equal frequency and magnitude in both groups under study would lead to an estimate of association that was diluted to the null, but it would not be biased. In this situation, however, the ability to generalize would be severely compromised.

Validity, taken broadly, refers to the "degree to which the inferences drawn from a study, including, or especially, generalizations beyond the study sample, are warranted when account is taken of the study methods, representativeness of the sample, and nature of the source population."

Two types of validity are commonly considered: internal and external. **Internal validity** addresses the extent to which observed differences in outcome between groups may be attributed **only** to the hypothesized exposure under investigation (in which case some would say that a causal association has been "proven"). It asks this question: Is the conclusion drawn about an association based on these data correct, or may the association have occurred by chance? A related question asks whether the conclusion that there is no association is incorrect because there is insufficient power, i.e., too few subjects.

External validity (or generalization) exists if the results can "produce unbiased inferences regarding a target population beyond the subjects in the study." It addresses the extent to which seemingly valid findings can safely be applied more widely. This question arises because most studies are conducted on samples from a larger population. Clearly, the more unusual or atypical the sample, the more difficult it is to argue that the findings are widely applicable.

Validity is optimized when bias can be excluded. Estimating the magnitude and direction of potential biases, and the ways in which they can be controlled, eliminated, or minimized, is the essence of modern epidemiology. The task is not only to recognize when they occur but also to identify their sources: sampling, measurement, other problems in data collection, weak design, inappropriate analyses, or even unconscious prejudice. Although some texts provide a shopping list of biases, most can be classified as various forms of selection bias, information bias, or confounding, although these categories are not always distinctive.

As Rothman (1986) explains, **selection bias** arises when two or more groups are being compared for disease or exposure frequency. In this context, selection bias "is a distortion of the effect measured; it results from procedures used to select subjects that lead to an effect estimate among subjects included in the study different from the estimate obtainable from the entire population theoretically targeted for study." Examples include self-selection and diagnostic bias.

Information bias originates from errors in obtaining the information needed to compare groups. "Information bias can occur whenever there are errors in the classification of subjects, but the consequences of the bias are different depending on whether the classification error on one axis of classification (either exposure or disease) is independent of the classification on the other axis"—differential misclassification for those that are not independent, and nondifferential misclassification for those that are. Other forms of information bias include recall or reporting bias.

Confounding is, as Rothman asserts, a central concept in modern epidemiology. It arises from "a mixing of effects. Specifically, the estimate of the effect of the exposure of interest is distorted because it is mixed with the effect of an extraneous factor." To be confounding, the extraneous variable must have the following three characteristics: (1) it must be a risk factor for the disease, (2) it must be associated with the exposure, and (3) it must not be an intermediate step in the causal path between exposure and disease (Rothman, 1986).

These are the main categories of bias. However, Sackett (1979) has actually listed 57 biases, and no doubt many others remain to be elucidated. For, as has been stated, in many respects, the avoidance, detection, and correction of bias are central to epidemiology. Much of the art and science of epidemiologic research hinge on the appropriate use of sampling, design, measures, and analyses to minimize or eliminate as many as possible of these sources of error. Systematic error may lead to false conclusions about the presence of a significant association or the reverse, i.e., that of no association when in truth one exists. However, when one can predict the direction of a bias that cannot be controlled, it may be possible to adjust interpretations of the results to account for that bias. A conservative interpretation, for example, applies when bias diminishes differences and yet differences are found. The reverse, however, is of much greater concern, i.e., bias leading to conclusions about relationships that do not actually exist.

Even under the assumption of an internally valid study (i.e., results that are free from bias), any conclusions drawn from data must consider the potential for one of two errors of hypothesis testing. A type I or α error occurs when one rejects the null hypothesis, H_0, when in fact H_0 is true. That is, the observed statistically significant association is actually due to chance or random error. At a declared level of significance of 5%, a Type 1 error will occur on average once in 20 "significant" studies. A type II or β error occurs when one rejects the alternative hypothesis, H_A, when H_A is true. In this case the observed "null result" has occurred because the sample size is too small to be able to detect the true association. In statistical jargon, the study lacks "power."

Causality and Inference

Inference, as used in philosophy and specifically in logic, describes the "process of passing from observations and axioms to generalizations." Analogously, in statistics it refers to "the development of generalizations from sample data, usually with calculated degrees of uncertainty."

Inference is central to epidemiology because most epidemiologic research leads to inductive processes—reasoning about causality from observations generated to test hypotheses. Each study that supports a hypothesis provides evidence to confirm the conviction that a causal relationship has been established. This is taken as tantamount to the belief that a general principle of nature, or truth, has been characterized.

The study of disease in children proceeds with the goal of identifying causes of these diseases based on data gathered from nature. In this sense, the data, whether clinical observations, laboratory values, or epidemiologic results, are a window into nature. And, as with any window, what one initially sees through it may not be a true representation of what is on the other side.

Scientists quickly learn to appreciate the distinction between association and causality. Thus, most recognize that not all things that follow are caused by those that precede them—the ever-present trap of reasoning "post hoc, ergo propter hoc" (after this, therefore related to this). However, many remain unaware of the sophisticated level to which disagreements about the essence of causality have risen. Although the debate over when, if ever, a causal relationship can be *proven* is long standing, over the last few decades it has resurfaced. Because not all associations are causal and because causation is a matter of judgment not calculation, there remains disagreement about how such judgments should be formed.

Causality: The Traditional Paradigm

Most of the fundamental disagreements about causal inference are well described elsewhere. Readers who wish to gain a better understanding of this central issue in the philosophy of science are encouraged to consult one of several excellent sources, including *The Logic of Scientific Discovery* (Popper, 1968) and *Causal Inference* (Rothman, 1988). The contentious issues are as follows: Traditionally, epidemiology has used a linear paradigm to examine causal relationships. In other words, an exposure or agent is assumed to *cause* a particular outcome. A hypothesis is then formally stated in the null form; that is, "no relationship exists between maternal drug use of DES and subsequent vaginal carcinoma in an offspring." This general idea is restated in operational, measurable terms, and armed with a null hypothesis the investigator then designs a study and analytic approach to test it. The actual testing of the hypothesis requires data and statistical models to compare the data gathered to that expected under the assumption that the null hypothesis is true.

Statistical testing estimates the probability of obtaining the study result by chance alone given that the null hypothesis is true. This probability is then used to either "accept" or "reject" the null hypothesis, on the basis of an arbitrary level of "significance," usually a P value of less than 5%. Recently, however, researchers have been urged to express results using confidence levels—"a rate, constructed so that the range of values (confidence limits) has a specified probability of including the true value of the variable."

Each null hypothesis H_0 has a mirror alternative hypothesis H_A. In this example, the H_A states that maternal DES use is associated with childhood neoplasia. Rejection of H_0 (i.e., $P < 0.05$) therefore implies "acceptance" of the H_A; that is, that a statistical association between exposure and outcome exists. It is then inferred that a causal relation has been established.

Causality assessment is, however, much more complex than simple statistical testing. First, statistical tests assume the study findings to be internally valid—free from bias or systematic error. Thus, results from studies using designs that minimize the potential for bias are judged superior. In addition, broader criteria, which address the totality of evidence, are also used to determine the degree of belief in any assessment of causality.

Historically, the origins of criteria for causation may be traced to the canons formulated in 1856 in *A System of Logic* (Mill, 1856). Canons are strategies for thinking logically, and Mill intended them to be used as a basis from which causality could be inferred. These strategies describe formal ways to establish that two events are causally related.

The criteria currently in use are also based on the postulates that Koch (1884) specified

> should be met before a causative relationship can be accepted between a particular bacterial parasite or disease agent and the disease in question: 1. The agent must be . . . present in every case of the disease by isolation in pure culture. 2. The agent must not be found in cases of other disease. 3. Once isolated, the agent must be capable of reproducing the disease in experimental animals. 4. The agent must be recovered from the experimental disease produced (Last, 1988).

In their modern expression, the criteria used owe much to Sir Austin Bradford Hill, the British statistician (Hill, 1965). Although frequently modified, their essence remains unchanged despite the fact that they are often overinterpreted.

Hill's list was only intended to help in the synthesis of evidence that a relationship could reasonably be viewed as causal. He never proposed a formal scoring system for use by the researcher to gauge how close the data came to "proving causality." Consequently, any such criteria serve best as elements that investigators need to keep in mind when considering the conclusiveness of their own work or that of others. Only one is truly a *sine qua non* for causality—temporality, that a cause must always precede its effect. The others include strength, consistency, specificity, biologic gradient, plausibility, coherence, experimental evidence, and analogy.

With these in mind, readers can assess the results summarized in this volume. Although in some circles formal systems have evolved based on these or similar considerations to facilitate a critical assessment of scientific reports, no such attempt is made in this text. The contributors, themselves experts in their respective fields, have exercised their best judgments about the validity of the conclusions from the studies they cite.

Alternative Causal Paradigms

As has been stated, not all subscribe to the traditional inferential or inductive approach. The main opposition comes from the hypothetico-deductive school, which denies that causality can ever be inferred from observations. It contends that only deductions from first principles (or axioms)—as are made by mathematicians—can provide such evidence and that in the real world of epidemiology this process rarely applies. Although the generals in this battle are philosophers of science, the foot soldiers include many distinguished epidemiologists.

Hypothetico-deductivists hold that, no matter how precise the measures, how elegant the design, nor how many of Hill's criteria (or those of others) have been met, causality can never be *proven*. This view was brought to the attention of epidemiologists by Buck (1975), who reminded them of the writings of Sir Karl Popper, the pre-eminent contemporary philosopher of science (1968). Put simply, "Popper argues that science advances by the process of deduction alone" (Susser, 1988). Buck's paper provoked many reactions, both favorable and critical, and since it appeared, a monograph edited by Rothman (1988) has expanded the debate.

Those convinced by Popper and Buck are simply following the position stated by Hume in his *Treatise of Human Nature* (1739) that "observers can only perceive events, not causes or associations." From this Popper asserts that we can only approach truth about causes by formulating testable hypotheses about associations of interest, testing them, and rejecting those that are false. This process may appear similar to the "traditional inductive" approach, but it differs in one critical respect: Popperians are strict "falsificationists." They are convinced that we cannot *prove* causes exist and that only false ideas can be disproved, or identified. For them, the process of disproof is incremental: the more and better the hypotheses we are able to falsify, the greater certainty that can be attached to those that remain. Nevertheless, hypotheses remain hypotheses, regardless of the degree of certainty attached to them. Any resolution of this debate will affect how epidemiologists conduct their work and, specifically, the nature of the conclusions they draw.

Many related ideas are found in discussions about causality. MacMahon, Pugh, and Ipsen (1960), for example, call attention to the distinction between necessary and sufficient causes and the divergence of effects that flow from a necessary cause. In an important, possibly seminal contribution, Rothman (1986) offers a general conceptual model that incorporates several of the fundamental ideas above. He suggests that causation can only be understood in relation to conceivable alternatives and adds that "causation and prevention are relative terms that should be viewed as two sides of the same coin." The notion of a sufficient cause—the set of minimal conditions and events that inevitably produce disease—is equivalent to the onset of disease when the cause is completed. Added to this are component causes, each constellation of which is viewed as minimally sufficient. Further account must then be taken of the strength of causes, interactions among them, their specificity, and the induction period, the time "from causal action until disease initiation," alongside the latent period, "the . . . interval between disease occurrence and detection."

For further discussion of issues related to causality see Elwood (1988), Susser (1973), and Rothman (1988).

Sources of Information

Although, as is described in a later section, in some studies the investigator must develop one or more new measures, for many purposes valuable data already exist. Indeed, many of the studies referred to in the chapters that follow draw heavily on existing sources of information.

The most widely available, and in some respects the most useful, of existing measures are population statistics drawn from censuses and related official surveys. Census data provide the much sought-after denominators required to enable numerator data to be expressed as rates. Vital statistics include information routinely and systematically collected in most countries about births, deaths, marriages, and divorces. These statistics are registered, tabulated, and analyzed annually. Mortality statistics are based on death certificates that include information about the causes of death and predisposing conditions. Morbidity statistics can be equally valuable when they are collected in a sufficiently systematic manner to permit meaningful comparisons, e.g., over time within the same country. One example is hospital discharge (or separation) data. These data usually include basic information about the patient (age, sex), a discharge diagnosis (usually using ICD codes), duration of stay, and major procedures.

Occasionally, community physicians (pediatricians, general practitioners, family physicians, or other primary care providers) are surveyed. In Britain, the General Practitioner Morbidity Survey, once a long-established tradition, has only been conducted sporadically in recent years. In the United States, the National Health Survey conducts a periodic study of a sample of practices—the National Ambulatory Medical Care Survey.

In addition, many countries require notification by practitioners of certain health conditions. Unfortunately, the quality of notifiable disease information varies, especially for infectious diseases (see Chapter 9). Even when notification is required by law, most conditions are greatly underreported. Abortions are usually notifiable, although their definition varies from one country to another. Some countries, such as the United States, conduct regular household surveys of morbidity. As well as the routine self-reported data obtained in the regular National Health Interview Surveys, supplementary data about childhood morbidity are also obtained from time to time. They are occasionally supplemented by the U.S. Health and Nutrition Examination Survey. In the United Kingdom similar health information is provided by the General Household Survey or by the Office of Population Censuses and Surveys (OPCS). Recently, national schemes have emerged to collect data from emergency departments to monitor injury occurrence (NISPP in Australia; CHIRPP in Canada).

Many countries have national disease registries, e.g., a register of congenital malformations is commonly found because of the thalidomide disaster. Some have attempted to maintain a broader register of birth defects and handicaps (see Chapter 4). In Canada, the British Columbia Register of Birth Defects is frequently used in such research (see Chapter 5), just as the Cancer Register in the United Kingdom is the source of much of the data described in Chapter 16. Occupational diseases, which affect some adolescents, are often recorded in separate data bases. All registers, although invariably imperfect, can be valuable tools in pediatric epidemiology.

In addition to these routine, large-scale data-gathering exercises, depending on the organization of services for school-aged and preschool children, health information may be obtained from school records and, in theory, from practitioners' records. However, it is rare that practitioner records are organized in such a manner that it is easy to obtain health information, even when such thorny problems as confidentiality and consent have been overcome.

Descriptive Statistics

Although the fundamental application of statistics is to describe data, statistics are also used to analyze relationships from which inferences are drawn. In each application there are two basic elements—the universe and the sample obtained from it—and statistics is about how the two are connected. Furthermore, data can be distributed in two main ways: those that have a normal (i.e., Gaussian) distribution and those that do not. This section deals only with data with a normal distribution, referred to as parametric; the latter, nonparametric, are more specialized (Siegel, 1956).

Descriptive statistics are "numbers intended to describe a study sample by summarizing and condensing a set of measurements on the individuals in that sample" (Kramer, 1988). To describe a sample in a manner that is scientifically useful requires only two numbers: one that specifies the central tendency of the distribution of values included and another that describes its dispersion, or spread. The most well known of the central tendency statistics is the mean, the average of all values, whereas the familiar "spread" statistic is variance, the sum of the squares of deviations from the mean divided by the number of degrees of freedom. Closely related and more commonly used in statistical tests is the standard deviation (SD), the positive square root of the variance, which should not be confused, as it often is, with the standard error (SE) (of the mean), i.e., the standard deviation divided by the square root of the sample size. Because the standard error depends on sample size, it can be misleading, and many investigators fall into the trap (perhaps intentionally) of reporting the standard error, which is invariably smaller than the standard deviation, when the latter is what is intended.

Quantifying the Occurrence of Disorders—Rates

At the heart of epidemiology is the need to quantify the occurrence of disease in a defined population in a manner that allows comparison across populations. This is best achieved by estimating rates of occurrence. Rates consist of three components: a numerator (events counts or occurrences), a denominator (a population), and a specified time period, e.g., 1 year. They are usually expressed using a multiplier that converts the resulting fractions to a whole number. Thus, 45 children who die of traffic accidents in a population of 12,000 in a given area over 1 year represent a prevalence rate of 3.75 per 1000 per year. Ratios are a special form of rates (the value obtained when dividing one quantity by another, e.g., the male:female ratio of 1:2), whereas *proportions* or *percentages* are simply special forms of ratios. The general term "rate" is, however, the parent of the two basic expressions used to describe occurrence—prevalence and incidence. These expressions, in turn, each have a number of increasingly specific offspring.

Special Types of Rates

Prevalence is "the number of occurrences of a disease or condition in a general population at a specified time." The specified time may represent a calendar date (e.g., December 19, 1962) or a point that may vary in real time across persons, e.g., the onset of puberty. Strictly speaking, therefore, a prevalence is a proportion, not a rate. A more precise use is **prevalence rate or ratio**—the total of individuals with a condition at a particular time or during a specified time period, divided by the population at risk of having the condition at that time, or midway through a period. We may have period prevalence, annual prevalence, lifetime prevalence, seasonal prevalence, or point prevalence—each of which differs only according to the time periods specified. Thus, measuring prevalence also provides the probability (or risk) that a person will be "diseased" at that point in time. This information is used to estimate the burden of disease in a population.

Prevalence rates are rarely used to determine etiology because of the heterogeneity of the "cases" reflected in the numerator: children who have had the disease for varying lengths of time. Therefore, the characteristics that define a prevalent case may, in fact, represent prognostic (i.e., leading to survival and thus inclusion in the numerator), rather than etiologic factors. In addition, if onset of disease leads to lifestyle changes, then these characteristics in prevalent cases may spuriously be thought to be antecedent (see length time bias).

These distinctions become important when we consider the other term, **in-**

cidence. The same ideas apply, with the important difference that incidence counts the number of illnesses, accidents, or the like that *begin* during a given period. Incidence rates estimate the probability (or risk) of developing the disease during a specified time period. Accordingly, incidence rates are preferred for etiologic analysis because the effect of survival is removed, and in addition, antecedent exposures are likely to be more valid.

The incidence rate parallels the prevalence rate. However, for clarity, some prefer **incidence density rate** or ratio (IDR), which uses person-duration in the denominator, in which case the specification of time period is no longer required (Kramer, 1988; Miettinen, 1986). In a follow-up study, a special term, **cumulative incidence rate** (CIR), is used to describe the number of new cases occurring in a specified period in relation to the size of the initial cohort. The distinction between IDR and CIR is based on the dynamic state of the population being studied. CIR is calculated on fixed cohorts, i.e., where all study subjects are followed from the beginning to the end of the study. In contrast, the IDR rate takes into account the fact that some cohorts are dynamic. That is, subjects enter the study group at different times and may leave the group for a variety of reasons—they die, withdraw, move away, etc. In order to use all available information, the IDR considers each child's contribution to the study in the context of person-time. For example, 20 children followed for 2 years equals 40 child-years of follow-up, as does 5 children followed for 8 years.

Relationship Between Prevalence and Incidence

The prevalence rate is driven by both the incidence rate and the average duration of disease, i.e., from onset to recovery, remission, or death. If the prevalence is low and both the incidence and average duration of the disease are stable, then prevalence = incidence × duration. Therefore, knowledge of any two components allows calculation of the third.

As stated in a previous section, accurate estimation of any rate of occurrence requires that the denominator represent only those truly "at risk." For example, when measuring the incidence rate of an infectious disease, those children who have already had the disease or are immune should be excluded from the denominator. In summary, underlying all epidemiologic rates is the person-time idea, and accordingly, with few exceptions, the notion of risk or exposure reflects not only the health of the child (susceptible, immune, etc.) but also the time over which exposures or at-risk-ness exists.

For example, the death rate is usually expressed as the proportion of a population that dies during a specified period, usually a year. This fraction is usually multiplied by 1000 or 100,000, depending on the specific application. The infant mortality rate is the yearly rate of deaths in children under 1 year of age and takes as its denominator the number of live births in the same year. In pediatric epidemiology there are a number of related terms that differ only in the age group in the denominator: neonatal (under 28 days of age), postneonatal (between 28 days and 1 year), fetal (from last menstrual period to birth), and perinatal (from 28 weeks conception to 7 days of age).

In child health the infant mortality rate is often of special interest because it is frequently viewed as a global index of the health status of the child population. Yet, death rates for specific causes can also be estimated and are often of equal importance. When these rates are expressed as all deaths relative to all known cases (at a given time and place), this statistic is referred to as the **case fatality** rate. Analogously, the **attack or case rate** is used to describe the number of new cases over a given time period in a specified population and is similar to a cumulative incidence rate. In infectious disease the term *inception rate* is often preferred because many illnesses (e.g., the common cold and otitis media) usually occur more than once during any specified period, especially during early childhood (see Chapter 9).

Adjustment

To compare rates it is often necessary to consider procedures that involve **adjustment**, which is "a summarizing procedure for a statistical measure in which the effects of differences in composition of the populations being compared are minimized by one of (several) methods." This notion is pivotal to both descriptive and analytic studies. It permits an investigator to make meaningful comparisons between x and y when he or she is unable to collect, or otherwise manipulate, the populations or groups being compared. In statistics, adjustment is often accomplished by regression procedures or analysis of covariance (see later section).

Any crude population rate (e.g., the annual Canadian pediatric cancer mortality rate) represents an average of category-specific mortality rates for children in various age groups. The crude estimate is therefore driven by the number of deaths and the proportion of the total population in each age category. If, however, cancer mortality varies with age, then a comparison of crude mortality rates in different populations must take account of differences in their population age distributions. (Alternatively, one could compare age-specific rates only, but this would be cumbersome, particularly if several populations are to be compared).

One technique used to provide comparable summary population rates is called **standardization**. It may be used for any variable that influences the rate and the distribution of which differs across the populations being compared. The most common approach is to calculate a weighted average of rates for the variable concerned (e.g., age) according to one of two methods, direct or indirect, the details of which are found in most textbooks.

Direct standardization takes specific rates in the study population and weights them by using as the denominator a selected *standard* population, e.g., the census population. This provides the "expected number of events" that would have occurred in the study group if it had the same age (or other variable) distribution as the standard. The adjusted summary rate is then calculated by dividing the sum of the expected number of events by the total study population. The other method, **indirect** standardization, is more complicated, but is based on the same principle and yields essentially similar results (see Rothman, 1986).

Before leaving this section on descriptive statistics, a special note is warranted regarding the approach to dichotomous discrete variables, the value of which is determined by chance. Unlike continuous measures with a Gaussian or "normal" distribution (and thus amenable to a variety of statistical procedures), the probability distribution, P, of dichotomous variables is binomial. Formulas for P, based "on the number of target outcomes, t, that can be expected among a number of individuals, n, when the probability of achieving the target in any one individual is π," are provided in most texts (Kramer, 1988). Under some circumstances (e.g., when π approaches 0 and the sample is large), the binomial distribution approximates the Poisson distribution.

Sampling

With few exceptions, epidemiologic observations are made on a subset or sample, rather than the entire population. This selected subset may either be random or nonrandom. Random sampling is probabilistic, in that all subjects in the population have a known and usually equal chance of being selected. A *probability sample* may be chosen by assigning a number to each subject and then selecting subjects randomly, e.g., using a table of random numbers. Studies using nonrandom sampling techniques (variously termed clutch, grab, or convenience) have limited, if any, inference because the various biases operating in the selection of subjects are unknown. Conversely, when samples are random, judgments about the conclusions derived from them can be attributed to the population sampled. As always, however, extrapolating findings to other populations requires caution.

A simple random (or probability) sample is one in which each person has an equal chance of being selected. A **stratified** sample involves "dividing the population into distinct subgroups according to some important characteristic such as age, or socioeconomic status and then selecting a random sample from each subgroup." Stratification is often used to control for the effects of confounding variables, although this also may be accomplished in the analysis; it is also used to sample a particular subgroup (see the section on confounding).

In contrast, a **systematic** sample involves selection according to some rule, e.g., names with specified alphabetic letters or by birth dates. Although probabilistic, such samples are frowned upon because they are more subject to bias. A **cluster** sample is one in which the unit selected is a group, rather than an individual. Although the cluster sample is a perfectly acceptable procedure and one that is frequently used in large population surveys, the statistical considerations involved are often complex, e.g., when calculations of sample size are being performed.

The idea of a representative sample is elusive. There is no official statistical definition of what is meant by representative, although in common parlance it refers to a sample that one believes represents well the population being studied. As Last points out, however, even random sampling should not be taken for granted: "A common fallacy lies in the unwarranted assumption that if a sample resembles a population closely on those factors that have been checked it is 'totally representative' and that no differences exist between the sample and the universe or reference population." Kendall and Buckman (1982) suggest that the word "representative be confined to samples that turn out to be so, however chosen, rather than applying it to those chosen with the object of being representative."

An important issue in sampling is the *response rate* achieved. Nonresponse can be due to deaths, removals, or refusals and, depending on the proportions, may introduce bias (see the section on bias). This is so because it should be assumed that nonparticipants, especially those who refuse to take part in a study, differ in some important respects from those who agree. Consequently, this difference should be elucidated whenever possible. The late Professor Cochrane suggested that response rates that were less than 90% were unacceptable. In pursuit of this he made a practice of visiting subjects on Christmas day and Sundays and even sought out those in prison!

Research Designs

Three broad groups of epidemiologic study have been described: descriptive, analytic, and experimental. Although this classification may at times be arbitrary and has been challenged, it nevertheless remains a useful system. **Descriptive** studies summarize data on population attributes, commonly on the basis of person, place, and time. As such, statistical (but not causal) inference is employed. **Analytic** studies implicitly examine relationships between variables, and thus causal inference is their main objective. In these studies, a hypothesis about the extent of an effect is formulated, and data are gathered to test the hypothesis. However, these designs may also be used to generate hypotheses—the usual domain of descriptive studies. The randomized trial, a form of experimental design, is regarded by many as the pinnacle of analytic studies. The hierarchical nature of these groupings is so ingrained that studies are often described in a derogatory manner, e.g., as being "only" descriptive. This pejorative judgment reflects a failure to fully appreciate the potential benefits of descriptive and analytic studies.

Analytic Designs

Kramer and Boivin (1988) proposed a classification of analytic research designs based on three axes: directionality, sample selection, and timing. **Directionality** refers to the order of inquiry; forward—from exposure to outcome (prospective); backwards—from outcome to exposure (retrospective); or the simultaneous determination of exposure and outcome status (cross-sectional, or prevalence). **Sample selection** refers to the criteria used in sampling, i.e., exposure, outcome, or "other." **Timing** is the temporal relationship between the study itself and the calendar time of exposure and outcome: historical (both in the past, before the study), concurrent, or mixed. For the purpose of this chapter, the axis of directionality is used as the major criterion for describing research designs.

The other fundamental dimension is whether the design is observational or experimental. The key distinction is that in the former the investigator has no opportunity to manipulate variables, whereas in the latter, the ability to do so bestows a host of powerful advantages that should make the interpretation of results more conclusive.

It is undoubtedly correct to assert that each component of the basic triad of research—design, measurement, and analysis—is equally essential, and hence that any study is only as strong as the weakest component. However, many view "design" as *primum inter pares*. More sins are committed when designs are poorly conceived than at any other stage of research. Although good measures and sound analyses may mitigate the consequences to some extent, inevitably it is design that matters most. It can, however, be argued that the most important threats to internal validity arise from analytic bias due to sampling and measurement issues (see Analytic Bias). In this case, the price paid for poor design is inefficiency, not bias.

The key component of design is the direction of inquiry. Does the question being asked begin with the outcome (e.g., the disease or "caseness" of the child), or does it begin with the putative risk factor to which the child may have been exposed? All epidemiologic research is in one direction, from cause to effect. However, this fundamental unidirectionality can be examined in a variety of ways. In a *cohort* study, the initial commitment is to a population in which events of interest will later occur, whereas in a *case-control* study, the commitment is first to events or outcomes.

Although in principle, any prospective design is always preferable because it permits the investigator to decide what to measure, how to do so, and when, such a design is frequently not possible because of time constraints, cost, or other less practical reasons. For example, when studying the consequences of maternal rubella infection, although it would be much preferable to be able to choose the biologic measures that determine the presence of infection (serology, etc.) and to specify precisely when, during the pregnancy, the infection occurred, this is only possible in a true prospective design. Inability to incorporate such features, however, hardly justifies ignoring retrospective data (or other, equally imperfect information).

Descriptive Designs

Descriptive surveys only describe variables and, in theory, do so without regard to hypotheses. As well as providing estimates of the magnitude of a health problem, they may, however, serve to generate many testable hypotheses.

Cross-sectional or prevalence surveys are intended to examine relationships between diseases and variables of interest in a defined population at one point in time; this may be a point in calendar time or a fixed point in the course of an event that may vary in real time from person to person, e.g., menarche. From data obtained in this manner, the results can be described in terms of the prevalence of disease in different subgroups, or the reverse—in terms of the presence or absence of variables in those with and without a disease. Prevalence surveys often provide strong "clues" about the relationship between variables and thus play an important role in generating hypotheses. However, no sense of cause and effect can be drawn from this design because the temporal relationship between exposure and outcome cannot be determined except with such variables as sex or blood group, whose status remains unchanged over time.

A *morbidity* survey is a special case of a prevalence or observational survey. Frequently cited examples include studies in which all children in a defined geographic area such as Monroe County, New York, or the Isle of Wight in the United Kingdom, were surveyed to determine the prevalence of all physical, mental, and behavioral problems. In each case an implicit secondary goal was to examine hypotheses about relationships between and among these variables. For more details about surveys, see Aday (1989).

Case-Control Design (Retrospective)

Case-control studies are the most powerful of the backward-looking, retrospective family. They begin with an outcome of interest (cases) and compare their past experiences with those who are not affected by the outcome (controls). The salient features are straightforward: cases and suitable controls are identified and the frequency of one or more attributes of interest compared in an identical, preferably blinded fashion. (A variation is to view case-ness as a function of severity and to compare those with a severe form of disease with those with milder manifestations).

The term "comparison group" in the broadest sense describes any group to which another is compared. Although distinctions between the terms "index" and "case" or "comparison" and "control" are small and often unimportant, they occasionally confuse even experienced researchers. When the index subset has a disease, it is preferable that it be described as a "case." Similarly, the term "control" is most appropriate when the comparison subject is matched in some way to the case.

Case-control studies are valuable and powerful tools, especially when cases are infrequent and investigators have neither the resources nor patience to wait until sufficiently large numbers have accumulated to permit the same question to be answered using a forward-looking design. Another advantage of this approach is that it is relatively inexpensive and can examine several putative risk factors for a single disease. The main disadvantage is the inability to estimate disease (outcome) risk directly (unless the study is population-based) and the ever-present possibilities of selection, recall bias, or both. The definitive text on case-control studies is that by Schlesselman (1982).

Cohort Designs (Prospective)

A cohort (the Latin word for "warriors" or one tenth of a Roman Legion) is, strictly speaking, a group *born* in the same time period and followed forward in time. Broadly, however, the term is also used for any group assembled at a given time and then followed or traced over a subsequent period. The essential feature of all such studies is that the time axis proceeds from exposure to outcome. Cohort studies often search for the causes of disorders by performing analyses that assess the role of specified attributes (risk factors or determinants).

The main problem for researchers is identifying groups large enough and that can be followed long enough (i.e., to provide a sufficient number of person-years) during which enough diseases (or other events of interest) can occur to permit meaningful analyses. Accordingly, a cohort study is a costly and often impractical approach.

One popular alternative is the **historical cohort** design. In it, a cohort defined in the past is identified, and past data are obtained (e.g., using existing records—medical, school, etc.) to classify children as to past exposure to a risk (or preventive) factor. For example, school records could be used to see if children were fully immunized at school entry and then their status with respect to the incidence of measles or complications of vaccines is determined. In this example, the investigator can only influence how the outcome is measured.

Another option is to take a cohort defined in the past and studied in the past, i.e., to perform secondary analyses of existing data (see Chapter 2). In a study of this kind, the researcher is able to choose the variables for analysis, but must accept how they are defined and when and how they were measured. It is possible to exercise some discretion about how subjects are selected in both groups, but as has been stated, data about risk factors (putative causes, etc.) must be accepted as "given." In some instances, this information is provided by the children (or their parents), whereas in others, it is found in medical or school records or in records of earlier laboratory test results. No matter how good any of these sources may be, rarely will they conform to all the investigator's preferences.

A **nested case-control** study in a sense combines the best of both worlds. In it, cases and controls are drawn from a cohort sample. This makes it possible to use data about both groups that are already available, and the effects of several forms of confounding may be reduced. This design is difficult to categorize because, although like a case-control it examines data looking back in time, by situating it in an ongoing cohort, it also provides an opportunity to view the data prospectively.

A critically important feature of all such studies is the need to "blind" those who assemble the data. Ideally, interviewers and raters must be unaware not only of the status of the subjects (case or control) but also of the hypotheses being examined. When data collectors, interviewers, testers, parents, or children are aware of the hypotheses, they may seek to please by giving information they think the researcher wants, rather than the truth.

Because cohort studies, especially birth cohorts, have played such an important role in the epidemiology of childhood disorders, an entire chapter (Chapter 2) is devoted to this topic.

Experimental Studies

In the designs so far described, the researcher is unable to manipulate variables, and accordingly, they are viewed as "observational." When manipulation *is* possible, the design falls into the other main, and usually preferable family of experimental (or quasi-experimental) designs. A true experiment (or random ized controlled trial; RCT) involves *both* random assignment and a comparison group. Quasi-experimental designs lack one of these essential features.

An experimental study is therefore one in which most design conditions are under the investigator's control. Those subjected to any maneuver have its effects compared with a group who receive another regimen, or none. The value of the comparison group is often enhanced by using a placebo or sham, so that both the subjects and investigators can be "blinded" to group status. Here again, the need for blinding the child or parents is essential. Still better is double-blinding, which further minimizes bias by concealing from researchers the identity of the group to which subjects belong until after the results are analyzed. We can go still further: when the analyst is also unaware of group assignment the study is referred to as a "triple blind."

The other essential element of experimental studies is random assignment. When this occurs and the numbers are sufficient, it is assumed that the groups being compared are similar, not only with respect to variables known to affect the outcome, such as age or sex, but also with respect to those not known or suspected. Yet, because randomization can fail for technical or probabilistic reasons, the careful researcher will always compare all measurable characteristics and, when substantial differences are found that cannot be corrected, will take these into account in the analyses. However, postrandomization testing does not warrant the use of statistical procedures; it is more a matter of eyeballing the data and making sensible judgments.

The main value of true experimental designs is the number and nature of threats to internal validity they are able to overcome. These threats, any of the many forms of bias described previously, are successively eliminated as we move closer and closer to the double- or triple-blinded RCT.

The ethics of true experiments are complex and occasionally controversial, but many safeguards have evolved to ensure the protection of children who participate in them. The usual defense is that when no one can genuinely know whether a new therapy will do more harm than good and because parents and children can refuse after they are fully informed of possible risks, the experimental approach is ethically acceptable.

Quasi-Experimental Designs

Unfortunately, an RCT is not always possible, although this approach is used far more widely in recent years than was thought possible in the past. The alternative is the gray zone of *quasi-experimental* designs. Their essence is that the investigator does not control the allocation or timing of the intervention. Such studies are usually considered better than those that are cross-sectional, but are much less powerful than genuinely experimental designs.

Investigators are often only able to obtain data from a single group once before and once after a maneuver has been introduced. Or, it may be possible to study the same subjects repeatedly, i.e., to make comparisons over time. The major quasi-experimental variant is one in which two groups are only compared after (but not before) one of the two was "treated."

Frequently, quasi-experimentation is used to assess a change arising from a "natural experiment." For example, when some states repealed motorbike helmet laws while others did not, researchers were able to compare subsequent head injuries or deaths among adolescent motorbikers in the repealed and nonrepealed states. Similarly, a historical event may have brought about a change of interest to researchers. To examine the effects of easier access to medical care, death rates among children were studied before and after the introduction of national health insurance in Canada (Hodge, Dougherty & Pless, unpublished).

A host of other variations lie between each of these examples of quasi-experimentation. These designs were fully described by Campbell and Stanley (1966) in a monograph that many regard as a classic. Although intended initially for psychologists, epidemiologists have adopted many of the terms and notations, as have evaluation researchers from a wide range of disciplines. Their popularity arises from the simple fact that the real world rarely provides ideal circumstances for investigators. The experienced and wise researcher makes the best of what is offered, knowing that it will contribute something of value to the store of knowledge if it is done well.

Measures

In a general sense, the selection of any measure or scale involves a similar series of steps. The investigator begins by deciding on a particular parameter, the "natural" scale for the parameter in question is characterized, and a particular measure is chosen that captures as much of the information sought as possible. Then, if necessary, there follows a data reduction step for convenience of analysis, or other purposes.

Some measures used in epidemiology are simple phenomena that can be assessed using "yes-no" questions. Others are counts of events, such as deaths or illnesses. At another level are indices that attempt to integrate an array of factors or variables. Sometimes the process of integration is arbitrary, and sometimes it uses such procedures as factor analysis or cluster analysis. Each of the latter procedures provides an empirical basis for weighting and grouping the ingredients of a proposed index or scale. Some measures are contentious because they represent attempts to assess abstract constructs, such as "patient satisfaction." Even such a commonly used measure as social class is not without its critics.

An important consideration involves knowing the nature of any scale being used because the distinctions affect how they may be used statistically. At one end are **nominal or categorical** measures—different forms of discrete data. With few exceptions these are not normally distributed, and accordingly, measures of this kind can only be analyzed using nonparametric statistics, such as the chi square test, because they cannot be added to give arithmetic averages or means. An exception is when a binary scale can be analyzed using the binomial distribution.

The next level includes **ordinal** measures, which involves "logically ordered categories like social class, occupational prestige, etc." The important distinction is that there is no "natural numerical distance" between values. For example, no sensible epidemiologist assumes that the "distance" between children from social class I and those in social class II is the same as that between III and IV. For the most part, ordinal measures are analyzed using parametric procedures, although doing so is not always acceptable.

At the other end are scales or measures that yield data in which there are no naturally occurring breaks, i.e., **continuous** data. Such parametric measures have a distribution, which, in theory at least, includes "a potentially infinite number of possible values along a continuum," e.g., height and weight. Closely allied are **interval** scales, which differ insofar as the units are discrete. (A ratio scale is a special case of an interval scale that has a true zero point). All these meet the requirements for parametric analyses.

Once the nature of a measure is clearly understood and the statistical implications appreciated, the next issue is to decide whether its (psychometric) properties are acceptable. Unfortunately, the scale for judging acceptability is itself relative and subjective. The properties that are important—for epidemiologists, as well as for social and behavioral scientists—are accuracy (or precision), validity, and reliability (often referred to as repeatability or reproducibility). Although the synonyms above are commonly used, several distinctions can be helpful.

Accuracy or validity is "how well a measure conforms to a standard or true value," whereas **precision** is the level of detail provided, e.g., the number of significant digits in the measurement. Another indicator of precision is the standard error of measurement (SEM)—the standard deviation of a series of replicate determinations of the same quantity. It must be emphasized, however, that precision does not imply accuracy or validity. Ideally, all measures should be both precise and valid. However, in general, precision is not a characteristic of most epidemiologic measures in contrast to the bench sciences. To make the distinction clear, consider an archer's target: the accurate archer hits the bullseye, whereas the precise archer may bunch all arrows closely together, but at the edge of the target. Thus, a **reliable** measure is one that is "sound and dependable" so that when repeated it yields the same results. A measure should give the same result when used by the same observer or by another (inter- and intra-observer reliability). Accordingly, poor reliability may arise from differences "between observers, instruments of measurement, or instability of the attribute being measured." For further details about measurement in general, see Norman and Streiner (1989).

Analysis

Of the three cornerstones of epidemiologic research, statistical analysis is the most respected, the most intimidating, and, paradoxically in some respects, perhaps the least important. One reason for this seemingly blasphemous statement is that, once a study is done, the measures and designs cannot be undone. The sins of poor measurement or poor design can rarely be corrected, even by the most talented and ingenious biostatistician. In contrast, if the data are properly assembled, statistical analyses that are incorrect or disputed can always be repeated.

The preceding paragraph is not intended to denigrate the importance of solid and sensible analysis; it simply helps one maintain a reasonable perspective on its relative importance. At the elementary level, several texts are invariably helpful, e.g., Swinscow (1980), Norman and Streiner (1986), and Phillips (1978). However, biostatistics has become much more complex in recent years. Readers who need more guidance should consult any of a number of more advanced texts for details that cannot be provided here. These texts include Kramer (1988),

Kleinbaum, Kupper, and Morgenstern (1982), Armitage (1971), Colton (1974); and Fleiss, 1981.

Inferential Statistics

Most statistics test whether the distribution of one or more variables may have occurred by chance and may be parametric or nonparametric. Parametric statistics involve dependent variables that have continuous distributions, whereas nonparametric statistics do not because, as explained above, they represent variables that are nominal or categorical—alive or dead, sick or well. Parametric statistics also assume that the data being analyzed are normally distributed, although in practice this requirement is often safely ignored.

Nonparametric statistics can be both simple and complicated. A familiar nonparametric statistic is the chi square test, which examines the probability that aggregated differences between a distribution of observed measures in a cross-tabulation ($n \times n$ table) exceeds what might be expected by chance. Other less familiar statistics often involve ranking procedures, e.g., the Mann-Whitney U-test, the sign test, the Wilcoxon signed rank test, and the Spearman correlation coefficient. These are dealt with extensively in Siegel (1956).

Comparing Means in Two or More Groups

Most inferential tests can be divided into two broad categories: those that compare means in two or more groups and those used for prediction. The two-group situation is handled by t tests, which may be paired or unpaired, depending on whether the data in each group are matched in any of several ways. The t test uses a statistic that, under the null hypothesis, has or would have a certain distribution—the t distribution. The probability of any t value being found by chance can be determined using tables that accompany most statistical texts.

When three or more means are compared, analysis of variance is required. In spite of the word "variance," the basic idea of this statistic is the same as in t tests—to consider how far apart the means in the groups being compared are while taking account of the variance in each group. Thus, between and within group variances are compared and the result expressed as an F statistic. An elaboration of this procedure is the analysis of covariance (ANCOVA), which takes account of the effects of other factors (covariates) that may influence the dependent measure.

Because the strange term **degrees of freedom** (df) has been used and recurs frequently in statistics, it seems wise to explain it, although Last notes that "this important concept in statistical testing cannot be defined briefly." Fortunately, it is easier to calculate than to explain. In a contingency table (e.g., a 3×2 table), the df is one less than the number of row categories, multiplied by one less than the number column categories. This essential component of statistics is needed to quantify the number of independent comparisons that can be made between members of a sample, i.e., how much freedom there is to do so.

Modeling Statistical Relationships

Reference has been made to independent or predictor (explanatory) variables, and to dependent or outcome variables. A causal path is assumed to flow from independent to dependent, and intermediate variables lie in between. Intervening variables are statistically associated with both independent and dependent variables. Typically, one goal of an analysis is to predict the latter from the former. Yet, life is rarely so simple, nor are statistical models.

The most important of the sources of confusion is the presence of a **confounding variable**. As described in an earlier section, confounding describes "a situation in which the effects of two processes are not separated, i.e., the distortion of an apparent effect of an exposure on risk brought about by (its) association with other factors that also influence the outcome." It addresses the relationship between the effects of two or more causal factors in a set of data—the relationship being such that it is not logically possible to separate the contribution of any one of the factors. It follows that, to estimate properly the effect of any risk factor, account must be taken of known confounders or they must somehow be controlled.

One example should help clarify the meaning of this pivotally important concept, which the reader will recall was introduced in the section on bias. If an investigator was studying the effects of maternal smoking on birthweight and failed to take account of maternal drinking and it had been shown that the latter also influences birthweight, drinking would confound the relationship. This is so because mothers who smoke heavily are also more likely to drink, and those who are teetotallers are likely to abstain from smoking, especially during pregnancy.

This completes the preparation needed to consider more fully the second major class of inferential statistics—that which involves regression analysis. In its simplest and most common form, a linear model is constructed that, given some data on a dependent variable y and one or more independent or predictor variables, seeks the "best" mathematical model to describe or predict y as a function of the x variables. A regression line diagrammatically presents the results of a regression equation (in the general form of $y = \beta x_0 + \beta x_1 + \beta x_2$), with the independent variable x shown on the abscissa or x axis, and the dependent variable y on the ordinate or y axis.

In epidemiology and biostatistics, several, often complex variations on this theme, such as logistic and proportional hazard models, are commonly used. Logistic models come into play when the dependent variable is categorical, i.e., life or death, ill or well. The proportional hazard model, also known as a Cox model, is used in survival (or life-table) analysis in which the time until an event or outcome occurs is a critical parameter.

A logistic regression is a statistical model of the probability of a categorical outcome (actually a logit transformation of any binary variable) as a function of one or more predictors or risk factors. (A logit is the logarithm of the ratio of frequencies of two different categorical outcomes, e.g., healthy versus sick). Logistic regression is used to model probabilities of such outcomes. The model can be extended to a multiple logistic form in which the x function is replaced by a linear term involving several factors, e.g., βx1, βx2, etc. The formula appears intimidating because it incorporates the natural exponential function, e, requires logarithmic arithmetic, and yields a range of values between zero and infinity.

Screening and Case-Finding

One way to determine the normal limits of a measure indicative of good health or disease is to compare its values when measurements are made in healthy and sick groups. If the two distributions fail to overlap, little problem in interpretation exists. When they do, however, as is more commonly the case, any value in the overlapping area can be interpreted differently. The choice of a cut-off, or what may be viewed as the limit of normality, depends on the relative importance attached to the correct identification of individuals as healthy or unhealthy. Shifting the cut-off point may improve either sensitivity or specificity; rarely, can it improve both.

The value of a test for diagnosis or screening depends initially on its sensitivity and specificity. The **sensitivity** of a test, whether used in the diagnostic context or screening, is estimated by comparing, in a 2 × 2 table, the proportion of diseased children who have a positive test result. **Specificity** is the opposite: the proportion of healthy children who have a negative test result. From a clinical and public health perspective, each of these is best judged from their respective predictive values. The **positive predictive value** of a test is the probability that a person with a positive test is a true positive; the negative predictive value is the opposite. The importance of these concepts arises because the values depend on the prevalence of the disease in the population being screened. Several examples in Chapter 4 make it clear that even a very good screening test may be of limited value if the prevalence of the disease is very low.

For some time, population screening was a popular approach to the early diagnosis of disease, which, in turn, was viewed as a way to improve outcomes. In some instances, screening has stood the test of time (see Chapter 5). However, the fundamental idea that early diagnosis leads to better, more effective therapy, and hence is more cost effective for society and the individual, has been seriously challenged. Consequently, many of the early zealous endeavors have been abandoned. It is nonetheless desirable to be familiar with the basic concepts employed in these programs. It is also important to understand the distinction between true population screening and the other situations in which the term is applied, albeit incorrectly. These include case-finding and diagnostic testing.

The main distinction is that true screening is aimed at the whole population or occasionally a vulnerable or high-risk subgroup within it. It is an outreach exercise that attempts to find those with disease in its early, preclinical phase. In contrast, case-finding involves similar procedures that occur in the context of a visit to the physician. When a child visits for an otitis media and the physician decides to search for an unrelated problem (e.g., to do a urinalysis to "screen" for asymptomatic renal disease), this activity is properly regarded as case-finding. The importance of the distinction is that in the context of population screening it is essential that specificity be as high as possible in order not to offer false reassurance that may actually delay diagnosis and treatment when symptoms occur. In the case-finding situation, it is assumed that contact with the physician will continue and should symptoms arise, they will be attended to promptly and properly. In this case, a lower level of specificity can be tolerated.

Much more can be said about screening, and those who wish a comprehensive and entertaining presentation of the additional issues are encouraged to consult the text by Sackett, Hayes, and Tugwell (1985).

Conclusion

This chapter makes no pretense at providing a comprehensive review. Its goal is to help the reader who may be unfamiliar with some of the terms or concepts used in the subsequent chapters to review their meaning. Many excellent texts are now available at both the basic and advanced levels. The level of detail provided here is deliberately limited because this chapter is intended to serve as a substantial aperitif to make the rich meal that follows more easily digestible.

Acknowledgments

I wish to acknowledge the wise counsel of students and colleagues, especially Colin Macarthur and Matthew Hodge, who read a draft of this chapter and made many detailed and important suggestions. Charles Pless also gave invaluable editorial and stylistic assistance. Others consulted in connection with later chapters included Richard Hamilton, Delip Mahalanabis, and Michael Kramer.

References

Aday LA. *Designing and Conducting Health Surveys: A Comprehensive Guide*. San Francisco: Jossey-Bass; 1989.

Armitage P. *Statistical Methods in Medical Research*. New York: John Wiley and Sons; 1974.

Buck C. Popper's philosophy for epidemiologists. *Int J Epidemiol* 1975; 121:343–350.

Campbell DT, Stanley JC. *Experimental and Quasi-Experimental Designs for Research*. Chicago: Rand McNally; 1963.

Colton T. *Statistics in Medicine*. Boston: Little, Brown; 1974.

Cook TD, Campbell DT. *Quasi-Experimentation: Design & Analysis Issues for Field Settings*. Chicago: Rand McNally; 1979.

Elwood JM. *Causal Relationships in Medicine—A Practical System for Critical Appraisal*. Oxford: Oxford University Press; 1988.

Fleiss JL. *Statistical Methods for Rates and Proportions*. New York: John Wiley & Sons; 1981.

Greenland S, ed. *Evolution of Epidemiologic Ideas: Annotated Readings on Concepts and Methods*. Chestnut Hill: Epidemiology Resources Inc; 1987.

Hill AB. The environment and disease: association or causation? *Proc Roy Soc Med* 1965; 58:295–300.

Hume D. *Treatise of Human Nature*. London: John Noon; 1739: revised and reprinted, Selby-Bigge LA, ed. Oxford: Clarendon Press; 1985.

Kelsey JL, Thompson WD, Evans AS. *Methods in Observational Epidemiology*. New York: Oxford University Press; 1986.

Kendall MG, Buckman AA. *A Dictionary of Statistical Terms*. 4th ed. London: Longman; 1982.

Kleinbaum DG, Kupper LL, Morgenstern H. *Epidemiologic Research: Principles and Quantitative Methods*. London: Lifetime Learning Publications; 1982.

Koch R. Die aetiologie der Tuberculose. *Meitteilungen aus dem Kasiserlichen Gsundheitsamte* 1884; 2:1.

Kramer MS. *Clinical Epidemiology and Biostatistics: A Primer for Clinical Investigators and Decision Makers*. New York: Springer-Verlag; 1988.

Kramer MS, Boivin J-F. Toward an "unconfounded" classification of epidemiologic research design. *J Chronic Dis* 1978; 40:683–688.

Last JM, ed. *A Dictionary of Epidemiology*. New York; Oxford University Press; 1988.

MacMahon B, Pugh TF, Ipsen J. *Epidemiologic Methods*. Boston: Little, Brown; 1960.

Mausner JS, Bahn AK, Kramer S. *Epidemiology—An Introductory Text*. Philadelphia: WB Saunders; 1985.

Miettinen OS. *Theoretical Epidemiology: Principles of Occurrence Research in Medicine*. New York: Wiley; 1986.

Mill JS. *A System of Logic*. London; 1856.

Norman GR, Streiner DL. *PDQ Statistics*. Toronto: BC Decker; 1986.

Norman GR, Streiner DL. *Principles of Measurement in Health Sciences*. Oxford: Oxford University Press; 1989.

Phillips DS. *Basic Statistics for Health Science Students*. San Francisco: WH Freeman and Co; 1978.

Popper KR. *The Logic of Scientific Discovery*. rev. ed. New York: Harper and Row; 1968.

Rothman KJ. *Modern Epidemiology*. Boston: Little, Brown & Co; 1986.

Rothman KJ, ed. *Causal Inference*. Chestnut Hill: Epidemiology Resources Inc; 1988.

Sackett DL. Bias in analytic research. *J Chronic Dis* 1979; 32:51–63.

Sackett DL, Haynes RB, Tugwell P. *Clinical Epidemiology: A Basic Science for Clinical Medicine*. Boston: Little, Brown & Co; 1985.

Schlesselman JJ. *Case-Control Studies*. New York: Oxford University Press; 1982.

Siegel S. *Nonparametric Statistics For The Behavioral Sciences*. New York: McGraw-Hill; 1956.

Streiner DL, Norman GR, Blum HM. *PDQ Epidemiology*. Toronto: BC Decker Inc; 1989.

Susser M. *Causal Thinking in the Health Sciences*. New York: Oxford University Press; 1973.

Susser M. Falsification, verification and causal inference in epidemiology: reconsideration in the light of Sir Karl Popper's philosophy. In: Rothman KJ, ed. *Causal Inference*. Chestnut Hill: Epidemiology Resources Inc; 1988.

Swinscow TDV. *Statistics at Square One*. London: British Medical Association; 1980.

2

The Special Role of Longitudinal Studies

CHRISTOPHER POWER

Longitudinal, follow-up, or cohort studies have a unique role to play in pediatric epidemiology (see Chapter 1). They are designed to collect information about a group of individuals exposed to a suspected risk factor and a group of nonexposed individuals, and usually this is done prospectively. Disease outcomes (mortality, morbidity, or disability) are compared according to category of exposure. It is therefore necessary to collect information on at least two time points, i.e., on exposure and at subsequent disease occurrence. In some instances, however, it is possible to take advantage of pre-existing records of disease outcome (e.g., cancer registers) or of information on exposure, which may be available from historical records (Rothman, 1986). Another variation of the longitudinal design is the general population follow-up, which either uses routinely collected data (Fox, 1985; OPCS, 1988) or establishes regular contact with a group of subjects specially selected for the study (often referred to as a "panel study"). General population surveys are usually multipurpose, obtaining information about a variety of risk factors and disease outcomes. As has been explained in the previous chapter, a cross-sectional study, in contrast, does not obtain information on individuals over time; even if a repeat survey is undertaken, it involves a different group of subjects.

Birth follow-up studies are of particular interest for childhood conditions because they focus on early life. Such studies are increasingly relevant to current debates on the importance of childhood environment and other factors in the development of adult disease (Ciba Foundation, 1991). They have been undertaken in many developed countries and only rarely in less industrialized nations (Barros et al., 1990). Britain is unique in having three national longitudinal studies, started in 1946, 1958, and 1970, which have followed representative samples throughout their childhood and, in two instances, into adult life (Butler & Bonham, 1963; Chamberlain et al., 1975; Joint Committee, 1948; Power, 1992; Wadsworth, 1987). The two older studies now also include information about the children of cohort members and therefore offer an opportunity to develop a further understanding of intergenerational influences on health.

Longitudinal studies have several purposes in epidemiologic research. They are primarily used for prediction of outcomes, such as mortality, disability, or disease. In this regard they are particularly useful for testing, rather than generating, hypotheses. Large multipurpose follow-up studies can nevertheless have a hypothesis-generating role, suggesting factors that warrant further investigation in smaller, more detailed studies. Depending upon their design, longitudinal studies can also identify the consequences of morbidity and disability, assess continuity or changes over time, and describe age trends.

This chapter describes several important ways in which longitudinal studies have contributed to an understanding of the epidemiology of childhood disorders; hence, it emphasizes the birth cohort studies. It outlines advantages and disadvantages of the longitudinal approach in general and specifically in relation to the four main purposes mentioned above.

Advantages and Disadvantages

A major strength of follow-up studies is that they overcome difficulties of recall of past circumstances by obtaining contemporary information. Representative population-based follow-up studies have the added advantage over small and often selected groups, such as clinic samples, in that their findings are generally applicable even though in some instances they are cohort-specific. Also, in general population samples in which different sections of society are represented, it is possible to investigate between-group (e.g., social and regional) differences. Birth cohorts have the potential to cover the entire life course. Even though longitudinal follow-up studies are expensive (see below), it has been argued that where multipurpose objectives can be well coordinated such studies may prove to be cost effective (Fergusson et al., 1989).

In general, longitudinal studies require that a large number of subjects be followed over a relatively long period. Therefore, a major disadvantage is their cost. Establishing contact with cohort members is time consuming and expensive, particularly in less developed countries where tracing of subjects can be extremely difficult because of high mobility among low-income families (Barros et al., 1990). The sample size decreases over time as subjects are lost to follow-up through death, emigration, nonresponse, and tracing failure.

An example of this reduction in sample size is seen in the 1958 cohort (Table 2.1): 83.3% of the original cohort were retained in the sample up to age 11 (similar to the 82.8% achieved in the Christchurch Development Study by the same age, Table 2.2, Fergusson et al., 1989). Further attrition reduced the sample to 79.5% by age 16 (Fogelman, 1983). Because there is a greater tendency for disadvantaged groups to be lost to follow-up, which results in sample bias, most studies expend considerable efforts to retain the good will of their subjects. For example, several studies send letters and birthday cards to express their appreciation to participants and to communicate some of the findings (Silva, 1990). Missing information also substantially reduces the sample available for analysis and is a common problem in investigations requiring measures collected at several ages or from different sources.

Another disadvantage is that results from longitudinal studies are not quickly available. Consequently, by the time earlier conditions are evaluated they may be less relevant to current circumstances because of a variety of changes—in treatment, provision of services, environmental conditions, social and family

Table 2.1. National Birth Cohort Studies in Britain

Year (study week)	Sample Size	Sample Description	Follow-Ups* (ages)
1946 (March 3–9th)	5,362	Single, legitimate births only: all from non-manual‡ and agricultural families; 1 in 4 sample from blue-collar families	2, 4, 6, 7, 8, 9, 11, 13, 15, 16, 17, 19, 20†, 22†, 23†, 25†, 26, 31†, 36
1958 (March 3–9th)	17,733	All births: immigrants (born during study week) included at ages 7, 11 and 16	7, 11, 16, 23, 33
1970 (April 5–11th)	16,567	All births: immigrants (born during study week) included at ages 5 and 10	5, 10, 16

*Of full sample.

†Postal questionnaire.

‡Social class in Britain includes six strata categorized by the Registrar General using occupational status. Class I is leading professions and business, II is lesser professions and business, III is skilled workers (non-manual and manual), IV is part-skilled workers, and V is unskilled workers.

Table 2.2. Examples of Birth Cohort Studies that Focus Primarily on Child Health

Study Title	Country	Reference	Year	Sample Size	Follow-Ups
Newcastle Thousand Families Survey	Great Britain	Miller et al., 1972	1947 (May-June)	1142	1, 3, 5, 9, 13, 14, 15 subsamples at 22 and 3
California Child Health and Development Studies	USA	van den Berg, et al., 1988	1959–1966	7500	5, 9–11
Northern Finland Birth Cohort	Finland	Rantakallio, 1988	1966	12058	1, 14
Dunedin Multidisciplinary Health and Development Study	New Zealand	Silva, 1990	1972 (Apr)–1973 (Mar)	1037	3, 5, 7, 9, 11, 13, 15
Christchurch Child Development Study	New Zealand	Fergusson et al., 1989	1977	1262	4 (months), 1, 2, 3, 4, 5, 6, 7, 8, 9, 10, 11
Pelotas Birth Cohort Study	Brazil	Barros et al., 1990	1982	5914	12 (months) 20 (months) 43 (months)

structure, etc.—occurring in the intervening period. Further, it is invariably the case that multipurpose studies collect information on a range of topics at the cost of detail in any one subject (this can, of course, be advantageous for some purposes). Other weaknesses and strengths are discussed in relation to the specific purposes for which longitudinal studies are used.

Prediction of Disease

The literature includes many reports in which follow-up data are used to predict childhood mortality, morbidity, growth, and development. Approaches vary; some studies focus on multiple outcomes from a single risk factor, whereas others examine a single outcome in relation to numerous risk factors.

A major scientific advantage of prospective studies is that exposure to suspected risk factors is ascertained before later disease status is known, and as a result, information on exposure is collected in an unbiased manner. Longitudinal studies rely on the variation that occurs in risk factors, such as diet and physical activity. Thus, the degree of association can be quantified for different exposure levels. Such information is especially important because the potential for experimental or intervention studies, which provide stronger evidence for causality, is inevitably restricted in human populations. An important advantage of longitudinal studies is therefore to clarify the direction in which associations are likely to operate, although they cannot provide "proof" of causality.

It has been suggested that a disadvantage of prospective follow-up is that the very act of investigation may act as an intervention, thereby modifying the behavior of participants. This undesirable effect would be especially problematic in research aiming to identify predictors of disease. Furthermore, studies may not collect what is later regarded as essential information, and early measurement techniques may appear inadequate in the light of subsequent improvements. For rare conditions, especially those with a long induction period, the sample size needed to obtain an adequate number of cases may prohibit the use of a prospective follow-up study.

Notwithstanding these restrictions, a prospective design has considerable strength in the prediction of childhood disorders, as the extensive literature on the subject testifies. Much of this literature focuses on birth events and circumstances. For example, an adverse effect of maternal smoking during pregnancy on mortality or birthweight of the child has now been demonstrated in several population samples (Butler & Bonham, 1963; Fergusson et al., 1979; Rush & Cassano, 1983). Further follow-up reveals the persistence of an adverse maternal smoking effect on later growth (Elwood et al., 1987; Rantakallio, 1988), adult height, and educational achievement (Fogelman & Manor, 1988).

Predictive Factors

Low Birthweight

Low birthweight is itself predictive of several adverse health risks—cerebral palsy, sensory, learning and behavioral disorders, and respiratory problems (see

Chapter 3). Evidence has accumulated from follow-up studies, such as the Northern Finland birth cohort (Table 2.2, Rantakallio, 1988). These data suggest, for example, that birthweight is predictive of psychomotor development at 1 year (as characterized by standing and walking without support), other predictive factors being gestational age, sex, and maternal age (girls and children of young mothers showing faster development). Heavier birthweight also seems to be associated with more advanced speech, as are female sex, low parity of mother, and urban place of residence (Rantakallio, 1988).

In addition, low birthweight (<2500 g) babies and those of short gestation (<37 weeks) have poorer growth, as demonstrated by the California Child Health and Development Study (Table 2.2; Van den Berg et al., 1988) and the Pelotas (Brazil) birth cohort study (Table 2.2; Victora et al., 1987). Follow-up studies also illustrate that birthweight is only one of several factors that predict childhood height and weight. Other influential factors for height are family size, parental stature, and social class (Douglas & Simpson, 1964; Goldstein, 1971; Miller et al., 1972). Predictors of childhood obesity also include parental body size, but whereas socioeconomic background is predictive of obesity in early adulthood, it seems to be unrelated to childhood obesity (Braddon et al., 1986; Power & Moynihan, 1988).

Breast Feeding

The protective effects of breast feeding have been examined in longitudinal studies of birth cohorts in a manner that would be difficult to establish in cross-sectional studies that rely on recall. An important requirement in seeking associations is that confounding factors, such as birthweight, mother's age, or level of education, are taken into account (see Chapter 1). Several studies have attempted to accomplish that objective. Barros et al. (1986) explored the confounding effect of birthweight on the association between breast feeding and infant mortality. They argue that in some populations there is an excess mortality of more than twofold among babies who are not breast fed, which is ascribed to a greater prevalence of low birthweight in this group. Disentangling the confounding effects of maternal education and socioeconomic circumstances in studies examining the effects of breast feeding on intellectual functioning has been another important contribution of cohort studies. Adjustment for such confounding factors reveals an advantage for breast-fed children, even after a considerable period of follow-up of 15 years (Rodgers, 1978), 10 years (Pollock, 1993), and 7 years (Fergusson et al., 1982). An advantage for breast-fed children was also shown in a study of low birthweight babies (Lucas et al., 1992). Nonetheless, it is possible that other factors that cannot be taken into account (parental attitudes, style, or personality) may confound the association. Hence, the results available so far are suggestive of a causal relationship, but are not proof of one.

Outcomes

Respiratory Conditions

Longitudinal follow-up has improved the understanding of factors predictive of respiratory conditions (see Chapter 18). Air pollution and manual (blue-collar) class origins were identified as risk factors for lower respiratory illness in childhood among subjects in the 1946 birth cohort (Table 2.1) and subsequently for respiratory symptoms at age 25 (Douglas & Waller, 1966; Kiernan et al., 1976). Predictors of childhood asthma differed, however, in that poor home circumstances did not emerge as risk factors (Anderson et al., 1986; Fergusson et al., 1989). Even so, early lower respiratory illness was associated with increased risk of both later asthma and other respiratory symptoms.

Accidents

Childhood accidents have also been investigated using longitudinal data. Increased risk of injury between 5 and 10 years of age was associated with number of injuries before age 5, male sex, aggressive child behavior, young maternal age, and many older and fewer younger siblings (Bijur et al., 1988a, b, and c). Predictors of road traffic injuries (ages 7 to 16) included overcrowding at home, being placed in the care of a local authority, family difficulties (as defined by parents), and fidgety and abnormal behavior of the child (Pless et al., 1989).

Emotional and Cognitive Development

Much effort has been devoted to identifying factors that predict emotional and intellectual development. Longitudinal research has a strong tradition in this field. An extensive range of factors have been investigated, some of which (e.g., low birthweight and breast feeding) have already been mentioned. Although most inquiries focus on family and social circumstances, others have considered the physical environment. For example, exposure to low levels of lead has been shown to have a small adverse effect on children's school performance and behavior (Fergusson et al., 1989). Among family factors that have been studied is being an unwanted child (Rantakallio, 1988). Follow-up of these children suggests that they have poorer school performance, especially in writing, than other children, although this decrement was less likely to be due to emotional rejection than to the reduced socioeconomic resources of the mother. Divorce and separation have also been examined as risk factors for poor emotional adjustment and intellectual development. Longitudinal evidence suggests that some of the problems that have been attributed to divorce and separation in cross-sectional studies can be largely accounted for by pre-existing conditions; that is, children from divorced or separated families have poorer achievement and behavior before the break-up occurs (Cherlin et al., 1991; Elliot & Richards, 1991). Hence, circumstances leading to or preceding divorce or separation may influence child behavior and school achievement, rather than the event itself.

Many other factors influence intellectual and emotional development during childhood. For example, childhood chronic illness has been shown to affect later emotional adjustment, as is discussed briefly in the following section. Socioeconomic disadvantage, such as financial hardship, paternal unemployment, and poor housing amenities, has been consistently linked with emotional and behavioral difficulties during childhood. Longitudinal evidence was essential in establishing the direction of effects, for example, underlying the relationship between unemployment and psychological health. Thus, a prospective study by

Banks and Jackson (1982) shows a deleterious effect of unemployment on the psychological health of young men that could not be accounted for by pre-existing psychological problems.

Specificity of Effects

Multipurpose follow-up studies have been influential in demonstrating that, although some risk factors predict specific conditions, others have more general effects. Childhood socioeconomic environment has a pervasive influence, as is evident from the literature cited here on emotional and behavioral problems, respiratory symptoms, and obesity in early adulthood.

An interesting development in research on prediction of disease and disorder is the increased recognition, especially in the psychological literature, of the cumulative effects of diverse influences. In psychological research this has been conceptualized as an interaction between vulnerability factors, such as childhood adversities, or protective factors, such as social support, and stressors, such as important life events (Brown & Harris, 1978). Longitudinal studies are ideal for testing hypotheses based on such models and to demonstrate whether they have wider application in research on other conditions. With the exception, however, of psychological research, the investigation of accumulation of risk factors remains an undeveloped approach.

Consequences of Morbidity, Disability, or Physical Attributes

A second common use of longitudinal studies is in establishing whether there are long-term sequelae of particular childhood conditions. This area of inquiry has attracted considerable interest and is of increasing relevance as more children survive conditions, such as congenital heart disease and childhood cancers, from which earlier generations had died (Celermajer, 1991). In the future it is likely that there will be more research on long-term consequences of childhood disorder. Previous work (described below) suggests that such studies should not only consider the physical and psychological consequences that may arise but also problems that manifest in education, employment, social relationships, fertility, and other social and economic areas.

Cross-sectional evidence can, of course, be used to show that those with particular childhood conditions differ from others in various respects, e.g., psychological well-being. Although such studies may suggest that adverse outcomes are associated with childhood disorders, there are many inherent weaknesses in this approach. In some instances it will be necessary to limit the possibility that events or conditions being treated as outcomes did not precede the disorder under investigation. Cross-sectional data are almost invariably inadequate for this purpose. Furthermore, recall of age of onset, severity, or frequency of disease episodes, are more readily obtained from prospective follow-ups than from cross-sectional studies.

General population longitudinal studies have additional advantages for inquiries on long-term consequences of childhood disorders. Most importantly, they contain information on children without the condition of interest, and this group often provides an excellent reference or comparison group. As the follow-up period increases, such studies also offer the opportunity to establish whether there are any latent effects. However, general population follow-up studies are of limited value for studying rare conditions because the numbers affected are usually inadequate, even in the larger studies. Usually, the only practical option for follow-up of rare conditions is to select them from clinic populations, although such groups are rarely representative of children with the condition and, in addition, an appropriate comparison group may not be easily identified.

One of the research topics that exemplifies the strength of the longitudinal approach in assessing consequences of disease is the evaluation of psychosocial adjustment in children with chronic physical disorders. Although various study designs have been used, a longitudinal follow-up approach is especially important in this context because the possibility that psychological maladjustment preceded or even caused the physical disorder has to be discounted. Much early work on this topic used small, selective samples and lacked prospective information, although study designs have improved in recent years (Nolan & Pless, 1986; Pless & Nolan, 1991). An example of recent work considers long-term consequences for children in the 1958 birth cohort (Table 2.1) who had a chronic physical illness at any time during childhood. As Table 2.3 illustrates, these children had increased risk of psychosocial problems, such as poor emotional well-being, in their early adulthood years (Pless et al., in press).

Prospective inquiries on long-term sequelae of specific conditions, such as epilepsy and asthma, have also been conducted. Britten et al. (1986) investigated whether children with epilepsy uncomplicated by other disorders differed from controls in their educational and occupational achievement, marriage and parenthood, self-esteem, and psychiatric morbidity. No evidence of handicap was evident by age 26, but 10 years later economic and self-esteem handicaps had

Table 2.3. Risk of Adverse Psychosocial Sequelae at Age 23 in Subjects with Chronic Physical Disorder*

Sequelae	Males	Females
Abnormal malaise† score	1.52 (1.13, 2.05)	1.18 (0.99, 1.48)
Psychiatric attention	1.43 (1.00, 2.03)	1.32 (1.02, 1.71)
No academic qualifications	1.26 (1.08, 1.47)	1.08 (0.91, 1.31)
Social class IV, V‡	1.09 (0.91, 1.30)	1.10 (0.92, 1.33)
Unemployed or out of labor force	1.15 (0.94, 1.40)	0.98 (0.76, 1.28)
Unemployed > 7%	1.20 (1.03, 1.41)	1.07 (0.89, 1.27)
Drinks alcohol—rarely/never	1.36 (1.15, 1.60)	0.91 (0.78, 1.06)
Socializing—		
No parties in last month	1.18 (1.02, 1.36)	1.01 (0.87, 1.18)
No visits in last month§	1.03 (0.79, 1.34)	1.23 (0.81, 1.87)

*Relative risks (95%) confidence intervals; subjects with chronic physical disorders versus healthy subjects in the 1958 birth cohort.

†Indicating a tendency toward depression.

‡See Table 2.1 for definition of social class.

§To or from friends and/or relatives.

emerged. For children with asthma, only a small adverse effect on employment in early adulthood was detected (Sibbald et al., 1992).

Other long-term sequelae of childhood respiratory illness and symptoms have been examined. Studies of childhood whooping cough show no discernible effects either later in childhood (Holland et al., 1978) or by age 36 (Britten & Wadsworth, 1986), whereas long-term effects have been found for other respiratory problems. Children with bronchitis by age 5 were more likely to have respiratory symptoms by age 11 and 14 years than other children, although loss to follow-up was particularly pronounced in this study (Holland et al., 1978). However, Strachan et al. (1988) also demonstrated that early childhood respiratory problems, namely pneumonia and asthma or wheezy bronchitis by age 7, were associated with a significant excess in the prevalence of chronic cough in young adults aged 23, even after allowing for smoking habits.

Children with behavior disorders also have been followed up to establish whether they experience adverse outcomes, especially during the transition from school to work. Maughan (1989) documents poorer outcomes—early school leaving, unstable work histories, and unskilled work—for 14-year-olds identified as having behavior disorder, in an Inner London sample. (A persistent behavior disorder was associated with high rates of delinquency). Similarly, as Table 2.4 shows, 16-year-olds with behavioral problems were more likely to be downwardly mobile from their social class of origin than their contemporaries in the 1958 birth cohort (Power et al., 1991). Other groups of children, particularly those with learning difficulties because of a physical, behavioral, or intellectual handicap, also face employment disadvantages on entering the labor market (Walker, 1982).

In addition to the many follow-up studies of childhood disorder, others investigate long-term consequences of childhood and adolescent body size and shape. Some studies extend over a considerable period into adulthood. For example, one Danish study followed up draftees (most of whom were aged 18 years) for an average of 12.5 years. The obese adolescents subsequently had lower attainment of social class than the nonobese, even after accounting for social class background and educational achievement (Sonne-Holme & Sorenson, 1986). Similarly, short stature was associated with downward social mobility from class of origin in young adults in the 1958 birth cohort (Power et al., 1986).

Table 2.4. Intergenerational Social Mobility* and Behavior Rating of 16 Year Olds in the 1958 Birth Cohort Study

	Mobility Between Social Class in Childhood (Age 16) and Age 23					
	Men			Women		
Behavior Rating at Age 16	Upward (n=245)	Stable (n=760)	Downward (n=319)	Upward (n=282)	Stable (n=801)	Downward (n=352)
Normal	68.6	44.2	32.9	68.1	60.9	37.8
Intermediate	25.7	41.2	42.9	25.9	33.6	44.0
Deviant	5.7	14.6	24.1	6.0	5.5	18.2

*From social class IIIM of origin. See Table 2.1 for definition of social classes.

Source: Adapted from Power et al., 1991.

Clearly, the literature cited above illustrates how ill health influences subsequent life circumstances, as well as the reverse. Each of these effects contributes to disparities in the occurrence of morbidity between different social and regional groups. Longitudinal studies, in contrast to cross-sectional studies, offer an opportunity to distinguish between social causation of such disparities (whereby the occurrence of disease is affected by conditions prevailing in different social or regional groups) and selective processes (by which individuals are sorted into social or regional groups on the basis of their health status). This distinction is especially useful in relation to later life problems, such as psychiatric disorder (Dohwenrend, 1990), it is also important for disparities at younger ages. Although much of the evidence described above suggests that certain childhood conditions prejudice subsequent employment opportunities, these selective effects may not be so strong as to provide the main explanation for social differences in ill health in early adulthood (Power et al., 1991).

Longitudinal studies with several years of follow-up also offer an opportunity to investigate whether the consequences observed for specific childhood conditions are mediated by other influences. In general, this research approach is relatively underdeveloped, even though longitudinal studies are ideal for studying pathways through to adult life.

Continuity and Change Over Time

There are many reasons for studying the persistence over time of specific illnesses and disorders and also of salient risk factors for later disease. Studying the former provides useful information on the prognosis of different conditions; the latter offers the potential for preventive action if formative stages can be identified. It is especially important to have information on continuity of salient risk factors for which treatment in later life is difficult and/or unsuccessful. To some extent, the topic of continuities and change could have been included under prediction of disease or consequences, because earlier disease and risk factor status can be predictive of the same measures in later life. An example of this phenomenon is the relationship between early respiratory problems and later respiratory symptoms described in the previous section (see Chapter 18).

Because it is rarely possible to obtain relevant information from cross-sectional surveys, longitudinal tracking of individual subjects is commonly used for such purposes. It is particularly useful for studying factors and illnesses for which recall is poor, either because information is unknown or because it is difficult to remember accurately. Furthermore, discrepancies in the motivation of diseased and nondiseased groups to recall the past can introduce bias into studies that rely on memory. An advantage of prospective follow-up is that it provides an unbiased assessment of a disease or risk factor over a defined period. For example, a prospective design would be preferable for assessing continuities in diet, blood pressure, or obesity.

There are numerous examples of studies tracking blood pressure and obesity because of their implications for disease in later life (see Chapter 18). One such study followed the blood pressure of children from 6 months of age to 10 years to identify the age at which children consistently appeared in one part of the distribution of blood pressure values for the population (de Swiet et al., 1992). Correlations of blood pressure measurements increased progressively with age, from between the first and last to the penultimate and last measurement, when the correlation was at its highest. Despite these correlations, most of the variability of blood pressure at age 10 was not associated with earlier measurements. This pattern is similar to that reported for childhood obesity. As might be expected, correlations between measures of overweight decrease as the interval between measurements increases (Peckham et al., 1983). Although obese children have a higher than expected risk of obesity in later life, it has now been consistently shown that most obesity in adolescence and early adulthood is not a continuation of obesity earlier in childhood (Hawk & Brook, 1979; Miller et al., 1972; Power & Moynihan, 1988; Sorenson & Sonne Holme, 1988; Stark et al., 1981).

Several longitudinal studies have investigated whether emotional and behavioral problems persist throughout childhood and into adult life (see Chapter 11). One difficulty is that transient emotional and behavioral disturbance is common during childhood (Ghodsian et al., 1980; Rutter, 1991). For example, 30% of the Dunedin study sample (Table 2.2) were identified as having problem behaviors at age 7, but only 9% of these cases were considered to represent a stable problem (McGee et al., 1984). Added to this is the complication, identified by Rutter (1991), that "psychopathological continuities are stronger than was usually supposed in the past, their strength having been concealed by a change in the form of the disturbance." It is not surprising, therefore, that, although there seems to be an increased risk of later psychological problems among those identified as maladjusted in childhood or adolescence (Power et al., 1991; Rodgers, 1990), conclusive evidence for strong continuities is still not available. Nonetheless, continuities in antisocial disorder are considered to be stronger than for anxiety and emotional disorder (Robins, 1978).

Another childhood condition for which long-term study of continuity and change has yielded important information is asthma. Prospective studies suggest that most children with symptoms before age 7 improve during adolescence (Anderson et al., 1986; McNicol & Williams, 1973). Follow-up studies restricted to children who are affected by a specific age (Martin et al., 1980; McNicol & Williams, 1973) cannot identify those children with later onset. This limitation is overcome in general population follow-ups as opposed to those involving clinic samples. Anderson et al. (1986) describe one such study in which the natural history of asthma was examined from the first year of life to 16 years in the 1958 birth cohort: 24.7% of children were affected during this period, the majority (18.3%) before age 8; 3.6% had onset between ages 8 and 11 and 2.8% between 12 and 16 years (see Chapter 18).

Age Trends

As the above studies illustrate, longitudinal samples provide information on prevalence of different conditions, development, and behavior at different ages. This information can be obtained more quickly and cheaply from cross-sectional surveys, and although data obtained from longitudinal studies have the advantage of avoiding generation (or cohort) effects, it is acknowledged that apparent trends with age may be influenced by changes over time (or period effects). Another disadvantage, mentioned earlier in relation to the prediction of disease, is that some characteristics under investigation (e.g., behavior) may be modified as a result of participation in the study.

Although it is not a primary aim of a longitudinal study to provide information on prevalence of childhood conditions, that provision of data is an important additional advantage and is often stated as a secondary aim. Some studies also use data on other relevant measures (e.g., blood pressure) to determine population norms at different ages during childhood. In many countries, including Britain, such data are not collected routinely; use of health services for various childhood disorders is often the only available data, and this information is distorted by availability and differential use by different sectors of the community. Descriptive information from cohort studies can therefore be useful in this context. Usually, the data are limited to common medical conditions ascertained at different ages, including asthma (Anderson et al., 1986; Fergusson et al., 1989), visual defects (Tibbenham et al., 1978), enuresis (Butler & Golding, 1986; Douglas, 1973), convulsions (Ross et al., 1980; van den Berg et al., 1988), hearing problems (Richardson et al., 1977), chronic illness (Pless & Douglas, 1971), eczema and hay fever (Butler & Golding, 1986), obesity (Peckham et al., 1983), and injuries (Chalmers et al., 1989; Pless et al., 1989). With large samples, it has also been possible to document the incidence of rarer conditions, such as cerebral palsy (Emond et al., 1989; Rantakallio, 1988) and CNS infections (Rantakallio, 1988).

The information provided by longitudinal studies can permit an estimation of *both* prevalence and incidence for different disorders if contact with the sample is fairly frequent. In contrast, cross-sectional studies are usually limited to estimates of prevalence because it is not always possible to obtain a reliable retrospective report of age of onset. For example, it was necessary to obtain longitudinal data before the incidence of stuttering could be estimated (Andrews & Harris, 1964).

Conclusions

Opinions about the value of longitudinal studies vary. Clearly, there are numerous shortcomings—expense, sample attrition and associated biases, the potential modification of behavior, and the time lag in obtaining results. Furthermore, some longitudinal designs are unsuitable for particular purposes, such as the study of rare conditions in general population samples. These shortcomings should be acknowledged and steps taken, wherever possible, to reduce their impact. Nevertheless, as this chapter illustrates, the advantages of longitudinal studies are also considerable. Advances in many research areas can only be achieved with such data. In particular, these studies are especially important in demonstrating the accumulation of risk over time and in identifying latent effects. Consequently, follow-up studies have now been initiated in several countries, only a few of which have been mentioned here. Inter-cohort comparison has been limited, mainly because of different study designs and measurements. Recently, however, there has been an attempt to enhance the potential for comparison by a European coordinating group (ELSPAC, 1989), but other comparisons are likely to remain on an ad hoc basis.

Longitudinal studies initiated in early life contribute to an understanding of the epidemiology of childhood conditions and also have the potential to contribute to research on disease in later life. They are especially valuable in disentangling the relative effects of early and later influences on adult disease. This area of research presents new challenges in the design and analysis of longitudinal studies. A primary concern is the recognition and treatment of confounding factors—an important issue for prospective research on childhood conditions because as the length of follow-up extends, it is likely that an even wider range of confounding factors will be introduced. Disadvantages and advantages of different longitudinal approaches will therefore become apparent in this type of research inquiry (Barker & Martyn, 1982; Elford et al., 1991) as they have in others.

References

Anderson HR, Bland JM, Patel S, Peckham C. The natural history of asthma in childhood. *J Epidemiol Comm Health* 1986; 40:121–129.

Andrews G, Harris M. *The Syndrome of Stuttering*. London: Spastics Society/Heinemann; 1964.

Banks MH, Jackson PR. Unemployment and risk of minor psychiatric disorder in young people: cross-sectional and longitudinal evidence. Psychol Med 1982; 12:789–798.

Barker DJP, Martyn CN. The maternal and fetal origins of cardiovascular disease. *J Epidemiol Comm Health* 1992; 46:8–11.

Barros FC, Victora CG, Vaughan JP, Smith PG. Birth weight and duration of breast feeding: are the beneficial effects of human milk being overestimated. *Pediatrics* 1986; 78:656–661.

Barros FC, Victora CG, Vaughan JP. The Pelotas (Brazil) birth cohort study 1982–1987: strategies for following up 6000 children in a developing country. *Paed Perinat Epidemiol* 1990; 4:205–220.

Bijur P, Golding J, Haslum M, Kurzon M. Behavioral predictors of injury in school-age children. *Am J Dis Child* 1988a; 142:1307–1312.

Bijur PE, Golding J, Haslum M. Persistence of occurrence of injury: can injuries of preschool children predict injuries of school-aged children? *Pediatrics* 1988b; 82:707–712.

Bijur PE, Golding J, Kurzon M. Childhood accidents, family size and birth order. *Soc Sci Med* 1988c; 26:839–843.

Braddon FEM, Rodgers B, Wadsworth MEJ, Davies JMC. Onset of obesity in a 36-year birth cohort study. *Br Med J* 1986; 293:299–303.

Britten N, Wadsworth J. Longterm respiratory sequelae of whooping cough in a nationally representative sample. *Br Med J* 1986; 292:441–444.

Britten N, Morgan K, Fenwick PBC, Britten H. Epilepsy and handicap from birth to age 36. *Dev Med Child Neurol* 1986; 28:719–728.

Brown GW, Harris TO. *Social Origins of Depression: A Study of Psychiatric Disorder in Women*. London, Tavistock; 1976.

Butler NR, Bonham DG. *Perinatal Mortality*. Edinburgh: Livingstone; 1963.

Butler, NR, Golding J. *From Birth to Five*. Oxford: Pergamon Press; 1986.

Celermajer DS, Deanfield JE. Adults with congenital heart disease. *Br Med J* 1991; 303:1413–1414.

Chalmers DJ, Cecchi J, Langley JD, Silva PA. Injuries in the 12th and 13th years of life. *Aust. Paediatr J* 1989; 25:14–20.

Chamberlain R, Chamberlain G, Howlett B, Claireaux A. *British Births 1970. Vol 1: The First Week of Life*. London: Heinemann Medical, 1975.

Cherlin AJ, Furstenberg FF, Case-Lansdale PL, et al. Longitudinal studies of effects of divorce on children in Great Britain and the United States. *Science* 1991; 252:1386–1389.

Ciba Foundation Symposium 156. *The Childhood Environment and Adult Disease*. Chichester: J Wiley; 1991.

de Swiet M, Fayers P, Shinebourne EA. Blood pressure in first 10 years of life: the Brompton study. *Br Med J* 1992; 304:23–26.

Dohrenwend BP. Socioeconomic status (SES) and psychiatric disorders: are the issues still compelling? *Soc Psychiatry Psychiatr Epidemiol* 1990; 25:41–47.

Douglas JWB. Early disturbing events and later enuresis. In: Kolvin I, MacKeith RC, Meadow ST, eds. *Bladder Control and Enuresis*. London: Spastics International Medical Publishers; 1973.

Douglas JWB, Simpson HR. Height in relation to puberty, family size and social class. A longitudinal study. *Milbank Mem Fund Q* 1964; 42:20–35.

Douglas JWB, Waller RE. Air pollution and respiratory infection in children. *Br J Prev Soc Med* 1966; 20:1–8.

Elford J, Whincup P, Shaper AG. Early life experience and adult cardiovascular disease: longitudinal and case-control studies. *Int J Epidemiol* 1991; 4:833–844.

Elliot J, Richards PM. Children and divorce: educational performance and behavior before and after separation. *Int J Law Family* 1991; 5:258–276.

ELSPAC. Research protocol: European longitudinal study of pregnancy and childhood. *Paed Perinat Epidemiol* 1989; 3:460–469.

Elwood PC, Sweetnam PM, Gray OP, Davies DP, Wood PDP. Growth of children from 0–5 years: with special reference to mother's smoking in pregnancy. *Ann Human Biol* 1987; 14:543–557.

Emond A, Golding J, Peckham CS. Cerebral palsy in two national cohort studies. *Arch Dis Child* 1989; 64:848–852.

Fergusson DM, Horwood LJ, Shannon FT. Smoking during pregnancy. *NZ Med J* 1979; 89:41–43.

Fergusson DM, Beautrais AL, Silva PA. Breast-feeding and cognitive development in the first seven years of life. *Soc Sci Med* 1982; 16:1705–1708.

Fergusson DM, Horwood LJ, Shannon FT, Lawton JM. The Christchurch Child Development Study: a review of epidemiological findings. *Paed Perinat Epidemiol* 1989; 3:302–325.

Fogelman K, ed. *Growing Up in Great Britain*. London, Macmillan; 1983.

Fogelman K, Manor O. Smoking in pregnancy and development into early adulthood. *Br Med J* 1988; 297:1233–1236.

Fox AJ. *Longitudinal Study: Social Class and Occupational Mobility 1971–77*. LS No. 2. London: HMSO; 1985.

Ghodsian M, Fogelman K, Lambert L, Tibbenham A. Changes in behavior ratings of a national sample of children. *Br J Soc Clin Psychol* 1980; 19:247–256.

Goldstein H. Factors influencing the height of seven-year-old children. Results from the National Child Development Study (1958 cohort). *Human Biol* 1971; 43:92–111.

Hawk LJ, Brook CGD. Influence of body fatness in childhood on fatness in adult life. *Br Med J* 1979; 1:151–152.

Holland WW, Bailey P, Bland JM. Long-term consequences of respiratory disease in infancy. *J Epidemiol Comm Health* 1978; 32:256–259.

Joint Committee of the Royal College of Obstetricians and Gynaecologists and the Population Investigation Committee. *Maternity in Great Britain*. Oxford: Oxford University Press; 1948.

Kiernan KE, Colley JRT, Douglas JWB, Reid DD. Chronic cough in young adults in relation to smoking habits, childhood environment and chest illness. *Respiration* 1976; 33:236–244.

Lucas A, Morley R, Cole TJ, Lister G, Leeson-Payne C. Breast milk and subsequent intelligence quotient in children born preterm. *Lancet* 1992; 339:261–264.

Martin AJ, McLennan LA, Landau LI, Phelan PD. The natural history of childhood asthma to adult life. *Br Med J* 1980; 280:1397–1400.

Maughan B. Growing up in the inner city: findings from the Inner London longitudinal study. *Paed Perinat Epidemiol* 1989; 3:195–215.

McGee R, Silva PA, Williams S. Behavior problems in a population of seven-year-old children: prevalence, stability and types of disorder—a research report. *Child Psychol Psychiat* 1984; 25:251–259.

McNicol KN, Williams HB. Spectrum of asthma in children. I. Clinical and physiological components. *Br Med J* 1973; 4:7–11.

Miller FJW, Billewicz WZ, Thomson AM. Growth from birth to adult life of 442 Newcastle Upon Tyne children. *Br J Prev Soc Med* 1972; 26:224–230.

Nolan T, Pless IB. Emotional correlates and consequences of birth defects. *J Pediatr* 1986; 109:201–216.

OPCS. *LS Census Link 1971–1981*. London: HMSO; 1988.

Peckham CS, Stark O, Simonite V, Wolff OH. Prevalence of obesity in British children born in 1946 and 1958. *Br Med J* 1983; 286:1237–1242.

Pless IB, Douglas JWB. Chronic illness in childhood: Part 1, epidemiological and later clinical characteristics. *Paediatrics* 1971; 47:405–414.

Pless IB, Peckham CS, Power C. Predicting traffic injuries in childhood: a cohort analysis. *J Pediatr* 1989; 115:932–938.

Pless IB, Nolan T. Revision, replication and neglect—research on maladjustment in chronic illness. *J Child Psychol Psychiat* 1991; 32:347–365.

Pless IB, Power C, Peckham C. Long term psychosocial sequelae of chronic physical disorders in childhood. *Pediatrics* 1993; in press.

Pollock JI. Longterm associations with infant feeding in a clinically advantaged population of babies. *Dev Med Child Neurol* 1993; in press.

Power C. A review of child health in the 1958 birth cohort: National Child Development Study. *Paed Perinatal Epidemiol* 1992; 6:81–110.

Power C, Moynihan C. Social class and changes in weight-for-height between childhood and early adulthood. *Int J Obesity* 1988; 12:445–453.

Power C, Fogelman K, Fox AJ. Health and social mobility during the early years of life. *Q J Soc Affairs* 1986; 2:397–413.

Power C, Manor O, Fox AJ. *Health and Class: The Early Years*. London: Chapman & Hall; 1991.

Rantakallio P. The longitudinal study of the Northern Finland birth cohort of 1966. *Paed Perinat Epidemiol* 1988; 2:59–88.

Richardson K, Hutchison D, Peckham C, Tibbenham A. Audiometric thresholds of a national sample of British sixteen year olds: a longitudinal study. *Dev Med Child Neurol* 1977; 19:797–802.

Robins LN. Sturdy childhood predictors of adult antisocial behavior: replications from longitudinal studies. *Psych Med* 1978; 8:611–622.

Rodgers B. Feeding in infancy and later ability and attainment: a longitudinal study. *Dev Med Child Neurol* 1978; 20:421–426.

Rodgers B. Behaviour and personality in childhood as predictors of adult psychiatric disorder. *J Child Psychol Psychiat* 1990; 31:393–414.

Ross EM, Peckham C, West P, et al. Epilepsy in childhood: findings from the National Child Development Study. *Br Med J* 1980; 200:207–210.

Rothman KJ. *Modern Epidemiology*. Boston: Little, Brown and Co: 1986.

Rush D, Cassano P. Relationship of cigarette smoking and social class to birthweight and perinatal mortality among all births in Britain, 5–11 April 1970. *J Epidemiol Comm Health* 1983; 37:249–255.

Rutter M. Childhood experiences and adult psychosocial functioning. In: Ciba Foundation 156, ed. *The Childhood Environment and Adult Disease*. Chichester: J Wiley; 1991.

Sibbald B, Anderson HR, McGuigan S. Asthma and unemployment in young adults. *Thorax* 1992; 47:19–24.

Silva PA. The Dunedin Multidisciplinary Health and Development Study: a 15 year longitudinal study. *Paed Perinat Epidemiol* 1990; 4:76–107.

Sonne-Holm S, Sorensen TIA. Prospective study of attainment of social class of severely obese subjects in relation to parental social class, intelligence, and education. *Br Med J* 1986; 292:586–589.

Sorensen TIA, Sonne-Holm S. Risk in childhood of development of severe adult obesity: retrospective, population-based case-cohort study. *Am J Epidemiol* 1988; 127:104–113.

Stark O, Atkins E, Wolff OH, Douglas JWB. Longitudinal study of obesity in the National Survey of Health and Development. *Br Med J* 1981; 283:13–17.

Strachan DP, Anderson HR, Bland JM, Peckham C. Asthma as a link between chest illness in childhood and chronic cough and phlegm in young adults. *Br Med J* 1988; 296:890–893.

Tibbenham A, Peckham C, Gardiner P. Vision screening in children tested at 7, 11 and 16 years. *Br Med J* 1978; 1:1312–1314.

van den Berg BJ, Christianson RE, Oechsli FW. The California Child Health and Development Studies of the School of Public Health, University of California at Berkeley. *Paed Perinat Epidemiol* 1988; 2:265–282.

Victora CG, Barros FC, Vaughan JP, Martines JC, Beria JU. Birthweight, socioeconomic status and growth of Brazilian infants. *Ann Human Biol* 1987; 14:49–57.

Wadsworth MEJ. Follow-up of the first national cohort: findings from the Medical Research Council National Survey of Health and Development. *Paed Perinat Epidemiol* 1987; 1:95–117.

Walker A. *Unqualified and Underemployed: Handicapped Young People and the Labour Market*. London: Macmillan; 1982.

PART I

PERINATAL DISORDERS

3

Low Birthweight and Prematurity

Eva Alberman

Babies who are born unexpectedly early or with an unusually low birthweight are at immediate and continuing high risk of mortality and of acute and long-term morbidity. It is well known that in developed countries they may account for more than half of infant deaths and perhaps a third of the cases of cerebral palsy, even when they are treated intensively with all the tools of modern medical technology (see Chapter 17). Survivors are also at increased risk of sensory, learning, or behavior disorders; respiratory problems; and health hazards in adult life.

The study of the epidemiology of prematurity presents a variety of challenges. Fundamental to it is the understanding of the biologic, social, environmental, and behavioral influences that act together to determine the distributions of birthweight, gestational age, and of birthweight for gestational age that are characteristic of the population under consideration. More directly related to the subject of this chapter is the study of the lower end of these distributions—the distinction between normal and abnormally low weight or gestation and, for the latter, their incidence, prediction, and primary prevention.

Additionally, it is of importance to study the factors that influence the risk of mortality and morbidity; to monitor the outcome of the affected births; to define as precisely as possible different types of adverse outcomes; and to pursue methods of preventing, palliating, or minimizing these outcomes. Finally, this is a field in which advances in medical technology have certainly resulted in steep increases in survival, but at a considerable cost in terms of health services resources and with a consequent small rise in the prevalence of impairment in the survivors. Questions have been asked about the degree to which it is cost effective or humane to strive for improved survival of extremely immature infants, and what methods can be used to enable society to contribute sensible answers to such questions.

In this chapter the discussion of these questions must necessarily be at a superficial level and, where possible, concentrates on the opportunities for the prevention of the morbidity to be described.

Biologic Considerations

Until recently, the focus of comparative epidemiologic studies has been largely limited to prematurity as defined by a birthweight below an arbitrary cut-off point. Birthweight is the only measure that has been collected on national and international levels, and it has the advantage of few problems of definition and thus the possibility of repeatable and reliable measurement. However, it is becoming clear that further advances in the understanding of this subject will require full use of all available information on the gestational age, as well as birthweight; their joint relationship in the populations under consideration; and the factors that influence them, particularly at the lower tails of the distributions.

Birthweight is the result of two determinants: the length of time the fetus remains in utero and the velocity of fetal growth. The curtailment of either causes some form of prematurity: the former causes preterm birth and the latter, fetal growth retardation. Often the two conditions coexist. It is, however, important to distinguish between their effects, for preterm birth exposes the infant to all the hazards of extrauterine life on immature lungs and other organs and therefore to a high risk of neonatal death. Fetal growth retardation may reflect prenatal impairment, but it is often compatible with extrauterine life. There is interaction between the two measures, so that babies who are both preterm and growth retarded have particularly high health risks.

Birthweight

The proportion of births defined by arbitrary cut-off points as being of low birthweight depends on the median, shape, and variance of the whole birthweight distribution from which they are derived. The median of these distributions is largely determined by the median weight at term. In Western populations, full term is defined as 40 weeks, and the median weight usually lies between 3000 and 4000 g. However, one hindrance to arriving at a common definition of prematurity, whether by gestation or birthweight, is that, as with measured intelligence, both are distributed in the population as a near-Gaussian or "normal" distribution. Particularly for birthweight, it is difficult to arrive at a cut-off point that discriminates between a baby at the lower end of the normal range and one who is significantly below its expected weight.

This difficulty is compounded by the fact that the means and spread of the distributions themselves vary with such biologic factors as plurality, sex, ethnic origin, and birth order. All these factors should be allowed for when estimating expected weight. These and other influences have been recently reviewed in some detail (Alberman & Evans, 1989). Within populations, birthweight distributions tend to remain remarkably stable over time because many of the demographic and other factors influencing birthweight tend to change slowly, except under conditions of great social evolution, such as in postwar Japan. However, small drifts over time of the median birthweight, both toward higher and lower birthweights, have been demonstrated (Evans & Alberman, 1989). In recent years there has also been a tendency toward an increased registration of extremely low weight births, who may previously have been regarded as miscarriages (Alberman & Botting, 1991).

One change that has occurred in the epidemiology of prematurity is the marked increase in the number of multiple births, particularly higher order births, as a consequence of artificially inducing ovulation or the implantation of multiple embryos after in-vitro fertilization. This increase has contributed to the rise that has been observed in the very lowest birthweight groups and brings with it the additional risks of multiple pregnancy (Botting et al., 1987). A recent trial of a nutrition intervention program suggests that some reduction in birthweight of twins can be achieved (Dubois et al., 1991), but his finding needs confirmation. Sadly, there has also been a trend toward an increase in very low birthweight babies in some inner cities, which is probably associated with the abuse of drugs. Joyce (1990) has reported an upward trend of such births in New York City between 1984 and 1988.

Several criteria have been used to define the point below which birthweight may be regarded as being low. The most commonly used cut-off point is that of 5½ pounds (2500 g) or less, a weight that in the early part of this century in populations of European descent, was likely to define a group at high risk of mortality or morbidity. In such populations, this weight is close to the cut-off point defined by the mean minus two standard deviations. The latter is another measure that has been used to define low birthweight, although it is generally acknowledged to be unsatisfactory because of the skew toward low birthweights at each gestational age. This fact has led to the more common adoption of a percentile—the third, fifth, or tenth—as the cut-off point. The advantage of using such a definition is that it allows for differences in the position of the median and variability of birthweight distribution that characterize populations of different genetic and sociobiologic constitution (see Table 3.2 below for the effect of using this on ranking mortality).

It is still commonplace to define low birthweight as a weight below 2500 g, as is recommended in the Ninth Revision of the WHO International Classification of Diseases (ICD). Births of a weight below 2000 g or, more often, below 1500 g are described as very low birthweight (VLBW) and those below 1000 g as extremely low birthweight (ELBW). It is increasingly the case that, although babies born with a birthweight between 1500 and 2499 g are at a disadvantage compared to those with heavier weights, in part because of the close relationship between this birthweight group and poor socioeconomic circumstances, the major medical problems arise in babies under 1500 g, and particularly in those under 1000 g birthweight.

The use of an arbitrary value for the definition of low birthweight or gestational age always begs the question of the appropriateness of that value for different populations. It is unfortunate that most of the research on long-term outcomes of premature births is based on this type of definition of prematurity, because this limits comparisons between populations with different birthweight and gestational age distributions.

Secondary or Residual Distributions

As stated earlier, even within homogeneous groups, the distribution of birthweight always seems to be skewed toward the lower tail. There is a school of thought that ascribes this skew to the presence of a secondary or residual distribution that is characterized by extremely high morbidity or mortality rates. This group is probably largely made up of babies who are of low weight for the gestational age they had achieved because of social disadvantages or maternal or fetal pathology. It has been recommended that, for the comparison of birthweight curves, only the parameters of the main distribution of births be used. Several mathematical methods have been proposed to discriminate between the residual and main distributions, and this question is discussed by Willcox and Russell (1986).

Birthweight and Gestation

There are several ways of using birthweight and gestational age jointly to arrive at definitions of different types of prematurity, and a variety of terms have been used to describe deviations from the norm. Fetal growth retardation exists when the birthweight is below that expected for gestational age. It may be expressed as being (1) a fixed point, (2) a given number of standard deviations below the mean, or (3) a given percentile. Affected births are described as small-for-dates (SFD), sometimes as light-for-dates (LFD), or as small-for-gestational-age (SGA).

Fetal Growth Retardation

Predisposing factors for low birthweight secondary to retarded fetal growth, after allowing for such physiologic influences as female sex, plurality, and low birth order, include social and economic disadvantage; pregnancy in adolescent or unsupported mothers; intrauterine exposure to tobacco, alcohol, or drugs; maternal ill health, including hypertension of pregnancy; and intrauterine infection or fetal anomaly. Low parental stature and weight are also associated with low birthweight, but may themselves be abnormally low because of long-standing socioeconomic disadvantages. It can be argued that an adjustment for the latter may conceal the extent of individual fetal growth retardation. Most of these factors interact with each other, and it is difficult to tease out the primary pathways through which they act.

Additional problems are posed by the absence of information on the actual time of conception and therefore the true length of gestation. Moreover, these problems are enhanced by the increasing use of ultrasound dating which is a measure of developmental, rather than chronologic age. The use of ultrasound may lead to an underestimate of true gestational age and therefore of expected growth. Objective methods of detecting abnormalities in fetal growth velocity include the charting of sequential ultrasound measures, such as the biparietal diameter (Campbell, 1989), to find babies whose growth unexpectedly deviates from an established track. However, these problems have not yet been resolved, and debate continues on the anthropometric indices that may best reflect growth anomalies (Colley et al., 1991).

Once pregnancy has occurred, our ability to prevent fetal growth retardation is extremely limited, except by stopping or reducing maternal smoking, drug, or alcohol consumption. There are indications from the literature that maternal work, if it involves long hours or heavy physical labor (Launer et al., 1990; Peoples-Sheps et al., 1991), may cause fetal growth retardation or preterm labor, but reports are not entirely consistent on these points. Almost certainly, the outcome will depend on the general health of the women concerned, the precise nature of the work, and whether there are additional complications of pregnancy, such as multiple births or pregnancy hypertension.

Many attempts have been made to reduce the incidence of low birthweight in mothers known to be at high risk. It had previously been thought that bed rest would be effective in increasing the weight of the babies, but this intervention has now been shown to be ineffective. In contrast, a meta-analysis of results of recently published trials on the effect of giving low-dose aspirin to mothers with pregnancy-induced hypertension suggests that this treatment may lead to reductions in the incidence of very low birthweight (Imperiale & Petrulis, 1991). However, a definitive view on the effectiveness of this treatment must await the results of large-scale trials currently underway (Collins, 1992).

Increasingly attention is being directed to the long-term antecedents of fetal growth retardation and at improving our understanding of the pathways through which social disadvantage limits growth rate.

Preterm Delivery

Remarkably little is known about the causes of preterm delivery, which certainly include multiple pregnancy, infection of the fetal membranes, and placental abruption, usually of unknown cause. It follows that the repertoire of primary preventive action is very limited. Secondary preventive actions include the attempt to stop the labor by the administration of beta-mimetic agents, but the success of this and other treatments is not as yet proven. The up-to-date results of recent relevant trials are available in the electronic *Oxford Database of Perinatal Trials* (1992).

Mortality

High-risk neonatal problems, as well as impairments, whether prenatally or postnatally caused, are associated with high mortality rates. There is always a steeply rising gradient of risk as birthweight falls. This relationship is illustrated in Figure 3.1, which is based on 100 g weight groups. In conducting comparative studies it is important to match for even small differences in distributions below 2500 g. In the lowest weight groups, mortality is highest in the first days of life, and the probability of survival then levels off rapidly (Powell et al., 1986).

The relationship of mortality to birthweight and gestational age depends on the cause under consideration, as is shown in Table 3.1 which is derived from 6 years of data from over 5 million white births in the United States. As expected, deaths certified as due to immaturity are most frequent where both birthweight and gestational age are low; deaths due to congenital malformations are also associated with low birthweight, but within this group, they are more common

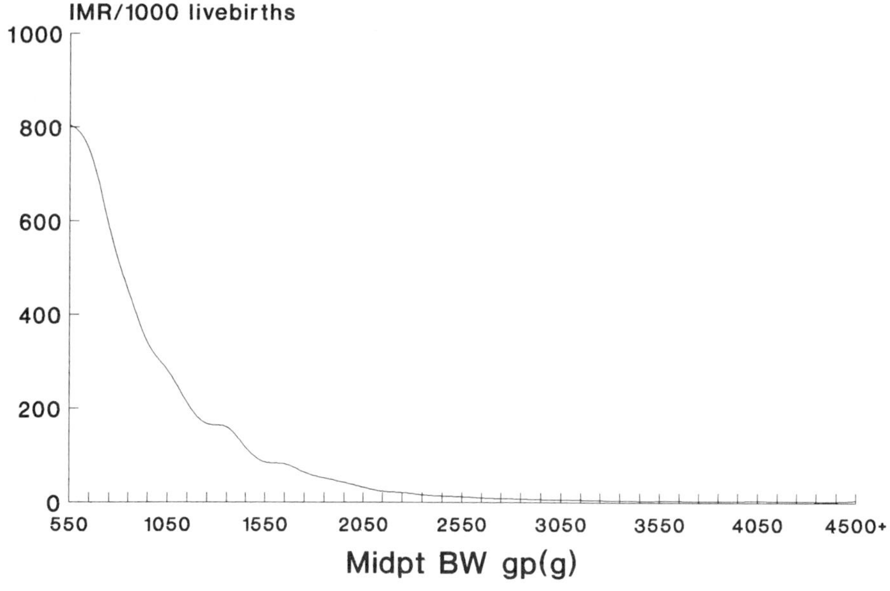

Fig. 3.1. Infant mortality by birthweight in England and Wales: Singletons, 1987. Source: OPCS unpub.

Table 3.1. Selected Causes of Infant Deaths by Birthweight and Gestational Age Groups (Unknowns Excluded)*

	Infant Deaths/100 Livebirths		
Birthweight (g)	≤33 wks	34–36 wks	≥37 wks
Immaturity			
<1500	200.4	40.0	64.7
–2499	13.2	2.5	1.2
>2499	2.9	0.6	0.1
Congenital malformations			
<1500	23.4	71.6	56.6
–2499	14.9	11.4	12.7
>2499	3.9	2.7	1.3
Sudden infant deaths			
<1500	2.4	3.26	2.9
–2499	4.9	2.91	2.6
>2499	2.2	1.81	1.2

*White births in the United States, 1980 to 1985.

Source: International Collaborative Effort (ICE) 2nd Generation (unpublished).

with increasing gestational age. Risk of sudden infant death is also increased in the lowest birthweight and gestational age groups and is least where birthweight is over 2500 g and gestational age over 36 weeks.

Trends in Mortality

In contrast to the consistent incidence of low birthweight within populations, the associated mortality risks vary sharply over time, as well as by place of occurrence. Although over recent years there has been some postponement of death among very low birthweight infants—from the neonatal to the postneonatal period—total infant survival in this group has risen fairly consistently in all developed countries (Alberman & Evans, 1989). Figure 3.2 gives an indication of the rise that occurred in Mersey, England (and also of morbidity trends to be discussed below). These increases in infant survival have been related to advances in medical technology and quality of neonatal care (Paneth et al., 1982).

Differences that exist between birthweight-specific mortality risks in different countries or different populations are in part related to the medical facilities available and in part are explicable by the appropriateness of the cut-off point of 2500 g to that particular population. In the United States, the birthweight distribution of black births is markedly shifted toward lower weights compared to that of white babies. However, the mortality risk of black infants is consistently less than that of white babies, but only at low weights (Table 3.2), although almost certainly black babies have less access to excellent neonatal care than do the white babies. When a percentile birthweight is used (for instance, the fifth), the differences between whites and blacks at the low centiles are reversed. Now

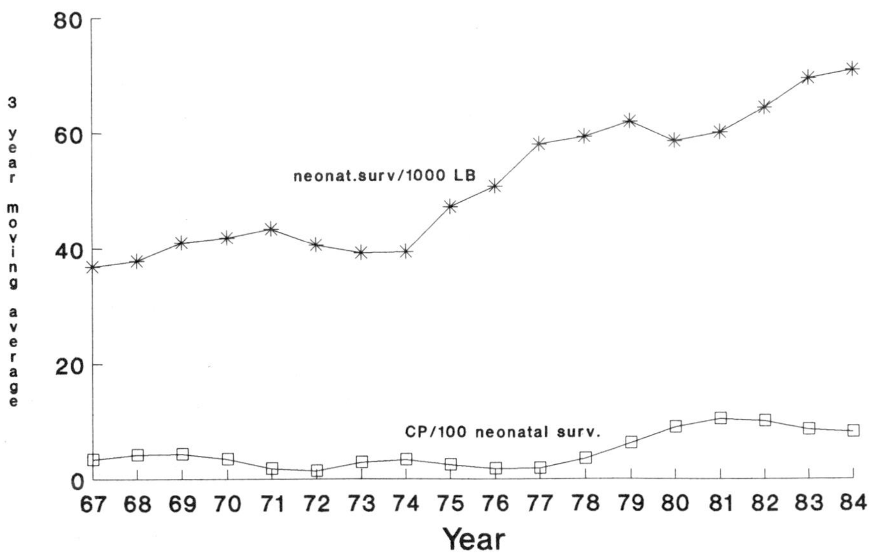

Fig. 3.2. Neonatal survivors of <1501 g in Mersey, England, 1967–1984.

Table 3.2. Different Birthweight Measures for Selected Countries and their Birthweight-Specific Mortality Rates (Stillbirths Plus Infant) per 1000 births: Singleton births, 1980

	Live & Stillbirth		Stillbirth & Infant Deaths/ 1000 Births at		
Country	% <2500 g	5th %tile(g)	5th %tile(g)	1500–1999 g	2000–2499 g
US (black)	11.6	2028	86.5	89.6	37.5
Israel (tot)	6.5	2330	89.9	172.9	47.8
Eng. & Wales	5.9	2385	89.8	206.3	55.3
Scotland	5.9	2384	80.1	183.2	49.6
US (white)	4.8	2505	44.4	139.1	44.8
Sweden	3.5	2566	46.8	157.9	52.1
Norway	3.5	2571	57.5	192.7	64.0

Source: International Collaborative Effort (ICE) 1st Generation.

Derived from Alberman & Evans (1989).

black babies in the United States have higher mortality rates (in this case stillbirth plus infant) than babies in the most privileged of the other countries and twice as high mortality rates as U.S. white babies at the same centile. Similarly, multiple births tend to have lower mortality rates than singletons at low birthweights, although this too is reversed at weights over about 1500 g, when the mortality risks of multiple births show an increase over those of singletons.

Morbidity

Over recent years the greatest concern in this field has been the risk of long-term morbidity in the increasing proportion and number of low birthweight survivors. Figure 3.2 from Mersey (England), referred to earlier, shows the relationship observed between trends of cerebral palsy and mortality in low birthweight, and similar findings have been reported elsewhere (Mutch et al., 1992). This pattern is not necessarily related causally to the immaturity. As stated earlier, babies with prenatally or genetically caused defects also tend to be preterm and are often also small-for-dates, so that their presence adds to the high rate of long-term disability found in births of low birthweight. The important difference between the congenital and the perinatally caused deficits are that in the latter there is the expectation that improvements in neonatal care will reduce their risk pari passu with that of reductions in mortality. In babies with prenatally caused defects, reductions in mortality risk can only increase the prevalence of morbidity in survivors. The crude rate must be a balance between prenatally and postnatally caused impairment. However, it must not be forgotten that, as mortality falls, the gain in healthy survivors has outweighed the increase in survivors with disabilities (Hagberg et al., 1982), and it is to be hoped that this trend will increase.

There are many problems in monitoring such patterns over time. The best clinical information tends to come from tertiary referral centers, which have access to the most up-to-date methods of early diagnosis and which usually carry out careful follow-up of survivors. However, this information tends to be biased both by the inclusion of the sickest infants and by the excellent care they are given. Reports on the condition of extremely young survivors may also be misleading because unexpected improvement may occur in early childhood in apparently neurologically damaged infants (Ford et al., 1990).

In recent years we have begun to receive regular reports of follow-up of population-based groups of low birthweight infants, often analyzed by gestational age, sex, and multiple birth. Although some are meticulously documented, Verloove-Vanhorick's (1989) careful review and evaluation of such studies from centers all over the world demonstrated that sometimes the data are incomplete and not comparable.

Interestingly, the patterns of neurologic deficit follow those of mortality. When common birthweight cut-off points are used, the outcome in low birthweight is better in girls who are gestationally more mature than in boys of the same birthweight. A similar situation pertains in low weight multiple compared to single births.

Impairments

The prevalence of most recognized impairments at or shortly after birth rises very sharply as birthweight and gestational age fall. Unfortunately, there are no good data on the prevalence of even visible impairments over the whole birthweight or gestational age range. Figure 3.3, derived from a survey of preschool survivors of 2000 g or less born in the Mersey region, England in 1979 to 1981, gives a good indication of the risks at these low weights and how they interact with gestational age. However, the consistent rise in prevalence of cerebral palsy

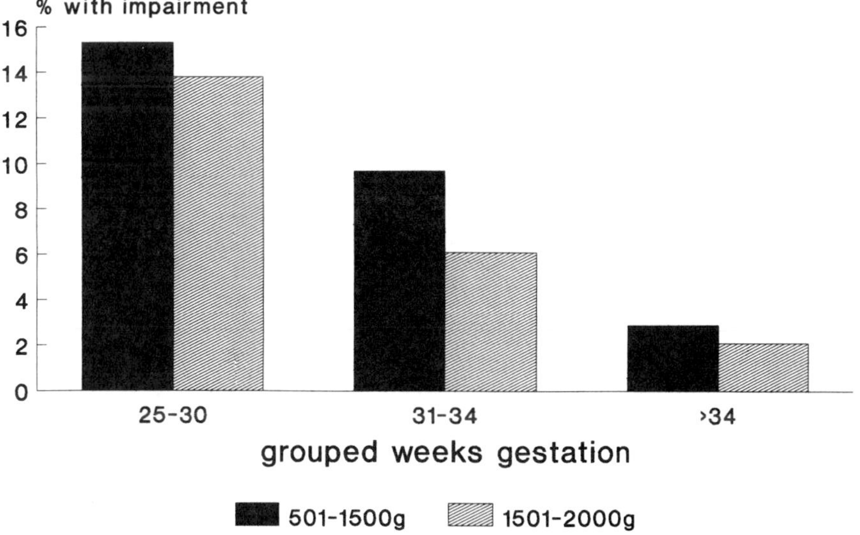

Fig. 3.3. Impairment rates in low birth weight survivors in Mersey, England, 1979–1981 (derived from Powell et al., 1986).

with falling birthweight and gestational age is well known, and Figure 3.4, using data from England, Sweden, and Western Australia, shows that the pattern is widespread and consistent. When babies are both preterm and small for gestational age, many of the impairments are due to obvious prenatal causes (Alberman et al., 1985; van Zeben-van der Aa et al., 1989a), including chromosomal anomalies, such malformations as neural tube defects, and established cerebral lesions due to a vascular accident or to intrauterine infections.

In extremely preterm infants there is also an excess of developmental anomalies, such as inguinal hernias and undescended testes, presumably because their normal migration was arrested. In the presence of hypoxia the ductus arteriosus may fail to close. There are also impairments, often occurring together, that are a direct consequence of functional or immunologic immaturity: respiratory distress partly due to lack of surfactant and immaturity of the lung structure; metabolic and kidney abnormalities; and vulnerability to infections that may lead to septicemia, necrotizing enterocolitis, or meningitis. Most importantly, central nervous system lesions may stem from weaknesses in the cerebral circulation. These defects include hemorrhages that frequently disappear without sequelae but may lead to obstructive hydrocephalus and ischemic lesions that may cause periventricular leukomalacia and in severe cases result in the formation of periventricular cysts.

There are numerous accounts of the complications found among preterm infants. The best studies are population based. These include a national study of preterm and very low birthweight babies born in the Netherlands in 1983 (van Zeben-van der Aa, 1989b); accounts of babies referred to the Mersey, England, regional center (Cooke, 1988); and reports that demonstrate trends over time from Melbourne, Australia (the Victorian Infant Collaborative Study Group, 1991).

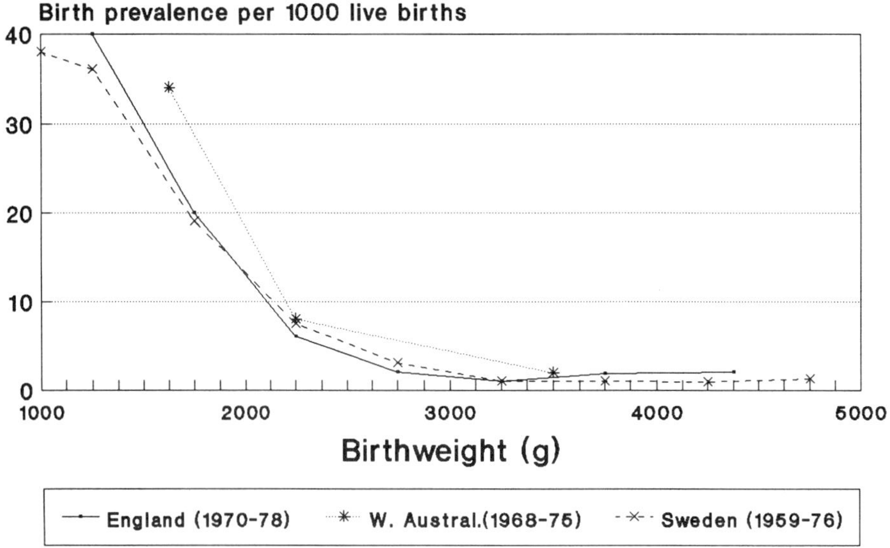

Fig. 3.4. Birth prevalence rates of the cerebral palsies from England, West Australia, and Sweden (derived from Stanley & Alberman, 1984).

New developments in brain imaging are beginning to increase our understanding of the pathologic nature and timing of the lesions that may cause long-standing brain damage. A recent report of children selected for magnetic resonance imaging examination because they were suffering from cerebral palsy (Truit et al., 1992) suggested that most of those who had been preterm had a pattern of periventricular damage considered to be characteristic of perinatal lesions. However, a small number of the preterm cerebral palsy infants had lesions that must have occurred in the mid-trimester or earlier. This finding fits in well with epidemiologic studies that suggest that, in a proportion of preterm deliveries, the size of which is still unknown, the early onset of labor was a consequence and not the cause of cerebral damage.

Sequelae

Respiratory Function

The most immediate need in the preterm baby is to safeguard respiratory function. There are now effective ways of reducing respiratory distress secondary to lack of surfactant in the extremely immature baby, either by the administration of corticosteroids to the mother before the birth or by the treatment of the baby with surfactant after the birth. Up to the present, results of randomized trials of surfactant treatment suggest that it increases survival of extremely preterm infants and that in the small number of treated survivors who have been followed no excess of neurodevelopmental abnormalities has yet been reported (*Oxford Database of Perinatal Trials*, 1992). The cost effectiveness of these preventive measures has been calculated: the cost per survivor is reduced between 5% and 16%, even though for babies under 31 weeks who are treated the total costs increase because of increased survival (Mugford et al., 1991).

If these treatments also reduce the incidence of chronic lung disease, as it seems they may, this effect would also be of great importance. In recent years there have been increases in very low birthweight "graduates" surviving with chronic lung disease, sometimes needing oxygen treatment for months, possibly in association with early parenteral lipid administration (Cooke, 1991). The significance of this long-term complication relates both to the distress caused to the infants and to their parents and the expense of their care, as well as to the possibility that affected infants also have an increased risk of neurologic damage (Skidmore et al., 1990; Vohr et al., 1991).

Retinopathy of Prematurity

The presence of retinopathy of prematurity (ROP) also rises very steeply with falling birthweight and more so with falling gestational age, although the long-term sequelae may be becoming less common. There have been several recent population-based surveys of this condition, which have taken advantage of the recent international agreement on standardization of the retinal signs and the distinction between the early and later stages of the acute condition. A report covering all very low birthweight births in New Zealand in 1986 shows that, on multiple logistic regression, three factors contribute significantly and independently to the risk of any stage of acute ROP: gestational age, principal hospital caring for the infant, and the administration of indomethacin. Only the first two contributed independently to the more severe degrees of the condition—stages 2 or higher (Darlow et al., 1992). In general the literature confirms the high prevalence of the acute disease in preterm infants, which is possibly reduced in centers of excellence, but the expected new epidemic of blindness as their survival increases has fortunately not emerged. Gibson et al. (1990) found no cases of blindness in their well-studied series of 127 cases, although there was an excess of persisting ophthalmic abnormalities, particularly in the presence of cystic periventricular leukomalacia. The suggestion that vitamin E might be a protective factor has not been confirmed (Law et al., 1990).

Neurologic Damage

It has already been stated that in the case of neurologic damage it is often difficult to distinguish between babies affected in the prenatal period and those affected in the perinatal or neonatal period. Even in those babies with an ultrasound picture of periventricular leukomalacia that may be characteristic of perinatal damage, it seems that the onset may have occurred days before delivery. This means that it is difficult to interpret the almost universal finding that surviving babies with long-term neurological damage have had a stormier neonatal course, in nearly all aspects, than have normal survivors. Particularly poor outcomes have been noted in babies with hydrocephalus, much of which is secondary to intracranial hemorrhage or infection.

Sensory Defects

All follow-up studies of low birthweight babies have found an excess prevalence of visual (over and above retinopathy of prematurity) and hearing defects. Again, some are attributable to prenatal damage, as is sometimes the case for cortical blindness in association with spastic quadriplegia, and some are due to neonatal events, such as deafness secondary to infection.

Growth

Taken as a group, low birthweight infants tend to grow less well than infants of normal weight or gestation; that is, they do not fully catch up, even when adjustment is made for gestational age. It is known that infants who were small-for-dates are particularly growth retarded, and it may be that new methods of disaggregating this group, using as indicators patterns of atypical fetal growth, may throw further light on this question. It is, however, encouraging that recent randomized controlled nutritional trials have demonstrated that low birthweight babies receiving breast milk have a more rapid growth velocity and an improvement in developmental outcome compared with controls (Lucas et al., 1989). This finding suggests that less severe forms of damage may be palliated with appropriate care.

Scarring

Most graduates of neonatal intensive care carry through life the scars secondary to their treatment. These include scars resulting from intravenous cannulation or from the treatment of pneumothoraces. Although most would agree that these scars are an acceptable price to pay for a good outcome, those in charge of the acute care nurseries should be aware that these scars can be quite disfiguring and, in the case of girls, may interfere with normal breast development.

Dentition

Various anomalies are seen in the primary dentition of premature infants; largely, these are defects of the enamel (Fearne et al., 1990). They are related to the gestational age and perinatal course, being more common in births before 32 weeks and where there has been a stormy course.

Behavioral and Learning Problems

The evidence from the literature is fairly clear on the increased risk of learning problems, hyperactivity, and clumsiness associated with very low birthweight, even when preschool development has proceeded well. Most reports suggest, however, that a majority of these effects are confounded by social disadvantage (Saigal, 1990).

Hospitalization

Most studies on the follow-up of preterm and low birthweight infants include as a poor outcome an excess of hospitalization, particularly in the first year of life. Much of this hospitalization is attributable to treatment for inguinal hernias or for respiratory infections. Because parents of graduates of neonatal intensive care are usually advised to bring their infants to the hospital if they are at all worried and the threshold for their admission is low, it is difficult to know how to interpret data on frequent hospitalization. It may be performing a preventive function, or it may be indicative of the vulnerability of the infants.

Social Class Effects and Social Interventions

It has been known for many years that low birthweight babies born into homes that were socially advantaged fared better in the long term than those in families living in deprivation, and this finding has been reinforced in a recent report (Pfeiffer & Aylward, 1990). More recently, there have been trials of the effects on the development of low birthweight children of providing social and educational support to the families, showing that such interventions can lead to improvements (The Infant Health and Development Programme, 1990).

Effects on Adult Health

In recent years there have been a spate of reports on the association between retardation of intrauterine growth and adult health, particularly cardiovascular and obstructive lung disease (Barker, 1992; see Chapter 18). On the whole the evidence for these associations is convincing, although doubt has been expressed about the relative importance of intrauterine growth retardation compared with later health behavior and social circumstances. Similarly, there is evidence that, even allowing for later influences, retardation of the mother's own intrauterine growth rate, particularly in early pregnancy, affects the birthweight of her children (Emanuel et al., 1992; Klebanoff et al., 1989). This area of long-term effects of reproductive health is likely to become of increasing interest as we learn more about the mechanisms involved.

Ethical Issues

In addition to the various preventive modalities described throughout this chapter, there has been much debate about the ethics and social value of using limited health care resources to help VLBW infants survive. This debate has extended to ways of conveying the public view to the professionals (Sinclair et al., 1981). Boyle and his colleagues (1983) in Canada conducted an important survey of the public's perception of the importance they attached to different impairments and related the findings to the costs of providing intensive neonatal care. In regard to individual choice, there has also been debate on the ethics of removing life support from infants in whom clinical and ultrasound evidence point to irreversible and disastrous brain damage, as well as the role played by parents and professionals in these difficult decisions. These issues will become more acute as developments in scanning improve the prediction of long-term damage (Ng & Dear, 1990).

Conclusion

Prematurity, especially very low birthweight, remains a major health problem in terms of distress and health care costs. Ironically, its importance has increased since medical advances have improved survival rates. Primary prevention still largely eludes us, and the development of secondary prevention of the large variety of adverse consequences has been a hard path, occasionally interrupted by iatrogenic disasters. The reward lies in the gain in the number of healthy survivors of very low birthweight, comprising some 80% of their total; the current cost is a small increase in absolute numbers of survivors with disability. There is still much to be learnt about the causes and timing of the latter, and some hope that the future will bring the means to reduce this number.

References

Alberman E, Benson J, Kani W. Disabilities in survivors of low birthweight. *Arch Dis Child* 1985; 60:913–919.

Alberman E, Botting B. Trends in prevalence and survival of very low birthweight infants, England and Wales: 1983–7. *Arch Dis Child* 1991; 66:1304–1308.

Alberman E, Evans S. The epidemiology of prematurity: aetiology, prevalence and outcome. *Ann Nestle* 1989; 47:69–88.

Barker DJP, ed. *Fetal and Infant Origins of Disease*. London: British Medical Journal; 1992.

Botting BJ, MacDonald Davies I, Macfarlane AJ. Recent trends in the incidence of multiple birth and associated mortality. *Arch Dis Child* 1987; 62:941–950.

Boyle MH, Torrance CW, Sinclair JC, Horwood, SP. (1983) Economic evaluation of neonatal intensive care of very low birthweight infants. *N Engl J Med* 1983; 308:1330–1337.

Campbell S. The detection of intrauterine growth retardation. In: Sharp F, Fraser RB, Milner RDG, eds. *Fetal Growth*. London: Royal College of Obstetricians and Gynaecologists; 1989:251–261.

Colley NV, Tremble JM, Henson GL, Cole TJ. Head circumference/abdominal circumference ratio (HC/AC), ponderal index and fetal malnutrition. Should head circumference/abdominal ratio be abandoned? *Br J Obstet Gynaecol* 1991; 98:524–527.

Collins R. Overview of antiplatelet agents for IUGR and pre-eclampsia. In: Chalmers I, ed. *The Oxford Database of Perinatal Trials*. Oxford: Oxford University Press; 1992.

Cooke RWI. Outcome and costs of care for the very immature infant. *Br Med Bull* 1988; 44:1135–1151.

Cooke RWI. Factors associated with chronic lung disease in preterm infants. *Arch Dis Child* 1991; 66:776–779.

Darlow BA, Horwood LJ, Clemett RS. Retinopathy of prematurity: risk factors in a prospective population based study. *Paed Perinat Epidemiol* 1992; 6:62–80.

Dubois S, Dougherty C, Duquette MP, Hanley JA, Moutquin JM. Twin pregnancy: the impact of the Higgins Nutrition Intervention Program on maternal and neonatal outcomes. *Am J Clin Nutr* 1991; 53:1397–1407.

Emanuel I, Filakti H, Alberman E, Evans SJW, Williams S. Intergenerational studies of human birth weight from the 1958 Birth Cohort. I. Evidence for a multigeneration effect. *Brit J Obst Gynaecol* 1992; 99:67–74.

Evans S, Alberman E. International Collaborative Effort (ICE) on Birthweight, Plurality, and Perinatal and Infant Mortality. II: Comparisons between birthweight distributions of births in member countries from 1970 to 1984. *Acta Obstet Gynecol Scand* 1989; 68:11–17.

Fearne JM, Bryan EM, Elliman AM, Brook AH, Williams DM. Enamel defects in the primary dentition of children born weighing less than 2000 g. *Br Dent J* 1990; 168:433–437.

Ford GW, Kitchen WH, Doyle LW, Rickards AL, Kelly E. Changing diagnosis of cerebral palsy in very low birthweight children. *Am J Perinatol* 1990; 7:178–181.

Gibson NA, Fielder AR, Trounce JQ, Levene MI. Ophthalmic findings in infants of very low birthweight. *Dev Med Child Neurol* 1990; 32:7–13.

Hagberg B, Hagberg G, Olow I. Gains and hazards of intensive neonatal care: an analysis from Swedish cerebral palsy epidemiology. *Dev Med Child Neurol* 1982; 24:13–19.

Imperiale TF, Petrulis AS. A meta-analysis of low-dose aspirin for the prevention of pregnancy induced hypertensive disease. *JAMA* 1991; 266:260–264.

Joyce T. The dramatic increase in the rate of low birthweight in New York City: an aggregate time-series analysis. *Am J Pub Health* 1990; 80:682–684.

Klebanoff MA, Meirik O, Berendes HW. Second-generation consequence of small-for-dates. *Pediatrics* 1989; 84:386–401.

Launer LJ, Villar J, Kestler E, de-Onis M. The effect of maternal work on fetal growth and duration of pregnancy: a prospective study. *Br J Obst Gynaecol* 1990; 97:62–67.

Law MR, Wijewardene K, Wald NJ. Is routine vitamin E administration justified in very low-birthweight infants? *Dev Med Child Neurol* 1990; 32:442–450.

Lucas A, Morley R, Cole TJ, Gore SM, Davis JA, Bamford MF, Dossetor JF. Early diet in preterm babies and developmental status in infancy. *Arch Dis Child* 1989; 64:1570–1578.

Mugford M, Piercy J, Chalmers I. Cost implications of different approaches to the prevention of respiratory distress syndrome. *Arch Dis Child* 1991; 66:757–764.

Mutch L, Alberman E, Hagberg B, Kodama K, Perat MV. Cerebral palsy epidemiology: where are we now and where are we going? *Dev Med Child Neurol* 1992; 34:547–555.

Ng PC, Dear PR. The predictive value of a normal ultrasound scan in the preterm baby—a meta-analysis. *Acta Paediatr Scand* 1990; 79:286–291.

Paneth N, Kiely JL, Wallenstein S, Marcus M, Pakter J, Susser M. Newborn intensive care and neonatal mortality in low-birth-weight infants. *N Engl J Med* 1982; 307:149–155.

Peoples-Sheps MD, Siegel E, Suchindran CM, Origasa H, Ware A, Barakat A. Characteristics of maternal employment during pregnancy: effects on low birthweight. *Am J Pub Health* 1991; 81:1007–1012.

Pfeiffer SI, Aylward GP. Outcome for preschoolers of very low birthweight: sociocultural and environmental influences. *Percept Mot Skills* 1990; 70:1367–1378.

Pharoah PO, Cooke T, Cooke RW, Rosenbloom L. Birthweight specific trends in cerebral palsy. *Arch Dis Child* 1990; 65:602–606.

Powell TG, Pharoah POD, Cooke RW. Survival and mortality in a geographically defined population of low birthweight infants. *Lancet* 1986; 1:539–543.

Saigal S. Follow-up of high-risk infants. Methological issues, current status, and future trends. In: Kiely M, ed. *Reproductive and Perinatal Epidemiology*. Boca Raton: CRC Press; 1990:337–355.

Sinclair JC, Torrance GW, Boyle MH, Horwood SP, Saigal S, Sackett DL. Evaluation of neonatal-intensive-care programmes. *N Engl J Med* 1981; 305:489–494.

Skidmore MD, Rivers A, Hack M. Increased risk of cerebral palsy among very low-birthweight infants with chronic lung disease. *Dev Med Child Neurol* 1990; 32:325–332.

Stanley F, Alberman E. Birthweight, gestational age and the cerebral palsies. In: Stanley F, Alberman E, eds. *The Epidemiology of the Cerebral Palsies*. Oxford: Spastics International Medical Publications; 1984:57–68.

The Infant Health and Development Programme. Enhancing the outcomes of low-birthweight, premature infants. A multisite, randomized trial. *JAMA* 1990; 263:3025–3042.

The Oxford Database of Perinatal Trials, edited by Iain Chalmers. Oxford: Oxford University Press; 1992.

The Victorian Infant Collaborative Study Group. Improvement of outcome for infants of birthweight under 1000g. *Arch Dis Child* 1991; 66:765–769.

Truit CL, Barkovich AJ, Koch TK, Ferrierro DM. Cerebral palsy: MRI findings in 40 patients. *Am J Nuclear Radiol* 1992; 13:67–78.

van Zeben van der Aa TM, Verloove Vanhorick SP, Brand R, Ruys JH. Morbidity of very low birthweight infants at corrected age of two years in a geographically defined population. Report from Project on Preterm and Small for Gestational Age Infants in The Netherlands. *Lancet* 1989; 1:253–255.

van Zeben-van der Aa, DM. (1989b) Outcome at two years of age in very preterm and very low birthweight infants in the Netherlands, (POPS, 1983) 's-Gravenhage, Pasmans Offsetdrukkerij B.V. Thesis, State University, Leiden.

Verloove-Vanhorick SP. Perinatal care delivery systems. In: Kaminski M, Breart G, Buekens P, Huisjes HJ, McIlwaine G, Selbmann HC, eds. *Review of Evaluative Studies on Intensive Care for Very Low Birthweight Infants—Medical Aspects*, Oxford Medical Publications; 1986; 212–243.

Vohr BR, Coll CG, Lobato D, Yunis KA, O'Dea C, Oh W. Neurodevelopmental and medical status of low birthweight survivors of bronchopulmonary dysplasia at 10 to 12 years of age. *Dev Med Child Neurol* 1991; 33:690–697.

Willcox AJ, Russell IT. Birthweight and perinatal mortality; towards a new method of analysis. *Int J Epidemiol* 1986; 15:188–196.

4

Structural Birth Defects

IAN LECK

The defects discussed in this chapter are macroscopic abnormalities of structure attributable to faulty development or deformation. With a few exceptions, they are present at birth. The exceptions are patent ductus arteriosus, which only becomes a defect when it persists after birth; "congenital" dislocation of the hip; and infantile hypertrophic pyloric stenosis. The last two conditions have traditionally been regarded as congenital, although in most cases they may not become fully established until after birth.

Most birth defects are laid down early in pregnancy and may cause a miscarriage, so that only a proportion of those affected—no more than the "tip of the iceberg" in the case of some malformations—survive long enough to be born. The proportion of liveborn and stillborn infants affected by these malformations (commonly termed "birth prevalence") is therefore less than the incidence (the proportion of embryos or fetuses in whom the malformations are laid down).

The first part of this chapter considers the birth prevalence of defects and then their incidence and mortality. A discussion of risk factors follows, which distinguishes between specific teratogens and other factors. Known teratogens are only responsible for a small proportion of cases of structural birth defects. In a much larger proportion, other risk factors, such as gender, birth rank, or mother's age, have been identified. These findings provide a basis for plausible hypotheses regarding the etiology of several such defects. One of these hypotheses is the proposal that folic acid intake affects the risk of neural tube defect. This hypothesis has recently led to a promising preventive intervention (MRC Vitamin Study Research Group, 1991). This intervention is discussed toward the end of the chapter, together with aspects of screening.

Patterns of Occurrence—Birth Prevalence

To obtain a complete picture of the birth prevalence of malformations in a community, it is necessary to have records that (1) cover all births in a community, as opposed to only those in particular hospitals; (2) document all defects observed; and (3) include both data collected at the time of birth and follow-up information covering the next year or longer. Records made at the time of birth, even if they document everything that has been observed, inevitably underreport some conditions (for example, congenital heart disease, which is often not diagnosed until later), whereas they may give an exaggerated impression of the impact of other defects, e.g., talipes and congenital dislocation of the hip, the diagnosis of which in the newborn is often based on findings that later disappear spontaneously. Follow-up information alone, on the other hand, misses cases of stillbirth and early death and also those defects corrected shortly after birth, e.g., pedunculated post-minimus, the commonest type of polydactyly in the West, which is often treated by simple ligation.

There are large areas of the world in which the above three conditions cannot be met; these are mostly areas where many births occur outside hospital but the available data cover only perinatal findings in hospital births. In these areas, the only common malformations about which much has been inferred from studies of birth prevalence are neural tube defects (NTDs) and cleft lip. These defects are almost always apparent and recorded at birth. Accordingly, the variations in birth prevalence among communities that they exhibit can reasonably be assumed to be largely genuine, since they are much too great to be interpreted plausibly in terms of selection for hospital confinement (Leck, 1993).

The account that follows deals first with the birth prevalence of a wide variety of defects in places where relatively reliable data are available for major malformations in general, and then with the prevalence of cleft lip and NTD over the much greater area where usable data exist for these conditions.

Prevalence by Place and Ethnic Group in Developed Countries

Three important studies of the birth prevalence of all structural birth defects illustrate what can be learnt from good data collected both at birth and by follow-up. These studies, in Japan, the United States, and England, included people of African, European, Oriental, and "South Asian" (i.e., Indian, Pakistani, or Bangladeshi) origin. Studies using a comparable range of data have also been carried out on populations of European origin in other parts of Europe and North America, and in Australia, but only reveal a few convincing differences in prevalence between these populations and those studied in England and the United States. The most striking of these differences are, first, the effects that variations in thalidomide use had on the frequency of limb and ear defects in different countries around 1960 and, second, the contrasting prevalence of NTDs in different localities (see later section on worldwide prevalence).

The Japanese study (Neel, 1958) covered births in the two cities struck by atom bombs in 1945 and in one other city. It was originally established to search for effects of nuclear radiation on the offspring of those exposed. Infants were examined by physicians employed by the Atomic Bomb Casualty Commission, initially within 10 days of birth. Necropsy findings were also available for about 13% of stillbirths and neonatal deaths. Random samples, including about 25% of surviving children, were re-examined between 8 and 10 months of age. Prevalence statistics were calculated on the assumption that the results of these necropsies and follow-up examinations were representative. They refer to infants neither of whose parents had received an estimated radiation dose of 50 roentgen equivalents physical or more from the atom bombs.

The U.S. study (Heinonen et al., 1977) was part of the Collaborative Perinatal Project. It was not based on residents of a defined area, but on pregnancies booked for delivery at 12 university-affiliated medical centers. The resulting births are likely to have been reasonably representative of all births in the communities served by these centers, since hospital delivery was almost universal. Defects were detected by examining infants daily during the first week after delivery and again at 1 year and at death, if applicable, and by interviewing their mothers at other times.

The English study (Knox & Lancashire, 1991) covered births to residents of one city, Birmingham. Defects were ascertained from a variety of sources, including the forms that hospital staff (family physicians in the case of domiciliary births) use to record all births and to report malformations; obstetric hospital records of births for which the data on these notification forms were insufficiently precise; necropsy reports; records made by health visitors (public health nurses, who are expected to follow up all children to the age of 5); and discharge records of children admitted to Birmingham hospitals with a diagnosis of any malformation.

Severe Defects of All Types.

The above studies suggest that, in developed countries, about 1 in 40 or 2.5% of total (i.e., live and still) births are affected by severe structural defects, defined as those causing death or substantial handicap or requiring treatment to prevent such outcomes. The Japanese data yield this figure when conditions that are minor or not generally regarded as malformations are excluded. The same is true for English data based mainly on infants of European descent in Birmingham (Leck, 1983a). The proportions of children with severe defects of all kinds among the other major ethnic groups in Birmingham (Afro-Caribbeans and South Asians) have not been published. However, other studies suggest that in the United Kingdom severe defects are less common in Afro-Caribbean residents and are more common in South Asians than in Europeans (Little & Nicoll, 1988). The excess found in South Asians is due at least in part to autosomal recessive defects, which reflects the high frequency of consanguinity, especially in the Pakistani community (Bundey et al., 1990; Young & Clarke, 1987; see Chapter 5).

In the U.S. study, about 3.3% of white and 2.3% of black children were classified as having "major malformations." This category consisted mainly of potentially lethal and handicapping defects like those that occurred in 2.5% of births in the Japanese and English series, but there were a few discrepancies. For example, in the American study syndactyly was counted as a major defect, whereas talipes equinovarus was not. There may also have been a greater readiness to diagnose microcephaly in infants with below-average head circumference.

Specific Defects.

The birth prevalence of a variety of specific types of defects in the series described above is shown in Table 4.1. Infants with two or more of the defects listed are counted under each one that they exhibited, with the following exceptions: first, the English and Japanese figures given for clubfoot (talipes) do not include cases in which this was secondary to another defect (e.g., spina bifida); second, the figures for cleft palate do not include cases associated with cleft lip, because cleft palate and lip combined differ epidemiologically from cleft palate alone and more closely resemble cleft lip (Fogh-Andersen, 1942); and third, cases of anencephaly with spina bifida have only been counted as anencephaly, and cases of spina bifida with hydrocephaly as spina bifida. This was a departure from the practice followed in the American report, in which such cases were counted under each of the relevant defects. Estimates of the numbers of cases of spina bifida with anencephaly and of hydrocephaly with spina bifida were therefore deducted from the American totals for spina bifida and hydrocephaly, respectively, before the statistics in Table 4.1 were calculated.

All but 3 of the 20 types of defects listed in Table 4.1 showed significant variations ($P \leq 0.05$) among the six population groups examined: Japanese; black and white American; and English of European, South Asian, and Afro-Caribbean origin. The three exceptions were Down syndrome, limb reduction deformities, and accessory auricle. A recent overview of the epidemiology of Down syndrome (Bell, 1991) also suggests that its birth prevalence shows little variation with place or ethnic group beyond what can be attributed to differences in ascertainment, maternal age distribution, or the frequency of pregnancy termination after prenatal diagnosis.

The variations exhibited by three other defects—microcephaly, clubfoot, and malformations of the heart and great vessels—may well be largely due to differences in ascertainment or definition. The reason microcephaly was reported more than three times as often in both American ethnic groups as in the Japanese and English series may merely be that the limits of normal head circumference were defined more broadly in the latter two studies. Prevalence in the U.S. series is close to that expected on statistical grounds if the defect is equated with a head circumference at least three standard deviations below the mean. Many of the cases of clubfoot in the American and English series (where the figures for this defect were well over twice the 1.4/1000 rate given for Japan) are likely to have been only abnormalities of neonatal posture that would resolve spontaneously. The prevalence of persistent nonpostural talipes equinovarus requiring orthopedic treatment in England is only about 1.2 per 1000, although a figure of 2.9 per 1000 is obtained when cases considered to need neonatal strapping are also included (Pryor et al., 1991; Wynne-Davies, 1964). The main source of the difference between the prevalence of malformations of the heart and great vessels in the English series (about 4 per 1000) and the figures for America and Japan (above 7 per 1000) may be that the methods used in the former study were insufficient to ascertain some cases. A figure of 6.9 per 1000 was obtained by Kenna, Smithells, and Fielding (1975) in Liverpool, England, where ascertainment included hospital outpatient records (not used in the Birmingham study).

The variations exhibited by the other 14 conditions in Table 4.1 seem more likely to be genuine, at least in part. Among defects of the central nervous system (CNS), anencephaly was reported most often among peoples of mainly Caucasoid origin (Europeans and South Asians in Birmingham and, to a lesser extent, American whites) and least often among those of predominantly Negroid ancestry (American blacks, and Afro-Caribbeans in Birmingham). Spina bifida

Table 4.1. Birth Prevalence of Various Specific Types of Structural Birth Defects

Type of Birth Defect	Prevalence per 1000 Births*					
	Hiroshima, Nagasaki, and Kure, Japan[†]	12 centers, United States[‡]		Birmingham, England[§]		
		Black	White	European	South Asian	Afro-Caribbean
Central nervous system						
Anencephaly	0.63	0.17	0.83	1.39	1.49	0.51
Spina bifida aperta (without anencephaly	0.20	0.63[‖]	0.54[‖]	2.07	1.61	0.39
Hydrocephaly (without spina bifida aperta)	0.44	0.97[¶]	1.02[¶]	0.92	1.04	0.74
Microcephaly	0.35	1.71	1.40	0.42[#]	—	—
Alimentary system						
Cleft lip (± cleft palate)	2.24	0.67	1.36	1.01	1.25	0.59
Cleft palate (without cleft lip)	0.72	0.50	0.70	0.67	0.76	0.16
Tracheo-esophageal fistula	0.35	0.21	0.13	0.38	0.45	0.08
Infantile hypertrophic pyloric stenosis	—	0.83	3.20	3 to 4**	—	—
Anal atresia	0.32	0.50	0.61	0.58	0.72	0.27
Limbs						
Reduction deformities	0.34	0.54[††]	0.70[††]	0.50	0.55	0.47
Dislocation of hip	7.12	0.54	3.16	2.78	1.38	0.78

Clubfoot	1.38[‡‡]	4.24	3.55	5.32[‡‡]	7.84[‡‡]	4.82[‡‡]
Polydactyly	0.97	13.73	1.53	1.11	2.13	9.55
Syndactyly	0.53	1.08	4.08	1.29	0.76	0.51
			Other			
Cataract	0.09	0.71	1.01	0.16	0.21	0.39
Accessory auricle	—	0.83	0.48	0.65	0.77	0.59
Malformations of heart and great vessels	7.09	7.49	8.64	3.86	4.48	3.56
Hypospadias[§§]	0.36	6.89	8.08	3.09[‖‖]	3.70[‖‖]	1.29[‖‖]
Down syndrome	0.87	1.21	1.32	1.38	1.47	1.33
Omphalocele	0.12	0.58	0.35	0.30	0.34	0.39
Number in related population	64,569[¶¶]	24,030	22,811	255,918	52,928	25,542

*Including stillbirths at 28 or more weeks in England and 20 or more weeks elsewhere.

[†]Estimated from data for nonconsanguineous pregnancies registered from 1948 to 1954 (Neel, 1958) on the assumption that infants who underwent necropsy after stillbirth or neonatal death and those followed up at 9 months were representative, respectively, of all who died before 4 weeks after birth (including stillbirths) and all who survived to this age.

[‡]Single births following pregnancies booked in 1959 to 1965 (Heinonen et al., 1977).

[§]1964 to 1984 births (Knox & Lancashire, 1991).

[‖]Estimated on the assumption that cases of spina bifida combined with anencephaly were distributed among ethnic groups in the same proportions as all cases of anencephaly.

[¶]Estimated on the assumption that cases of hydrocephaly combined with spina bifida were distributed among ethnic groups in the same proportions as all cases of spina bifida.

[#]1964 to 1981 births.

**Figures for various parts of England and Wales in the late 1970s (Knox et al., 1983; Walsworth-Bell, 1983; Webb et al., 1983).

[††]Absence of limb or part (not including hemimelia/phocomelia).

[‡‡]Clubfoot not secondary to another malformation.

[§§]Prevalence per 1000 male births.

[‖‖]Includes epispadias.

[¶¶]Number examined externally shortly after birth. Necropsy and follow-up data were available, respectively, for about 13% of stillbirths and neonatal deaths and 25% of survivors.

showed a similar trend among the English births, but not among the Americans. However, statistics based on larger populations suggest that both spina bifida and anencephaly affect whites more often than blacks in the United States, but are less common there than among whites in England (Division of Birth Defects and Developmental Disabilities, 1989; Erickson, 1976). In the Japanese study, the figure for anencephaly was between those in Caucasoids and Negroids. However, the figure for spina bifida was lower, as was that for hydrocephaly (for which the English and U.S. figures did not vary substantially).

The most common defects of the alimentary system are cleft lip and infantile hypertrophic pyloric stenosis. Cleft lip occurred most often among Japanese births and least often among the two Negroid populations. Pyloric stenosis was only included in the U.S. series, in which it was much more common among whites than blacks. The figures shown in Table 4.1 for pyloric stenosis in England are taken from studies which suggest that it is as common in England as it is among American whites. It was only one-third as prevalent among Japanese as among Caucasoid infants in Hawaii (Shim et al., 1970). The most striking feature of the less common alimentary defects—cleft palate without cleft lip, tracheo-esophageal fistula, and anal atresia—is that each was less than half as prevalent among Afro-Caribbeans as among other ethnic groups in Birmingham, although there were no differences of this magnitude between black and white Americans.

The trends for hip dislocation, polydactyly, and syndactyly may all be distorted by errors of ascertainment, but they also show features that are likely to be genuine. Most cases of polydactyly and syndactyly are of little functional importance, which may result in underascertainment. However, the trend for polydactyly to be many times more prevalent in blacks than whites is well established. Syndactyly was more than twice as common in whites as blacks in both the American and the English studies, which suggests that this trend is also real.

Unlike these two defects, dislocation of the hip tends to be overascertained. This is because in much of the West neonatal screening for hip joint instability is practiced and cases of instability tend to be ascertained and enumerated as "dislocation." The prevalence of these cases is several times as high as the prevalence that established dislocation attains in the absence of screening (generally 0.8–1.5 per 1000 in populations of Northern European descent). This implies that most hips that exhibit neonatal instability would stabilize and not progress to dislocation if untreated (Leck, 1986). Yet, although the U.S. and English figures for hip dislocation in Table 4.1 are likely to be inflated, the main trends they exhibit—risks that are lower than in Japan and higher for whites than blacks—are consistent with findings in children who have not been screened and treated at birth (Robinson, 1968; Salter, 1968; Yamamuro & Ishida, 1984).

The other defects listed—cataract, hypospadias, and omphalocele—were all of low prevalence in the Japanese series. For two of them (cataract and hypospadias) the U.S. figures were consistently higher than the English. As omphalocele is much the most obvious of these malformations, its low prevalence in the Japanese series is more likely to be a genuine finding than the trends in cataract and hypospadias. These trends could be due to between-series variations in thoroughness and duration of follow-up and hence in ascertainment. Other factors may, however, have contributed to these trends. For example, the relatively high prevalence of cataract in the American series and in Afro-Caribbean children in Birmingham may be related to maternal rubella, a well-known cause of this defect. A massive epidemic of rubella occurred in the United States during the period covered by the American study (although known cases of infection were excluded from this study). Migrants from the tropics to the United Kingdom, as were many of the Afro-Caribbean mothers, are less often immune to rubella than native Britons (Peckham et al., 1983; see Chapter 6). No such explanation can be offered for the Anglo-American difference in the prevalence of hypospadias, but support for the reality of this difference is provided by studies examining severity as well as prevalence in the two countries (Roberts & Lloyd, 1973; Sweet et al., 1974). Not only was the American prevalence higher overall but also its ratio to the British prevalence was almost as high for the more severe cases (those in which the urethra opened proximal to the corona) as for the milder. One would have expected the contrast to apply mainly to the milder cases had the difference been due only to the fact that the American data were more complete.

Worldwide Prevalence: Neural Tube Defects and Cleft Lip

Estimates of the birth prevalence of cleft lip and neural tube defects (NTDs) from a large number of studies (some hospital-based and some area-based) are plotted in Figure 4.1. The type of point plotted for each estimate gives a broad indication of place, and its horizontal alignment shows the predominant primary race. (Latin Americans described as Mestizo or European have been aligned separately since they are of mixed Caucasoid and American Indian ancestry).

The reason for selecting these particular estimates was that each was based on a denominator of more than 10,000 liveborn and stillborn infants (15,000 for each estimate for cleft lip) who could all, or almost all, be inferred to belong to one broad ethnic group and who had been examined by methods that should have ascertained most cases, including those associated with stillbirth or other malformations (Leck, 1984). To avoid confusion between differences in the prevalence of NTDs that could be of etiologic significance and differences due to antenatal screening and induced abortion, none of the NTD estimates in Figure 4.1 relates to the period since the introduction of screening. Many of the studies from which the estimates were taken classified NTDs in only two categories: anencephaly, which includes craniorachischisis, and "spina bifida," which comprises meningocele, myelocele, and encephalocele. This convention is followed in Figure 4.1. The figures shown for spina bifida therefore differ from those in Table 4.1 in including cases of encephalocele.

The figures can be criticized for including cases in which cleft lip or NTDs were accompanied by other malformations not secondary to them, since such cases may differ in their epidemiology from cases of NTD or cleft lip alone. However, the reports of some of the studies did not distinguish between cases with and without other defects, and it would have destroyed the comparability of the figures if some but not all had excluded the former.

The birth prevalence of cleft lip varies relatively little between places with populations of the same racial group, but much more between races. The low,

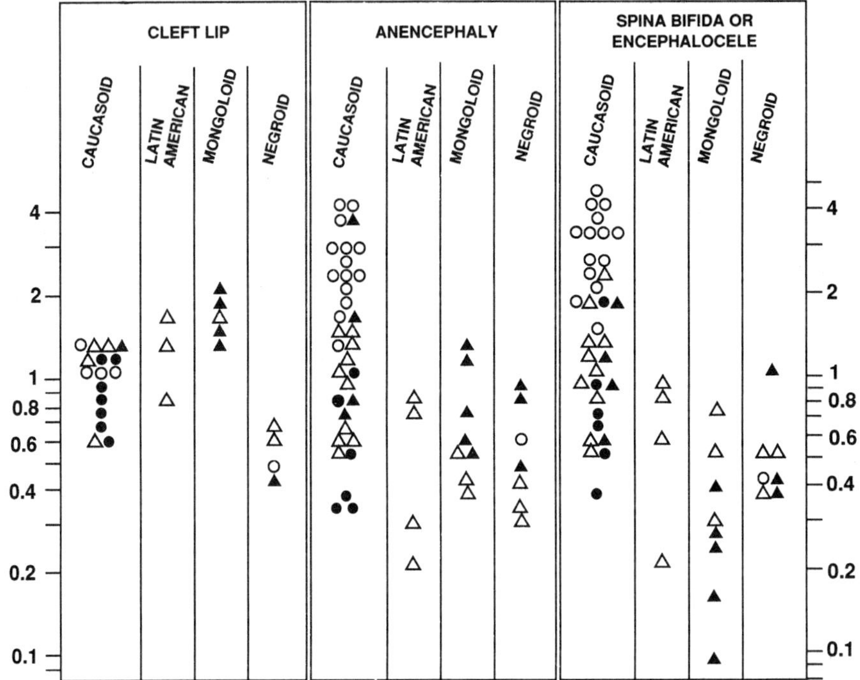

Fig. 4.1. Birth prevalence of cleft lip and neural tube defects per 1000 total births (log scale) in series of cases of relatively uniform racial origin. The alignment of the point plotted for each estimate of prevalence shows the predominant primary race of the population concerned, and the type of point shows its location (*open circles* = Great Britain and Ireland; *open triangles* = the Americas (including Hawaii); *closed circles* = mainland Europe; *closed triangles* = other continents).

moderate, and high figures given in Table 4.1 for black, white, and Japanese infants, respectively, are seen in Figure 4.1 to be typical of Negroid, Caucasoid, and Mongoloid populations. The range for Latin Americans, whose ancestors on the American Indian side were, of course, probably of Mongoloid origin, lies between the Caucasoid and Mongoloid ranges. Live birth statistics indicate that cleft lip is even more common in some North American Indian populations (Lowry & Trimble, 1977; Niswander & Adams, 1967) than in the Mongoloid populations represented in Figure 4.1, which were of Western Pacific origin. The Negroid-Caucasoid-Mongoloid gradient tends to persist even among those living in the same place, as is exemplified by figures for black and white communities in England and the United States (including those in Table 4.1) and for white infants and those of Western Pacific origin in Hawaii and California (Leck, 1984). All these findings can be interpreted as evidence that the birth prevalence of cleft lip is affected much less by the environment than by the genetic differences among racial groups, e.g., the differences that the orofacial characteristics of these groups reflect (Chung & Kau, 1985).

The pattern for NTDs is much more complex. Before antenatal screening and pregnancy termination for them became widespread, both anencephaly and spina bifida varied in prevalence by a factor of more than ten between places with Caucasoid populations. The lowest birth prevalence ratios shown in Figure 4.1 for this racial group came from mainland Europe, whereas the highest were from Great Britain and Ireland, especially in the areas around the Irish sea. There is also some evidence that India and the Eastern Mediterranean (excluding the Jewish population of Israel) are covered by a belt of high birth prevalence and that in this belt, unlike the West, anencephaly is substantially more common than spina bifida. In Caucasoid populations that have migrated from one place to another (e.g., people of South Asian and Irish origin in England and the descendants of migrants from mainland Europe and Ireland to North America), the birth prevalence of NTDs tends to be closer to the norm for the place to which they have come than is the birth prevalence in their countries of origin (Knox & Lancashire, 1991; Leck, 1984). This finding suggests that the variation between Caucasoids in different places is due at least in part to environmental differences (although the migrants could theoretically have been selected in some way that affected their genetic predisposition to bear offspring with NTDs).

The non-Caucasoid birth prevalence ratios for NTDs shown in Figure 4.1 are comparable to the lower Caucasoid ratios except that spina bifida (but not anencephaly) is much less common in the Mongoloid populations shown. However, this is not true of all Mongoloids. Data published since the material in Figure 4.1 was assembled indicate that the Northeast of China includes areas where the prevalence of NTDs is among the highest known and where anencephaly and spina bifida are almost equally common (Chinese Birth Defects Monitoring Program, 1990; Lian et al., 1987).

In places in England and the United States to which people from low-prevalence Mongoloid or Negroid populations have migrated, the total prevalence of NTDs in their descendants tends to be lower than in the white population and not consistently higher than in the immigrants' countries of origin. These findings suggest that genetic factors are largely responsible for NTDs being less common in the Mongoloid and Negroid populations from which the migrants came than in English and U.S. Caucasoids. However, migrant studies also suggest that environmental factors may influence whether the type of NTD exhibited by affected Mongoloid and Negroid children is anencephaly or spina bifida (Leck, 1993).

In summary, comparisons between populations thus reveal markedly different patterns for cleft lip and NTDs. The pattern for cleft lip is largely one of differences between primary racial groups, which invites a genetic explanation. The birth prevalence of NTDs, by contrast, varies markedly within as well as between these groups, and both environmental and genetic factors are likely to be involved in this pattern.

Temporal Variations

It was a variation in prevalence over time—an epidemic of cases of cataract—that led Gregg (1941) to discover that maternal rubella was teratogenic, and another epidemic, this time of limb and ear defects, prompted Lenz (1961) to carry out his inquiries incriminating thalidomide. More recently, declines in the prevalence of defects due to congenital rubella have demonstrated the benefits of rubella immunization in childhood (Menser et al., 1984; Smithells et al., 1991). There are, however, many unexplained seasonal and secular trends in the prevalence of other birth defects.

Seasonal Trends

In several countries, anencephaly and/or spina bifida fluctuate in birth prevalence between a peak and a trough among spring and autumn conceptions, respectively. The most extensive data come from the United Kingdom (e.g., Knox & Lancashire, 1991; Maclean & MacLeod, 1984; Rogers & Weatherall, 1976) where the prevalence of anencephaly tends to peak in conceptions in early spring, and late spring conceptions tend to be at highest risk of spina bifida. These trends do not repeat themselves every year, but when national figures for many years are combined, the ratio between the highest and lowest monthly prevalence averages around 5:4 for each type of defect. Most of the comparable trends reported from other countries are restricted to defects of one type only, e.g., anencephaly in Newfoundland (where prevalence peaked among winter conceptions) and Westphalia (West Germany), and spina bifida in Hungary (Czeizel & Révész, 1970; Fraser et al., 1986; Tünte, 1964, 1968). In contrast, most studies in the United States (e.g., Khoury et al., 1982) find no seasonal variation in defects of either type, although a significant bimodal seasonal trend, with a principal peak among winter conceptions, has been reported for anencephaly in Utah (Jorde et al., 1984).

Congenital dislocation of the hip (CDH) has repeatedly been reported to occur most commonly in infants born in autumn and winter. As already suggested, it is important to distinguish between two groups of hips that are commonly referred to as cases of CDH—those that appear unstable at neonatal screening and those that, in screened and unscreened populations alike, present beyond the neonatal period with established dislocation. The association with autumn or winter birth is a consistent feature of established dislocation, and there are several reports of it also applying to neonatally unstable hips (Chen et al., 1970; Dunn et al., 1985; Record & Edwards, 1958; Robinson, 1968; Wynne-Davies, 1970a). However, no excess of autumn and winter births was found in several other series in which most or all the cases had neonatal instability (Artz et al., 1975; Bower et al., 1987; Knox & Lancashire, 1991; Xilinas & Lagarde, 1975).

There is also some evidence that the prevalence of clubfoot may be increased in winter or spring births. In a large U.S. study, clubfoot was reported most frequently in the first quarter of the year in regions with moderate winters and hot summers, and a month or two later in areas where cold winters and hot summers occurred (Wehrung & Hay, 1970). However, no seasonal variation was seen in Birmingham, England, where the weather is less extreme (Knox & Lancashire, 1991). Clubfoot was not analyzed by type in these studies. Talipes equinovarus, the most important type, occurred more often in winter than summer births in a smaller English series (Pryor et al., 1991).

In England, two studies of PDA revealed increases in frequency among females (but not males) born in late summer and early autumn (Polani & Campbell, 1960; Record & McKeown, 1953), whereas a third found an excess of cases among early summer births (Bound et al., 1989). Yet, other British and American studies detected no such trends (Leck, 1977).

Secular Trends

Substantial secular trends involving both anencephaly and spina bifida have been reported from many countries. For example, prolonged waves of high prevalence, each with a peak higher by two-thirds or more than the level before and after passage of the wave, seem to have built up during the 1920s and fallen away during the 1940s in both England and the northeastern United States. During the next two decades, England experienced a further wave with a peak in 1954 to 1955 but then little change after this wave had passed, whereas prevalence declined in the northeastern United States (Leck, 1983b). Since the early 1970s, a substantial further decline has been observed in many countries. Data for England and Wales on cases ascertained from stillbirth and death certificates or, for liveborn infants with spina bifida, birth notification forms are summarized in Figure 4.2. They show that among births in 1990 spina bifida was only 8.5% as common and anencephaly 2.7% as common as in 1972. The reductions reported from the United States have been more modest. In Atlanta, for example, the reported prevalence in 1988 to 1989 was 40% as high for spina bifida and 30% as high for anencephaly as in 1970 to 1971 (Yen et al., 1992).

One factor in the decline since the early 1970s has been the growing use of antenatal screening for NTDs by ultrasound and maternal serum alphafetoprotein (MSAFP) assay. If the MSAFP test is positive and no NTD is visible ultrasonically, an amniotic fluid alphafetoprotein (AFAFP) assay is used as a diagnostic test. Pregnancy termination is offered when NTD is diagnosed. In England and Wales, notification of medical termination of pregnancy is mandatory, and the data collected on the notification form include medical reasons for termination. The numbers of terminations for which each medical reason (e.g., CNS malformation) is given at notification are published annually, but a comparison of these data and information from other sources for the year 1985 (Cuckle et al., 1989) suggested that the number of terminations actually carried out for NTDs was 1.9 times as great as the number of notified terminations for CNS malformations. Figure 4.2 includes a comparison of the observed trend in birth prevalence of anencephaly and/or spina bifida in England and Wales (*solid circles*) with the estimated trend in **natural birth prevalence** (the prevalence had no pregnancies been terminated for NTDs—*open circles*). In calculating the latter trend it was assumed that there was the same undernotification of terminations for NTDs in other years as in 1985 and that if these terminations had not been carried out the affected pregnancies would all have ended in livebirths or stillbirths. The resulting figures suggest that, even in the absence of antenatal diagnosis and termination, the birth prevalence of NTDs in 1990 would only have been 37% of what it was in 1972. Data from the European Registration of Congenital Anomalies and Twins (EUROCAT) program, a network of malformation registries in Europe, suggest that during the 1980s the natural birth prevalence of NTDs also fell in Scotland and Ireland (including the Irish Republic,

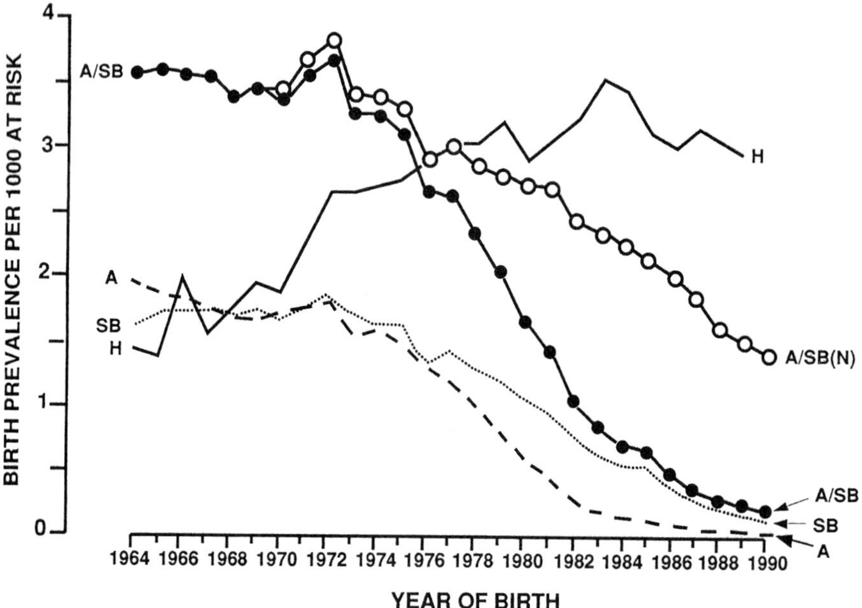

Fig. 4.2. Observed prevalence at birth of hypospadias or epispadias (H) per 1000 male births and of anencephaly (A), spina bifida without anencephaly (SB), and anencephaly and/or spina bifida (A/SB) per 1000 total births, and estimated natural birth prevalence of anencephaly and/or spina bifida (A/SB(N)) per 1000 total births and pregnancy terminations for NTDs.

[Cases were total births with hypospadias and live births with spina bifida reported under the national scheme for notification of malformations (Rogers & Weatherall, 1976; Office of Population Censuses and Surveys, 1983–92b; Matlai & Beral, 1985); total births with anencephaly and stillbirths with spina bifida reported on stillbirth and death certificates (General Register Office, 1968 and 1970; Office of Population Censuses and Surveys, 1971–92a); and pregnancy terminations for which the reasons included malformation of the central nervous system (CNS) according to statutory notification forms (Cuckle & Wald, 1987; Office of Population Censuses and Surveys, 1987–91). Numbers of pregnancy terminations for anencephaly and spina bifida were estimated by multiplying reported numbers of pregnancy terminations for central nervous system (CNS) malformations by 1.875 (the ratio between the number of pregnancies estimated by Cuckle et al. (1989) to have been actually terminated for anencephaly or spina bifida in 1985 and the number terminated for CNS malformations that year according to statutory notification forms). Natural birth prevalence was estimated on the assumption that if the pregnancies terminated for anencephaly or spina bifida had continued, two-thirds would have resulted in birth in the same calendar year as the termination and one-third in the next year.]

where pregnancy termination is illegal), but not in mainland Europe where NTDs were previously much less common (EUROCAT Working Group, 1991).

The birth prevalence of cases of hypospadias and epispadias (mostly hypospadias) reported on birth notification forms in England and Wales more than doubled between 1967 and 1983, although it has since declined somewhat (Figure 4.2). Increases during the 1970s and decreases more recently have also been reported from centers within the United Kingdom that ascertained cases from hospital admission records as well as birth notification forms (EUROCAT Working Group, 1991; Knox & Lancashire, 1991; Simpkin et al., 1985). Reports from other countries describe increases during the 1970s in Norway (Bjerkedal & Bakketeig, 1975), Sweden (Källén & Winberg, 1982), and Hungary (Czeizel, 1985), but not in British Columbia (Baird, 1985). Decreases during the 1980s were reported in part of the Netherlands, but not in the other non-British registers covered by EUROCAT (EUROCAT Working Group, 1991).

The prevalence of cryptorchidism (a condition beyond the scope of this chapter) is increased in boys with hypospadias (Shima et al., 1979; Svensson, 1979), and in England and Wales there is some evidence that cryptorchidism became more common during the years when the birth prevalence of notified cases of hypospadias was increasing (Matlai & Beral, 1985). Also, the risks of hypospadias and cryptorchidism may be increased by exposure to exogenous sex hormones in pregnancy (Aarskog, 1979; Dupue, 1984). The birth prevalence of these conditions may therefore have altered because of changes in the prescribing of these hormones. However, comparisons of the birth notification statistics for England and Wales with figures from other sources suggest that the notification of male genital tract malformations is incomplete and biased (Swerdlow & Melzer, 1988). This seems to imply that the changes in the numbers reported could be artifacts.

The evidence of secular trends in the incidence of infantile hypertrophic pyloric stenosis comes largely from records of hospital admissions. (Incidence is a better term than birth prevalence to use in this context because the defect does not normally present until after birth). Studies in the United Kingdom suggest that its incidence was about 2 per 1000 in the 1960s but was rather higher in previous decades (Leck, 1977) and that during the 1970s it rose to between 3 and 5 per 1000 depending on place (Grant & McAleer, 1984; Knox et al., 1983; Walsworth-Bell, 1983; Webb et al., 1983). A more recent British report (Tam & Chan, 1991) described an increase between the late 1970s and the late 1980s, but the initial figure was so low as to cast doubt on the reliability of the data.

Little is known about trends in pyloric stenosis in other countries, although a decrease was found between 1930 and 1959 in Gothenburg, Sweden, (Wallgren, 1960) and an increase between 1950 and 1984 among males in Olmsted County, Minnesota (Jedd et al., 1988). No change in incidence was detected in British Columbia in 1966 to 1977 (Walpole, 1981), or in Funen County, Denmark, in 1955 to 1984 (Rasmussen et al., 1989). The last two studies enumerated all infants with infantile pyloric stenosis or pylorospasm found in hospital records, whereas most of the others included only those in whom the presence of hypertrophy was confirmed, e.g., by pyloromyotomy. It is therefore possible that the trends observed in these other studies were not changes in prevalence but reflected changes in medical practice, e.g., increases and decreases in the proportion of affected children who were not ascertained because they were treated medically—perhaps at home—rather than undergoing pyloromyotomy.

The above secular trends were detected by inspecting annual rates and applying simple statistical tests. Knox and Lancashire (1991) used several more sophisticated methods to search for temporal variations in the frequency of different types of birth defects over the 21 years covered by their study in

Birmingham, England (see above). Among these methods were (1) tests for cyclical variations with periodicities of up to 70 months, (2) Knox's test for space-time interaction, and (3) polynomial curve fitting and a comparison of the resulting curves with the trends exhibited by indices of prevalence of various infectious diseases.

Significant cyclical variations, mostly with periodicities of the order of 4 or 5 years, were detected for many types of malformations. Hydrocephaly, polydactyly, accessory auricle, bile duct atresia, and several cardiac defects gave the most significant results. In the test for space-time interaction, the evidence that cases arising at about the same time tended to be separated by short distances was most convincing for two of the above conditions—hydrocephaly and accessory auricle. Also, there were more instances than would be expected by chance of hydrocephalic infants being born shortly before infants with accessory auricle who lived in the same locality. It was therefore postulated that an infection that tends to be widespread at different times in different places may cause accessory auricle when exposure occurs early in pregnancy, and hydrocephaly when it occurs later.

Several of the polynomial curves that were fitted to the distributions of defects over time showed similarities to trends in the numbers of cases of infection with members of the *Coxsackie* group of enteroviruses reported by public health laboratories in England and Wales (see Chapter 6). There were, for example, similarities between the trends for coxsackie-virus A and hydrocephaly, for coxsackie-virus B4 and cleft palate (without cleft lip), and for coxsackie-virus B3 and B5 and syndactyly. The association between coxsackie-virus A and hydrocephaly seems the most likely to be causal, because an infectious etiology for hydrocephaly is also suggested by the space-time interaction analysis and by an association between hydrocephaly and low maternal age that was observed in the same study. The findings should encourage case-control comparisons of stored serum samples from pregnant women whose offspring had any of the defects associated with *Coxsackie* infection in this study.

Incidence and Prenatal Mortality

The incidence of birth defects (i.e., the proportion of embryos in which they are laid down) and the prenatal mortality experienced by these embryos have been explored by direct and indirect methods. The direct method takes as a proxy for incidence the prevalence of defects in embryos and early fetuses removed at medical abortion. The indirect method determines the prevalence of defects in embryos and fetuses that have miscarried (i.e., aborted spontaneously), multiplies this by the proportion of known pregnancies that end in miscarriage, and estimates incidence by adding the resulting figure to the product of the birth prevalence of defects and the proportion of known pregnancies that end in birth. If one was applying the indirect method to a population in which antenatal diagnosis and termination of affected pregnancies were practiced, one would use the natural birth prevalence of defects and the proportion of pregnancies that would have ended in birth if these terminations had not taken place, in preference to the observed birth prevalence and proportion of pregnancies ending in birth.

Neither method is entirely accurate, for various reasons. By considering only induced abortions, the direct method misses cases in which miscarriage occurs before the time at which abortion would have been induced. Its data base is also unlikely to be representative of all pregnant women in terms of age, social circumstances, or even health (although the reasons for most induced abortions are not strictly medical). The indirect method also misses early losses, since it can only take note of miscarriages for which the products of conception are available for examination (generally hospital cases). Both methods rely on data based on embryos or small fetuses, which are often insufficiently well preserved to establish whether malformations are present. Thus, the best that the investigator may be able to do is to estimate the frequency of malformations some time after their inception, after making the somewhat shaky assumption that the material from miscarriages at each stage of gestation that was fit to study was representative of all the miscarriages that occurred at that stage.

Despite these limitations, the resulting figures for malformations that are visible in late embryos and early fetuses are likely to give a better estimate of incidence than can be inferred from birth prevalence statistics. The section that follows focuses mainly on results obtained when the direct and indirect methods were applied, respectively, to data on early induced abortions in Kyoto, Japan, and on miscarriages in London, England. The incidence and prenatal mortality of all morphologically and chromosomally abnormal concepti are considered first, followed by the findings for specific defects.

All Abnormal Concepti

In the Kyoto series of induced abortions, localized external malformations were observed in 4.2% of undamaged embryos aged between 6 and 8 weeks from conception (Nishimura, 1970). Chorionic sacs that contained no embryo seem to have occurred even more often (Shiota, 1989). Chromosomal anomalies were found in 1.9% of 4- to 8-week embryos in this series (Nishimura, 1970), and in 6.9% of 5- to 8-week concepti (including empty chorionic sacs) from another Japanese center (Yamamoto & Watanabe, 1979). In a recent English study of induced abortions, numerical chromosomal anomalies were found in chorionic material from 4.7% of cases (Burgoyne et al., 1991), which is broadly consistent with the latter Japanese figure. Some of the cases of chromosomal anomalies in these two series may well have been mosaics in which the abnormal cell line was confined to the chorion. This type of mosaicism has been reported in 2% of 9- to 12-week pregnancies submitted to chorionic villus sampling. Studies of miscarriages suggest that it may be even more common (Kalousek et al., 1992).

The London study (Creasy et al., 1976) covered miscarriages at gestational ages of 8 to 28 weeks, i.e., 6 to 26 weeks from conception. From the results, it has been estimated that external abnormalities that might be detected in a miscarried embryo or early fetus (including absence of embryo) are present in 6.3% of 6-week concepti and that the proportion of 6-week concepti with chromosomal anomalies is also 6.3% (Leck, 1993). Other studies of miscarriages

(Hassold et al., 1978, 1980) suggest that chromosomal anomalies occur in approximately 7% to 9% of 6-week concepti. None of these figures allows fully for the occurrence of mosaics in which the abnormal cell line is confined to the chorion, most cases of which are likely to have been missed in the studies quoted.

As noted previously, even estimates such as the above—whether based on induced abortions or miscarriages—fail to show the total impact of maldevelopment, both because they do not take account of very early miscarriages and because even the later abortions on which they are based are unlikely to be representative of all such abortions. In addition, the figures quoted for structural malformations cover only those diagnosed by external inspection and are based on embryos and fetuses many of which were too young for some defects to be apparent. Some of these limitations were partially overcome in a study in Seattle. Embryos and fetuses not affected by severe disorganization and that miscarried at ages from 2 weeks after conception were examined for structural malformations by methods including the use of a dissecting microscope (Shepard et al., 1989). Using the results of this study, major structural maldevelopment (absence of the embryo, severe disorganization, or severe structural defects) was estimated to be the fate of 13% of concepti alive 2 weeks after fertilization (Leck, 1993).

The above estimates agree in indicating that most concepti with major developmental abnormalities die during the first two trimesters of pregnancy. The 0.7% birth prevalence reported for abnormal karyotypes is of the order of one tenth as great as most of the above estimates for concepti a few weeks old. This suggests that about 90% of chromosomally abnormal concepti who survive the first few weeks miscarry later. The figures for structural maldevelopment are not closely comparable with each other, but again all point to low survival rates during the first two trimesters. Among estimates of the birth prevalence of external malformations that might be detected in the embryonic period in Japan (0.5%—Neel, 1958) and in England (0.8%—Leck et al., 1968), the former figure was about one eighth as high as the proportion of intact embryos in which localized external malformations were observed in Kyoto, and the latter was about one eighth as high as the proportion of 6-week concepti exhibiting severe external maldevelopment of any kind (including anembryony) as estimated from the London data. The birth prevalence of all severe structural defects is about one fifth as high as the Seattle-based estimate of the proportion of 2-week concepti who are, or will become, seriously maldeveloped.

Even the proportion of concepti alive a few weeks after conception in which maldevelopment occurs is probably small in comparison to the proportion of all concepti that develop abnormally. This suggests that even more affected concepti are lost during the very early weeks than subsequently. Among the evidence for this assertion is that (1) two fifths of concepti recovered by Hertig and coworkers (1956) from women who underwent hysterectomy 2–17 days after conception were morphologically abnormal and (2) in studies of ova fertilized in vitro, between 23% and 40% were chromosomally abnormal (Zenzes & Casper, 1992).

Specific Defects

The data for induced abortions in Kyoto and miscarriages in London have been used elsewhere (Leck, 1983a) to estimate the frequency of specific types of defects in late embryos or early fetuses. The results were then compared with birth prevalence statistics from the same countries (Figure 4.3). Except for spina bifida in London, this comparison suggests that the defects shown are some two or more times as common in early pregnancy as at birth. In three more recent series from predominantly white localities (MacHenry et al., 1979; McFadden & Kallousek, 1989; Shepard et al., 1989), spina bifida was reported in at least three times as high a proportion of miscarriages as in the London series, suggesting that some cases in the latter series may have been overlooked.

The studies on which Figure 4.3 is based also indicate that various anomalies, such as cyclopia, polydactyly, and abnormal karyotypes other than Down syndrome, which do not pose enough of a problem among infants to be included in this Figure, are ten or more times as common in embryos as in fetuses that survive to the last trimester. Indeed, most of the anomalies seen in early concepti are of types seldom or never seen at birth. Even those that are morphologically similar to malformations observed in the newborn may often differ from them in etiology: for example, most miscarried embryos (as opposed to fetuses) with NTDs have chromosomal anomalies (McFadden & Kallousek, 1989), which is true of hardly any infants (including stillbirths) with these defects. However, by no means do all the cases of malformations in which miscarriage occurs differ in etiology from infant cases. For example, Down syndrome has the same immediate cause (triplication of most or all of autosome 21) in miscarried and born cases alike.

When a high proportion of cases of a type of malformation miscarry, it cannot

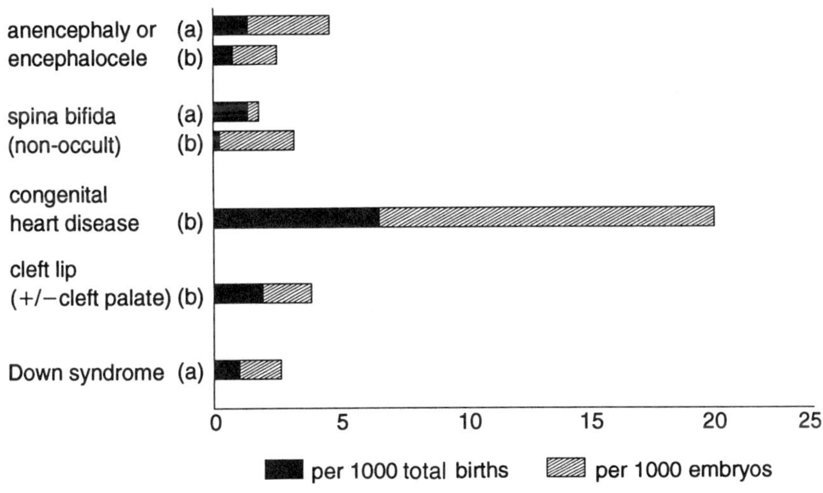

Fig. 4.3. Estimated frequency of common malformations per 1000 total births (*solid blocks*) and embryos (*total blocks*). Estimates are based on data for births and miscarriages in England (blocks labeled *a*) and births and induced abortions in Japan (blocks labeled *b*).

be taken for granted that this defect's incidence is above average in groups of pregnancies in which its birth prevalence is high; a high birth prevalence may alternatively point to a reduced frequency of miscarriage in the group concerned. There are at least two generally applicable ways of exploring which of these two possible explanations for a high birth prevalence is more likely to be correct. The more direct approach is to use data either for miscarriages and births or for induced abortions to estimate the incidence of malformations in different groups of embryos and then to compare the results, e.g., the findings for NTDs in Japan and England in Figure 4.3. The other main approach is to look for variations in the proportion of *all* pregnancies ending in miscarriage, on the assumption that in groups where this proportion is lowest the impact of miscarriage on malformation frequency is likely to be least. If, therefore, this proportion is found to be particularly low in a group of pregnancies among which the birth prevalence of a type of malformation is high, the reason for the high birth prevalence is postulated to be that relatively few cases have been lost by miscarriage (Stein et al., 1975).

Although not widely used, these two approaches have been followed to a limited extent in investigating two of the variations in the birth prevalence of malformations described earlier in this chapter—the geographical and seasonal differences in the prevalence of NTDs. Only one of the two approaches—the study of the total frequency of miscarriages—seems to have been used to study the seasonal fluctuation, and the results suggest that this fluctuation is *not* secondary to any variation in the risk of miscarriage (Leck, 1977). Figure 4.3 explores a geographical difference—that between Japan and England—by comparing estimates of the incidence in embryos. The results suggest that the differences between these countries in the birth prevalence of anencephaly and spina bifida have different explanations—a higher incidence in England in the case of anencephaly, and more miscarriages in Japan in the case of spina bifida (although as stated earlier, some instances of spina bifida in miscarriages in the London series may well have been missed). Within the United Kingdom, where the birth prevalence of NTDs increases as one goes north and west from the London area, an opposite trend in the frequency of miscarriages has been reported. Yet, against this evidence that the variation in birth prevalence is due to different proportions of cases miscarrying must be weighed surveys of NTDs in miscarriages that suggest that Northern Ireland (in the northwest of the United Kingdom) experiences a substantially higher incidence of anencephaly and spina bifida than London, as well as a higher birth prevalence (Leck, 1983b). It therefore seems from the limited evidence available that trends in the birth prevalence of defects may reflect variations both in incidence and in the proportion of cases miscarrying.

Mortality Beyond Midpregnancy

More extensive mortality data are available for the period beyond midpregnancy than for the first few months from conception. This is due to the existence in most developed countries of a requirement to notify particulars, including cause of death, for "late" fetal deaths, as well as deaths after birth. The time beyond which delivery must occur for a fetal death to be considered "late" is defined as the 20th week from onset of the last menstrual period (LMP) in some jurisdictions, including most of the United States, and as the 28th week in others, e.g., the United Kingdom until very recently.

Impact on the General Population

According to death registration data for 1990 (Table 4.2), approximately 2.3 per 1000 infants (including stillbirths) born in England and Wales die from malformations by the age of 5 years. This figure includes 1.6 per 1000 who die during the first year after birth. Infants whose deaths were attributed to anomalies of the respiratory tract are excluded from these numerators because the problem in most of these cases is incomplete development of the lungs, which is generally due to immaturity, rather than malformation. By comparison, the proportion of infants certified as dying during the first year after birth from nonrespiratory malformations in 1985 was 2.2 per 1000 in England and Wales, Scotland, and Sweden and 2.0 per 1000 in the United States (Powell-Griner & Woolbright, 1990).

Malformations can be entered on death certificates not only as principal causes of death but also as associated conditions. Although some certificates list malformations in both categories, there may well be more on which no malformations are recorded, although some were present. Despite some double counting, the total number of entries of malformations on death certificates (as estimated in the second row of figures in Table 4.2) is therefore likely to constitute

Table 4.2. Estimated Mortality of Subjects with Malformations Reported on Stillbirth and Death Certificates, per 1000 Total Births (Malformed and Not Malformed): England and Wales, 1990

	Stillbirths	First-Week Deaths	Deaths at 1–4 Weeks	Deaths at 4–52 Weeks*	Deaths at 1–5 Years (Cumulative Mortality)*
Malformations (all types†) recorded as principal causes of death	0.33	0.78	0.33	0.51	0.32
Malformations recorded as principal causes of death or associated conditions					
All types†	0.53	1.32	0.58	0.87	0.55
Malformations of heart and great vessels	0.08	0.45	0.37	0.51	0.32

*In calculating these figures, it was assumed (1) that infants who died aged before 6 months and those who died aged 6–12 months were born in 1990 and 1989, respectively; (2) that children who died at each year of age from 1 onward were equally divided as to year of birth between the 2 years in which they could have been born; and (3) that the ratio between the numbers of malformations recorded as principal causes of death and as associated conditions was the same for deaths beyond 4 weeks (for which the latter number was not recorded) as it was for neonatal deaths.

†Anomalies of respiratory system are excluded.

Basic data primarily from Office of Population Censuses and Surveys (1992a).

a more accurate estimate of the total number of deaths of malformed individuals than is the number of deaths ascribed principally to malformations. According to the former estimate, nearly 3.9 per 1000 infants (including stillbirths) are malformed and die within 5 years of birth, including 0.5 per 1000 before birth, 1.3 during the next week, 0.6 between 1 and 4 weeks, and 0.9 during the rest of the first year. The estimates for stillbirths and deaths in the first week after birth may be compared with hospital-based data from European and North American centers aggregated by Kalter (1991). These figures suggest that malformed infants accounted for 1.1 stillbirths and 0.8 first-week deaths per 1000 total births in European centers in 1980 to 1989. The corresponding North American figures were 0.6 and 1.1 per 1000. Although the three sets of figures for stillbirths and first week deaths considered separately vary, those for the two categories combined (perinatal deaths) are very similar.

Kalter (1991) also drew attention to increases in the percentage of perinatal deaths reported to be associated with malformations. The increases were especially marked in his European series, where the percentage of stillbirths in this category rose from 5.4% to 18.3% and the percentage of first-week deaths from 6.5% to 36.3% between the 1940s and the 1980s. In his North American series the figure for stillbirths remained at about 12% and that for first-week deaths only rose from 16.4% to 31.4%. The increases reflect the fact that the fall in perinatal mortality over the last few decades has been less steep for malformed infants than for others. Why this should be more true for Europe than for North America is a question that calls for further study.

The group of malformations most commonly associated with death in early life is cardiovascular anomalies. From late fetal life to 4 years of age, these anomalies account for about 45% of all malformations recorded on stillbirth and death certificates; beyond the perinatal period this proportion is about 60% (Table 4.2).

Impact on the Malformed

Given that 2.5% of all infants (including stillbirths) have severe malformations, it can be estimated from the figures in Table 4.2 that in England and Wales approximately 15% of those affected die within 5 years of birth, although death may only be certified as due to a malformation in about 9%—three fifths of those who die (Table 4.3). The cumulative proportion estimated to have died rises from 2% at birth to 7% after 1 week and to 10% after 4 weeks. For the United States, estimates of 4%, 11%, and 12% for the numbers dead by these ages were given by Kalter (1991). The two sets of figures differ mainly because the proportion of stillborn infants in whom malformations were reported was higher in Kalter's series. This may be because deliveries of dead fetuses between 20 and 28 weeks from the LMP were counted as stillbirths in the United States but not in England and Wales, and/or because malformations in stillbirths may have been less completely reported on the registration documents on which the British figures are based than in the hospital records on which Kalter relied. Previous work (Leck, 1983a) suggests that in England and Wales the reporting

Table 4.3. Estimated Cumulative Mortality per 100 Still- or Liveborn Malformed Individuals

	Mortality before				
Type of Malformation	Birth	One week	Four weeks	One year	Five years
Severe malformations of any kind					
Mortality for which malformations were recorded as principal cause*	1	4	6	8	9
Mortality for which malformations were recorded as principal cause or associated condition*	2	7	10	13	15
Specific defects[†]					
Anencephaly[‡]	59	100	100	100	100
Spina bifida aperta[‡]	12	23	37	50	54
Malformations of heart and great vessels*	1	8	13	20	25
Down syndrome	4[§]	8[§]	10[‖]	16[‖]	22[‖]

*Calculated from statistics in Table 4–2 on the assumptions that 2.5% of all infants (including stillbirths) have severe malformations of any kind and that 0.69% (as in Kenna et al., 1975) have malformations of heart and great vessels.

[†]Figures based on all deaths in Down syndrome and on deaths in individuals with other conditions where the condition concerned was recorded as the principal cause of death or as an associated condition.

[‡]Calculated from 1990 mortality statistics and 1985 to 1990 birth statistics for England and Wales (Office of Population Censuses and Surveys, 1992a and b) on the assumptions (1) that all cases born in each relevant year were reported on stillbirth certificates or (if liveborn) under the national scheme for notification of malformations; (2) that infants dying in 1990 were born in 1990 if aged less than 6 months at death and in 1989 if aged 6–12 months; (3) that children who died in 1990 at each year of age from 1 onward were equally divided as to year of birth between the 2 years in which they could have been born; and (4) that the ratio between the numbers of malformations recorded as principal causes of death and as associated conditions was the same for deaths beyond 4 weeks (for which the latter number was not recorded) as it was for neonatal deaths.

[§]Data of Fryers & Mackay (1979).

[‖]Data of Bell et al. (1989), adjusted for stillbirths by assuming that the same proportion of cases in Bell's population as in that of Fryers and Mackay (1979) was stillborn.

of malformations on registration documents is less complete for stillbirths than for postnatal deaths.

As for mortality in the whole of the first year after birth, Lynberg et al. (1991) reported that in Atlanta, Georgia, 8% of malformed infants died during this period. Because about 3.8% of infants were counted as malformed in this study it seems likely that some nonsevere defects were included. If the birth prevalence of severe malformations had been 2.5%, as is usual, and if the same proportion of infants with nonsevere malformations as of all infants (1.3%) had died in the first year, it can be calculated that 12% of those with severe malformations would have done so. This is similar to the 11% suggested by the data for England and Wales (Table 4.3).

This section concludes by considering the frequency of death in early life among infants with specific types of defects, estimated from the figures in Table 4.2 in the case of malformations of the heart and great vessels and from similar sources (some indicated in the footnotes to Table 4.3) for other conditions. Table 4.3 includes estimates for four conditions that are or (in the case of the NTDs) used to be relatively common and that are still of high mortality—anencephaly, spina bifida aperta, malformations of the heart and great vessels

(CHD), and Down syndrome. Anencephaly is always rapidly fatal. Approximately half of all children with spina bifida die within 5 years of birth, but this proportion is much higher if active treatment is restricted to infants whose sphincters and lower limbs are not completely paralyzed (Lorber, 1973). Death during or before early childhood also seems to be the outcome in a quarter of all infants with CHD and in a somewhat lower proportion of those with Down syndrome. Within these groups there are, of course, considerable variations in mortality between those with and without additional defects and between those in the cardiovascular group whose malformations are of different types. For example, the proportion of liveborn children with Down syndrome who died within 5 years of birth varied in one series between 37% for those who also had heart defects and 13% for those who did not (Baird & Sadovnick, 1987).

Risk Factors

Specific Teratogens

No agent or deficiency should be accepted as a teratogen, unless birth defects have not merely occurred in some individuals who have been exposed to the agent or deficiency but have also been shown to be more common in the exposed than in the general population (see Chapter 1). This guideline might seem obvious, but it has been ignored repeatedly. For example, the drug marketed in the United Stages as Bendectin and in the United Kingdom as Debendox was widely accused of being teratogenic when a number of malformed children were born to mothers who had taken Bendectin/Debendox. Yet, both case-control and cohort studies carried out later suggested that there were no more such cases than would have been expected to occur in the large number of infants born to users of the drug (Orme, 1985).

Even evidence that a defect is more common than average in those exposed to an agent or deficiency should not be accepted uncritically as proof of causation. When based on retrospective interviews with parents, such evidence may simply reflect recall bias. An apparent association between an exposure and a defect may also be produced by selection bias or by confounding—by selection bias if, for example, a control group in which exposed individuals are underrepresented has been used and by confounding if exposure tends to occur in individuals who are at increased risk of the defect for some other reason. As is described in Chapter 1, an exposure associated with an above-average frequency of malformations should not normally be considered teratogenic unless the following four conditions are met:

1. The association appears unlikely to be caused by bias or confounding, e.g., because the odds ratio or relative risk of malformation in the exposed is very high—perhaps in double figures—or because several analytic studies using different methods and data bases have yielded similar risk estimates.
2. The malformations responsible for the excess of cases among exposed offspring are largely of one or a few specific types, as opposed to being distributed by type in the same way as cases seen in the general population.

3. The time in pregnancy at which the cases involved in the excess have been exposed is no later than the time at which the defects would have originated.
4. Experience in fields other than epidemiology (e.g., animal experiments or—in the case of micro-organisms—laboratory evidence of fetal infection in humans) makes it plausible that the exposure and malformations could be causally related.

Bearing in mind these criteria, some 20 factors can reasonably be assumed to cause malformations in humans. These factors are listed in Table 4.4, together with the defects mainly associated with them and (where obtainable) an estimate to one significant figure of the risk difference (exposed), i.e., the amount by which the birth prevalence of defects in those exposed to each factor exceeds the birth prevalence in the unexposed (see Chapter 1). Where the data on which the risk differences are based were analyzed by intensity, time of exposure, or both, these risk differences refer to infants exposed to the highest intensities and/or at the times of highest risk that it seems reasonable to consider separately. However, time and intensity of exposure were not given in all data sets, and even when given they are likely to have been distorted by unreliable recording. Accordingly, and because most of the risk difference estimates are based on small numbers, these estimates should not be regarded as entirely accurate or comparable, but they do indicate the orders of magnitude of the hazards concerned.

The first six entries in Table 4.4 are infections. For the more important of these—cytomegalovirus infection, rubella, and toxoplasmosis—the most useful available data on the frequency of defects differ in two ways from the sources of the risk differences cited lower down in Table 4.4. First, the risks of defects caused by the three main infectious diseases have generally been estimated for children for whom there is serologic or virologic evidence that they have themselves been infected. Second, in the best studies of defects in children with evidence of prenatal infection, the children have been expertly examined when several years old, with the result that chronic conditions that are not malformations in the strict sense of the word—notably retinopathy and defects of hearing and intelligence—have been included when the prevalence of defects has been estimated. For Table 4.4, the teratogenic risk if the *mother* is infected (the analogue of the estimated risks given for other teratogens) was estimated for each of the main infections, by multiplying the risk to prenatally infected children by the prevalence of prenatal infection among all children whose mothers appear from serologic studies to have been infected during pregnancy. The resulting figures cover the risk of the chronic defects mentioned, as well as of true malformations, whereas the other figures in Table 4.4 do not.

The need for caution in interpreting these figures is illustrated by the fact that in Britain the number of cases of symptomatic toxoplasmosis reported in infants is much lower in relation to the frequency of maternal toxoplasmosis than the risk of lasting damage after maternal seroconversion given in Table 4.4 (30% to 40%) would lead one to expect (Hall, 1992). The latter range may therefore be an overestimate.

The risks to infants of mothers first infected by cytomegalovirus and *Toxoplasma* during pregnancy in Table 4.4 are based on reports that did not include

Table 4.4. Teratogens and Their Effects on the Frequency of Malformations in Humans*

Teratogen	Main Defects Caused	Estimated Risk Difference (Exposed)[†]
	Infections	
Cytomegalovirus infection	Deafness; brain damage; eye disorders	8% after maternal seroconversion in pregnancy (according to estimates that 40% of infants from affected pregnancies have been infected and that 20% of their infections lead to handicap; Stagno, 1990)
Herpes simplex	Brain damage; eye disorders; cutaneous scars	Not known
Rubella	Eye and heart defects; deafness; brain damage	90% after serologically confirmed infection of mother in first 10 weeks of pregnancy (Miller et al., 1982)
Toxoplasmosis	Brain damage; eye disorders; deafness	30%–40% after maternal seroconversion in pregnancy without treatment (according to estimates that 40%–50% of infants from affected pregnancies have been infected and that among infected infants 10% show severe effects at birth or during infancy and 70% first show sequelae later; Hall, 1992)
Varicella-zoster	Brain damage; eye disorders; cutaneous scars	2% after clinical varicella infection of mother in first trimester (Preblud et al., 1986); not known for zoster
Venezuelan equine encephalitis	Brain damage	Not known
	Other Maternal Diseases	
Phenylketonuria	Brain damage; cardiac defects	Microcephaly in 80% of infants of phenylketonurics with blood phenylalanine ≥ 1.2 mmol/L (Lipson et al., 1984)
Insulin-dependent diabetes mellitus	Cardiovascular and central nervous defects; caudal regression	Major defects in 8% of infants of affected women who did not receive special care during early pregnancy
	Medications	
Androgens and progestins	Anomalies of external genitalia	Mild clitoridal hypertrophy in 20% and more marked virilization in 9% of female infants after norethindrone (20 mg+/day) in first trimester; risks with other drugs not known but seem to be lower. Hypospadias in 0.6% of male infants after progestins in early pregnancy
Anticonvulsants	Spina bifida (after valproate; Lammer et al., 1987); oral clefts; cardiovascular defects	4% overall (Janz, 1982), but varies with number and nature of anticonvulsants used (Nakane et al., 1980)
Coumarin derivatives	Nasal hypoplasia; epiphyseal stippling on x-rays; brain damage	Nasal hypoplasia/epiphyseal stippling in 8% after use in first trimester; brain damage in 5% after use in second trimester

Table 4.4. (Continued)

Teratogen	Main Defects Caused	Estimated Risk Difference (Exposed)[†]
Diethylstilbestrol	Genital anomalies	Testicular anomalies, epididymal cysts, or penile hypoplasia in 20% of males, and ridges in cervix and/or vagina in 40% of females (generally combined with anomalies of corpus uteri) after dose increasing from 5 to 150 mg between 7 and 34 weeks gestation
Folic acid antagonists (aminopterin, methotrexate)	Craniofacial defects	40% after aminopterin in first 10 weeks of pregnancy; not known for methotrexate
Lithium	Cardiac defects, especially Ebstein's anomaly	3% (based on pregnancies in most of which there was first trimester lithium use; Jacobson et al., 1992; Källén & Tandberg, 1983)
Retinoids	Microtia/anotia; central nervous, cardio-aortic, and thymic defects	20% after isotretinoin in first trimester (Lammer et al., 1988); not known for other retinoids (Rosa, 1991)
Thalidomide	Reduction deformities of limbs and ears	50% after use in first 8 weeks of pregnancy
	Other Chemical Agents	
Cocaine	Urinary tract defects	Major defects in 5% of users of cocaine ± other drugs (cohort studies reviewed by Lutiger et al., 1991)
Ethyl alcohol	Brain damage; cardiac and joint defects	30% of infants (excluding perinatal deaths) of women with manifest chronic alcoholism
Methylmercury	Brain damage	6% of infants in fishing villages where seafood was contaminated
	Miscellaneous Influences	
Hypoxia	Persistant ductus arteriosus; perhaps atrial septal defect	1–5% of schoolchildren born and living ≥ 4 km above sea level (Miao et al., 1988; Peñalosa et al., 1964)
Iodine deficiency	Brain damage; deafness	40% of surviving infants in iodine-deficient area whose mothers' blood total thyroxine was <25 ng/mL (Pharoah et al., 1976)
Ionizing radiation	Brain damage	Microcephaly in 70% after estimated dose ≥ 1.5 gray from atomic bombs in first 18 weeks of pregnancy

*Supporting references are as given by Leck (1983a), except where stated.

[†]Based on series of all infants, including stillbirths, except where stated.

analyses by time of infection. Other data suggest that the chance of toxoplasmosis being transmitted to an offspring is greatest when the mother is infected late in pregnancy, but that if an embryo or fetus acquires this infection early in pregnancy its risk of suffering severe damage is greater than if infected later (Desmonts & Couvreur, 1979). For women first infected by cytomegalovirus during pregnancy, it is less clear how the child's risks vary with the time during gestation when infection occurs (Best, 1987). Infants whose mothers have first been infected with either organism before pregnancy occasionally exhibit defects due to infection, but are much less likely to do so than those whose mothers seroconvert during pregnancy (Griffiths et al., 1991; Hall, 1992).

The entries for noninfectious teratogens in Table 4.4 are largely self-explanatory. The risk differences given for these teratogens relate almost entirely to defects generally regarded as malformations. They do not relate to other signs of impaired prenatal development, such as dysmorphic facies, hypoplastic distal phalanges, and retarded growth. These are described in considerable proportions of infants exposed to some of the teratogens listed, e.g., alcohol and several anticonvulsants.

There are probably only three noninfectious agents or deficiencies in Table 4.4 of which it might arguably be said that their causal relationship to the defects listed is doubtful. These are lithium, cocaine, and hypoxia, for which the estimated risk differences do not exceed 5%. The overall risk difference quoted for anticonvulsants is just as low, but the case against these drugs is based on much more extensive data, and subsets of these data yield substantially higher risk differences, e.g., 9% and 21% for the offspring of women on three and four anticonvulsants, respectively, in one large series (Nakane et al., 1980) when epileptics on no drugs are taken as the referent group.

Support for lithium being a human teratogen is provided by the international Register of Lithium Babies. Among 225 infants on this register, 11% had major malformations. Ebstein's anomaly (a condition reported in only about one in 20,000 births) was present in almost one quarter of these malformed infants, and other cardiac anomalies were found in another half (Jacobson et al., 1992). It could well be that the percentage of malformed babies was so high because they were more likely than normal infants to be registered, but it is difficult to see why cardiac defects (especially the rare Ebstein's anomaly) should have been present in a much higher proportion of the malformed than is usual, unless lithium increases their frequency. However, it is doubtful whether the association should be regarded as proven without more data from other sources. The two studies cited in Table 4.4, which do not include the Register of Lithium Babies because of its possible unrepresentativeness, covered 165 exposed infants of whom 10 were malformed (4 with heart defects), as well as 15 exposed fetuses from induced abortions (1 with Ebstein's anomaly).

The risk difference for cocaine in Table 4.4 is based on a larger number of exposed infants (437), who were assembled from six cohort studies that Lutiger et al. (1991) included in a meta-analysis. They concluded that malformations of the genitourinary (GU) tract but not of other systems showed a statistically significant increase in birth prevalence among the infants of cocaine users, although a recent brief report based on 1324 exposed infants suggests that exposure does not increase the risk of GU malformation (Rajegowda et al., 1991). If the association between GU malformations and cocaine use is real, there is some evidence that the malformations mainly involved are urinary. These predominated over genital defects in the cohort studies, and a statistically significant association between urinary but not genital malformations and maternal cocaine use was also observed by Chávez, Mulinare, and Cordero (1989) in a case-control study that was nested within the Metropolitan Atlanta Congenital Defects Program, probably the foremost American resource for epidemiologic studies of malformations.

Hypoxia seems likely to increase the risk of persistence of the ductus arteriosus and possibly of the foramen ovale, both of which normally close after birth. Studies in two countries where people live at very varying altitudes—Peru (Alzamora-Castro et al., 1960; Peñaloza et al., 1964) and China (including Tibet; Miao et al., 1988)—suggest that the prevalence beyond infancy of PDA increases with altitude until above 4 km it is many times as high as at sea level. The Chinese data show a similar trend for atrial septal defect (ASD). Support for attributing the trend for PDA to variations in oxygen tension (low at high altitudes) is provided by the fact that the ductus of the newborn tends to dilate when blood oxygen is low and to constrict when it is high, both in humans and in other animals (Dawes, 1961; Moss et al., 1964). If ASD is also more common at high altitudes, a possible reason is that oxygen deficiency delays the fall in pulmonary vascular resistance in the newborn and may in this way raise right atrial pressure and impede closure of the foramen ovale (Miao et al., 1988). This is an example of evidence from fields other than epidemiology supporting an etiologic hypothesis by providing a biologic rationale for it (see Chapter 1). There is no such evidence to suggest why cocaine should be particularly harmful to the urinary tract or lithium to the tricuspid valve (the site of Ebstein's anomaly).

Two general points about the list of teratogens in the table should be noted. First, prenatal exposure to some of the teratogens listed causes not only defects but also diseases, e.g., diabetes after congenital rubella (Menser et al., 1978) and vaginal adenocarcinoma after maternal use of diethylstilbestrol (Herbst et al., 1971). Second, several factors that others might call teratogens have not been listed. Some of these—e.g., assisted conception (Lancaster, 1991), chorionic villus sampling (Dolk et al., 1992), cigarette smoking (Hartsfield & Hudson, 1991) and hyperthermia (Milunsky et al., 1991)—are omitted because although the evidence of their teratogenicity merits serious consideration it was felt on balance to be less strong than in the case of the factors listed. Other factors are not listed because their established transplacental effects are limited to conditions other than anatomic malformations—e.g., abnormal coloration of teeth (tetracycline, Cohlan, 1977) and of skin (polychlorinated biphenyls; Miller, 1971), cutis laxa (D-penicillamine; Schardein, 1985), scalp ulcers (methimazole; Milham, 1986), deafness (streptomycin; Snider et al., 1980), hydrops (parvovirus B19; Public Health Laboratory Service Working Party on Fifth Disease, 1990) and inflammation that does not affect organogenesis (syphilis, for example; Ingall et al., 1990).

This account of specific environmental teratogens concludes by considering what proportions of all major malformations can be attributed to these teratogens and to monogenic and chromosomal abnormalities (see Chapter 5). Kalter and Warkany (1983) estimated that major malformations due to environmental teratogens occurred in 1.5 per 1000 births in the United States. This figure is equivalent to 5% of affected infants if one assumes, as these workers did, that the birth prevalence of major malformations is 3% (a figure broadly consistent with the study by Heinonen et al. (1977) described previously). The figure of 1.5 per 1000 was largely based on estimates of the contributions made by rubella, cytomegalovirus infection, toxoplasmosis, diabetes mellitus, and anticonvulsants. No other teratogen was considered widespread enough to contribute much to the total figure apart from alcohol, the effects of which Kalter and Warkany did not attempt to quantify.

With the addition of alcohol, the teratogens mentioned are still likely to be responsible for most malformations of known environmental origin, but the estimates of how much each contributes that Kalter and Warkany made for the United States need to be revised. Congenital rubella is now a very rare event. Congenital toxoplasmosis, which used to occur in 1 to 2 per 1000 infants in the United States (Wilson & Remington, 1979) also seems to have become less common there: the most recent work quoted by Remington and Desmonts (1990) suggests a figure of 0.2 per 1000 or less. Although most of those infected may eventually develop sequelae, such as chorioretinitis, no more than 10%—0.02 or less per 1000 births—are likely to have severe malformations as usually understood (Table 4.4). Congenital cytomegalovirus infection occurs in many more infants—about 1%, of whom one eighth may be born with clinical cytomegalic inclusion disease and one fifth may develop lasting defects (Stagno, 1990). However, even the lasting defects that arise in clinically diseased neonates (who are most at risk of these defects) are almost all conditions such as deafness, rather than severe anatomic malformations. For the latter, it seems reasonable only to allow a figure of 0.1 per 1000 births (see Chapter 6).

Kalter and Warkany (1983) assumed on the basis of earlier work that, among women giving birth, 4.7 per 1000 have insulin-dependent diabetes and 5.2 per 1000 are on anticonvulsant therapy. By multiplying these figures by the risk differences in Table 4.4, it is estimated that major malformations due to diabetes and to anticonvulsants occur in 0.38 per 1000 and 0.21 per 1000 infants, respectively. The impact of excessive alcohol consumption may be greater: the prevalence of the fetal alcohol syndrome in the United States is believed to be between 1 and 2 per 1000 infants (Clarren & Smith, 1978). Although the diagnostic criteria for this syndrome (a combination of growth retardation, central nervous system (CNS) involvement, and characteristic facies; Sokol and Clarren, 1989) can be satisfied without any major anatomic malformation being present, it seems reasonable to allow for 0.5 per 1000 infants having such malformations as part of the syndrome.

The sum of these prevalence estimates for major malformations caused by *Toxoplasma*, cytomegalovirus, diabetes, anticonvulsants, and alcohol is 1.21 per 1000. Rounding this total to 1.3 per 1000, to allow for the effects of the less common teratogens provides an estimate of 4.3% for the proportion of major malformations that may be attributed to known environmental causes. If the teratogenicity of cocaine (still debatable) were to be confirmed, this figure might need to be revised upward, because large numbers of women (possibly 10% to 15% of the urban poor in the United States; Singer et al., 1991) use this drug. However, it seems unlikely that known environmental causes account for a larger proportion of major malformations than the 5% originally estimated by Kalter and Warkany (1983).

Monogenic conditions were incriminated in 3%, and chromosomal abnormalities in 10% of a recent large U.S. series of infants (including stillbirths) with major malformations (Nelson & Holmes, 1989). Adding these percentages and a figure of 5% to cover the contribution of recognized environmental teratogens yields a total of only 18% for the proportion of major malformations attributable to a known specific cause.

Other Risk Factors

It is not practicable to review here all the ways in which the birth prevalence of malformations varies with factors other than specific teratogens—factors that include characteristics of infants (e.g., sex), of their parents (e.g., mother's age), and of the families to which they belong (e.g., presence or absence of affected relatives). Instead, the focus is on relationships between risk factors and five malformations—Down syndrome, cleft lip, NTDs, clubfoot, and hip dislocation. These examples have been selected because studies of their risk factors have facilitated screening and/or seem to shed light on their etiology.

Down Syndrome

Down syndrome differs in two major respects from the other four malformations listed. First, it arises in most cases from a preconceptional error (the presence of an extra autosome 21 in one gamete), whereas the laying down of the other malformations cannot be traced back before embryogenesis. Second, although it has well-established links with relatively few risk factors, these factors include two—older maternal age and a history of the syndrome in one of certain categories of relatives—with which it is associated much more strongly than the other four malformations are with their risk factors. It is because of the strength of these associations that diagnostic tests for Down syndrome are widely offered to older pregnant women and to those with certain family histories.

Over most of the maternal age range the birth prevalence of Down syndrome exhibits an exponential increase, starting from a baseline value of about 0.63 per 1000, rather than from 0 (Figure 4.4). This has led to the suggestion that affected individuals fall into two classes of similar size, one with a birth prevalence unrelated to mother's age and one in which prevalence increases exponentially. One model of how an exponential increase might arise is that each oocyte is at risk of experiencing deleterious random events of some kind throughout a period lasting from early in the mother's life until the oocyte becomes an ovum, and nondisjunction of the two number 21 autosomes is the outcome for oocytes that have experienced a large number of these random events (Smith & Berg, 1976).

Among the types of Down syndrome that can be distinguished by the cytogeneticist, the small group with translocations seems to be largely independent of maternal age (Wright et al., 1967). Conversely, among cases of regular trisomy, those in which nondisjunction occurs during the first meiotic division of the oocyte are the most likely on theoretical grounds to be maternal age-related, since each oocyte remains in an early stage of the first meiotic division from before the woman's birth until shortly before becoming an ovum—the period during which maternal age-related damage is envisaged as accumulating. It would not be surprising if cases due to nondisjunction in the second meiotic division of the oocyte were also maternal age-related. However, the prevalence of cases

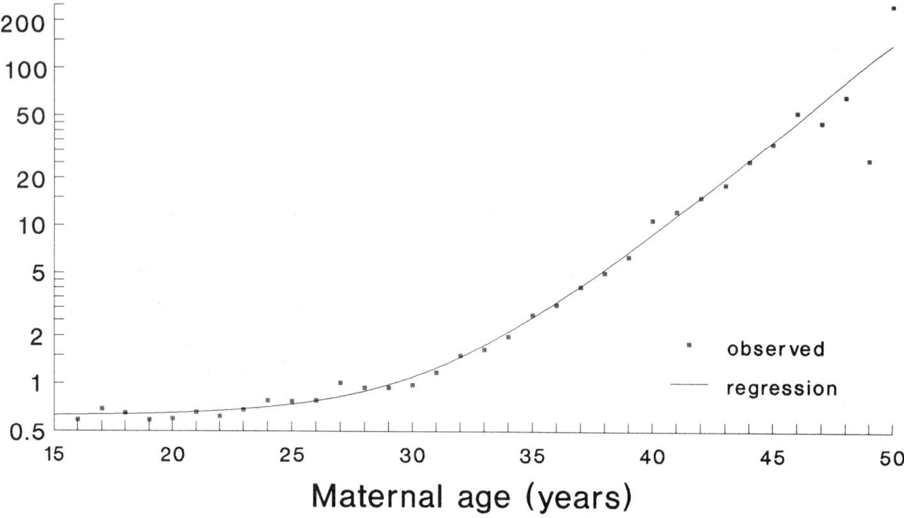

Fig. 4.4. Prevalence of Down syndrome per 1000 live births at each year of maternal age according to eight series (including a total of 4528 cases) pooled by Cuckle et al. (1987). The continuous line shows the prevalence (y) at each maternal age (x) predicted by the equation:

$$y = 0.000627 + e^{-16.2395 + 0.286x}$$

due to nondisjunction during spermatogenesis (i.e., those of paternal origin) would be expected to be independent of both parents' ages, because there seems to be no association between father's age and the risk of Down syndrome beyond what can be explained by the correlation between fathers' and mothers' ages (Cross & Hook, 1987; Ferguson-Smith & Yates, 1984). Nevertheless, when cases were divided into those that appeared from chromosomal banding analysis to be of maternal and paternal origin, those classified as of paternal origin were found to be almost as strongly maternal age-related as were those of maternal origin (Stein et al., 1986).

This similarity between maternal and paternal cases led these investigators to reason that the maternal age effect must arise after conception (when these two groups of cases are exposed to the same environment), rather than before. They therefore suggested that early prenatal mortality, rather than the risk of nondisjunction, was affected by maternal age. However, any variation in prenatal mortality with maternal age might be expected to affect cases in which the source of the extra chromosome is a lifelong abnormality in one parent's karyotype (regular or mosaic 21-trisomy or a 21-translocation), as well as those due to new mutations. In fact, the inherited cases show little variation in prevalence with maternal age (Hook, 1983; Peters et al., 1987). Also, recent studies using DNA analysis cast doubt on the accuracy with which the cases analyzed by Stein et al. (1986) were classified as to parental origin. It seems that many cases classified as paternal in chromosomal banding studies may, in reality, have been maternal (Antonarakis and Down Syndrome Collaborative Group, 1991; Sherman et al., 1991).

Cumulative damage to the oocyte and variations in prenatal mortality are not the only explanations put forward for the relationship of Down syndrome to maternal age. Another suggestion often made is that delayed fertilization (which declining coital frequency might render more common with advancing age) predisposes to chromosomal damage. A recent advocate of this suggestion is Sharav (1991), who reported that Down syndrome appeared to be relatively common among births to religious Jews and hinted that this might be because they restrict coitus to the latter part of the menstrual cycle. As evidence *against* a role for delayed fertilization in the causation of Down syndrome, Lilienfeld and Benesch (1969) and Sever et al. (1970) reported that neither acts of coitus nor pregnancies seemed to be separated by longer intervals for mothers of affected individuals than for controls. The most widely accepted explanation for the maternal age effect is still the view that older mothers' oocytes are more likely to suffer nondisjunction because they have been exposed to potential damage for a longer time before ovulation.

The second risk factor for Down syndrome is a family history of the disorder. Here, a distinction may be made between children whose parents or monozygotic twins have abnormal karyotypes and other relatives of affected individuals. In the first, relatively small group, genetic theory predicts that if affected gametes and zygotes with an extra autosome 21 were of normal viability the risks would be high: one third if a parent had a balanced translocation involving an autosome 21 and another type of chromosome, one half if a parent was affected by Down syndrome, and nearly 100% if a parent had a balanced 21:21 translocation or if a monozygotic twin of the child was affected. In practice, the predictions for monozygotic twins of cases and for children of parents with 21:21 translocations are fulfilled, but Down syndrome only occurs in about two fifths of the children of women with Down syndrome and in 10% to 15% and 2% to 3% of children whose mothers and fathers, respectively, have translocations between an autosome 21 and a chromosome of another type (Boué & Gallano, 1984; de Wolff et al., 1962; Frias, 1975; Gorlin, 1977; Stein et al., 1975). One reason for these figures being lower than predicted is presumably that affected concepti are at increased risk of prenatal death. The particularly low risk for children of fathers affected by translocations suggests that selection against male gametes with translocations also occurs.

The risks to children with a family history of Down syndrome but no affected parent or monozygotic twin cannot be predicted from genetic theory. The available data are consistent with the view that the risk of chromosomal anomaly is higher than normal (perhaps by about 1 per 100 births) in infants whose mothers have already borne children with Down syndrome, that this absolute excess does not increase with maternal age, and that those affected include almost equal numbers with Down syndrome and other chromosomal anomalies (Stene et al., 1984).

Another probable risk factor for Down syndrome is maleness. Excesses of males have been reported in many series of cases. The early reports of this kind were based mainly on cases ascertained a considerable time after birth, and the reason why males predominated among these cases was thought by some to be that early mortality was higher among females (Hay, 1971; Record & Smith, 1955). However, Down syndrome has also been found to be more common in males than females (by about 20%) in recent studies based on much more complete ascertainment, e.g., those of Iselius and Lindsten (1986) and Staples et al. (1991).

Cleft Lip and NTDs

A comparison of these conditions illustrates how epidemiologic studies can clarify the relative importance of genotype and environment in the etiology of birth defects. It has already been noted that differences between primary racial groups that invite a genetic explanation predominate in the pattern for cleft lip (with or without cleft palate), whereas the pattern for NTDs includes variations between racially similar populations in different places. These findings suggest that the latter pattern is influenced by environmental factors. That NTDs exhibit marked trends over time (both seasonal and secular) has also been shown earlier. This is further evidence that environmental factors have a role in their etiology that cannot be matched for cleft lip. Further clues to the etiology of NTDs and cleft lip have been sought by studying their relationship to family history, gender, maternal age, family size, and socio-economic status (SES). Associations with family size and SES are those most likely to point to the involvement of environmental factors in etiology. Associations with maternal age are more equivocal, since they may be caused by the effects of advancing age either on the intrauterine environment or on the frequency of genic or chromosomal mutation.

Except where stated, NTDs are treated as a single category in this section, because they have two features in common that suggest that they are etiologically similar: incomplete formation of the neural tube as their origin and a tendency to occur in the same groups of people, e.g., the same families, the same birth cohorts, and members of the same sex.

Cleft lip and NTDs show rather similar family patterns, with recurrence risks that amount to a few percent for infants with one affected sibling and that increase with the number of affected family members. The proportions affected by cleft lip among the monozygotic twins and first-, second-, and third-degree relatives of subjects with this defect are about 40%, 4%, 0.7%, and 0.25%, respectively, in Caucasoid populations (Carter, 1976). In Japan the recurrence risk of cleft lip seems to be lower than in Caucasoids—about 2% in first-degree relatives (Koguchi, 1975)—although the overall prevalence is higher (Table 4.1). None of these familial figures applies to cases' parents or grandparents, since relatively few malformed people reproduce.

For NTDs, reliable figures on the risks to second- and third-degree relatives are not available. The risk to first-degree relatives (confined to siblings in most series) tends to vary directly with population prevalence. It ranged from 1.3% in the Jewish population of Israel to 8.9% in Belfast, Northern Ireland, when the risks for all births in these populations were 1.4 and 8.7 per 1000, respectively (Naggan, 1971; Nevin & Johnston, 1980). The risk to monozygotic twins was estimated to be 20% in a group of populations in which the weighted mean prevalence of NTDs was 2.8 per 1000 (Leck, 1983a).

These trends are largely what would be expected if liability to each of these defects was determined by multiple genetic and environmental factors and if each defect occurred in individuals whose liability to it exceeded a threshold—the "multifactorial threshold model" (Carter, 1976). However, complex segregation analyses of several series (e.g., Chung et al., 1986; Marazita et al., 1986; Yang et al., 1991) suggest that the multifactorial threshold model on its own does not fit the distribution of cleft lip in Caucasoid families and that this pattern is more consistent with the hypothesis that at least some cases are due to a major gene with low penetrance. However, some of these analyses suggest that a multifactorial threshold effect also operates. Similar conclusions were drawn for a Chinese series of cleft lip cases (Marazita et al., 1991), although the multifactorial threshold hypothesis on its own fitted Japanese data (Chung et al., 1986).

The results of segregation analyses of NTD families also vary according to country. British data have been interpreted as being equally consistent with single gene and multifactorial models (Lalouel et al., 1979) and as favoring a mixture of both these effects (Shaffer et al., 1990). A single gene effect was supported by studies in Poland (Pietrzyk, 1980) and France (Demenais et al., 1982), although the results of the latter were also compatible with the hypothesis that cases cluster in families because of environmental factors that these families share.

Before leaving family studies, it should be recalled that many embryos affected by cleft lip and NTDs are lost by miscarriage (Fig. 4.3). It follows that these defects may arise much more commonly in the relatives of cases than the above birth prevalence figures suggest. Hypotheses based on these figures should therefore be treated with caution.

The birth prevalence of cleft lip varies with gender and shows an upward trend at high maternal ages. Generally the same is true of NTDs, although these defects affect more females than males, whereas cleft lip affects more males. In localities where the birth prevalence of NTDs is low, the increase in NTD prevalence with maternal age is sometimes absent, and the female excess among anencephalics (although not among cases of spina bifida) tends to be substantially less than where prevalence is high (Borman et al., 1986; Leck, 1977).

Family size and SES seem to differ from family history, gender, and maternal age in having little or no influence on the birth prevalence of cleft lip. NTDs, on the other hand, have been found in many British and North American studies to vary substantially in prevalence with these two attributes. The main variations are an increase as one passes from the more to the less socioeconomically privileged families and a birth rank trend that commonly has two components—a decrease between first-born and second-born infants and an increase with birth rank thereafter (Leck, 1983b). In low risk areas, however, prevalence often increases monotonically with birth rank and may sometimes be unrelated to SES (Borman et al., 1986; Bower et al., 1984; Leck, 1983b; Strassburg et al., 1983). There is evidence that the increase at high birth ranks occurs because the risk of NTD is elevated in births to women whose ultimate number of pregnancies will be high (women who inevitably account for larger proportions of births at higher parities than at lower) and that the average individual woman's chance of bearing an affected child lessens in each successive pregnancy even beyond the second (Elwood & Elwood, 1980).

This evidence linking NTDs but not cleft lip to family size and SES, like the studies relating prevalence to time, place, and ethnic group reviewed earlier, suggests that environmental factors are of greater etiologic importance in NTDs than in cleft lip. It has also been argued that environmental influences (including a cause of anencephaly to which females are more susceptible than males) may play a smaller role in the etiology of NTDs in low prevalence populations than they do where prevalence is high (Borman et al., 1986). The basis of this argument is the evidence that several risk factors for NTDs—conception in spring, high maternal age, primiparity, low socioeconomic status, and (in relation to anencephaly) femaleness—operate weakly or not at all in populations where birth prevalence is particularly low.

One group of environmental influences that has received special attention in the search for causes of NTDs is nutritional deficiencies. Prominent among the reasons for attention being focused in this way were two of the above findings: that the risk factors for NTDs included both low SES and conception in spring (when the body's reserves of some nutrients may be lowered). Other considerations were the occurrence of anomalies including NTDs in human fetuses whose mothers had taken a folic acid antagonist (Thiersch, 1952, 1956) and in the offspring of laboratory animals subjected to various vitamin deficiencies by Hale (1935), Warkany (1947), Giroud (1955) and their successors. Following on from this work, Hibbard and Smithells (1965) observed that at around the time of delivery the mothers of infants with malformations of the CNS were many times more likely than other mothers to be positive to the formiminoglutamic acid excretion test for folate deficiency. In addition, Smithells, Sheppard, and Schorah (1976) found when they tested maternal blood vitamin levels in early pregnancy that the mean levels of erythrocyte folate and leukocyte ascorbic acid were only about two thirds as high in pregnancies where the fetus had an NTD as in other pregnancies.

These findings have encouraged many more observational studies and some interventions in which hypotheses linking NTDs to vitamin deficiency in general and folate deficiency in particular have been tested. Most of these inquiries have been reviewed by Leck (1993). The observational studies were concerned with a variety of exposure variables, including overall quality of the diet (Laurence et al., 1980, 1983), folate content of the diet as a whole (Bower & Stanley, 1989), intake of supplements containing folate (Bower & Stanley, 1992; Mills et al., 1989; Milunsky et al., 1989; Winship et al., 1984), and intake of vitamin supplements irrespective of whether they contained folate (Bower & Stanley, 1992; Mills et al., 1989; Milunsky et al., 1989; Mulinare et al., 1988). In most of these studies a reduced birth prevalence of NTDs was associated with the exposure variables considered. The association was stronger with intake of supplementary folate than with intake of all vitamin supplements in two of the three studies in which both were considered (Bower & Stanley, 1992; Milunsky et al., 1989). The third of these three studies (Mills et al., 1989) revealed no association with either of these factors; but this study was based on a low prevalence population, which suggests that environmental factors may play a relatively small part in etiology there. The association between NTDs and vitamin intake is discussed further in the final section of this chapter where interventions are reviewed.

Clubfoot and Hip Dislocation

These conditions provide examples of how epidemiologic findings can support theories about the mechanisms by which defects are produced. In established dislocation of the hip and nonpostural talipes equinovarus, the most severe forms of the two conditions, familial risks resembling those already described for cleft lip and NTDs have been reported (Leck, 1977). These risks can be interpreted as evidence of the involvement of multiple genetic and environmental factors in causation. Several epidemiologic observations suggest that clubfoot and hip dislocation may each occur when the relevant parts of the fetus or infant fail to proffer adequate resistance to the physical pressure on them and that resistance is affected particularly by the genotype and pressure by the environment (Figure 4.5).

In hip dislocation, the evidence linking the genotype to fetal resistance includes reports that not only cases but also their relatives are affected much more often than controls by shallowness of the acetabulum and a generalized laxity of connective tissue, both of which might be expected to render the hips more liable to dislocate (Czeizel et al., 1975; Wynne-Davies, 1970a and b). Apart from these two conditions, experimental work has suggested that there is a type of joint laxity to which the female genotype confers susceptibility. This, it was postulated, might be caused by relaxin secreted by the fetal uterus under the influence of maternal hormones (Wilkinson, 1963). If this happened, it would explain why hip dislocation is more common in females than males.

Connective tissue laxity of genetic origin has also been reported in about one sixth of children with talipes equinovarus or calcaneovalgus, and high ratios of female to male cases, perhaps attributable to hormone-induced joint laxity, occur in the less severe forms of clubfoot—talipes calcaneovalgus, metatarsus varus, and the "postural" type of talipes equinovarus (which may be self-correcting). However, nonpostural talipes equinovarus is more common in males (Leck, 1977).

Several circumstances that might be expected to involve increased pressure on the fetus seem to be associated with an above-average frequency both of hip dislocation and of clubfoot (at least in its less severe forms). They include primigravidity (in which the uterus is likely to be relatively "tight"), breech presentation, and oligohydramnios (Leck, 1977). Prolonged gestation, another possible source of increased pressure, is also associated with hip dislocation (Asher, 1986; Bower et al., 1987). The evidence that hip dislocation and clubfoot are most common in children born at around the coldest time of year (see above) may mean that wearing tight or heavy clothing during late pregnancy has a constricting effect.

Another possible explanation for the seasonal trend in hip dislocation is that it is in part a postnatal effect caused by the use in winter of tight or heavy bedclothes, which constrict young infants and, in particular, limit their hip flexion and abduction. Established hip dislocation also shows a pattern of variation

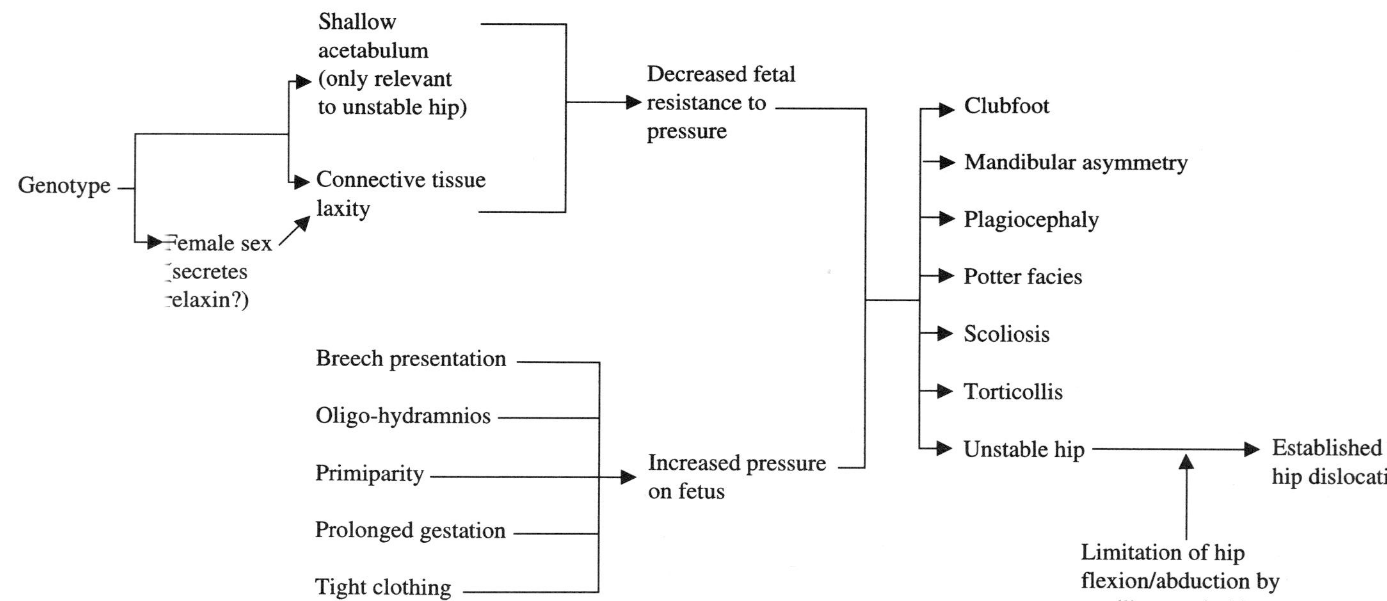

Fig. 4.5. Possible causes and consequences of imbalance between physical pressure upon the fetus/infant and its resistance to this pressure.

between different communities related to how babies are nursed. The condition is particularly common in cultures where infants are traditionally cradled with their hips extended and abducted, e.g., among the Lapps and various North American Indian tribes. Conversely, it is uncommon in societies where infants are characteristically nursed in a position of flexion and abduction (e.g., among Africans and Chinese) and in some although not all communities where screening and treatment of newborn infants for hip joint instability are practiced (Leck, 1986; Salter, 1968). All these practices may affect the frequency with which neonatal instability of the hip progresses to established dislocation.

As further evidence that both hip dislocation and clubfoot can result from imbalance between the physical forces to which the fetus or infant is exposed and the resistance it offers to these forces, defects of these types often occur in the same individuals, as do several deformities that seem likely to be caused by similar mechanisms—for example, mandibular asymmetry, plagiocephaly, Potter facies, postural scoliosis, and sternomastoid torticollis (Dunn, 1976).

Interventions

The interventions to reduce the impact of birth defects that have been carried out or recommended for use at a population level include rubella immunization (see Chapter 9) and vitamin supplementation to reduce incidence, antenatal screening to enable pregnancies complicated by major defects to be terminated (see Chapter 5), and neonatal screening to identify malformed infants who may benefit from treatment. Vitamin supplementation, antenatal screening for NTDs and Down syndrome, and neonatal screening for hip joint instability are considered here.

Vitamin Supplementation to Prevent NTDs

The link between vitamin supplementation and a reduced prevalence of NTDs, which was suggested by the observational studies mentioned earlier, has been further examined in several intervention studies.

Most of these studies explored whether women who had previously borne offspring with NTDs could reduce the risk of recurrences by improving their diet or taking vitamin supplements while trying to conceive and for 2 or 3 months after conception. In each of these studies, the intervention tested was associated with a reduction in the natural birth prevalence of NTDs. However, most of the studies are open to serious criticisms. In some, numbers were small and differences in outcome between the intervention group and the controls were not statistically significant (Laurence et al., 1980, 1981; Vergel et al., 1990), whereas in most of the larger series the pregnancies subjected to intervention and the control pregnancies differed in other respects that could have affected the outcome (Nevin & Seller, 1990; Smithells et al., 1981, 1983, 1989).

However, these criticisms do not apply to the most recently completed study of recurrence risks (MRC Vitamin Study Research Group, 1991). In this study, women with affected offspring who wished to conceive again were randomly allocated to receive daily tablets containing one of four formulations—folic acid (4 mg) and other vitamins, folic acid alone, other vitamins alone, or placebo—from the time of entry to the study until 12 weeks after onset of the LMP. In a series of nearly 1200 pregnancies the recurrence risk was 1.0% after taking folic acid and 3.5% after not doing so—a significant difference at the 1% level—whereas the taking of other vitamins was not significantly related to risk. This finding, and the earlier evidence that folic acid supplementation reduces the recurrence risk of NTDs in high-risk sibships, is enough to justify advising all women who have previously borne affected children to take folic acid periconceptionally, although some of the earlier studies (e.g., those of Smithells et al., 1981, 1983, 1989) suggest that the dose need not be as high as in the MRC Vitamin Study.

An intervention study of the effect of vitamin supplementation on the prevalence of NTDs and other defects in *firstborn* children has also been completed (Czeizel & Dudás, 1992). Women who wished to conceive for the first time were each randomly allocated to receive daily tablets containing one of two formulations—multiple vitamins (including folic acid, 0.8 mg) and essential metallic ions, or low doses of vitamin C and some of the metallic ions alone—from at least 1 month before conception until the date of the second missed menstrual period. NTDs occurred in none of about 2000 infants of women who were allocated the multivitamin preparation and in six (2.9 per 1000) of a similar number born after the other preparation had been allocated—a significant difference at the 5% level. Taken in conjunction with the observational study findings reviewed earlier, this finding suggests that it may not be only in high-risk families that folic acid protects against NTDs. However, this hypothesis needs to be tested further, and the mechanisms linking folic acid intake to NTD risk need to be explored at the molecular level.

Antenatal Screening for NTDs and Down Syndrome

For the sake of brevity, the comments on screening here and in the section on neonatal screening for hip instability that follows concentrate mainly on the accuracy of the tests. The main indices of accuracy considered are sensitivity (the proportion of cases of a condition in which screening is positive), specificity (the proportion of noncases in which screening is negative), and the predictive value of a positive result (the proportion of subjects with a positive test result who are cases, which is directly related to the frequency of the condition for which one is screening; see Chapter 1).

As with most well-developed screening programs, those for NTDs and Down syndrome involve screening tests for all who are eligible for screening and further diagnostic tests for those in whom the screening tests are positive. The most widely used laboratory-based screening test for NTDs is the measurement of maternal serum alphafetoprotein (MSAFP) at 16 to 18 weeks gestation. This test is commonly regarded as positive if it yields a figure at least 2.5 times the median for all pregnancies of the same gestation length. The diagnostic procedures mainly used in these circumstances are ultrasonography and (unless the scan clearly shows a NTD) amniocentesis with measurement of amniotic fluid alphafetoprotein (AFAFP). The latter is regarded as abnormal if it reaches a level of at least three times the median AFAFP value. In this case an acetylcholinesterase test may be done, and pregnancy termination is likely to be offered if this test too is positive.

This whole process has been estimated to detect 86% of anencephalics and 78% of cases of open spina bifida at the cost of causing death in between 0.1 per 1000 and 0.3 per 1000 normal fetuses (Wald & Cuckle, 1984). Almost all these deaths would be due to amniocentesis, which was assumed in calculating these figures to carry a 0.5% to 1.5% risk of miscarriage. Only in five per million normal subjects was it estimated that the MSAFP, AFAFP, and acetylcholinesterase tests would all be positive and termination be offered. It follows that the sensitivity of the whole process is 86% for anencephaly and 78% for open spina bifida, and the specificity (not counting cases of multiple pregnancy, incipient miscarriage, and exomphalos, in which the tests are often positive) is the difference between unity and 5 per 1,000,000—i.e., 99.9995%!

The screening test alone (MSAFP measurement) seems from the figures of Wald and Cuckle (1984) to have a sensitivity of 88% for anencephaly and 79% for open spina bifida, and a specificity of 96.7% in singleton pregnancies. In a community where the natural birth prevalence stood at 0.7 per 1000 for anencephaly and 0.6 per 1000 for open spina bifida (figures consistent with the most recent British experience, Figure 4.2), the above sensitivity and specificity estimates indicate that the predictive value of a positive MSAFP test result would be 3.2%. To obtain this proportion, the number of results in every thousand expected to be true positive $[(0.88\times0.7) + (0.79\times0.6)]$ was divided by the sum of this figure and the number expected to be false positive $[(1-0.967)(1000-0.7-0.6)]$. Among fetuses from a community like that described whose mothers were referred for diagnostic testing because of a positive screening test, the proportion found to have a NTD (3.2%) would thus be three times as great as the 1% in whom amniocentesis is reported to lead to miscarriage (Tabor et al., 1986). Many regard this as an acceptable balance of risks.

In screening for Down syndrome, maternal age has been used instead of a laboratory-based screening test to define a group of high-risk pregnancies—generally those in women aged 35 or older. The diagnostic test used in these pregnancies is to culture and karyotype fetal cells obtained by amniocentesis or chorionic villus sampling. The sensitivity and specificity of screening for Down syndrome by maternal age are variable. The higher the percentage of pregnant women above the cut-off point, the higher is the proportion of infants with Down syndrome who are born to these women (i.e., the sensitivity of screening by maternal age) and the lower is the proportion of normal infants born at younger maternal ages, i.e., the specificity. If pregnancies at maternal ages of 35 and over had been regarded as screen-positive in the population on which the figures for Birmingham, England in Table 4.1 are based, the sensitivity and specificity of the screen would have been 39% and 91%, respectively (Leck, 1993). These figures and the recorded prevalence of Down syndrome (1.4 per 1000) yield a proportion of 0.6% for the predictive value of a positive test. All these indices of the accuracy of a maternal age of 35 or older as a screen for Down syndrome compare unfavorably with the corresponding figures for an elevated MSAFP level as an initial screen for NTDs.

Numerous suggestions have recently been made for improving the accuracy of screening for Down syndrome by using various laboratory tests that tend to give higher or lower values than normal in pregnancies in which the fetus has Down syndrome, e.g., maternal serum concentrations of alphafetoprotein, unconjugated estriol, and human chorionic gonadotrophin (Wald et al., 1988). If the levels of such substances are measured in a pregnant woman, they can be used together with maternal age to predict the risk of her fetus having Down syndrome. Amniocentesis or chorionic villus sampling can then be offered if the risk exceeds a certain level. With this level set at 1:250, it was estimated that a sensitivity of 61% combined with a specificity of 95.0% could have been achieved if a combination of the above three laboratory tests and maternal age had been used to screen pregnancies in a British population where the natural birth prevalence of Down syndrome was 1.3 per 1000 (Wald et al., 1988). Given these figures, a positive result (i.e., a result implying a risk of 1:250 or more) would have a predictive value of 1.56%.

Although these figures compare favorably with those based on screening by maternal age alone, they imply that, among the women selected for diagnostic testing, the proportion in whom one would expect to find fetal Down syndrome (1.56%) would not be very different from the proportion in whom diagnostic testing would lead to miscarriage of a normal fetus—perhaps about 1% if the fetal cells for karyotyping were obtained by amniocentesis or transabdominal chorionic villus sampling and more if transcervical chorionic villus sampling was used (Smidt-Jensen et al., 1992). As with any screening test that is regarded as positive when a variable exceeds a threshold, the predictive value of a positive result could, of course, be increased by raising the level of risk that subjects must reach if they are to proceed to amniocentesis or chorionic villus sampling, but doing so would lower the sensitivity. For example, Wald et al. (1988) estimated that raising the threshold risk from 1:250 to 1:100 would increase the predictive value to 3.3%, but would decrease the sensitivity to 44%.

Neonatal Screening for Hip Joint Instability

The standard screening test for hip joint instability is the Ortolani-Barlow maneuver. For this test, the examiner holds each thigh of the neonate in midabduction and subjects it first to forward pressure on the greater trochanter and then to outward and backward pressure on the inner side. The test is regarded as positive if the femoral head is heard or felt to slip into the acetabulum when forward pressure is applied and/or to slip out of the acetabulum with backward pressure. The first of these two results should be obtained if the joint is dislocated but reducible, and the second if it is dislocatable.

When a positive result is obtained, it is not the usual procedure to carry out a diagnostic test in the same way that is done when screening for NTDs and Down syndrome. Instead, treatment by splinting to maintain the joint in a reduced position for several weeks or months is initiated, either in all those in whom the screening test is initially positive or at least in those in whom it remains positive for a few days or weeks.

In the absence of a diagnostic test, the accuracy of the Ortolani-Barlow maneuver as a means of detecting infants in whom established dislocation would arise if they were not splinted is best estimated from (1) the proportion of infants in whom this screening test is positive, (2) the proportion who pass the test but are later found to have established dislocation, and (3) the frequency of established dislocation in unscreened populations (probably about 1.25 per 1000 in populations of mainly northwestern European origin; Leck, 1986). In what is possibly the most carefully screened British population that has been reported, the test was positive in 19.35 per 1000 infants, and dislocation first presented late in 0.43 per 1000 (Dunn et al., 1985). This implies that the test results were truly positive in 0.82 (i.e., 1.25–0.43) per 1000, falsely positive in 18.53 (i.e., 19.35–0.82), falsely negative in 0.43, and truly negative in the remaining 980.22, i.e., 1000 - 0.82 - 18.53 - 0.43. It follows from these figures that in the hands of Dunn et al. (1985) the test had a sensitivity of 65.6% and a specificity of 98.1%, and the predictive value of a positive test was 4.2%.

In other hands, however, the test has yielded very different results. In the United Kingdom alone, the prevalence of positive test results has ranged from 1.6 per 1000 to 28.5 per 1000, and the proportion of infants in whom dislocation has first presented late has varied from 0.1 per 1000 to 1.3 per 1000 in populations described by different workers (Clarke et al., 1989; Finlay et al., 1967; Mackenzie & Wilson, 1981; Wilkinson, 1972).

These findings point to three limitations of the test. First, the variability of the prevalence of positive results suggests that observers differ in what they regard as a positive result, i.e., the test is not very reliable. Second, the occurrence of significant numbers of late cases in infants in whom the test has been negative indicates that cases are being missed by the test and/or arise later—the latter conceivably due in some instances to damage of the hip by the test itself (Moore, 1989; Sanfridson et al., 1991). Third, most of the infants who are splinted because the test is positive—an estimated 95.8% in the series of Dunn et al. (1985)—would not progress to established dislocation in the absence of treatment and may therefore be being treated unnecessarily. This last problem would of course be solved if infants in whom screening is positive could be subjected to a diagnostic test indicating whether their instability would progress to dislocation. A possible step in this direction is the introduction of ultrasonic examination of the hip in such cases (Gardiner & Dunn, 1990; Harcke & Kumar, 1991), but the impact of this test on the accuracy of screening has yet to be quantified.

Finally, it should be noted that some neonates who are splinted as a result of screening still need surgery later. For example, this was true of 0.22 per 1000 of the population covered by the above-quoted study of Dunn et al. (1985). This is a fairly typical figure (Leck, 1986) and suggests that splinting was not totally successful in about one quarter of the 0.82 per 1000 infants in this population in whom the screening test was estimated above to have been truly positive.

Conclusions

Structural birth defects in childhood remain one of the most tragic occurrences. It is perhaps because of this that so much epidemiologic research has concentrated on this problem. As is evident from the findings reviewed in this chapter, there is now an extensive body of knowledge that has illuminated many of the causes of these defects. More importantly, this knowledge has been applied in a number of promising modes of intervention. Given the continued interest in this fascinating area of study, it is likely that many more advances in understanding and control will occur in the near future.

References

Aarskog D. Maternal progestins as a possible cause of hypospadias. *N Engl J Med* 1979; 300:75.

Alzamora-Castro V, Battilana G, Abugattas R, et al. Patent ductus arteriosus and high altitude. *Am J Cardiol* 1960; 5:761.

Antonarakis SE, Down Syndrome Collaborative Group. Parental origin of the extra chromosome in trisomy 21 as indicated by analysis of DNA polymorphisms. *N Engl J Med* 1991; 324:872.

Artz TD, Levine DB, Wan Ngo Lim et al. Neonatal diagnosis, treatment and related factors of congenital dislocation of the hip. *Clin Orthop* 1975; 110:112.

Asher MA. Screening for congenital dislocation of the hip, scoliosis, and other abnormalities affecting the musculoskeletal system. *Pediat Clin N Am* 1986; 33:1335.

Baird PA. Incidence of hypospadias. *Lancet* 1985; 1:1162.

Baird PA, Sadovnick AD. Life expectancy in Down syndrome. *J Pediat* 1987; 110:849.

Bell JA. The epidemiology of Down's syndrome. *Med J Aust* 1991; 155:115.

Bell JA, Pearn JH, Firman D. Childhood deaths in Down's syndrome. Survival curves and causes of death from a total population study in Queensland, Australia, 1976 to 1985. *J Med Genet* 1989; 26:764.

Best JM. Congenital cytomegalovirus infection. *Br Med J* 1987; 294:1440.

Bjerkedal T, Bakketeig LS. Surveillance of congenital malformations and other conditions of the newborn. *Int J Epidemiol* 1975; 4:31.

Borman GB, Smith AH, Howard JK. Risk factors in the prevalence of anencephalus and spina bifida in New Zealand. *Teratology* 1986; 33:221.

Boué A, Gallano P. A collaborative study of the segregation of inherited chromosome structural rearrangements in 1356 prenatal diagnoses. *Prenat Diagn* 1984; 4 (special issue):45.

Bound JP, Harvey PW, Francis BJ. Seasonal prevalence of major congenital malformations in the Fylde of Lancashire 1957–1981. *J Epidemiol Comm Health* 1989; 43:330.

Bower C, Stanley FJ. Dietary folate as a risk factor for neural tube defects: evidence from a case-control study in Western Australia. *Med J Aust* 1989; 150:613.

Bower C, Stanley FJ. Periconceptional vitamin supplementation and neural tube defects; evidence from a case-control study in Western Australia and a review of current publications. *J Epidemiol Comm Health* 1992; 46:157.

Bower C, Hobbs M, Carney A, et al. Neural tube defects in Western Australia 1966–81 and a review of Australian data 1942–81. *J Epidemiol Comm Health* 1984; 38:208.

Bower C, Stanley FJ, Kricker A. Congenital dislocation of the hip in Western Australia: a comparison of neonatally and postneonatally diagnosed cases. *Clin Orthop Rel Res* 1987; 224:37.

Bundey S, Alam H, Kaur A, et al. Race, consanguinity and social features in Birmingham babies: a basis for a prospective study. *J Epidemiol Comm Health* 1990; 44:130.

Burgoyne PS, Holland K, Stephens R. Incidence of numerical chromosome anomalies in human pregnancy: estimation from induced and spontaneous abortion data. *Hum Reprod* 1991; 6:555.

Carter CO. Genetics of common single malformations. *Br Med Bull* 1976; 32:21.

Chávez GF, Mulinare J, Cordero JF. Maternal cocaine use during early pregnancy as a risk factor for congenital urogenital anomalies. *JAMA* 1989; 262:795.

Chen R, Weissman SL, Salama R, et al. Congenital dislocation of the hip (CDH) and seasonality: the gestational age of vulnerability to some seasonal factor. *Am J Epidemiol* 1970; 92:287.

Chinese Birth Defects Monitoring Program. Central nervous system congenital malformations, especially neural tube defects in 29 provinces, metropolitan cities and autonomous regions of China. *Int J Epidemiol* 1990; 19, 978.

Chung CS, Kau MC. Racial differences in cephalometric measurements and incidence of cleft lip with or without cleft palate. *J Craniofac Genet Dev Biol* 1985; 5:341.

Chung CS, Bixler D, Watanabe T, et al. Segregation analysis of cleft lip with or without cleft palate: a comparison of Danish and Japanese data. *Am J Hum Genet* 1986; 39:603.

Clarke NMP, Clegg J, Al-Chalabi AN. Ultrasound screening of hips at risk for CDH: failure to reduce the incidence of late cases. *J Bone Joint Surg* 1989; 71B:9.

Clarren SK, Smith DW. The fetal alcohol syndrome. *N Engl J Med* 1978; 298:1063.

Cohlan SQ. Tetracycline staining of teeth. *Teratology* 1977; 15:127.

Creasy MR, Crolla JA, Alberman ED. A cytogenetic study of spontaneous abortions using banding techniques. *Hum Genet* 1976; 31:177.

Cross PK, Hook EB. An analysis of paternal age and 47, +21 in 35,000 new prenatal cytogenetic diagnosis data from the New York State Chromosome Registry: no significant effect. *Hum Genet* 1987; 77:307.

Cuckle HS, Wald N. The impact of screening for open neural tube defects in England and Wales. *Prenat Diagn* 1987; 7:91.

Cuckle, HS, Wald NJ, Thompson SG. Estimating a woman's risk of having a pregnancy associated with Down's syndrome using her age and serum alpha-fetoprotein level. *Br J Obstet Gynaecol* 1987; 94:387.

Cuckle HS, Wald NJ, Cuckle PM. Prenatal screening and diagnosis of neural tube defects in England and Wales in 1985. *Prenat Diagn* 1989; 9:393.

Czeizel AE. Increasing trends in congenital malformations of male external genitalia. *Lancet* 1985; 2:462.

Czeizel AE, Révész C. Major malformations of the central nervous system in Hungary. *Br J Prev Soc Med* 1970; 24:205.

Czeizel AE, Dudás I. Prevention of the first occurrence of neural-tube defects by periconceptional vitamin supplementation. *N Engl J Med* 1992; 327:1832.

Czeizel AE, Tusnády G, Vaczó G, et al. The mechanism of genetic predisposition to congenital dislocation of hip. *J Med Genet* 1975; 12:121.

Dawes GS. Changes in the circulation at birth. *Br Med Bull* 1961; 17:148.

Demenais F, Le Merrer M, Briard ML, et al. Neural tube defects in France: segregation analysis. *Am J Med Genet* 1982; 11:287.

Depue RH. Maternal and gestational factors affecting the risk of cryptorchidism and inguinal hernia. *Int J Epidemiol* 1984; 13:311.

Desmonts G, Couvreur J. Congenital toxoplasmosis: a prospective study of 542 women who aquired (sic) toxoplasmosis during pregnancy. Pathophysiology of congenital disease. In: Thalhammer O, Baumgarten K, Pollak A, eds. *Perinatal Medicine: Sixth European Conference, Vienna 1978.* Stuttgart: Thieme; 1979:51.

de Wolff E, Schärer K, Lejeune J. Contribution à l'etude des jumeaux mongoliens. Un cas de monozygotisme hétérocaryote. *Helv Paediat Acta* 1962; 17:301.

Division of Birth Defects and Developmental Disabilities. *Communication to Neural Tube Defects Etiology Research Conference, Wilmington, Delaware.* 1989.

Dolk H, Bertrand F, Lechat MF. Chorionic villus sampling and limb abnormalities. *Lancet* 1992; 339:876.

Dunn PM. Congenital postural deformities. *Br Med Bull* 1976; 32:71.

Dunn PM, Evans RE, Thearle MJ, et al. Congenital dislocation of the hip: early and late diagnosis and management compared. *Arch Dis Child* 1985; 60:407.

Elwood JM, Elwood JH. *Epidemiology of Anencephalus and Spina Bifida.* Oxford: Oxford University Press; 1980.

Erickson JD. Racial variations in the incidence of congenital malformations. *Ann Hum Genet* 1976; 39:315.

EUROCAT Working Group. *EUROCAT Report 4: Surveillance of Congenital Anomalies 1980–1988.* Brussels: EUROCAT Central Registry; 1991.

Finlay HVL, Maudsley RH, Busfield PI. Dislocatable hip and dislocated hip in the newborn infant. *Br Med J* 1967; 4:377.

Fogh-Andersen P. *Inheritance of Harelip and Cleft Palate.* Copenhagen: Busck; 1942.

Fraser FC, Frecker M, Allderdice P. Seasonal variation of neural tube defects in Newfoundland and elsewhere. *Teratology* 1986; 33:299.

Frias JL. Prenatal diagnosis of genetic abnormalities. *Clin Obstet Gynecol* 1975; 18:221.

Fryers T, Mackay RI. Down syndrome: prevalence at birth, mortality and survival. A 17-year study. *Early Hum Dev* 1979; 3:29.

Furguson-Smith MA, Yates JRW. Maternal age specific rates for chromosomal aberrations and factors influencing them: report of a collaborative study of 52965 amniocenteses. *Prenat Diagn* 1984; 4 (special issue):5.

Gardiner HM, Dunn PM. Controlled trial of immediate splinting versus ultrasonographic surveillance in congenitally dislocatable hips. *Lancet* 1990; 336:1553.

General Register Office. *Registrar General's Annual Review of England and Wales, Part 1, 1967* and *1968.* London: Her Majesty's Stationery Office; 1968, 1970.

Giroud A. Les malformations congénitales et leur causes. *Biol Méd* 1955; 44:1.

Gorlin RJ. Classical chromosomal disorders. In: Yunis JJ, ed. *New Chromosomal Syndromes.* London: Academic Press; 1977:59.

Grant GA, McAleer JJA. Incidence of infantile hypertrophic pyloric stenosis. *Lancet* 1984; 1:1177.

Gregg N McA. Congenital cataract following German measles in the mother. *Trans Ophthal Soc Aust* 1941; 3:35.

Griffiths PD, Baboonian C, Rutter D, et al. Congenital and maternal cytomegalovirus infections in a London population. *Br J Obstet Gynaecol* 1991; 98:135.

Hale F. The relation of vitamin A to anophthalmos in pigs. *Am J Ophthalmol* 1935; 18:1087.

Hall SM. Congenital toxoplasmosis. *Br Med J* 1992; 305:291.

Harcke HT, Kumar SJ. The role of ultrasound in the diagnosis and management of congenital dislocation and dysplasia of the hip. *J Bone Joint Surg* 1991; 73A:622.

Hartsfield JK, Hudson TC. Meta-analysis in clinical teratology: maternal cigarette smoking and oral clefting. *Teratology* 1991; 43:471.

Hassold TJ, Matsuyama A, Newlands IM, et al. A cytogenetic study of spontaneous abortions in Hawaii. *Ann Hum Genet* Lond 1978; 41:443.

Hassold TJ, Chen N, Funkhouser J, et al. A cytogenetic study of 1000 spontaneous abortions. *Ann Hum Genet* (Lond) 1980; 44:151.

Hay S. Sex differences in the incidence of certain congenital malformations: a review of the literature and some new data. *Teratology* 1971; 4:277.

Heinonen OP, Slone D, Shapiro S. *Birth Defects and Drugs in Pregnancy*, Littleton, MA: Publishing Sciences Group; 1977.

Herbst AL, Ulfelder H, Poskanzer DC. Adenocarcinoma of the vagina: association of maternal stilbestrol therapy with tumor appearance in young women. *N Engl J Med* 1971; 284:878.

Hertig AT, Rock J, Adams EC. Description of 34 human ova within first 17 days of development. *Am J Anat* 1956; 98:435.

Hibbard ED, Smithells RW. Folic acid metabolism and human embryopathy. *Lancet* 1965; 1:1254.

Hook EB. Down syndrome rates and relaxed selection at older maternal ages. *Am J Hum Genet* 1983; 35:1307.

Ingall D, Dobson SRM, Musher D. Syphilis. In: Remington JS, Klein JO, eds. *Infectious Diseases of the Fetus and Newborn Infant*. 3rd ed. Philadelphia: WB Saunders; 1990:367.

Iselius L, Lindsten J. Changes in the incidence of Down syndrome in Sweden during 1968–1982. *Hum Genet* 1986; 72:133.

Jacobson SL, Jones K, Johnson K, et al. Prospective multicentre study of pregnancy outcome after lithium exposure during first trimester. *Lancet* 1992; 339:530.

Janz D. On major malformations and minor anomalies in the offspring of parents with epilepsy: review of the literature. In: Janz D, Dam M, Richens A, et al., eds, *Epilepsy, Pregnancy, and the Child*. New York: Raven Press; 1982:211.

Jedd MB, Melton LJ, Griffin MR, et al. Trends in infantile hypertrophic pyloric stenosis in Olmsted County, Minnesota, 1950–84. *Paediat Perinat Epidemiol* 1988; 2:148.

Jorde LB, Fineman RM, Martin RA. Epidemiology of neural tube defects in Utah, 1940–1979. *Am J Epidemiol* 1984; 119:487.

Källén B, Tandberg A. Lithium in pregnancy: a cohort study on manic-depressive women. *Acta Psychiat Scand* 1983; 68:134.

Källén B, Winberg J. An epidemiological study of hypospadias in Sweden. *Acta Paediat Scand* 1982; 293 (suppl).

Kalousek K, Barrett IJ, Gärtner AB. Spontaneous abortion and confined chromosomal mosaicism. *Human Genet* 1992; 88:642.

Kalter H. Five-decade international trends in the relation of perinatal mortality and congenital malformations: stillbirth and neonatal death compared. *Int J Epidemiol* 1991; 20:173.

Kalter H, Warkany J. Congenital malformations: etiologic factors and their role in prevention. *N Engl J Med* 1983; 308:424 (Part 1) and 491 (Part 2).

Kenna AP, Smithells RW, Fielding DW. Congenital heart disease in Liverpool: 1960–69. *Q J Med* 1975; 44:17.

Khoury MJ, Erickson JD, James LM. Etiologic heterogeneity of neural tube defects: clues from epidemiology. *Am J Epidemiol* 1982; 115:538.

Knox EG, Lancashire RJ. *Epidemiology of Congenital Malformations*. London: Her Majesty's Stationery Office; 1991.

Knox EG, Armstrong E, Haynes R. Changing incidence of infantile hypertrophic pyloric stenosis. *Arch Dis Child* 1983; 58:582.

Koguchi H. Recurrence rate in offspring and siblings of patients with cleft lip and/or cleft palate. *Jpn J Hum Genet* 1975; 20:207.

Lalouel JM, Morton NE, Jackson J. Neural tube malformations: complex segregation analysis and calculation of recurrence risks. *J Med Genet* 1979; 16:8.

Lammer EJ, Sever LE, Oakley GP. Teratogen update: valproic acid. *Teratology* 1987; 35:465.

Lammer EJ, Hayes AM, Schunior A, et al. Unusually high risk for adverse outcomes of pregnancy following fetal isotretinoin exposure. *Am J Hum Genet* 1988; 43:A58.

Lancaster PAL. Congenital malformations after assisted conception. *Teratology* 1991; 44:477.

Laurence KM, James N, Miller M, et al. Increased risk of recurrence of pregnancies complicated by fetal neural tube defects in mothers receiving poor diets, and possible benefit of dietary counselling. *Br Med J* 1980; 281:1592.

Laurence KM, James N, Miller MH, et al. Double-blind randomised controlled trial of folate treatment before conception to prevent recurrence of neural-tube defects. *Br Med J* 1981; 282:1509.

Laurence KM, Campbell H, James NE. The role of improvement in the maternal diet and preconceptional folic acid supplementation in the prevention of neural tube defects. In: Dobbing J, ed. *Prevention of Spina Bifida and Other Neural Tube Defects*. London: Academic Press; 1983:85.

Leck I. Correlations of malformation frequency with environmental and genetic attributes in man. In: Wilson JG, Fraser FC, eds. *Handbook of Teratology*. Vol. 3. New York: Plenum; 1977:243.

Leck I. Fetal malformations. In: Barron SL, Thomson AM, eds. *Obstetrical Epidemiology*. London: Academic Press; 1983a:263.

Leck I. Epidemiological clues to the causation of neural tube defects. In: Dobbing J, ed. *Prevention of Spina Bifida and Other Neural Tube Defects*. London: Academic Press; 1983b:155.

Leck I. The geographical distribution of neural tube defects and oral clefts. *Br Med Bull* 1984; 40:390.

Leck I. An epidemiological assessment of neonatal screening for dislocation of the hip. *J Roy Coll Phys Lond*. 1986; 20:56.

Leck I. The contribution of epidemiologic studies. In: Stevenson RE, Hall JG, Goodman R, eds. *Human Malformations*. New York: Oxford University Press; 1993.

Leck I, Record RG, McKeown T, et al. The incidence of malformations in Birmingham, England, 1950–59. *Teratology* 1968; 1:263.

Lenz W. Kindliche Missbildungen nach Medikament-Einnahme während der Gravidität? *Dtsch Med Wschr* 1961; 86:2555.

Lian Z-H, Yang H-Y, Li Z. Neural tube defects in Beijing-Tianjin area of China: urban-rural distribution and some other epidemiological characteristics. *J Epidemiol Comm Health* 1987; 41:259.

Lilienfeld AM, Benesch CH. *Epidemiology of Mongolism*. Baltimore: Johns Hopkins Press; 1969.

Lipson A, Beuhler B, Bartley J, et al. Maternal hyperphenylalaninemia fetal effects. *J Pediat* 1984; 104:216.

Little J, Nicoll A. The epidemiology and service implications of congenital and constitutional anomalies in ethnic minorities in the United Kingdom. *Paediat Perinat Epidemiol* 1988; 2:161.

Lorber J. Early results of selective treatment of spina bifida cystica. *Br Med J* 1973; 4:201.

Lowry RB, Trimble BK. Incidence rates for cleft lip and palate in British Columbia 1952–71 for North American Indian, Japanese, Chinese and total populations: secular trends over twenty years. *Teratology* 1977, 16.277.

Lutiger B, Graham K, Einarson TR, et al. Relationship between gestational cocaine use and pregnancy outcome: a meta-analysis. *Teratology* 1991; 44:405.

Lynberg MC, McClearn AB, Edmonds LD, et al. Mortality among infants with birth defects, Metropolitan Atlanta, 1983–1989. *Am J Epidemiol* 1991; 134:776.

MacHenry JCRM, Nevin NC, Merrett JD. Comparison of central nervous system malformations in spontaneous abortions in Northern Ireland and south-east England. *Br Med J* 1979; 1:1395.

Mackenzie IG, Wilson JG. Problems encountered in the early diagnosis and management of congenital dislocation of the hip. *J Bone Joint Surg* 1981; 63B:38.

Maclean MH, MacLeod A. Seasonal variation in the frequency of anencephalus and spina bifida births in the United Kingdom. *J Epidemiol Comm Health* 1984; 38:99.

Marazita ML, Goldstein AM, Smalley SL, et al. Cleft lip with or without cleft palate: reanalysis of a three-generation family study from England. *Genet Epidemiol* 1986; 3:335.

Marazita ML, Hu DN, Spence MA, et al. Genetic analysis of cleft lip with or without cleft palate in Shanghai, China. *Am J Hum Genet* 1991; 49 (suppl):475.

Matlai P, Beral V. Trends in congenital malformations of external genitalia. *Lancet* 1985; 1:108.

McFadden DE, Kallousek DK. Survey of neural tube defects in spontaneously aborted embryos. *Am J Med Genet* 1989; 32:356.

Menser MA, Forrest JM, Bransby RD. Rubella infection and diabetes mellitus. *Lancet* 1978; 1:57.

Menser MA, Hudson JR, Murphy AM, et al. Impact of rubella vaccination in Australia. *Lancet* 1984; 1:1059.

Miao C-Y, Li W-X, Geng D, et al. Effect of high altitude on prevalence of congenital heart disease. *Chinese Med J* 1988; 101:415.

Milham S. Scalp defects in infants of mothers treated for hyperthyroidism with methimazole or carbimazole during pregnancy. *Teratology* 1986; 32:321.

Miller E, Cradock-Watson JE, Pollock TM. Consequences of confirmed maternal rubella at successive stages of pregnancy. *Lancet* 1982; 2:781.

Miller RW. Cola-colored babies: chlorobiphenyl poisoning in Japan. *Teratology* 1971; 4:212.

Mills JL, Rhoads GG, Simpson JL, et al. The absence of a relation between the periconceptional use of vitamins and neural-tube defects. *N Engl J Med* 1989; 321:430.

Milunsky A, Jick H, Jick SS, et al. Multivitamin/folic acid supplementation in early pregnancy reduces the prevalence of neural tube defects. *JAMA* 1989; 262:2847.

Milunsky A, Ulcickas ME, Willett W, et al. Hyperthermia and neural tube defects. *Pediat Res* 1991; 29:71A.

Moore FH. Examining infants' hips—can it do harm? *J Bone Joint Surg* 1989; 71B:4.

Moss AJ, Emmanouilides GC, Adams FH, et al. Response of ductus arteriosus and pulmonary and systemic arterial pressure to changes in oxygen environment in newborn infants. *Pediatrics* 1964; 33:937.

MRC Vitamin Study Research Group. Prevention of neural tube defects: results of the Medical Research Council Vitamin Study. *Lancet* 1991; 338:131.

Mulinare J, Cordero JF, Erickson JD, et al. Periconceptional use of multivitamins and the occurrence of anencephaly and spina bifida. *JAMA* 1988; 260:3141.

Naggan L. Anencephaly and spina bifida in Israel. *Pediatrics* 1971; 47:577.

Nakane Y, Okuma T, Takahashi R, et al. Multi-institutional study on the teratogenicity and fetal toxicity of antiepileptic drugs: a report of a collaborative study group in Japan. *Epilepsia* 1980; 21:663.

Neel JV. A study of major congenital defects in Japanese infants. *Am J Hum Genet* 1958; 10:398.

Nelson K, Holmes LB. Malformations due to presumed spontaneous mutations in newborn infants. *N Engl J Med* 1989; 320:19.

Nevin NC, Johnston WP. A family study of spina bifida and anencephalus in Belfast, Northern Ireland (1964 to 1968). *J Med Genet* 1980; 17:203.

Nevin NC, Seller MJ. Prevention of neural-tube-defect recurrences. *Lancet* 1990; 335:178.

Nishimura H. Incidence of malformations in abortions. In: Fraser FC, McKusick VA, eds. *Congenital Malformations: Proceedings of the Third International Conference (International Congress Series No 204)*. Amsterdam: Excerpta Medica; 1970:275.

Niswander JD, Adams MS. Oral clefts in the American Indian. *US Publ Health Rep* 1967; 82:807.

Office of Population Censuses and Surveys. *Registrar General's Annual Review of England and Wales, Part I, 1969* to *1973; Mortality Statistics: Childhood, 1974* to *1990: Series DH3, nos. 1–6, 8, 10–12, 16*, and *19*, and *Series DH6, nos. 1–4*. London: Her Majesty's Stationery Office; 1971–92a.

Office of Population Censuses and Surveys. *Congenital Malformations Statistics: Notifications, 1971–80* to *1990: Series MB3, nos. 1–6*. London: Her Majesty's Stationery Office; 1983–92b.

Office of Population Censuses and Surveys. *Abortion Statistics: Legal Abortions Carried Out Under the Abortion Act in England and Wales, 1986* to *1990: Series AB, nos. 13–17*. London: Her Majesty's Stationery Office; 1987–91.

Orme ML'E. The Debendox saga. *Br Med J* 1985; 291:918.

Peckham CS, Tookey P, Nelson DB, et al. Ethnic minority women and congenital rubella. *Br Med J* 1983; 287:129.

Peñaloza D, Arias-Stella J, Sime F, et al. The heart and pulmonary circulation in children at high altitudes. *Pediatrics* 1964; 34:568.

Peters GB, Ford JH, Nicholl JK. Trisomy 21 mosaicism and maternal age effect. *Lancet* 1987; 1:1202.

Pharoah POD, Ellis SM, Ekins RP, et al. Maternal thyroid function, iodine deficiency and fetal development, *Clin Endocrinol* 1976; 5:159.

Pietrzyk JJ. Neural tube defects: complex segregation analysis and recurrence risk. *Am J Med Genet* 1980; 7:293.

Polani PE, Campbell M. Factors in the causation of persistent ductus arteriosus. *Ann Hum Genet* 1960; 24:343.

Powell-Griner E, Woolbright A. Trends in infant deaths from congenital anomalies: results from England and Wales, Scotland, Sweden and the United States. *Int J Epidemiol* 1990; 19:391.

Preblud SR, Cochi SL, Orenstein WA. Varicella-zoster infection in pregnancy. *N Engl J Med* 1986; 315:1416.

Pryor GA, Viller RN, Ronen A, et al. Seasonal variation in the incidence of congenital talipes equinovarus. *J Bone Joint Surg* 1991; 73-B:632.

Public Health Laboratory Service Working Party on Fifth Disease. Prospective study of human parvovirus (B19) infection in pregnancy. *Br Med J* 1990; 300:1166.

Rajegowda B, Lala R, Nagaraj A, et al. Does cocaine (CO) increase congenital urogenital abnormalities (CUGA) in newborns? *Pediat Res* 1991; 29:71A.

Rasmussen L, Green A, Hansen LP. The epidemiology of infantile hypertrophic pyloric stenosis in a Danish population, 1950–84. *Int J Epidemiol* 1989; 18:413.

Record RG, Edwards JH. Environmental influences related to the aetiology of congenital dislocation of the hip. *Br J Prev Soc Med* 1958; 12:8.

Record RG, McKeown T. Observations relating to the aetiology of patent ductus arteriosus. *Br Heart J* 1953; 15:376.

Record RG, Smith A. Incidence, mortality, and sex distribution of mongoloid defectives. *Br J Prev Soc Med* 1955; 9:10.

Remington JS, Desmonts G. Toxoplasmosis. In: Remington JS, Klein JO, eds. *Infectious Diseases of the Fetus and Newborn Infant. 3rd ed.* Philadelphia: WB Saunders; 1990:89.

Roberts CJ, Lloyd S. Observations on the epidemiology of simple hypospadias. *Br Med J* 1973; 1:768.

Robinson GW. Birth characteristics of children with congenital dislocation of the hip. *Am J Epidemiol* 1968; 87:275.

Rogers SC, Weatherall JAC. *Anencephalus, Spina Bifida and Congenital Hydrocephalus: England and Wales 1964–1972 (Studies on Medical and Population Subjects No. 32)*. London: Her Majesty's Stationery Office; 1976.

Rosa F. Detecting human retenoid embryopathy. *Teratology* 1991; 43:419.

Salter RB. Etiology, pathogenesis and possible prevention of congenital dislocation of the hip. *Can Med Assoc J* 1968; 98:933.

Sanfridson J, Redlund-Johnell I, Udén A. Why is congenital dislocation of the hip still missed? Analysis of 96,891 infants screened in Malmö 1956–1987. *Acta Orthop Scand* 1991; 62:87.

Schardein JL. Current status of drugs as teratogens in man. *Progr Clin Biol Res* 1985; 163C:181.

Sever JL, Gilkeson MR, Chen TC, et al. Epidemiology of mongolism in the Collaborative Project. *Ann NY Acad Sci* 1970; 171:328.

Shaffer LG, Marazita ML, Bodurtha J, et al. Evidence for a major gene in familial anencephaly. *Am J Med Genet* 1990; 36:97.

Sharav T. Aging gametes in relation to incidence, gender and twinning in Down syndrome. *Am J Med Genet* 1991; 39:116.

Shepard TH, Fantel AG, Fitzsimmons J. Congenital defect rates among spontaneous abortions: twenty years of monitoring. *Teratology* 1989; 39:325.

Sherman SL, Takaesu N, Freeman SB, et al. Trisomy 21: association between reduced recombination and nondisjunction. *Am J Hum Genet* 1991; 49:608.

Shim WKT, Campbell A, Wright SW. Pyloric stenosis in the racial groups of Hawaii. *J Pediat* 1970; 76:89.

Shima H, Ikoma F, Terakawa T, et al. Developmental anomalies associated with hypospadias. *J Urol* 1979; 122:619.

Shiota K. Maternal fertility, reproductive loss, and defective human embryos. *J Epidemiol Comm Health* 1989; 43:261.

Simpkin JM, Owens JR, Harris F. Incidence of hypospadias. *Lancet* 1985; 2:384.

Singer LT, Garber R, Kliegman R. Neurobehavioural sequelae of fetal cocaine exposure. *J. Pediatr* 1991; 119:667.

Smidt-Jensen S, Permin M, Philip J, et al. Randomised comparison of amniocentesis and transabdominal and transcervical chorionic villus sampling. *Lancet* 1992; 340:1237.

Smith GF, Berg JM. *Down's anomaly*. 2nd ed. Edinburgh: Churchill Livingstone; 1976.

Smithells RW, Sheppard S, Schorah CJ. Vitamin deficiencies and neural tube defects. *Arch Dis Child* 1976; 51:944.

Smithells RW, Sheppard S, Schorah CJ, et al. Apparent prevention of neural tube defects by vitamin supplementation. *Arch Dis Child* 1981; 56:911.

Smithells RW, Nevin NC, Seller MJ, et al. Further experience of vitamin supplementation for prevention of neural tube defect recurrences. *Lancet* 1983; 1:1027.

Smithells RW, Sheppard S, Wild J, et al. Prevention of neural tube defect recurrences in Yorkshire: final report. *Lancet* 1989; 2:498.

Smithells R, Sheppard S, Holzel H, et al. Congenital rubella in Great Britain 1971–1988. *Health Bull* 1991; 49:266.

Snider DE, Layde PM, Johnson MW, et al. Treatment of tuberculosis during pregnancy. *Am Rev Resp Dis* 1980; 122:65.

Sokol RJ, Clarren SK. Guidelines for use of terminology describing the impact of prenatal alcohol on the offspring. *Alcohol Clin Exp Res* 1989; 4:579.

Stagno S. Cytomegalovirus. In: Remington JS, Klein JO, eds. *Infectious Diseases of the Fetus and Newborn Infant*. Philadelphia: WB Saunders; 1990:241.

Staples AJ, Sutherland GR, Haan EA, et al. Epidemiology of Down syndrome in South Australia, 1960–89. *Am J Hum Genet* 1991; 49:1014.

Stein Z, Susser S, Warburton D, et al. Spontaneous abortion as a screening device: the effect of fetal survival on the incidence of birth defects. *Am J Epidemiol* 1975; 102:275.

Stein Z, Stein W, Susser M. Attrition of trisomies as a maternal screening device: an explanation of the association of trisomy 21 with maternal age. *Lancet* 1986; 1:944.

Stene J, Stene E, Mikkelsen M. Risk for chromosomal abnormality at amniocentesis following a child with a non-inherited chromosome aberration: a European collaborative study on prenatal diagnosis 1981. *Prenat Diagn* 1984; 4 (special issue): 81.

Strassburg MA, Greenland S, Portigal LD, et al. A population-based case-control study of anencephalus and spina bifida in a low-risk area. *Dev Med Child Neurol* 1983; 25:632.

Svensson J. Male hypospadias, 625 cases, associated malformations and possible etiological factors. *Acta Paediat Scand* 1979; 68:587.

Sweet RA, Schrott HG, Kurland R, et al. Study of the incidence of hypospadias in Rochester, Minnesota, 1940–70, and a case-control comparison of possible etiologic factors. *Mayo Clin Proc* 1974; 49:52.

Swerdlow AJ, Melzer D. The value of England and Wales congenital malformation notification scheme data for epidemiology: male genital tract malformations. *J Epidemiol Comm Health* 1988; 42:8.

Tabor A, Philip J, Madsen M, et al. Randomised controlled trial of genetic amniocentesis in 4606 low-risk women. *Lancet* 1986; 1:1282.

Tam PKM, Chan J. Increasing incidence of hypertrophic pyloric stenosis. *Arch Dis Child* 1991; 66:530.

Thiersch JB. Therapeutic abortions with a folic acid antagonist, 4-aminopteroyl-glutamic acid (4-amino P.G.A.) administered by the oral route. *Am J Obstet Gynecol* 1952; 63:1298.

Thiersch JB. The control of reproduction in rats with the aid of antimetabolites and early experiences with antimetabolites as abortifacient agents in man. *Acta Endocrinol* 1956; 23 (suppl 28):37.

Tünte W. Zur Häufigkeit der Anencephalie und Spina bifida aperta im Regierungsbezirk Münster. *Zschr Menschl Verebungs- und Konstitutionslehre* 1964; 37:525.

Tünte W. Zur Frage der jahreszeitlichen Häufigkeit der Anencephalie. *Humangenetik* 1968; 6:225.

Vergel RG, Sanchez LR, Heredero BL, et al. Primary prevention of neural tube defects with folic acid supplementation: Cuban experience. *Prenat Diagn* 1990; 10:149.

Wald NJ, Cuckle HS. Open neural tube defects. In: Wald NJ, ed. *Antenatal and Neonatal Screening*. Oxford: Oxford University Press; 1984:25.

Wald NJ, Cuckle HS, Densem JW, et al. Maternal serum screening for Down's syndrome in early pregnancy. *Br Med J* 1988; 297:883.

Wallgren A. Is the rate of hypertrophic pyloric stenosis declining? *Acta Paediatr* 1960; 49:530.

Walpole IR. Some epidemiological aspects of pyloric stenosis in British Columbia. *Am J Med Genet* 1981; 10:237.

Walsworth-Bell JP. Infantile hypertrophic pyloric stenosis in Greater Manchester. *J Epidemiol Comm Health* 1983; 37:149.

Warkany J. Etiology of congenital malformations. *Adv Pediat* 1947; 2:1.

Webb AR, Lari J, Dodge JA. Infantile hypertrophic pyloric stenosis in South Glamorgan 1970–9: effects of change in feeding practice. *Arch Dis Child* 1983; 58:586.

Wehrung DA, Hay S. A study of seasonal incidence of congenital malformations in the United States. *Br J Prev Soc Med* 1970; 24:24.

Wilkinson JA. Prime factors in the etiology of congenital dislocation of the hip. *J Bone Joint Surg* 1963; 45B:268.

Wilkinson JA. A post-natal survey for congenital displacement of the hip. *J Bone Joint Surg* 1972; 54B:40.

Wilson CB, Remington JS. Prevention of congenital toxoplasmosis: a viewpoint from a laboratory in the United States. In: Thalhammer O, Baumgarten K, Pollak A, eds. *Perinatal Medicine: Sixth European Congress, Vienna 1978*. Stuttgart: Thieme; 1979:76.

Winship KA, Cahal DA, Weber JCP, et al. Maternal drug histories and central nervous system anomalies. *Arch Dis Child* 1984; 59:1052.

Wright SW, Day RW, Muller H, et al. The frequency of trisomy and translocation in Down's syndrome. *J Pediat* 1967; 70:420.

Wynne-Davies R. Family studies and the cause of congenital club foot. Talipes equinovarus, talipes calcaneovalgus and metatarsus varus. *J Bone Joint Surg* 1964; 45B; 445.

Wynne-Davies R. Acetabular dysplasia and familial joint laxity: two aetiological factors in congenital dislocation of the hip. A review of 589 patients and their families. *J Bone Joint Surg* 1970a; 52B; 704.

Wynne-Davies R. A family study of neonatal and late-diagnosis congenital dislocation of the hip. *J Med Genet* 1970b; 7:315.

Xilinas ME, Lagarde D. Congenital dislocation of the hip in Brittany. *Lancet* 1975; 1:863.

Yamamoto M, Watanabe G. Epidemiology of gross chromosomal anomalies at the early embryonic stage of pregnancy. In: Klingberg MA, Weatherall JAC, eds. *Epidemiologic Methods for Detection of Teratogens* (*Contributions to Epidemiology and Biostatistics. Vol. 1*). Basel: Karger; 1979:101.

Yamamuro T, Ishida K. Recent advances in the prevention, early diagnosis, and treatment of congenital dislocation of the hip in Japan. *Clin Orthop Rel Res* 1984; 184:34.

Yang P, Hecht J, Murray J, et al. Complex segregation analysis of cleft lip and palate. *Am J Hum Genet* 1991; 49 (suppl):486.

Yen IH, Khoury MJ, Erickson JD, et al. The changing epidemiology of neural tube defects: United States, 1968–1989. *Am J Dis Child* 1992; 146:857.

Young ID, Clarke M. Lethal malformations and perinatal mortality: a 10 year review with comparison of ethnic differences. *Br Med J* 1987; 295:89.

Zenzes MT, Casper RF. Cytogenetics of human oocytes, zygotes and embryos after in vitro fertilisation. *Hum Genet* 1992; 88:367.

5

Genetic Disorders

JOSEPH T.R. CLARKE

Although single-gene disorders as causes of disease in children tend individually to be uncommon, as a group they are important to pediatric medicine (Scriver et al., 1989). They account for a diverse range of disorders that cause pathologic changes varying in severity and involving every system or tissue of the body. As infant and childhood morbidity and mortality due to nutritional and infectious diseases have declined over the past 20 years, the proportional contribution of genetic disease to pediatric pathology has grown markedly. Furthermore, improvements in the diagnosis of single-gene defects have contributed to an apparent increase in the incidence of genetic disease.

Genetic disease in general is characterized by marked clinical variability, even among members of the same family bearing the same gene defect. In some cases the presence of the defect cannot be demonstrated at all, despite unambiguous evidence from the pattern of inheritance that the family members carry the defective gene. These characteristics, when added to the difficulty in some instances of differentiating a genetic disease from an acquired condition it closely resembles, contribute to the problem of variable and incomplete ascertainment that pervades much of the descriptive epidemiology of genetic disorders. Although the impact of molecular genetics on the determination of total incidence or prevalence may be small, these technological advances have had a profound effect on the definition and classification of the disorders, particularly in identifying asymptomatic individuals in a population who carry a specific gene. Improvements in medical management have decreased the immediate mortality due to many genetic diseases and have almost certainly therefore contributed to an increase in prevalence of various conditions. The net impact of these advances has yet to be subjected to systematic investigation.

The objective of this chapter is to review some of the fundamental concepts of population genetics, to outline the methodology and summarize the results of some studies on the incidence of single-gene disorders, and to review measures to decrease the burden of single-gene disorders as causes of disease in children.

Biologic Considerations

Principles of Genetics

For a comprehensive overview of human genetics in general and of the genetics of populations in particular, the reader is advised to consult one of several excellent reviews (Crow, 1986; Morton, 1982; Scriver et al., 1989; Thompson et al., 1991; Vogel & Motulsky, 1986). Our understanding of the pattern of occurrence of disease due to single-gene defects in human populations is based primarily on concepts developed by Gregor Mendel, who described the transmission of heritable characteristics from parents to offspring by discrete genetic units passed from generation to generation independently of each other. The unit of inheritance is the gene. The genetic information contained in genes is encoded in deoxyribonucleic acid (DNA). DNA is located in the nuclei of cells and is made up of four subunits, called nucleotides. They are covalently linked together in very large linear molecules in which the instructions for the synthesis of proteins by the cell, and therefore the physical characteristics of the organism, are determined by the sequence of the four nucleotides taken three at a time. The location of each gene in relation to other genes is called its locus. Variants of a gene located at the same locus are called alleles, and the properties of each allele determine the characteristics of the gene product. For example, the β-globin gene codes for the production of the β-globin polypeptide of hemoglobin. The most common β-globin allele, β^A, codes for the production of normal adult hemoglobin A. Another β-globin allele, β^S, characterized by a single nucleotide substitution in the structure of the DNA of the β-globin gene, codes for the synthesis of hemoglobin S, which in homozygous form causes sickle cell anemia. Alleles are transmitted from parents to children according to Mendel's laws of inheritance.

Genes transmitted through succeeding generations of a freely mating population are redistributed independently and randomly in the offspring in proportions predictable by the terms of the binomial theorem. This random reassortment of genes during passage from one generation to another is the result of extensive recombination between homologous parental chromosomes. The probability of two genes on the same chromosome becoming separated by the process of recombination during gametogenesis (the formation of oocytes and spermatocytes during embryogenesis) is related in part to the physical distance between them. Genes with little likelihood of recombination occurring between them because they are very close to each other are said to be closely linked. The distance between them is estimated by **linkage analysis** (Ott, 1991), the principal means by which the locations of specific genes are determined. This linkage is expressed as a **lod score**, the logarithm to the base 10 of the odds that two loci are linked.

When the contribution of mutation to the production of new alleles is small and constant, the distribution of alleles in a randomly mating, demographically stable population as a whole approaches the Hardy-Weinberg (HW) equilibrium. For a two-allele system at HW equilibrium, the proportion of individuals bearing one or other of the two alleles is given by the formula: $p^2 + 2\,pq + q^2 = 1$, in which p is the relative frequency of one allele (A) in the population and q ($= 1 - p$) is the relative frequency of the other (B). The proportion of individuals homozygous for the A allele (i.e., carrying two A alleles) is given by the first term (p^2); the proportion homozygous for the B allele is given by the last term (q^2). The middle term, 2pq, describes the proportion of individuals who are heterozygous for the two alleles, i.e., carrying one A allele and one B allele. From this brief explanation, it should be clear why the HW concept is central to the understanding of the epidemiology of these disorders.

Common causes of deviations from the HW equilibrium in human populations include the tendency for human mating to occur nonrandomly within culturally or racially defined subgroups of the larger population (**stratification**), the tendency to choose mates with particular characteristics (**assortative mating**), inbreeding (**consanguinity**), environmental **selection** in favor of or against a specific allele, migration (**gene flow**), and random fluctuations in gene frequencies in relatively small populations occurring by chance alone (**genetic drift**). The increased prevalence of a specific genetic condition in a demographically isolated population as a result of the introduction of the mutation by a founder is called a **founder effect**. The HW equilibrium and factors causing departures from it are discussed in some detail in the text by Vogel and Motulsky (1986).

Although ionizing radiation and many chemicals are mutagenic, the majority of mutations are spontaneous or occur without any identifiable proximate cause. The rates of spontaneous mutation of many autosomal dominant and X-linked recessive genes have been estimated from the incidence of sporadic cases, coupled with estimates of the fitness (i.e. relative fertility) of affected individuals (Vogel & Motulsky, 1986). Potential sources of error in these estimates include small sample size, illegitimacy, errors in diagnosis, incomplete penetrance, and errors in estimates of fertility. For some well-defined autosomal dominant conditions, such as achondroplasia, and for some X-linked recessive diseases, such as Duchenne muscular dystrophy, estimates of mutation rates are generally accepted to be quite reliable. In contrast, estimates of the mutation rates for other dominantly inherited conditions, such as tuberous sclerosis and osteogenesis imperfecta, are confounded by marked variability of expression of the mutation and genetic heterogeneity. Estimates of mutation rates for some autosomal dominant and X-linked recessive conditions are presented in Table 5.1. Some of the conditions listed are genetic lethals, meaning that the mutations are not transmitted by individually carrying them to their offspring, usually because procreation by these individuals does not occur. Spontaneous mutation is in these cases a major contributor to the incidence of the diseases, and changes in mutation rates would be expected also to affect disease incidences. The limitations of the past methods for estimating mutation rates make current estimates for autosomal recessive genes unreliable.

In structural terms, mutations are variations in the sequence of nucleotides comprising a gene. The DNA of the human haploid genome (the sequence of nucleotides making up the total genetic information in each oocyte or spermatocyte) is composed of approximately 3×10^9 nucleotide pairs, of which less than 1% represent sequences coding for the specific amino acids in the polypeptide products of gene expression. The remaining nucleotide pairs represent

Table 5.1. Representative Spontaneous Mutation Rates Expressed as Mutations per Locus per Generation

Disease	Mutation Rate
Autosomal Dominant	
Achondroplasia	$0.6 - 4 \times 10^{-5}$
Aniridia	$2.5 - 5 \times 10^{-6}$
Retinoblastoma	$0.5 - 1.2 \times 10^{-5}$
Osteogenesis imperfecta	1×10^{-5}
Neurofibromatosis, type I	1×10^{-4}
Polycystic disease of the kidneys	$0.6 - 1.2 \times 10^{-4}$
X-Linked Recessive	
Duchenne muscular dystrophy	1×10^{-4}
Hemophilia A	$3 - 6 \times 10^{-5}$
Hemophilia B	$2 - 3 \times 10^{-6}$
Incontinentia pigmenti	$0.6 - 2 \times 10^{-5}$
Orofaciodigital syndrome	5×10^{-6}

Source: Modified from Vogel & Motulsky, 1986.

noncoding intervening sequences (IVS; introns) interspersed with the coding sequences (exons) of each gene; regulatory sequences flanking each gene; large numbers of repetitive sequences of various lengths scattered throughout the genome; specialized structures, such as those at the telomeres and centromeres; and sequences of unknown structure and function. The structure, properties, and organization of genetic information are reviewed in an excellent text by Singer & Berg (1991).

Whether or not a given mutation results in disease depends on the effect that the change in nucleotide sequence of the gene or flanking regulatory regions has on the production and function of a gene product; marked variations of the nucleotide sequence in many of the noncoding regions of the genome have little apparent impact on either. Benign variations in noncoding sequence are, for the most part, subject to the same rules of inheritance as genes themselves. That is, they are transmitted from parents to offspring according to Mendel's laws of inheritance, and variations that are closely linked to each other tend to pass from generation to generation (i.e., segregate) together. This makes them particularly useful for tracing the transmission of specific sequences of DNA through several generations of one family or within genetically distinct populations. Because they do not affect the genetic fitness of the organism, they accumulate and provide the basis for marked genetic variability (Jeffreys, 1979).

The potential for variations in the genome occurring as a result of random mutation is enormous. Variations that occur in the population with a frequency greater than that which would be expected to be maintained by mutation alone, operationally defined as greater than 1%, are called **polymorphisms**. There are many examples of polymorphisms. They include the blood group antigens, HLA antigens, certain variant hemoglobins, immunoglobulins, and numerous other serum proteins (Harris, 1980). Some have been shown to be associated with relative susceptibility or resistance to disease; most are probably genetically neutral. The ability to identify and track them in populations is extremely important in genetic epidemiology.

Molecular Genetics

Whereas the study of genetic variations was formerly dependent on the detection of variations in gene products, such as electrophoretic variants of serum proteins, our current ability to identify variations at the level of the nucleotide sequence of genomic DNA, whether the polymorphic sequence is expressed or not, has revolutionized the science of human population genetics.

Southern Analysis

The analysis of variations in DNA structure was greatly facilitated by the discovery of bacterial enzymes (restriction endonucleases) that cleave DNA at specific sites defined by the nucleotide sequence in the region. Sequence variations involving the short sequences of nucleotides (recognition sites) where DNA is cleaved by specific restriction endonucleases result in systematic variations in the size of fragments produced by digestion of DNA—restriction fragment length polymorphisms (RFLP; Antonarakis, 1989; Antonarakis et al., 1982; Jeffreys, 1979; Kan & Dozy, 1978; Lawn et al., 1978). The presence of specific RFLPs in a sample of DNA is commonly demonstrated by Southern blot analysis, named after the British scientist, Edward Southern, who described it in 1975 (Southern, 1975). In this technique, DNA is isolated, digested with a specific restriction endonuclease, and its fragments separated according to size by electrophoresis through a suitable gel. The DNA fragments are transferred by blotting to a nylon or nitrocellulose membrane, and the membrane is exposed to a solution of an appropriate radioisotopically labeled probe consisting of a relatively short sequence of DNA complementary to the nucleotide sequence spanning the polymorphism. The membrane is washed, and the location of the probe is established by exposing it to x-ray film. The specific polymorphic allele is identified by the presence or absence of bands on the autoradiogram corresponding to fragments of specific lengths.

The usefulness of RFLPs is limited because a restriction site can only be either present or absent, so that the maximum heterozygote frequency for any allele is 50%. A more informative system of DNA polymorphism consists of the numerous repetitive noncoding sequences of nucleotides in the genome, such as variable number tandem repeats (VNTR; Nakamura et al., 1987) and short tandem repeats (STR; Edwards et al., 1991), in which the alleles differ from each other in the number of repetitions of the sequence. These sequences are proving to be much more useful for the study of genomic variation because several different alleles are possible at a given locus, each allele corresponding to a different number of repeats, and the frequency of heterozygotes in the population may approach 100%.

The usefulness for epidemiologic studies of a specific RFLP depends not only on the degree of variability of the polymorphism in the population but also on its relationship to the gene of interest. It is most useful if it is located very close (in genetic terms) to the gene or mutation, with the result that there is little likelihood of recombination occurring between them during gametogenesis. In cases in which the exact location and characteristics of the gene of interest are unknown, RFLP analysis, in association with appropriate linkage studies, is the principal means by which the inheritance of mutations in specific families is determined (Johnson, 1988). Figure 5.1 shows an autoradiogram of a Southern blot that illustrates the existence and pattern of inheritance of RFLPs on the X chromosome and the application of the analysis to carrier identification and thus the prenatal diagnosis of Duchenne muscular dystrophy in a case in which the specific mutation is unknown.

Haplotype Analysis

When, as is often the case, the structure or precise location of a disease-related mutant allele is unknown, the likelihood that an individual related to a child affected with the disease carries the same mutation may be estimated by tracing the inheritance of one or more polymorphisms that are closely linked to it. The pattern of closely linked polymorphisms provides a molecular genetic background (**haplotype**); identification of specific haplotypes has been found to be useful in the elucidation of the probable history of specific mutations in different human populations. A review of RFLP haplotypes in the context of the β-globin locus and specific β-thalassemia mutations has been provided by Orkin and Kazazian (1984).

One of the most thoroughly studied systems of haplotypes is that associated with phenylketonuria (PKU; Daiger et al., 1989a and b; Konecki & Lichter-Konecki, 1991; Woo, 1989). By determining the presence or absence of one or more of eight different polymorphic restriction enzyme recognition sites, within or closely adjacent to the gene for phenylalanine hydroxylase (PAH), a total of 46 possible haplotypes were observed (Daiger et al., 1989a). However, in northern European populations, in which the incidence of PKU is relatively high, four haplotypes (haplotypes 1–4) alone were found to account for over 80% of PKU-bearing chromosomes, and two of the four haplotypes (haplotypes 2 and 3) accounted for over 40% of the PKU chromosomes. The latter two haplotypes occurred on only 12.6% of the normal chromosomes studied. When the association between a disease gene, such as PKU, and the pattern of closely linked RFLPs (haplotype) constituting the genetic background of the mutation is significantly different from what would be expected on the basis of the HW equilibrium (see Principles section), the disease gene and haplotype are said to be in **linkage disequilibrium**. Each mutation is presumed to have occurred at some time, on some chromosome, with a particular haplotype. Over several generations, the relationship between the original mutation and haplotype is gradually changed as a result of recombination. Given enough time and random mating, the nonrandom association between the mutation and the original haplotype will eventually break down. The existence of linkage disequilibrium is interpreted as evidence that the mutation causing the disease of interest occurred only once, and relatively recently, in evolutionary terms.

Two point mutations associated with classical PKU are particularly common among Caucasians; one of them is in strong linkage disequilibrium with haplotype 2, and the other is in nearly complete linkage disequilibrium with haplotype 3. In Asiatic populations, haplotype 4 accounts for more than 80% of all normal and PKU-bearing chromosomes (Daiger et al., 1989b). Only two Oriental PKU mutations have been characterized, and neither is present in Caucasians (Wang

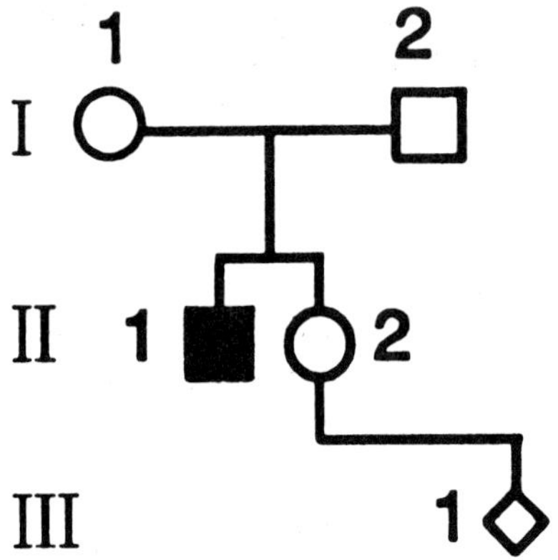

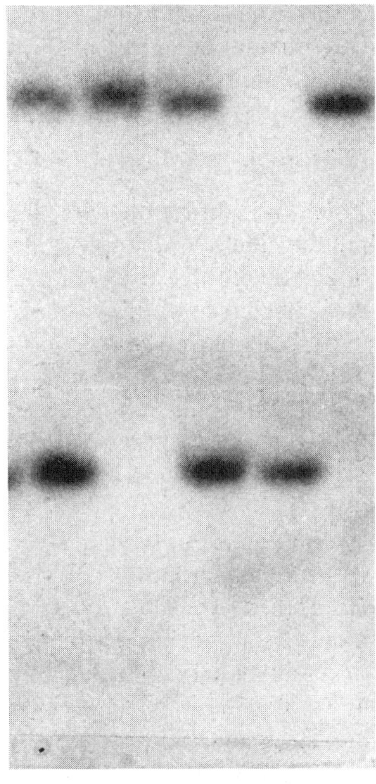

Fig. 5.1. Southern blot analysis. DNA extracted from peripheral blood lymphocytes of the individuals shown in the pedigree at the top of the figure was digested with the restriction endonuclease, *Msp*I, and the fragments were separated according to size by agarose gel electrophoresis, transferred to a nylon membrane, and reacted with a short radiolabeled nucleotide sequence, PERT87, which binds specifically to a site closely linked to the Duchenne muscular dystrophy gene. The autoradiogram obtained by exposure of the membrane to x-ray film shows bands corresponding to different alleles of a specific restriction fragment length polymorphism (RFLP) on the X chromosome. The results indicate that the individual, I-1, who is heterozygous for Duchenne muscular dystrophy (DMD), has two alleles, one 4.0 kb (*upper band*) and one 1.8 kb (*lower band*). The son, II-1, is affected with the disease. The analysis shows that the mutation causing the disease in II-1 is on the same X chromosome as that carrying the higher molecular weight PERT87 allele. His sister, II-2, has inherited the 1.8 kb allele from her father, I-2, and the 4.0 kb allele from her mother. Since this is the same maternal allele as that carried by her affected brother, she is presumed also to be a carrier of the mutation. The results of prenatal testing of the fetus she is carrying, III-1, show that, assuming no recombination has occurred within the gene itself, the fetus inherited the grandmaternal X chromosome bearing the mutation that caused DMD in II-1 and is affected with the disease. (Courtesy of PN Ray, Toronto.)

et al., 1991). Taken together, these and other observations on various PKU mutations and associated haplotypes in different populations support the notion that PKU arose as a result of multiple independent mutations in different peoples (Konecki & Lichter-Konecki, 1991), though the possibility of some selective advantage for carriers of the gene has also been postulated (see National Differences section).

Mutation Analysis

In many Mendelian conditions affecting children, several specific mutations have been identified. In general, autosomal dominant or X-linked recessive mutations tend to include a wide variety of distinct alleles of which a high proportion are large deletions, duplications, or other rearrangements. In many cases, the genetic fitness (i.e. relative fertility) of affected individuals is impaired, and a large proportion of abnormal alleles occur as a result of new mutations. Disease-related mutations of this type tend to involve major structural disruptions or to cluster around functionally important parts of the gene (Worton & Thompson, 1988). Figure 5.2 shows some of the mutations identified in males with Duchenne muscular dystrophy and the milder variant of the disease, Becker muscular dystrophy.

In contrast, analysis of mutations associated with autosomal recessive conditions, such as PKU, cystic fibrosis, Tay-Sachs disease, and other disorders, shows that single base changes or other relatively small structural alterations predominate, and a few specific mutations, each resulting in the production of little or no normally functional gene product, tend to account for a high proportion of the abnormal alleles. The presence of a normal allele is sufficient to compensate completely for the defect in the mutant, and the genetic fitness (relative fertility) of carriers of the mutation is generally not affected. The high frequency of a few specific mutant alleles would seem to be the final result of a complex interaction among the molecular environment, the role of the sequence in the structure and function of the gene product, and factors disturbing the random segregation of alleles in the population, such as inbreeding, migration, genetic drift, and natural selection.

The detection of specific mutations is facilitated by the application of allele-specific oligonucleotide (ASO) probing (Landegren et al., 1988). By this technique, total genomic DNA or, more commonly, DNA amplified by the polymerase chain reaction (PCR, see below) is applied to an adherent membrane and reacted with relatively short, radiolabeled oligonucleotide probes that exactly match either the normal or the mutant allele. The specific binding of probe to the DNA adsorbed to the membrane indicates the presence of the corresponding allele; no binding signals its absence. This is a technically easy, sensitive, and highly specific test for the presence, in any sample of DNA, of any allele for which labeled, allele-specific oligonucleotide probes are available.

Polymerase Chain Reaction

Progress in the investigation of mutations and molecular polymorphisms in populations has been facilitated greatly by the invention of the polymerase chain

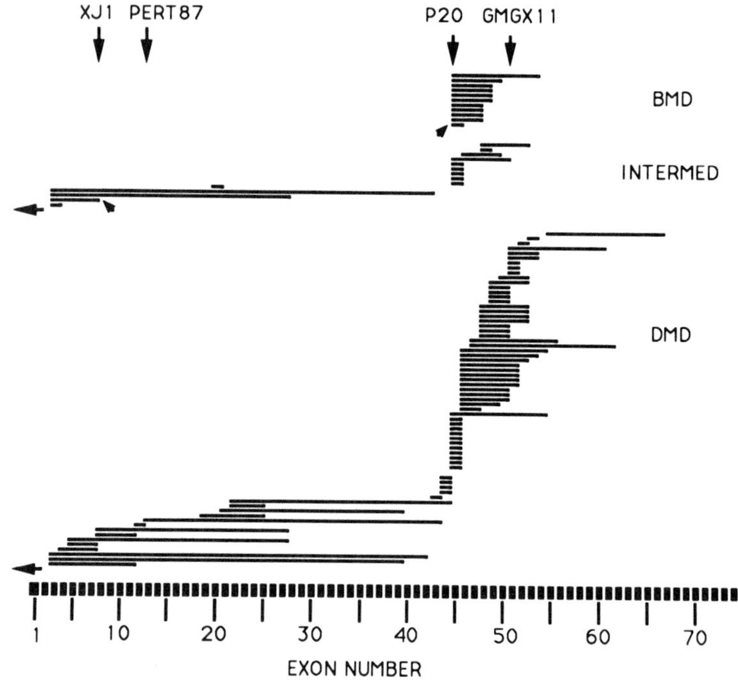

Fig. 5.2. Deletions account for 60% of the mutations of the dystrophin gene in boys with clinically severe Duchenne muscular dystrophy (DMD), relatively mild Becker muscular dystrophy (BMD), and clinically intermediate forms of muscular dystrophy (INTERMED). The 74 fragments of DNA (exons) making up the dystrophin gene are shown at the bottom of the figure. The extent of each deletion is shown by a horizontal bar. The arrows at the top show the location of RFLPs detectable by the probes, XJ1, PERT87, P20, and GMGX11. The arrows at the left indicate deletions of the first exon that extend into the regulatory region of the gene, causing complete disruption of the production of gene product. (Courtesy of R.G. Worton, Toronto.)

reaction (PCR; Eisenstein, 1990; Saiki et al., 1985, 1988). By this technique, selected regions of extremely small samples of DNA can be amplified by several orders of magnitude to generate enough DNA for Southern blot analysis or, more commonly, analysis of specific alleles by ASO probing (Landegren et al., 1988).

Mitochondrial Genome

Mitochondrial DNA (mtDNA) represents a special class of DNA from the standpoint of variation and inheritance (Wallace, 1989). The mutation rate of mtDNA is several-fold higher than the mutation rate of nuclear DNA; mutation-derived variation is particularly marked in the short, noncoding D loop of the mitochondrial chromosome. Several disorders attributable to mtDNA mutations have been described (Menkes, 1987), but they seem to be very rare and at present do not contribute significantly to the overall disease burden attributable to single-gene defects in children. Since the mtDNA of an individual is derived entirely from the mother, the inheritance of mutations or polymorphisms is matrilineal. The combination of a high mutation rate and matrilineal inheritance has made mitochondrial mutations particularly important to studies on evolution. However, the study of the epidemiology of pediatric diseases attributable to mitochondrial mutations, including clinical definition of the diseases and estimates of their incidence, is still in its infancy.

Patterns of Occurrence

Estimation of Incidence

The estimation of the incidence of disease in children that occurs as a result of single-gene defects is complicated because the conditions are individually rare and their diagnosis is often difficult and also because the distributions of specific genotypes in the total population are likely not to be homogeneous. The specific population and methods chosen depend on the objective of the study: the detection of disease for the purpose of medical intervention, the development of screening programs, resource allocation, or the elucidation of the distribution of specific alleles.

Three approaches have been taken to determine the incidence of genetic diseases in populations: retrospective surveys, population-based screening, and genetic registries (see Chapter 1). Each form of ascertainment is subject to biases.

Retrospective Surveys

Retrospective enumeration of the occurrence of genetic conditions has been widely employed to estimate the incidence and spectrum of genetic disease occurring in selected, controlled environments, such as in hospitals or in specific geographic regions. The data are derived predominantly from a review of relevant hospital or clinic records. Surveys of this type are vulnerable to incomplete ascertainment and for the most part have been confined to surveys of the incidence of specific, well-defined disorders in discrete populations in which the diagnosis is obvious and all affected individuals are likely to funnel through a common diagnostic gate where counting is most likely to be accurate and complete. Complete ascertainment in this type of study depends on appropriate documentation, which is more often achieved in surveys of specific, well-defined conditions than it is in more general surveys. This approach has been used to determine the scope of the contribution of single-gene defects to admissions to hospitals (Day & Holmes, 1973; Hall et al., 1978; Polani, 1973; Reich et al., 1974; Roberts et al., 1970; Scriver et al., 1973), as well as the incidence of specific diseases, such as cystic fibrosis in New England (Kramm et al., 1962) and β-thalassemia in Quebec (Kaplan et al., 1991).

Incidence data derived from hospital records are also subject to bias introduced as a result of the variability in the type and degree of morbidity associated with different disorders; the likelihood of hospitalization, which may vary from center to center and from time to time; and the duration of hospitalization (Roberts et al., 1978). Reliable interpretation of the data requires careful consideration of these variables and may limit the value of the results, depending on the intended application.

Population Screening

Population screening for specific mutant phenotypes has also yielded information on the incidence of particular monogenic disorders (i.e., disorders caused by mutations in one gene) in the population screened. In this case, the completeness and accuracy of ascertainment depend on the degree of compliance (e.g., in submitting samples for testing) and the sensitivity and specificity of the screening test. Most population genetic screening programs have been undertaken with the objective of identifying infants affected with treatable disorders for the purpose of initiating treatment before irreparable damage due to the mutation has occurred (see Screening section below). Few programs have been launched only to determine the prevalence of particular mutations or biochemical phenotypes in the population, and these have tended to be small in scale.

Screening tests applied with the goal of medical intervention are often selected on the basis of high sensitivity and technical simplicity at the potential cost of specificity because it is assumed that infants identified by the test would subsequently be subjected to more thorough diagnostic investigation. Raw incidence data obtained by this process may overestimate the true incidence of a genetic disease unless care is taken to follow up the screening with more specific testing of individuals identified as being at high risk for the allele under investigation. An example of a large-scale, prospective screening program undertaken for epidemiologic purposes is the province-wide program for the identification of amino aciduria in Quebec (Laberge et al., 1975; Lemieux et al., 1988; Scriver et al., 1978). Other examples of epidemiologic applications of genetic screening, made possible by advances in molecular genetics, are the multinational collaborative studies of the frequency in various subpopulations of specific mutations and related haplotypes associated with cystic fibrosis (Romeo & Devoto, 1990), PKU (Kalaydjieva et al., 1991), and thalassemia (Kazazian, 1990).

Genetic Registries

Prospective genetic disease or birth defect registries have the potential to provide reliable information on the total incidence of mutant phenotypes (i.e., genetic load) in particular populations (Cordero, 1992; see Chapter 1). An example of such a registry is the Health Surveillance Registry (HSR) of the province of British Columbia, established in 1952 (Baird, 1987; Baird et al., 1988; Lowry et al., 1975). Initially, any child under 21 years of age who had a disability severe enough to interfere with normal living, obtaining an education, or later earning a living was considered eligible for registration. Since 1962, eligibility has been expanded to include any person with a familial condition or congenital malformation that is not disabling. Registration in the HSR is voluntary, but to minimize the possibility of incomplete ascertainment, data are accumulated from more than 60 sources. Each case is assigned an identifying number and an etiology code. Etiology codes for genetic conditions include autosomal dominant, recessive, X-linked, chromosomal, multifactorial, and unspecified genetic, as well as various environmental causes. An important aspect of the HSR is the commitment, embedded in appropriate legislation, to confidentiality. The robustness of registry data on genetic conditions is ensured by the formal involvement of medical geneticists, clinical genetics services, and diagnostic laboratories involved in the investigation of genetic disorders.

Factors Affecting Incidence Estimates

In the context of genetic disease, the term "incidence" may be applied to the frequency of a clinical phenotype, a biochemical phenotype, or a particular genotype. For example, a significant proportion of cases of mental retardation (the clinical phenotype) in a population may be traceable to genetic defects. In a small fraction of cases, mental retardation is associated with persistent elevation of phenylalanine concentrations in plasma (the biochemical phenotype); in some of these cases, it is associated with a genetic defect in the enzyme, phenylalanine hydroxylase (PAH; the genotype). However, hyperphenylalaninemia also occurs as a result of benign PAH mutations, which are not associated with mental retardation, and as a consequence of mutations affecting pterin cofactor metabolism, in which mental retardation occurs in spite of treatment. These conditions represent examples of **genetic heterogeneity**—the situation when mutations of completely different genes or different mutations of one gene produce similar biochemical or clinical phenotypes. Some acquired diseases mimic known genetic diseases so closely (**phenocopies**) that they are impossible to distinguish without biochemical or molecular genetic analysis, adding to the difficulty of estimating the true incidence of diseases due to single-gene defects. It follows that the reliability of estimates of the incidence of these defects as causes of disease in children is influenced directly by the accuracy of diagnosis, and the accuracy of diagnosis depends in turn on elucidating the relationship between clinical and biochemical phenotypes and relevant genotypes. The elucidation of mutations by the application of molecular genetic techniques has improved the definition of genotypes. However, the relationship between a specific mutation (genotype) and clinical outcome is not always clear. In some cases, the putative mutation may be discovered to be a benign polymorphism; in others, the relationship is complex, involving poorly understood gene-gene or gene-environmental interactions. Although the number of genetic diseases for which the genotype-phenotype relationship is known is growing rapidly, in the majority of cases, the relationship is uncertain.

Estimates of incidence are also influenced by completeness of ascertainment. Failures of sampling or reporting tend to result in an underestimation of the incidence of specific genetic disorders. Newborn screening programs commonly report close to 100% compliance based on the number of samples tested compared with the number of births, ignoring those instances when an infant may have been tested twice. Efforts to improve completeness by legislating participation in screening programs have produced variable results. In one large study of PKU screening programs in the United States, there was no relationship between the existence of prescriptive legislation in a particular state and the completeness of screening (National Academy of Sciences, 1975). Similarly, the failure to report individuals eligible for registration by a surveillance registry results in underestimation of the defect in question.

Programs designed to determine incidence are most likely to succeed if the data are derived from a number of sources. However, the provision for multiple entry points also increases the likelihood that any child would be inadvertently entered more than once.

Single-Gene Disorders

The total incidence of some relatively common genetic disorders in children is shown in Table 5.2 (see Chapter 4). In most cases, the rates were established by surveys.

National Differences

National, ethnic, or racial differences in the incidence of single-gene disorders in children mirror closely the overall genetic and evolutionary histories of the populations (Adams et al., 1990; Bowman & Murray, 1990; Goodman, 1979; Polednak, 1989). The same factors that contribute to the racial and, to a lesser extent, cultural characteristics of a population, affect the gene pools and therefore the genetic burdens of the populations. Migration is a major and well-known contributor to changes in the genetic characteristics of geographically confined populations (gene flow). Coupled with geographic or cultural isolation, it results in circumstances conducive to significant alterations in the genetic profile of relatively small subpopulations by inbreeding and by chance alone

Table 5.2. Incidence of Some Common Single-Gene Disorders

Disorder	Estimated Incidence per 100,000 Births
Autosomal Dominant	
Familial hypercholesterolemia	200
Hereditary spherocytosis	20
von Willebrand's disease	12.5
Marfan disease	5
Achondroplasia	2
Autosomal Recessive	
Sickle cell anemia (U.S. blacks)	153
Cystic fibrosis (Caucasians)	40
Tay-Sachs disease (Ashkenazi Jews)	33
α_1-antitrypsin ZZ genotype	28
Phenylketonuria (average)	8
Mucopolysaccharidoses (all types)	4
Glycogen-storage disease (all types)	2
X-Linked Recessive	
Duchenne muscular dystrophy (males)	28
Hemophilia A (males)	10
Fragile X mental retardation (males)	50
Fragile X mental retardation (females)	33

Source: Modified from Scriver et al., 1989.

(genetic drift). Examples of situations in which the frequent occurrence of specific autosomal recessive disorders in certain populations has been attributed to migration and geographic or demographic isolation include Tay-Sachs and Gaucher disease among Ashkenazi Jews (Goodman, 1979), congenital nephrosis among Finns (Eriksson et al., 1980), familial Mediterranean fever among Armenians (Schwabe & Peters, 1974), and hereditary tyrosinemia among French-Canadians (Laberge, 1969; Table 5.3).

Natural selection has had a marked effect on the genetic characteristics of some populations, including the frequency of certain alleles for genetic diseases. The high incidence of thalassemia in Mediterranean and Asiatic peoples and of sickle cell anemia in African blacks has been traced to the relative resistance of asymptomatic carriers of the mutations to malaria (Bowman & Murray, 1990). The examples of thalassemia and sickle cell disease have spurred efforts to determine whether the high frequency of other mutant alleles may also be due to heterozygote advantage. Although the high incidence of PKU in some European subpopulations is explainable in part on the basis of a founder effect, the prevalence of the disease, the variety of mutations involved, and the strong linkage disequilibrium between specific mutations and certain haplotypes suggest the possibility of some selective advantage to carriers of PKU mutations (Kidd, 1987). The same observations with respect to cystic fibrosis (CF), the commonest lethal autosomal recessive disease in humans, has led to speculation that heterozygous carriers of CF mutations also enjoy some subtle selective advantage (Tsui & Buchwald, 1991). Some have suggested that CF carriers may be relatively resistant to bacterial toxin-mediated diarrhea (Baxter et al., 1988). Confirmation of selection or any other putative advantage in the case of CF or PKU awaits further investigation.

Interventions: Screening

Large-scale screening is a well-established means of identifying members of a population, such as infants, affected by a specific genetic condition at a pre-

Table 5.3. Racial Variations in the Incidence of Single-Gene Disorders

Disease	Race	Estimated Incidence per 100,000 Births
Porphyria variegata	South African (White)	300
	Caucasians (general)	1
Huntington chorea	Tasmania	17
	Japan	2.9
Adrenogenital syndrome	Yupik Eskimos	200
	North Americans	25
Cystic fibrosis	North Americans	40
	African-Americans	1
Tay-Sachs disease	Ashkenazi Jews	33
	Sephardi Jews, Gentiles	0.3
β-Thalassemia	Mediterraneans	153
Sickle cell anemia	Africans	153

Source: Modified from Weatherall, 1985.

symptomatic stage with the objective of initiating therapeutic measures that would prevent serious disability. The initiative for the screening process rests with the health care system, rather than with the subject to be tested, who is generally well and may not even be aware that testing is being done. In some jurisdictions, screening is mandated by law. In most cases, consent to be tested is considered to be implied unless the subject or parent specifically objects. By testing in this manner, the state assumes responsibility for ensuring that resources are available to provide appropriate investigation and management of children identified by the testing program to be at high risk for disease (Scriver et al., 1978). The decision to introduce screening for a specific disorder requires consideration of the goal of the undertaking, the nature of the disease, the availability of a suitable test, and the characteristics of the population to be screened (National Academy of Sciences, 1975).

Screening to Enhance Medical Intervention

The introduction of screening for PKU in early infancy marked an important milestone in the application of public health measures to the primary prevention of disability (e.g., mental retardation) caused by a genetic defect—phenylalanine hydroxylase mutations (Scriver, 1982; Scriver et al., 1978). Early experience with the treatment of affected infants indicated that the severe mental retardation characteristic of the condition could be prevented by the early initiation of careful dietary phenylalanine restriction—before the manifestation of clinical signs of the disease (Scriver & Clow, 1980). The development of a simple, inexpensive, and reliable blood test for hyperphenylalaninemia (Guthrie & Susi, 1963) led to rapid and widespread adoption of screening for PKU throughout Europe and North America. In spite of incomplete participation and a high frequency of false-positive screening tests (Holtzman et al., 1974a and b), these screening programs resulted in a sharp decrease in the prevalence of mental retardation due to the disease (MacCready, 1974). Subsequently, guidelines emerged for the establishment and general operation of genetic screening programs (National Academy of Sciences, 1975). However, the apparent success of screening for PKU in newborn infants in the prevention of mental retardation has tended to obscure the fact that the screening process has produced its own problems. Inappropriate or overzealous treatment has been reported to cause illness and even death in some infants (Hanley et al., 1970); even the need to subject infants with false-positive test results to further testing may generate long-term parental concern about the health of their children (Holtzman, 1991; Sorenson et al., 1984).

Neonatal screening for other single-gene defects, such as galactosemia, congenital adrenogenital hyperplasia, sickle cell anemia, and cystic fibrosis, was developed despite the fact that the benefits of presymptomatic detection and treatment were not as well established as in the case of PKU. The importance of adequate public education and the availability of the resources needed to deal with children with positive test results has been stressed repeatedly (Bowman, 1977; Scriver, 1985; Wilfond & Fost, 1990), as has the need for rigorous, randomized, controlled trials of the value of presymptomatic detection and intervention (Holtzman, 1991). However, few sound studies of the effectiveness of genetic screening programs have actually been undertaken.

Screening for Reproductive Planning

Screening techniques have been applied to the identification of couples at risk for having children affected with certain autosomal recessive conditions because both parents are carriers of mutant genes that occur with high frequency in the population (Kaback, 1981). The goal of this type of screening is qualitatively different from that of screening for affected individuals. Whereas the rationale for screening for affected individuals is based on the availability of specific treatment that can reasonably be expected to improve significantly the natural course of the disease (e.g., dietary phenylalanine restriction in PKU), screening for carriers is based on the availability of measures to prevent the disease, usually prenatal diagnosis and selective termination of pregnancy, in the expectation that couples identified to be at high risk for having an affected child would avail themselves of these services.

Experience with early sickle cell screening programs in the United States has shown that screening for carriers of an autosomal recessive gene is potentially harmful (Bowman, 1991). Although many of the difficulties encountered were related to the prevalence of sickle cell disease among blacks, most were qualitatively similar to problems that might be anticipated in any such screening program. They included difficulties with the test used to screen for sickle hemoglobin—a test that did not differentiate sickle cell trait from sickle cell disease—and flaws in the educational material used in the promotion of the programs (Bowman, 1977). When combined with misguided discrimination by insurance companies and employers against individuals with the harmless sickle cell trait, the hasty introduction of legislation mandating sickle cell screening in a number of states, the distasteful nature of the only options available to those discovered to be at risk for having affected children, and confusion among medical practitioners and public health officials, these difficulties resulted in widespread public resistance to the programs. In contrast to this experience, prenatal thalassemia screening programs in Italy (Cao et al., 1984, 1989) and Greece (Loukopoulos, 1985) have met with a high level of acceptance and have resulted in sharp decreases in the incidence of the disease in these areas. Notably, in situations where this strategy has been most effective, intensive population educational programs have been undertaken along with the screening.

The development in the late 1960s of a biochemical test for carriers of the Tay-Sachs disease gene, coupled with the high frequency of the disease among Ashkenazi Jews, sparked the organization of a number of large-scale community screening clinics in the United States and Canada directed at identifying couples at risk for having offspring with the disease. The success of these voluntary clinics, organized and run primarily by members of the Jewish communities involved, led to a sharp decline in the incidence of this disease (Kaback, 1982). Since the mid-1970s, two additional approaches to Tay-Sachs carrier detection have evolved. In Montreal, Scriver and his associates began to screen high-school students (Clow & Scriver, 1974), an approach that was associated with high rates of participation without apparent stigmatization (Zeesman et al., 1984). Other centers developed case-finding approaches to Tay-Sachs carrier detection.

Case-Finding

Case-finding, rather than population screening, is another approach taken by most programs directed at the detection of carriers of recessive disease mutations (see Chapter 1). It is the process by which a health care professional carries out certain tests on selected individuals presenting to them for care, regardless of the problem that generated the consultation. The goal is the same as for screening: the detection of the risk of disease at an early stage when specific intervention might be expected to prevent it.

In case-finding, however, the fact that the process is initiated by the subject (in this case a parent), who is concerned about the possibility of some other illness, the nature of the contract between the individual and the health care system is different. The parties of the contract are the patient (or his or her parents) and the health care professional; although the health care professional may be personally held responsible for failing to provide what might be regarded as good general medical care as a result of having failed to examine the patient for the risk of some high-incidence, preventable, or treatable condition, the state is generally not involved. The responsibility for following up on the results of testing rests with the individual and the private physician, and the state would not normally be held responsible for ensuring that resources are available to provide further investigation or management, regardless of the implications to the patient, or to the state, for that matter.

A case-finding approach to the identification of individuals at high risk for genetic disease has worked well to reduce perinatal morbidity and mortality due to Rh disease (Zimmerman, 1973). In this instance, the acceptability of the preventive intervention (i.e., administration of immune globulin to Rh-negative women at the time of parturition) to both physician and patient is high. However, most case-finding programs aimed at identifying carriers of recessive genes, such as Tay-Sachs disease, involve complex counseling, and the options available for prevention—prenatal diagnosis and selective abortion—are not regarded with the same level of societal acceptance as administration of immune globulin. The Health Belief Model of Rosenstock (1966) has been applied in studies undertaken to determine what motivates individuals to present for testing for preventable genetic disease. According to the model, the decision by healthy individuals to seek preventive testing in the absence of symptoms of disease depends on their psychological readiness to take action with respect to a particular health condition; their belief that (1) the testing is feasible and appropriate and (2) it would reduce either their perceived susceptibility or the perceived severity of the health condition; and the lack of serious psychological barriers to the proposed action. Conventional variables in the Health Belief Model played a highly significant part in predicting the participation of partners of pregnant women who were being tested to determine if they were carriers of hemoglobinopathies (Rowley et al., 1991). On the other hand, in the case of Tay-Sachs carrier detection, none of the conventional motivating variables seemed to play a major role in the decision to undergo testing in one of the first metropolitan screening programs in the United States (Goldstein et al., 1977); identification as Jewish seemed to be the most important motivator, but the effect was weak.

Carrier detection by case-finding seems in general to have been regarded by those undergoing testing as an aspect of reproductive care, rather than part of reproductive planning. Its success requires the cooperation of primary care physicians—cooperation that has proved uncertain at best in the case of Tay-Sachs carrier detection (Beck et al., 1974; Clarke et al., 1989; Lowden et al., 1974), but which has been more successful in the case of programs aimed at detecting thalassemia carriers in Montreal (Scriver et al., 1984).

The advent of molecular genetic techniques has drastically altered the potential for screening for genetic disease (Clarke et al., 1990). The identification of common mutations, coupled with sensitive and highly specific molecular tests that can be applied to extremely small samples of blood or even saliva, has now made it possible to identify carriers of a wide variety of genotypes for which screening tests did not previously exist. As in any form of screening, this form of testing assumes a close and predictable correlation between genotype and disease phenotype. Although this assumption is usually sound in the case of mutations that have been shown to result in the production of no gene product, the majority of autosomal recessive diseases for which the mutations have been characterized are due to more subtle changes, and the relationship between mutation and phenotype is not as obvious. Some single base changes result in severe alterations in the production or stability of the gene product, whereas other mutations of this type are harmless. Before this type of screening is applied on any scale, it would be necessary to prove by appropriate expression of the mutant gene, clinical studies, and pedigree analyses that a specific mutation is responsible for the disease phenotype.

Studies have shown that, in specific populations, a relatively small number of specific mutations account for the majority of disease alleles for several relatively common diseases (Table 5.4).

In the case of cystic fibrosis, the most common lethal autosomal recessive disease affecting Caucasian children, testing for four to seven mutations would detect about 85% of CF carriers (Beaudet, 1990). Hence, the potential exists to prevent the disease by identifying couples at risk for having affected children and offering them prenatal diagnosis and the option to terminate the pregnancy should the fetus be found to be affected. However, there is considerable difference of opinion with regard to the advisability of proceeding with large-scale population screening (Wilfond & Fost, 1990). Hesitancy stems from the inability to test for a sufficient number of CF mutations, differences in the frequency of specific CF mutations in different subpopulations, uncertainties concerning the relationship between specific mutations and severity of the disease in affected infants, and the requirement for abortion as the only means of preventing the disease. For these and other reasons, in the United States it has been recommended that population-based carrier testing for CF not be implemented at this time (Caskey et al., 1990; Workshop on Population Screening for the Cystic Fibrosis Gene, 1990). Recently published studies of the attitudes of participants in a pilot program to screen for CF carriers in the United Kingdom suggested

Table 5.4. Common Mutations in Specific Populations

Disease	Ethnic Group	Mutation	%	Reference
Cystic fibrosis	Danish	ΔF508	87	Romeo & Devoto, 1990
	German	ΔF508	62–77	Romeo & Devoto, 1990
	French	ΔF508	67–75	Romeo & Devoto, 1990
	British	ΔF508	70	Romeo & Devoto, 1990
	Italian	ΔF508	42–54	Romeo & Dovoto, 1990
	Israeli Jews	ΔF508	32	Romeo & Devoto, 1990
	Turkish	ΔF508	27	Romeo & Dovoto, 1990
PKU	Hungarian	R408W	55	Romeo & Devoto, 1990
		IVS-12, splice	5	Romeo & Devoto, 1990
	Danes	R408W	20	Romeo & Devoto, 1990
		IVS-12, splice	38	Romeo & Devoto, 1990
	Scots	R408W	11	Romeo & Devoto, 1990
		IVS-12, splice	5	Romeo & Devoto, 1990
	Japanese	R413P	27	Wang et al., 1991
	Yemenite Jews	Exon 3 del	100	Avigad et al., 1990
β-thalassemia	Italian	IVS-1, nt 110	31	Cao et al., 1989
		Nonsense 39	27	Cao et al., 1989
	Greek	IVS-1, nt 110	8	Cao et al., 1989
		Nonsense 39	67	Cao et al., 1989
	Asian Indian	IVS-1, nt 5	36	Kazazian et al., 1984
Tay-Sachs disease	Ashkenazi Jews	Exon 11, 4 bp ins	70	Triggs-Raine et al., 1990
		IVS-12, splice	30	Triggs-Raine et al., 1990
Gaucher's disease	Ashkenazi Jews	N370S	73	Zimran et al., 1991

that fears concerning the potentially harmful psychological effects of screening may be exaggerated (Mennie et al., 1992; Watson et al., 1992). However, the results must be considered preliminary; screening in such situations should be undertaken cautiously with ample regard for the many social and psychological issues involved (Editorial, 1992).

Factors Influencing the Decision to Screen

A general consensus on the indications and conditions for genetic screening was achieved some years ago (Scriver; 1985). These indications include the following:

The specific rationale for genetic screening should be defined; namely, whether the goal is medical intervention, family planning, or research.

Population screening for medical intervention should not be performed outside an integrated program capable of information dispersal, screening, retrieval of persons with positive tests, diagnosis, counseling, medical management, and outcome evaluation.

The screening procedure should maximize specificity (by counting false-positive tests), sensitivity (by counting false-negative tests), and predictive efficiency (ratio of true-positive to false-positive tests) of the test. Proficiency testing should be implemented to monitor performance.

The contribution of ethnic and geographic factors to variation of the phenotype should be considered when designing and implementing programs.

Participation should be informed and in keeping with the relevant mores of the society; participants should acquire accurate information relevant to their needs.

Information about the rationale and goal of the program and the meaning of test results should be available to participants, physicians, and all other personnel affected by the program.

The outcome and impact of the program, whether for service or research in medical, economic, social, and legal contexts, should be evaluated. Its policy should be sufficiently flexible so that practice can be modified in keeping with developments and findings.

The availability of a simple, reliable, and inexpensive screening test is a necessary, though not sufficient, condition for screening. For genetic conditions, the test should be easy to perform and preferably adaptable to automation. The accuracy and precision must be satisfactory under the conditions of screening. The sensitivity, specificity, and predictive value of positive and negative tests should be known and acceptable. The specimen required for testing should be easily and safely obtainable and be stable under potentially adverse conditions of transport and storage.

Severity and the availability of treatment that demonstrably improves the natural course of the disease have been generally accepted criteria for screening for individuals affected with any condition. Moreover, the benefits of early detection and treatment, in terms of life-span and productivity gained, should generally exceed the costs of the screening process, including the costs dealing with subjects with false-positive test results. Put another way, the costs of screening and early management of high-risk subjects identified by the process should be less than the costs of not screening in terms of suffering, lost productivity, and hospitalization. These conditions have been met with regard to neonatal screening for PKU (Holtzman et al., 1981) and congenital hypothyroidism (Scriver, 1985) and for carrier testing for β-thalassemia (Ostrowsky et al., 1985).

Although there is currently no treatment available that has been shown unambiguously to alter significantly the course of Duchenne muscular dystrophy (DMD), presymptomatic screening for boys with the disease has been suggested as a means of identifying carriers of the mutation in order to prevent recurrence in subsequent sons (Plauchu et al., 1980; Smith et al., 1989). Whether or not this has been achieved in any of the few large-scale DMD screening programs has not been rigorously tested. The ethical propriety of screening newborn infants for the potential benefit of others when the infant being tested will not benefit has been questioned (Knoppers & Laberge, 1990).

The characteristics of the candidate population to be considered include the incidence of the disease, the perception of risk among those screened, and the acceptance of screening—including acceptance of the management options available to them (Bowman, 1977; Hastings Center, 1972; National Academy of Sciences, 1975). Experience with screening for the sickle cell trait underscored the dangers of stigmatization of individuals identified as carriers of the sickle cell gene and the potential for fueling racial tensions (Bowman, 1977; Kenen & Schmidt, 1978; Whitten & Fichoff, 1974). The same concerns existed with respect to Tay-Sachs carrier screening among Jews. However, unlike sickle trait screening programs, the initial drive for early Tay-Sachs screening programs in the United States and Canada developed from within the target communities, and participation was generally good. Community participation in the planning and operation of genetic screening programs of this type seems to be critical to their success.

Other Interventions

Prenatal Diagnosis

Although effective treatment may not be available for the majority of single-gene defects causing disease in children, many are preventable by early prenatal diagnosis and selective termination of pregnancy. Table 5.5 shows a list of prenatal diagnostic modalities and some selected examples of the application of the procedures.

Coupled with screening for carriers, the application of prenatal diagnosis has decreased the incidence of Tay-Sachs disease among Ashkenazi Jews and of β-thalassemia in some regions of the Mediterranean basin. In other instances, the impact has not been as great. Although the parents of children with PKU seen in the PKU Clinic of the Hospital for Sick Children have been counseled routinely over the past 5 years concerning the availability of prevention of the disease in

Table 5.5. Prenatal Diagnosis of Single-Gene Defects Causing Disease in Children

Disease	Modality	Abnormality
	Structural Abnormality	
X-linked hydrocephalus	Ultrasound	Demonstration of enlarged head
Meckel-Gruber syndrome	Ultrasound	Demonstration of neural tube defect
	Cellular Abnormality	
Mucolipidosis IV	Amniocentesis	Ultrastructural abnormality in cultured amniotic fluid cells
Batten disease	Amniocentesis	Ultrastructural abnormality in amniotic fluid cells
	Metabolite Analysis	
Hereditary tyrosinemia	Amniocentesis	Succinylacetone in amniotic fluid
	Enzyme Analysis	
Lysosomal storage diseases	CVS or amniocentesis	Deficiency of enzyme activity
	Secondary Biochemical Abnormality	
Cystic fibrosis	Amniocentesis	Elevated levels of intestinal enzymes in amniotic fluid
Meckel-Gruber syndrome	Amniocentesis	Elevated levels of α-fetoprotein in amniotic fluid
	DNA Analysis	
Cystic fibrosis	CVS	Haplotype analysis ± demonstration of specific mutation
Tay-Sachs disease	CVS	Demonstration of specific mutation
β-Thalassemia	CVS	Demonstration of specific mutation
Phenylketonuria	CVS	Haplotype analysis ± demonstration of specific mutation

Source: Adapted from Scriver et al., 1989.

future offspring by prenatal diagnosis, only one couple has requested the service. Over the same period, a total of 22 children have been born to these couples; 7 were affected with the disease, 12 were unaffected, and three pregnancies ended in miscarriage (WB Hanley, unpublished observations). The apparent lack of interest in pursuing prenatal diagnosis is likely attributable to the fact that the condition is treatable.

A survey in the United Kingdom, which sampled the attitudes of individuals with no family history of cystic fibrosis, showed that participation in carrier testing depended greatly on the setting in which the offer was made, from a high of 87% among those seen personally in a family planning clinic setting to as low as 10% among those contacted solely by mail (Watson et al., 1991). The survey also confirmed that the general level of understanding of the genetic principles involved in the prevention of CF through carrier detection and prenatal diagnosis was low. The reported attitudes toward prenatal diagnosis showed a great deal of uncertainty among those questioned, which probably reflected how little the respondents knew about the disease and the genetic risks involved. Another survey in the United States of parents of children with cystic fibrosis (CF) showed that the majority felt the availability of prenatal diagnosis provided an important reproductive option for families at risk for the disease (Kaback et al., 1984).

In contrast, in three of the nine cases over the past 4 years in which fetuses were found by prenatal diagnosis at the Hospital for Sick Children to be affected with CF, the couple elected not to terminate the pregnancies (E. Hutton, personal communication). Others have reported a similar experience; at Baylor College of Medicine in Houston, 7 couples out of 14 who were found, by prenatal diagnosis, to be carrying affected fetuses elected to continue the pregnancies (AL Beaudet, personal communication). All the couples concerned had living children affected with CF. The preliminary analysis of the outcomes of a Canadian neonatal screening program for Duchenne muscular dystrophy indicated that many women identified as carriers of DMD subsequent to the birth of an affected infant chose not to undergo prenatal diagnosis during their next pregnancy. A total of 14 DMD carriers were identified as a result of the detection of five infant boys with presymptomatic disease. There were seven pregnancies among five of these women after they were identified and counseled as carriers. Prenatal diagnosis was sought for only one of the pregnancies, and two of the other six yielded affected male infants (C Greenberg, personal communication). The adult siblings and other relatives of children who have died of CF or DMD apparently seem more likely to pursue the possibility of prenatal diagnosis and to terminate a pregnancy if the fetus is found to be affected. This had led to speculation that experience with the later, more debilitating stages of the diseases is a major factor for those contemplating prevention of the disease by this approach. More research is required to identify the factors affecting decision making in these and other similar situations. In the meantime, although testing to identify carriers and the availability of prenatal diagnosis will permit couples to make informed decisions about reproduction, considerable additional information about the implications of test results and a better understanding of reproductive options available would be necessary before widespread population screening for carriers of specific mutations is undertaken (Wilfond & Fost, 1990).

Environmental Manipulation

The environmental approach to the management of single-gene defects in children requires acknowledgment of the fact that mutant gene expression is ultimately the outcome of interaction between all genes, including the mutant allele, and the environment. Each individual possesses genetic variations that affect the balance between adaptive and maladaptive genetic and environmental influences; the extent to which environmental pressures are responsible for departures from wellness may determine the responsiveness of the condition to therapeutic environmental manipulation. General strategies with some examples are shown in Table 5.6.

In many inherited metabolic diseases, the damage occurring as a result of the mutation is due either to accumulation of toxic metabolites proximal to the reaction affected, deficiency of products of the reaction, or a combination of both. In the first case, accumulation of toxic metabolites may be prevented by dietary restriction of the metabolites themselves or of their precursors, as long as endogenous biosynthesis of the metabolites is relatively insignificant. This is the basis for the treatment of hereditary disorders of essential amino acid metabolism, such as phenylketonuria, by dietary protein restriction. If the deleterious effects of the mutation are due to deficiency of the product of the reaction affected, replacement of the product often results in near normalization. Treatment of vitamin B_{12}-responsive methylmalonic aciduria with pharmacologic doses

Table 5.6. Treatment of Genetic Disease

Strategy	Disease	Treatment
	Clinical Phenotype	
Avoidance	Pseudocholine esterase deficiency	Avoidance of depolarizing muscle relaxants
Pharmacologic manipulation	Neurodegenerative disorders	Anticonvulsants
Surgical correction	Familial polyposis coli	Colectomy
	Metabolite	
Substrate restriction	Phenylketonuria	Dietary phenylalanine restriction
Alternative pathway	Urea cycle enzyme defects	Benzoate and phenylacetate
Metabolic inhibition	Familial hypercholesterolemia	HMG-CoA reductase inhibitors
Product replacement	Congenital adrenal hyperplasia	Cortisol and mineralocorticoids
	Dysfunctional Protein	
Activation	Homocystinuria	Pyridoxine
Replacement	Hemophilia	Factor VIII
	Organ Transplantation	
Source of gene product	β-thalassemia	Bone marrow transplantation
Replacement of damaged organ	Fabry disease	Kidney transplantation

Source: Adapted from Scriver et al., 1989.

of the vitamin is an example of reversal of the metabolic consequences of the defect in organic acid metabolism. Other examples are shown in Table 5.7.

In some cases, the pathogenesis of the disease caused by an inborn error of metabolism is not known, or the accumulating toxic metabolites or areas of the body damaged by deficiency of the product of an enzyme reaction are not accessible. In these instances, effective treatment has yet to be developed.

Mutant Gene Product Replacement

In many cases, reversal of the clinical consequences of a protein deficiency caused by mutation of the gene coding for its synthesis is achievable by simple replacement of the protein. The treatment of hemophilia A with exogenous Factor VIII is an example of successful management of the bleeding diathesis by replacement of the gene product.

Another area in which replacement of the gene product is proving to be particularly promising is enzyme replacement therapy. However, for this process to work, there must be an adequate supply of purified exogenous enzyme, it must be safe to administer, it must be distributed to areas of the body where it is needed, it must have a reasonable biologic half-life after ingestion or injection, it must not raise an immune response, and it should be reasonably inexpensive because treatment is likely to be lifelong. The treatment of adenosine deaminase (ADA) deficiency by infusion of exogenous polyethylene glycol-treated enzyme has been shown to be effective in restoring the immune system in children affected with severe combined immunodeficiency disease (SCID; Hershfield & Chaffee, 1991). More recently, the periodic administration of modified human placental lysosomal glucocerebrosidase has been shown to be effective in reversing some aspects of Gaucher's disease (Barton et al., 1991).

Allogeneic bone marrow transplantation is effective in the treatment of severe

Table 5.7. Inherited Metabolic Diseases that Respond to Cofactor/Enzyme Therapy

Coenzyme/Vitamin	Disorder	Enzyme Defect
	Coenzyme Binding Defects	
Pyridoxine	Cystathioninuria	Cystathionase
	Classical homocystinuria	Cystathionine β-synthase
	Hyperornithinemia with gyrate atrophy	Ornithine α-aminotransferase
	Xanthurenic aciduria	Kynureninase
	B_6-dependent seizures	Glutamic acid decarboxylase
	Coenzyme Synthesis Defects	
Cobalamin	Methylmalonic acidemia (cbl A, B)	Methylmalonyl-CoA mutase
	Homocystinuria and methylmalonic aciduria (cbl C, D, F)	Methionine synthase and methylmalonyl-CoA mutase
	Homocystinuria (cbl E, G)	Methionine synthase
Folate	Methylenetetrahydrofolate reductase deficiency	Methionine synthase
Biopterin	Hyperphenylalaninemia	Aromatic amino acid hydroxylases
Biotin	Multiple carboxylase deficiency	Carboxylases
Riboflavin	Glutaric acidemia, type II	Electron-transfer flavoprotein

Source: Adapted from Levy, 1991.

combined immunodeficiency syndrome (SCIDS) due to adenosine deaminase deficiency and of the hematopoietic defect in β-thalassemia (Lucarelli et al., 1987). However, this form of treatment is expensive and involves high morbidity and significant risk of mortality. More recently it has been employed as a means of introducing a continuing supply of enzyme for the replacement therapy of some lysosomal storage diseases (Krivit & Shapiro, 1991). Some promising preliminary results have been reported. However, determining the long-term role of this approach to treatment in the management of lysosomal storage diseases will require further study.

Gene Transfer Therapy

Several genetic defects in mice have been corrected successfully by germline gene therapy (Desnick & Schuchman, 1991). Research is currently in progress to explore the feasibility of somatic cell gene therapy in animal models of human disease and ultimately in primary human genetic diseases. Inborn errors of metabolism affecting primarily hematopoietic tissues, such as adenosine deaminase deficiency, are particularly promising candidates for gene therapy. The need for targeting a relatively inaccessible tissue (i.e. the brain) and tissue-specific gene expression make the outlook for gene therapy of such diseases as Tay-Sachs disease less promising. The total impact of this form of treatment on the prevalence of single-gene defects in human populations is unlikely to be significant in the foreseeable future.

Evaluation of Interventions

Although some of the above strategies have been shown to be dramatically successful in their short-term effect on gross mortality, few have been subjected to rigorous evaluation of long-term outcomes. This is due in part to the relative rarity of the individual conditions and the marked clinical heterogeneity within each class of disorders.

The evaluation of the treatment of phenylketonuria merits detailed review for it underscores some of the difficulties encountered in the assessment of treatment of rare genetic diseases in general. It is one of the few single-gene defects affecting children for which there are sufficient numbers of cases to generate statistically significant comparison groups. Even so, the condition is uncommon enough to require participation of several collaborating centers, which introduces the potential for variations in the selection of patients and controls and their management. Other confounding variables include variations in commitment to the treatment, which is itself technically difficult for the subjects and their parents, and clinical and genetic heterogeneity. The evaluation of other treatments, such as bone marrow transplantation, for rarer, more heterogeneous conditions, such as the lysosomal storage diseases, is likely to be even more difficult (Krivit & Shapiro, 1991).

In spite of the apparent benefit, which was evident by the mid-1960s, of dietary phenylalanine restriction for the prevention of mental retardation in children with PKU, some investigators continued to challenge the effectiveness of the treatment (Bessman, 1966). In the course of a large, multicenter study undertaken to resolve the issue, a group of infants identified through screening in the newborn period was studied prospectively (Williamson et al., 1977). However, dietary therapy by then was sufficiently widely accepted that a randomized on-diet/off-diet study was considered to be unethical. Therefore, all infants with the disease were studied on therapeutic diets and their growth and development compared with that of untreated older affected siblings and that of unaffected siblings. Unfortunately, although all the treated children did well, the untreated, affected control group was too small to permit meaningful statistical comparisons. By the time the study was completed, however, the evidence supporting the benefit of dietary treatment was considered to be overwhelming. Attention turned instead to the evaluation of the effect of termination of the therapeutic diet.

Although the results of early studies had indicated that diet termination at age 5 to 6 years was safe (Holtzman et al., 1975), there was considerable anecdotal and experimental evidence suggesting that termination of dietary phenylalanine restriction was associated with subtle, though significant, intellectual deterioration in at least some affected individuals. Formal evaluation of the problem, by the same multicenter group that undertook the original evaluation of the efficacy of dietary phenylalanine restriction (Williamson et al., 1977), was flawed by the way the subjects redistributed themselves after randomization. At age 6, each child in the original study was randomly assigned to one of two groups: one to continue and the other to discontinue the therapeutic diet. Unfortunately, only 46% of those originally randomized remained in their assigned groups through age 8 years when the results were analyzed (Koch et al., 1982). The study was further confounded by the variable dietary control achieved by those children assigned to the diet continuation group. Yet, further analysis of the data, along with the results of other studies (Smith et al., 1978), seemed to confirm the suspicion that discontinuation of dietary phenylalanine restriction in later childhood was associated with intellectual deterioration in at least some children with phenylketonuria (Holtzman et al., 1986).

Conclusions

Recent and continuing advances in molecular biology have added a great deal to what is known about the epidemiology of single-gene disorders in children. By relatively simple testing, it has become possible to identify a large number of specific mutations, to determine their frequency in various populations, and to estimate their total contribution to morbidity and mortality. The techniques for the rapid and accurate detection of infants affected with various common genetic disorders, and the identification of those at high risk for having children affected with these diseases, are now available and are being applied, in some cases on a large scale, in the prevention of the diseases or disability arising from them. However, there remain a large number of social and ethical issues to resolve before the full impact of screening and preventive intervention can be realized. The current treatment of most specific genetic diseases is based primarily on environmental manipulation, though effective enzyme replacement therapy seems now to be available for some disorders. In only a few instances has the effectiveness of treatment of any single-gene disease in children been evaluated systematically.

References

Adams J, Lam DA, Hermalin AI, Smouse PE, eds. *Convergent Issues in Genetics and Demography*. New York: Oxford University Press; 1990.

Antonarakis SE. Diagnosis of genetic disorders at the DNA level. *N Engl J Med* 1989; 320:153–163.

Antonarakis SE, Phillips IJA, Kazazian HH. Genetic diseases: diagnosis by restriction endonuclease analysis. *J Pediatr* 1982; 100:845–856.

Avigad S, Cohen BE, Bauer S, Schwartz G, Frydman M, Woo SLC, Niny Y, Shiloh Y. A single origin of phenylketonuria in Yemenite Jews. *Nature* 1990; 344:168–170.

Baird PA. Measuring birth defects and handicapping disorders in the population: the British Columbia Health Surveillance Registry. *Can Med Assoc J* 1987; 36:109–110.

Baird PA, Anderson TW, Newcombe HB, Lowry RB. Genetic disorders in children and young adults: a population study. *Am J Hum Genet* 1988; 42:677–693.

Barton NW, Brady RO, Dambrosia JM, Di Bisceglie AM, Doppelt SH, Hill SC, Mankin HJ, Murray GJ, Parker RI, Argoff CE, Grewal RP, Yu K-T, et al. Replacement therapy for inherited enzyme deficiency—macrophage-targeted glucocerebrosidase for Gaucher's disease. *N Engl J Med* 1991; 324:1464–1470.

Baxter PS, Goldhill J, Hardcastle J, Hardcastle PT, Taylor CJ. Accounting for cystic fibrosis. *Nature* 1988; 335:211.

Beaudet AL. Carrier screening for cystic fibrosis. *Am J Hum Genet* 1990; 47:603–605 (editorial).

Beck E, Blaichman S, Scriver CR, Clow CL. Advocacy and compliance in genetic screening. Behavior of physicians and clients in a voluntary program for testing for the Tay-Sachs gene. *N Engl J Med* 1974; 291:1166–1170.

Bessman SP. Legislation and advances in medical knowledge: acceleration or inhibition? *J Pediatr* 1966; 69:334–338.

Bowman JE. Genetic screening programs and public policy. *Phylon* 1977; 38:117–142.

Bowman JE. Prenatal screening for hemoglobinopathies. *Am J Hum Genet* 1991; 48:433–438.

Bowman JE, Murray JRF, eds. *Genetic Variation and Disorders in Peoples of African Origin*. Baltimore: Johns Hopkins University Press; 1990.

Cao A, Pintus L, Lecca U, et al. Control of homozygous β-thalassemia by carrier screening and antenatal diagnosis in Sardinians. *Clin Genet* 1984; 26:12–22.

Cao A, Gossens M, Pirastu M. β-Thalassemia mutations in Mediterranean populations. *Br J Haematol* 1989; 71:309–312.

Caskey CT, Kaback MM, Beaudet AL. The American Society of Human Genetics statement on cystic fibrosis screening. *Am J Hum Genet* 1990; 46:393.

Clarke JTR, Skomorowski MA, Zuker S. Tay-Sachs disease carrier screening: follow-up of a case-finding approach. *Am J Med Genet* 1989; 34:601–605.

Clarke JTR, Gravel RA, Mahuran DJ. Carrier screening for Tay-Sachs disease: prospects for direct mutation analysis. In: Knoppers BM, Laberge CM, eds. *Genetic Screening: from Newborns to DNA Typing*. Amsterdam: Elsevier Science Publishers; 1990:179–195.

Clow CL, Scriver CR. Knowledge about and attitudes towards genetic screening among high-school students—Tay-Sachs experience. *Pediatrics* 1974; 59:86–91.

Cordero JF. Registries of birth defects and genetic diseases. *Ped Clin North Am* 1992; 39:65–77.

Crow JF. *Basic Concepts in Population, Quantitative and Evolutionary Genetics*. New York: W.H. Freeman & Co; 1986.

Daiger SP, Chakraborty R, Reed L, Fekete G, Schuler D, Berenssi G, Nasz I, Brdicka R, Kamaryt J, Pijackova A, Moore S, Sullivan S, Woo SLC. Polymorphic DNA haplotypes at the phenylalanine hydroxylase (PAH) locus in European families with phenylketonuria (PKU). *Am J Hum Genet* 1989a; 45:310–318.

Daiger SP, Reed L, Huang S-S, Zeng Y-T, Wang T, Lo WHY, Okano Y, Hase Y, Fukuda Y, Oura T, Tada K, Woo SLC. Polymorphic DNA haplotypes at the phenylalanine hydroxylase (PAH) locus in Asian families with phenylketonuria (PAH). *Am J Hum Genet* 1989b; 45:319–324.

Day N, Holmes LB. The incidence of genetic disease in a university hospital population. *Am J Hum Genet* 1973; 25:237–246.

Desnick RJ, Schuchman EH. Human gene therapy: strategies and prospects for inborn errors of metabolism. In: Desnick RJ, ed. *Treatment of Genetic Diseases*. New York: Churchill Livingstone; 1991:239–259.

Editorial. Screening for cystic fibrosis. *Lancet* 1992; 340:209–210.

Edwards A, Civitello A, Hammond HA, Caskey CT. DNA typing and genetic mapping with trimeric and tetrameric tandem repeats. *Am J Hum Genet* 1991; 49:746–756.

Eisenstein BI. The polymerase chain reaction. A new method of using molecular genetics for medical diagnosis. *N Engl J Med* 1990; 322:178–183.

Eriksson AW, Forsius H, Nevanlinna HR, Workman PL, Norio RK, eds. *Population Structure and Genetic Disorders*. London: Academic Press; 1980.

Goldstein MS, Greenwald S, Nathan T, Massarik F, Kaback MM. Health behavior and genetic screening for carriers of Tay-Sachs disease: a prospective study. *Soc Sci Med* 1977; 11:515–520.

Goodman RM. *Genetic Disorders among the Jewish People*. Baltimore: Johns Hopkins University Press; 1979.

Guthrie R, Susi A. A simple phenylalanine method for detecting phenylketonuria in large populations of newborn infants. *Pediatrics* 1963; 32:338–343.

Hall JG, Powers EK, McIlvaine RT, Ean VH. The frequency and familial burden of genetic disease in a pediatric hospital. *Am J Med Genet* 1978; 1:416–436.

Hanley WB, Linsao L, Davidson W, Moes CAF. Malnutrition with early treatment of phenylketonuria. *Pediatr Res* 1970; 4:318–327.

Harris H. *The Principles of Human Biochemical Genetics*. 4th ed. Amsterdam: North-Holland; 1980.

Hastings Center. Ethical and social issues in screening for genetic disease. *N Engl J Med* 1972; 186:1129–1132.

Hershfield MS, Chaffee S. PEG-enzyme replacement therapy for adenosine deaminase deficiency. In: Desnick RJ, ed. *Treatment of Genetic Diseases*. New York: Churchill Livingstone; 1991; 169–182.

Holtzman NA. What drives neonatal screening programs? *N Engl J Med* 1991; 325:802–804.

Holtzman NA, Meek AG, Mellits ED. Neonatal screening for phenylketonuria. I. Effectiveness. *JAMA* 1974a; 229:667–670.

Holtzman NA, Meek AG, Mellitts ED. Neonatal screening for phenylketonuria. IV. Factors influencing the occurrence of false positives. *Am J Publ Health* 1974b; 64:775–779.

Holtzman NA, Welcher DW, Mellits ED. Randomized controlled study of diet termination in phenylketonuria. *N Engl J Med* 1975; 293:1121–1124.

Holtzman NA, Leonard CO, Farfel MR. Issues in antenatal and neonatal screening and surveillance for hereditary and congenital disorders. *Annu Rev Pub Health* 1981; 2:219–251.

Holtzman NA, Kronmal RA, van Doorninck W, Azen C, Koch R. Effect of age at loss of dietary control on intellectual performance and behavior of children with phenylketonuria. *N Engl J Med* 1986; 314:593–598.

Jeffreys AJ. DNA sequence variants in the Gg-, Ag-, δ- and β-globin genes of man. *Cell* 1979; 18:1–10.

Johnson JP. Genetic counseling using linked DNA probes: cystic fibrosis as a prototype. *J Pediatr* 1988; 113:957–964.

Kaback MM. Screening for recessive gene carriers in clinical practice. In: Kaback MM, ed. *Genetic Issues in Pediatric and Obstetric Practice*. Chicago: Year Book Medical Publishers; 1981:489–500.

Kaback MM. Screening for reproductive counseling: social, ethical, and medicolegal issues in the Tay-Sachs disease experience. *Prog Clin Biol Res* 1982; 103B:447–459.

Kaback MM, Zippin D, Boyd P, Cantor R, Lewiston W, Davis B, Dooley R, Giammons S, Harwood I, Kagan B, Kurland G, Osher A, Rucker R, Stiehm R, Wang C. Attitudes toward prenatal diagnosis of cystic fibrosis among parents of affected children. In: Lawson D, ed. *Cystic Fibrosis Horizons. Proceedings of the 9th International Cystic Fibrosis Congress*. Chichester: John Wiley & Sons; 1984:15–28.

Kalaydjieva L, Dworniczak B, Kucinskas V, Yurgeliavicius V, Kunert E, Horst J. Geographic distribution gradients of the major PKU mutations and the linked haplotypes. *Hum Genet* 1991; 86:411–413.

Kan YW, Dozy AM. Polymorphism of DNA sequence adjacent to human β-globin structural gene: relationship to sickle mutation. *Proc Natl Acad Sci USA* 1978; 75:5631–5635.

Kaplan F, Kokotsis G, Capua A, Scriver CR. Quantitation of beta-thalassemia genes in Quebec immigrants of Mediterranean, Southeast Asian, and Asian Indian origins. *Clin Invest Med* 1991; 14:325–330.

Kazazian JHH. The thalassemia syndromes: molecular basis and prenatal diagnosis in 1990. *Sem Haematol* 1990; 27:209–228.

Kazazian JHH, Orkin SH, Antonarakis SE, Sexton JP, Boehm CD, Goff SC, Waber PG. Molecular characterization of seven β-thalassemia mutations in Asian Indians. *EMBO J* 1984; 3:593–596.

Kenen RH, Schmidt RM. Stigmatization of carrier status: social implications of heterozygote genetic screening programs. *Am J Pub Health* 1978; 68:1116–1120.

Kidd KK. Phenylketonuria: population genetics of a disease. *Nature* 1987; 327:282–283.

Knoppers BM, Laberge CM, eds. *Genetic Screening: from Newborns to DNA Typing*. Amsterdam: Elsevier Science Publishers; 1990.

Koch R, Azen CG, Friedman EG, Williamson ML. Preliminary report on the effects of diet discontinuation in phenylketonuria. *J Pediatr* 1982; 100:870–875.

Konecki DS, Lichter-Konecki U. The phenylketonuria locus: current knowledge about alleles and mutations of the phenylalanine hydroxylase gene in various populations. *Hum Genet* 1991; 87:377–388.

Kramm ER, Crane MM, Sirkin MG, Brown ML. A cystic fibrosis pilot survey in three New England states. *Am J Pub Health* 1962; 52:2041–2057.

Krivit W, Shapiro EG. Bone marrow transplantation for storage diseases. In: Desnick

RJ, ed. *Treatment of Genetic Diseases*. New York: Churchill Livingstone; 1991:203–221.

Laberge C. Hereditary tyrosinemia in a French-Canadian isolate. *Am J Hum Genet* 1969; 21:36–45.

Laberge C, Scriver CR, Clow CL, Dufour D. Le réseau de médecine génétique du Québec: un programme intégre de diagnostic, conseil et traitement des maladies métaboliques héréditaires. *Union Méd Can* 1975; 104:428–432.

Landegren U, Kaiser R, Caskey C, Hood L. DNA diagnostics—molecular techniques and automation. *Science* 1988; 242:229–237.

Lawn RM, Fritsch EF, Parker RC, Blake G, Maniatis T. The isolation and characterization of linked δ- and β-globin genes from a cloned library of human DNA. *Cell* 1978; 15:1157–1174.

Lemieux B, Auray-Blais C, Giguere R, Shapcott D, Scriver CR. Newborn urine screening experience with over one million infants in the Quebec Network of Genetic Medicine. *J Inher Metab Dis* 1988; 11:45–55.

Levy HL. Nutritional therapy in inborn errors of metabolism. In: Desnick RJ, ed. *Treatment of Genetic Diseases*. New York: Churchill Livingstone; 1991:1–22.

Loukopoulos D. Prenatal diagnosis of thalassemia and of the hemoglobinopathies: a review. *Hemoglobin* 1985; 9:435–459.

Lowden JA, Zuker S, Wilensky AJ, Skomorowski MA. Screening for carriers of Tay-Sachs disease: a community project. *Can Med Assoc J* 1974; 111:229–233.

Lowry RB, Miller JR, Scott AE, Renwick DHG. The British Columbia registry for handicapped children and adults: evolutionary changes over twenty years. *Can J Pub Health* 1975; 66:322–326.

Lucarelli G, Galimberti M, Polchi P, Giardini C, Politi P, Baronciani D, Angelucci E, Manenti F, Delfini C, Aureli G, Muretto P. Marrow transplantation in patients with advanced thalassemia. *N Engl J Med* 1987; 316:1050–1055.

MacCready RA. Admissions of phenylketonuric patients to residential institutions before and after screening programs of the newborn infant. *J Pediatr* 1974; 85:383–385.

Menkes JH. Genetic disorders of mitochondrial function. *J Pediatr* 1987; 110:255–259.

Mennie ME, Gilfillan A, Compton M, Curtis L, Liston WA, Pullen I, Whyte DA, Brock DJH. Prenatal screening for cystic fibrosis. *Lancet* 1992; 340:214–218.

Morton NE. *Outline of Genetic Epidemiology*. Basel: S. Karger AG; 1982.

Nakamura Y, Leppert M, O'Connell P, Wolff R, Holm T, Culver M, Martin C, et al. Variable number of tandem repeat (VNTR) markers for human gene mapping. *Science* 1987; 235:1616–1622.

National Academy of Sciences (National Research Council). *Genetic Screening. Programs, Principles, and Research*. Washington: National Academy of Sciences; 1975.

Orkin SH, Kazazian JHH. The mutation and polymorphism of the human β-globin gene and its surrounding DNA. *Annu Rev Genet* 1984; 18:131–171.

Ostrowsky JT, Lippman A, Scriver CR. Cost-benefit analysis of a thalassemia disease prevention program. *Am J Pub Health* 1985; 75:732–736.

Ott J. *Analysis of Human Genetic Linkage*. Rev ed. Baltimore: Johns Hopkins University Press; 1991.

Plauchu H, Dellamonica C, Cotte J, Robert JM. Duchenne muscular dystrophy: systematic neonatal screening and earlier detection of carriers. *J Genet Hum* 1980; 28:65–82.

Polani PE. The incidence of developmental and other genetic abnormalities. *Guy's Hosp Rep* 1973; 122:53–63.

Polednak AP. *Racial and Ethnic Differences in Disease*. New York: Oxford University Press; 1989.

Reich E, Wallace S, Ben-Yishay M, Schlesinger S, Marks J, Bloom A. Genetic disease in a pediatric hospital. *Am J Hum Genet* 1974; 26:71A.

Roberts DF, Chavez J, Court SDM. The genetic component in child mortality. *Arch Dis Child* 1970; 45:33–38.

Roberts RS, Spitzer WO, Delmore T, Sackett DL. An empirical demonstration of Berkson's bias. *J Chron Dis* 1978; 34:119–128.

Romeo G, Devoto M. Population analysis of the major mutation in cystic fibrosis. *Hum Genet* 1990; 85:391–445.

Rosenstock IM. Why people use health services. *Milbank Mem Fund* 1966; 44:94–127.

Rowley PT, Loader S, Sutera CJ, Walden M, Kozyra A. Prenatal screening for hemoglobinopathies. III. Applicability of the Health Belief Model. *Am J Hum Genet* 1991; 48:452–459.

Saiki RK, Scharf S, Faloona F, Mullis K, Horn G, Erlich H, Arnheim N. Enzymatic amplification of β-globin genomic sequences and restriction site analysis for diagnosis of sickle cell anemia. *Science* 1985; 230:1350–1354.

Saiki RK, Gelfand DH, Stoffel S, Scharf SJ, Higuchi R, Horn GT, Mullis KB, Erlich HA. Primer-directed enzymatic amplification of DNA with a thermostable DNA polymerase. *Science* 1988; 239:487–491.

Schwabe AD, Peters RS. Familial Mediterranean fever in Armenians. Analysis of 100 cases. *Medicine* 1974; 53:453–462.

Scriver CR. Screening for medical intervention: the PKU experience. *Prog Clin Biol Res* 1982; 103B:437–445.

Scriver CR. Population screening: report of a workshop. In: Marois M (ed) *Prevention of Physical and Mental Congenital Defects, Part B: Epidemiology, Early Detection and Therapy, and Environmental Factors*. New York: Alan R Liss Inc; 1985; 89–152.

Scriver CR, Clow CL. Phenylketonuria: epitome of human biochemical genetics. *N Engl J Med* 1980; 303:1336–1342 and 1394–1400.

Scriver CR, Neal JL, Saginur R, Clow A. The frequency of genetic disease and congenital malformation among patients in a pediatric hospital. *Can Med Assoc J* 1973; 108:1111–1115.

Scriver CR, Laberge C, Clow CL, Fraser FC. Genetics and medicine: an evolving relationship. *Science* 1978; 200:946–952.

Scriver CR, Bardanis M, Cartier L, Clow CL, Lancaster GA, Ostrowsky JT. Beta-thalassemia disease prevention: genetic medicine applied. *Am J Hum Genet* 1984; 36:1024–1038.

Scriver CR, Beaudet AL, Sly WS, Valle D, eds. *The Metabolic Basis of Inherited Disease*. 6th ed. New York: McGraw-Hill; 1989.

Smith I, Lobascher J, Stevenson J, Wolff OH, Schmidt H, Grubel-Kaiser S, Bickel H. Effect of stopping low-phenylalanine diet on intellectual progress in children with phenylketonuria. *Br Med J* 1978; 2:723–726.

Smith RA, Sibert JR, Wallace SJ, Harper PS. Early diagnosis and secondary prevention of Duchenne muscular dystrophy. *Arch Dis Child* 1989; 64:787–790.

Sorenson JR, Levy HL, Mangione TW, Sepe SJ. Parental response to repeat testing of infants with 'false-positive' results in a newborn screening program. *Pediatrics* 1984; 73:183–187.

Southern EM. Detecting of specific sequences among DNA fragments separated by gel electrophoresis. *J Mol Biol* 1975; 98:503–517.

Thompson MW, McInnes RR, Willard HF. *Genetics in Medicine*. 5th ed. Philadelphia: WB Saunders; 1991.

Triggs-Raine BL, Feigenbaum ASJ, Natowicz M, Skomorowski MA, Schuster SM, Clarke JTR, Mahuran DJ, Kolodny EH, Gravel RA. Screening for carriers of Tay-Sachs disease among Ashkenazi Jews—a comparison of DNA-based and enzyme-based tests. *N Engl J Med* 1990; 323:6–12.

Tsui L-C, Buchwald M. Biochemical and molecular genetics of cystic fibrosis. In: Harris H, Hirschhorn K, eds. *Advances in Human Genetics*. New York: Plenum Press; 1991:153–266.

Vogel F, Motulsky AG. *Human Genetics*. 2nd ed. Berlin: Springer-Verlag; 1986.

Wallace DC. Mitochondrial DNA mutations and neuromuscular disease. *Trends Genet* 1989; 5:9–13.

Wang T, Okano Y, Eisensmith RC, Harvey ML, Lo WHY, Huang S-Z, Zeng Y-T, Yuan L-F, Furuyama J-I, Oura T, Sommer SS, Woo SLC. Founder effect of a prevalent phenylketonuria mutation in the Oriental population. *Proc Natl Acad Sci USA* 1991; 88:2146–2150.

Watson EK, Mayall ES, Lamb J, Chapple J, Williamson R. Psychological and social consequences of community carrier screening programme for cystic fibrosis. *Lancet* 1992; 340:217–220.

Watson EK, Mayall E, Chapple J, Dalziel M, Harrington K, Williams C, Williamson R. Screening for carriers of cystic fibrosis through primary health care services. *Br Med J* 1991; 303:504–507.

Weatherall DJ. *The New Genetics and Clinical Practice*. 2nd ed. Oxford: Oxford University Press; 1985.

Whitten CF, Fichoff J. Psychosocial effects of sickle cell disease. *Arch Intern Med* 1974; 133:681–689.

Wilfond BS, Fost N. The cystic fibrosis gene: medical and social implications for heterozygote detection. *JAMA* 1990; 263:2777–2783.

Williamson M, Dobson JC, Koch R. Collaborative study of children treated for phenylketonuria: study design. *Pediatrics* 1977; 60:815–821.

Woo SLC. Molecular basis and population genetics of phenylketonuria. *Biochemistry* 1989; 28:1–7.

Workshop on Population Screening for the Cystic Fibrosis Gene. Statement from the National Institutes of Health. *N Engl J Med* 1990; 323:70–71.

Worton RG, Thompson MW. Genetics of Duchenne muscular dystrophy. *Annu Rev Genet* 1988; 22:601–629.

Zeesman S, Clow CL, Scriver CR. A private view of heterozygosity: eight-year follow-up study on carriers of the Tay-Sachs gene detected by high school screening in Montreal. *Am J Med Genet* 1984; 18:769–778.

Zimmerman DR. *Rh: The Intimate History of a Disease and Its Conquest*. New York: Macmillan; 1973.

Zimran A, Gelbart T, Westwood B, Grabowski GA, Beutler E. High frequency of the Gaucher disease mutation at nucleotide 1226 among Ashkenazi Jews. *Am J Hum Genet* 1991; 49:855–859.

PART II

INFECTIOUS DISORDERS

6

Congenital Infections

CATHERINE S. PECKHAM AND STUART LOGAN

Knowledge about the role of infections in pregnancy and the effects they may or may not have on the fetus and infant is of great practical importance for clinicians and policy makers. Accurate information is needed so that women exposed to specific infections can be informed about the implications of this exposure for their pregnancy and can then be offered the most appropriate management. In addition, decisions about the appropriateness of recommending the introduction of a screening program to detect a specific infection in pregnancy, with a view to treatment or the opportunity to offer termination of the pregnancy, must be based on sound epidemiologic information. This information should include data on the prevalence of the infection, the risk of maternal-infant transmission, the consequences of congenital or perinatal infection on pregnancy outcome and subsequent disability, and the benefits of treatment. Unfortunately, information is often derived from anecdotal experience or based on clinic populations that do not reflect the population at risk (see Chapter 1). In addition, the relevant issues may be clouded by media attention that then prompts campaigns for screening programs based on opinion, rather than on sound analyses of their risks and benefits.

Biologic Considerations

Infections in pregnancy are common. In one large prospective study of 30,000 pregnancies, over 5% were complicated by at least one clinically recognizable illness (Sever & White, 1968). Most infections are nonspecific or viral, and unless the infant has signs of infection at birth, it is unlikely that investigations for evidence of congenital infection will be performed. Fortunately, relatively few maternal infections have been shown to have a deleterious effect on the fetus or newborn infant (Table 6.1).

It is often difficult to establish whether a particular infection causes fetal infection and damage (Table 6.2). Not only are most maternal infections mild or asymptomatic and therefore unlikely to be diagnosed but also most congenitally infected infants are well at the time of birth with no stigmata of infection. As a result, data associating maternal infections with adverse outcome tend to

Table 6.1. Agents Causing Congenital Infection

Viruses	Bacteria	Protozoa
Rubella	*Trepenoma pallidum*	*Toxoplasma gondii*
Cytomegalic	*Listeria monocytogenes*	
HIV		
Varicella zoster		
Parvovirus		
HTLV-1		
Herpes simplex*		
Hepatitis B*		

*Intrauterine infection with these organisms has been reported.

be biased toward those whose infants present with symptoms in infancy. Prospective studies are required both to elucidate the possible causal relationships between infection and adverse outcome for the fetus or newborn infant and to estimate risk. They require follow-up of women throughout pregnancy so that those who become infected can be identified using the most appropriate investigations. As specific infections in pregnancy are relatively infrequent, large numbers of women need to be enrolled to achieve an adequate sample size. Even cytomegalovirus (CMV) infection, the commonest congenital infection, occurs in fewer than 1% of pregnancies, and only a proportion of these infections are transmitted to the fetus.

In many situations it is not possible to determine conclusively whether the young infant is infected. Passively acquired material IgG antibody may persist for some months and cannot be distinguished from antibody due to fetal infection. In addition, for many congenital infections there is no sensitive and specific laboratory test. In studies of such infections as toxoplasmosis, human parvovirus, or human immunodeficiency virus (HIV), infants may need to be followed clinically and serologically for many months before a definitive diagnosis of congenital infection can be made. Obviously, the effect of loss to follow-up is of critical importance in such studies. Children with symptoms may be seen more frequently and benefit from medical follow-up, whereas parents of children with no problems may be reluctant to continue seeking medical attention. In this situation, the risk of adverse outcome may be exaggerated.

The significance of a nonspecific outcome, such as abortion, prematurity, neurologic or sensory organ sequelae, or more subtle defects, can only be established by comparison with an appropriate control group. Because many of

Table 6.2. Problems in the Elucidation of Congenital Infections

Most infections are uncommon in pregnancy.
Maternal infections are often asymptomatic or nonspecific.
Infection in the infant is seldom obvious at birth.
It is often difficult to establish an early diagnosis of congenital infection.
Damage due to congenital infection may appear too late for a diagnosis of congenital rather than acquired infection.

the postulated effects of congenital infections do not manifest or develop for months or even years, long-term studies are required to characterize and quantify the full spectrum of these effects (Peckham, 1972). Large prospective studies are difficult to plan and coordinate, are by necessity lengthy and costly, and require continued close collaboration among epidemiologists, microbiologists, obstetricians, and pediatricians (see Chapter 1).

For infections that are uncommon in pregnancy, even if they are symptomatic, the numbers required for prospective studies may be unrealistic. Examples of such infections include mumps, chickenpox, and measles (see Chapter 9). In certain circumstances, a possible causal link between one of these infections and fetal damage may be inferred on the basis of case reports of damage in infants born to women who have had the infection during pregnancy. However, congenital defects are relatively common, and the apparent link could merely be a chance association. The likelihood that a real association exists is increased if the organism can be recovered from the fetus or damaged infant or if there is serologic evidence of transplacental infection. This does not necessarily establish a causal relationship, but if the pattern of damage is unusual and consistent with previous reports, such as the fetal varicella syndrome, the association becomes more likely. Unfortunately, in this situation the risk to an individual woman with the infection cannot be estimated.

Infections may be acquired in utero (congenital infection), at the time of birth (natal infection), or during the neonatal period (postnatal infection). Intrauterine infection often follows invasion of the maternal bloodstream by microorganisms. The placenta can be infected without fetal infection. Infections can also reach the fetus from the genital tract via the cervical amniotic route. Infection acquired by the infant during delivery may result from exposure to infected cervical secretions, maternal blood, or feces. In the neonatal period, possible sources of infection include breast milk, transfused blood, or infected contacts.

The consequences of a maternal infection include spontaneous abortion, stillbirth, premature labor, the birth of an infant with obvious abnormalities, the birth of a normal infant, or the late appearance of problems in a child who was normal at birth (Fig. 6.1). Although fetal damage in the form of congenital abnormalities may be apparent at birth, tissue destruction may continue after birth because of the persistence of viable organisms (Haywood, 1986). Such chronic infections occur with rubella, CMV, HIV, *Toxoplasma gondii*, and syphilis. It is often not possible to ascribe damage appearing after the neonatal period to congenital infection because microbiologic investigation at this stage often fails to distinguish congenital from postnatally acquired infection. The difficulty is compounded by the nonspecific nature of the signs and symptoms. For example, congenital CMV cannot be diagnosed in a 3-month infant presenting with fits and who is excreting the virus in the urine because the virus may have been acquired after birth (Peckham et al., 1987a).

In this chapter, some of the infections in pregnancy that may result in congenital infection with fetal damage are discussed. We do not attempt to be exhaustive but rather concentrate on those infections that are particularly common or that illustrate important epidemiologic points.

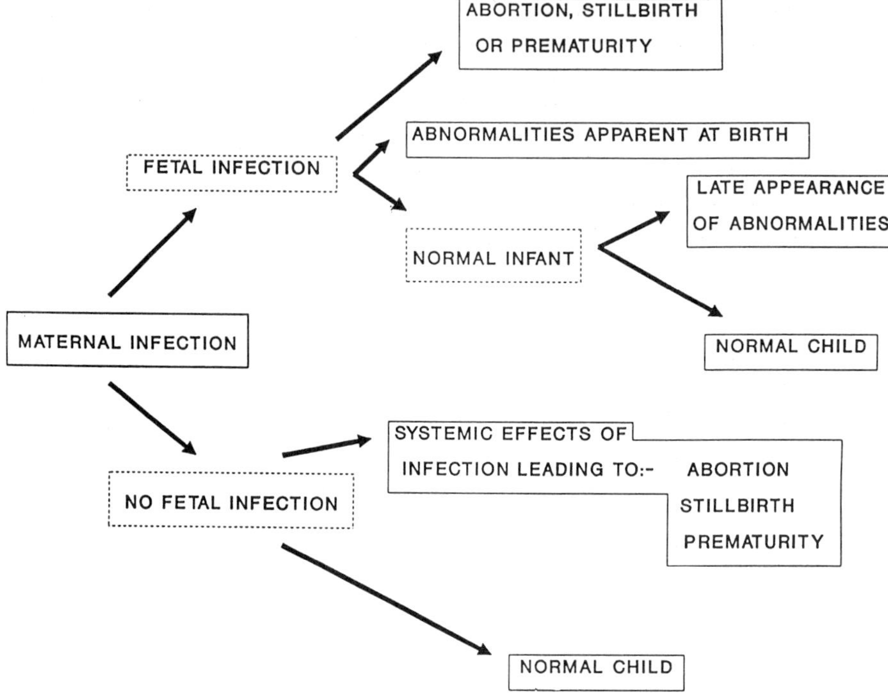

Fig. 6.1. Consequences of infection in pregnancy.

Patterns of Occurrence

Rubella

Congenital rubella defects were first reported in 1941 by Gregg, an Australian ophthalmologist, who observed congenital cataracts in babies born to mothers with a history of rubella in early pregnancy (Gregg, 1941). This observation was soon confirmed by other Australian ophthalmologists, and further defects, including congenital heart defects and severe hearing loss, were also reported in these children. The suggestion that such a mild disease as rubella could cause severe defects was treated with great skepticism. It was not until some years later, when studies had been repeated in other countries and similar defects had been reported, that Gregg's contribution was fully appreciated. The full spectrum of rubella defects was subsequently established in epidemiologic studies in the United States and Europe following epidemics in the 1960s and 1970s (Cooper, 1975; Miller et al., 1982; Peckham, 1972).

In contrast to other maternal infections that cause fetal damage, rubella virus is teratogenic and damages developing organs when acquired in the first trimester of pregnancy. Early prospective studies based on clinical recognition of maternal rubella and long-term follow-up of infants born to these mothers were carried out in the 1960s to characterize the abnormalities associated with congenital rubella and to estimate the risk of damage following maternal infection at different stages of gestation. Taken together, these studies suggested that the risk of damage was about 21% following infection in the first 8 weeks of pregnancy, declining to about 6% for infection in the fourth month (Dudgeon, 1976). Infection beyond 16 weeks gestation was only occasionally associated with defects, although cases of deafness have been reported following infection up to 22 weeks. Because these early studies relied on a clinical diagnosis of maternal infection, they are likely to have underestimated the true risk of damage because women presenting with rashes that were not due to rubella may have been included. Once laboratory tests for the diagnosis of rubella infection became available, it was no longer feasible to set up prospective studies because a confirmed diagnosis of rubella in pregnancy usually resulted in a therapeutic abortion. However, a recent study based on laboratory reports of confirmed infection reported substantially higher estimates of fetal damage than earlier studies (Miller, 1991). Over 1000 women in whom the dates of the last menstrual period and rash were known were followed up. More than 90% of those infected in the first trimester of pregnancy and half of those infected between 13 to 16 weeks chose to have a therapeutic abortion. Table 6.3 shows the risk of fetal infection by gestational age and Table 6.4 the risk of defects in infected infants and the overall risk of damage in a pregnancy complicated by rubella. Studies of children born after exposure to rubella late in pregnancy show no increased risk of defects (Grilner et al., 1983; Miller et al., 1982).

Although there have been isolated reports of possible congenital defects following maternal rubella before conception, in none of these cases was the maternal or fetal infection confirmed by adequate laboratory tests. In a prospective study Enders et al. (1988) found no risk associated with exposure to rubella before conception.

Some congenital rubella abnormalities, such as cataracts or congenital heart disease, are obvious shortly after birth, but others, such as hearing impairment, may not become apparent for years. Other forms of late-onset disease include diabetes mellitus and encephalopathy (Marshall, 1973). Exposure to maternal

Table 6.3. Outcome of Serologically Confirmed Symptomatic Maternal Rubella Cases, 1976–1988 and 1983–1987*

Stage of Pregnancy (number of completed weeks between rash & LMP)	Number of Infants Tested	Infected	
		(No.)	(%)
2–<11	20	20	100
11–12	22	16	73
13–14	30	19	63
15–16	53	24	45
17–18	56	21	38
19–22	82	76	32
23–26	57	14	25
27–30	52	20	38
31–36	36	21	58
>37	11	9	82
Total	419	190	45

*Cases reported to the PHLS Communicable Disease Surveillance Centre.

Table 6.4. Risk of Congenital Rubella Defects Following Confirmed Maternal Rubella at Successive Stages of Pregnancy

Stage of Pregnancy (number of completed weeks from LMP)	Number Followed Up	Defect present No.	Defect present (%)	Overall Risk of Pregnancy Resulting in Infant with Rubella Defect* (%)
2–10	20	18	90	90
11–12	12	6	50	34
13–16	36	12	33	17
17–18	15	1	7	3
>19	58	0	—	—

*Overall risk of defect = fetal infection rate (from table) × risk of defect if infected. All affected infants had sensorineural deafness; eight infants infected before 8 weeks also had congenital heart disease.

rubella infection in early pregnancy is likely to result in fetal infection with multiple defects, whereas damage following exposure to infection in the third or fourth month usually results in a single defect—sensorineural hearing impairment. This is the most frequent rubella effect, and the hearing loss, which may be unilateral or bilateral, is often associated with pigmentary retinopathy. Epidemiologic studies carried out in the United Kingdom before the introduction of rubella vaccine suggested that rubella accounted for at least 16% of cases of moderate to severe deafness and 2% of cases of congenital heart disease among British children (Peckham, 1985). These figures represent the birth of about 200 to 300 children with congenital rubella defects in England and Wales during a nonepidemic year—a birth prevalence of about 1 per 2000 births.

With the development of live attenuated rubella vaccines, congenital rubella has become a preventable condition. There are two possible strategies for immunization (see Chapter 9). The first, which was adopted in the United States, involves the immunization of all infants of both sexes to eliminate the risk of exposure of pregnant women to rubella by interrupting its transmission in the community. In the second approach of selective immunization, which was originally adopted in the United Kingdom, adolescent girls are immunized to eliminate the risk of rubella occurring in pregnancy. The vaccine is given after the peak age of infection, and the aim is not to interrupt the transmission of infection within the population but to "mop up" those who have escaped childhood infection. This approach allows for the boosting of vaccine-induced antibody by circulating wild virus.

Selective immunization is still used in a number of countries and is effective in reducing the number of children born with congenital rubella syndrome (CRS). However, a small number of women will escape both natural infection and immunization and remain susceptible to rubella infection in pregnancy. Universal immunization has a more immediate effect on the elimination of congenital rubella, but there is a potential danger. If high rates of vaccine coverage are not achieved and maintained, the program may slow the rate of viral transmission, resulting in an increase in the peak age of infection, with an increase in the proportion of susceptible women of child-bearing age.

In the United Kingdom rubella vaccine was introduced in 1970 for girls between 11 and 14 years and was soon extended to include susceptible women of child-bearing age. Women found to be susceptible in the antenatal period were also offered vaccine postpartum. In 1988 the program was augmented to include measles, mumps, and rubella (MMR) vaccine for boys and girls in the second year of life. Figure 6.2 shows the decline in notifications of CRS and terminations of pregnancy for maternal rubella since the introduction of vaccines in the United Kingdom. However, the need for continued surveillance is demonstrated by Figure 6.3, which shows the recent increase in congenital rubella in the United States, despite high uptake of MMR by the age of five years for the period 1970 to 1990 (CDC, 1991, 1992). In addition to the reduction in the percentage of susceptible pregnant women—from about 18% to 3%—that has occurred as a result of the selective vaccine programs, there has been a striking decrease in the incidence of rubella infection in the United Kingdom since the introduction of MMR in 1988.

Parvovirus B19 Infection

Parvovirus B19 infection has been associated with an increase in fetal death, both abortion and stillbirth (CDC, 1989). The virus may cause hydrops fetalis as a result of profound fetal anemia following replication of the virus in erythroid precursor cells, as well as congestive cardiac failure in the fetus. In children, parvovirus infection classically presents with fever and a facial rash—a "slapped cheek" appearance. In adults the presentation is often atypical and may be confused clinically with rubella infection. The correct diagnosis can only be established by serologic tests.

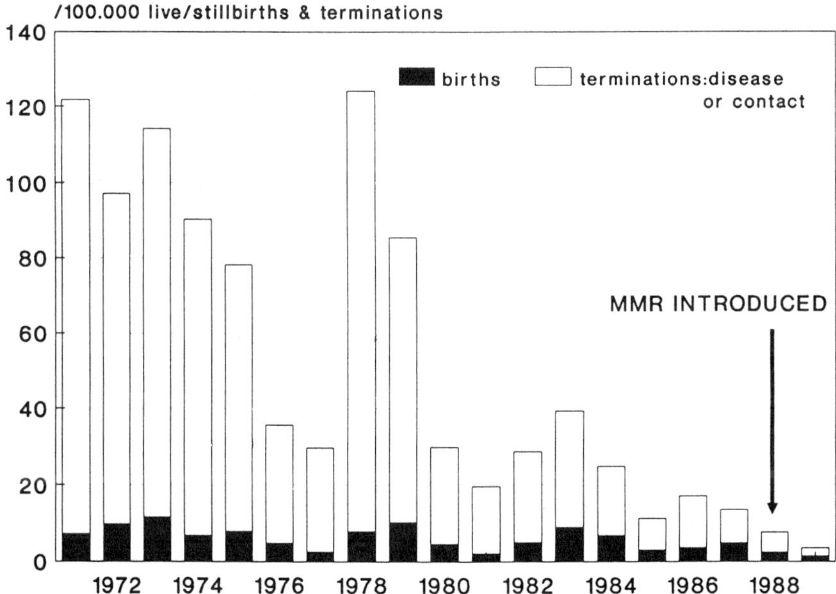

Fig. 6.2. Congenital rubella births and terminations for rubella, 1972 to 1989.

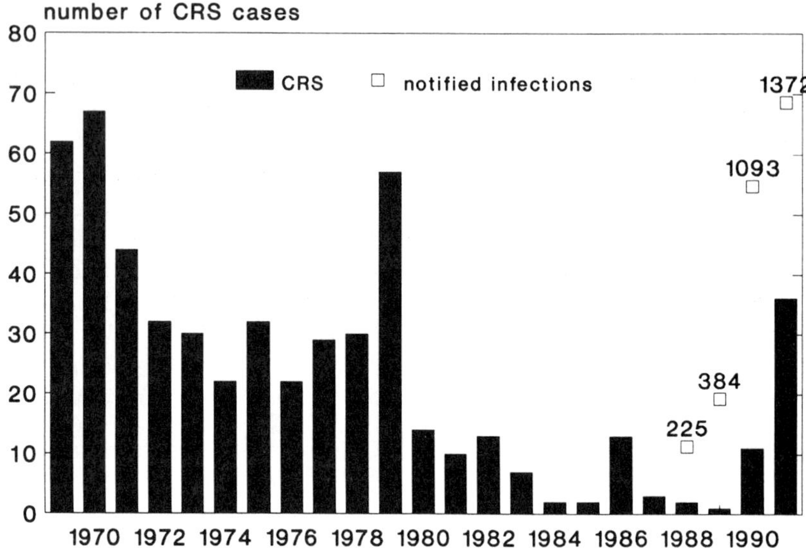

Fig. 6.3. Rubella in the United States, 1969 to 1991.

Early reports based on small case series of parvovirus infection in pregnancy suggested a high proportion of fetal loss caused by fetal hydrops. In one such study 42 pregnancies were complicated by B19 infection, and of the 39 pregnancies that the women elected to continue, fetal loss was reported in 7 (18%) and hydrops fetalis in 10 (26%; Schwartz et al., 1988). Although they provided useful information these studies cannot provide estimates of the risk of pregnancy loss due to B19 infection.

In a prospective study in the United Kingdom (PHLS, 1990), 190 pregnant women with serologically confirmed B19 infection were followed. Of the 186 who elected to continue the pregnancy to term, 156 (84%) delivered normal infants. No significant abnormalities were found in the 114 infants followed to 1 year of age, although 27 had serologic evidence of intrauterine infection—an estimated vertical transmission rate of 33%. The total fetal loss rate was 16% (30 cases), which was similar to that in an uninfected unmatched antenatal sample. There was an excess fetal loss, however, in the second trimester, and based on virologic findings in the aborted fetuses the risk of fetal death due to B19 infection in pregnancy was estimated to be 9%.

Preliminary data from a prospective study of 200 women in the United States with serologic evidence of B19 infection in pregnancy showed a 2% to 3% increase in fetal death compared with control and that the difference occurred in the first 20 weeks of pregnancy (Torok, 1990). No increase in abnormalities was found. On the basis of these two studies, Torok (1990) estimated that the risk of fetal death following B19 infection in pregnancy was less than 10% and that most of the excess risk was related to maternal infection in the first 20 weeks of pregnancy.

Because some of the animal parvoviruses are teratogens, it is reassuring that there have been no reports to date of liveborn infants with specific congenital anomalies linked to B19 infection in utero, and there is no evidence that the rate of congenital defects exceeds the background rate. Accordingly, parvovirus infection is not an indication for termination of pregnancy.

Varicella Zoster Virus Infection

Varicella, or chickenpox, in pregnancy is relatively rare because it is a highly contagious infection and in developed temperate regions is almost invariably acquired in childhood. In semitropical and tropical countries, infection occurs at an older age, and a higher proportion of adults are susceptible.

Varicella zoster is a DNA virus and a member of the herpes group. Large prospective follow-up studies carried out in the United States and in the United Kingdom in the 1960s were unable to demonstrate any association between chickenpox and fetal damage (Bradford Hill et al., 1968; Manson et al., 1960; Seigel, 1973). However, several case reports of infants born to mothers who had varicella in pregnancy in different parts of the world have suggested an association between chickenpox in early pregnancy and the "fetal varicella syndrome" (Enders, 1985). Although there have been only around 40 cases reported in the world literature, the constellation of abnormalities described is sufficiently distinctive to suggest that this is a causal association. The pathognomonic stigmata of the varicella syndrome include cicatricial scars that are often dermatomal in distribution and related to hypoplasia of the limbs and malformed digits. CNS damage may manifest itself by convulsions and mental retardation, and chorioretinitis and optic atrophy may be present. It has been suggested that a possible reason for the apparently low risk of damage and the finding that the abnormalities tend to occur in a dermatomal distribution is that problems only arise if the equivalent of intrauterine zoster occurs (Higa et al., 1987).

In a recent prospective study carried out in England and West Germany between 1980 and 1991, 918 women who had chickenpox in the first 36 weeks of pregnancy were followed to term; four infants had varicella embryopathy (Miller, 1992, personal communication). The risk of varicella embryopathy after maternal chickenpox in the first 27 weeks of gestation was 0.6% (CI 0.2–1.4), and no cases occurred after 28 weeks (Table 6.5). In this study, 521 infants were tested for the presence of V-Z specific IgM antibody in the neonatal period or persistent IgG at 1 year, and 63 (12%) showed evidence of subclinical congenital

Table 6.5. Risk of Varicella Embryopathy Following Maternal Chickenpox at Successive Stages of Pregnancy

Stage of Pregnancy (number of completed weeks of pregnancy from LMP)	Number of Pregnancies Followed to Term	Babies with Embryopathy (No.)	(% ± 95% CI)
1–13	347	1	(0.3, .006–1.6)
14–27	379	3	(0.8, 0.2–2.3)*
28–36	192	0	—
Total	918	4	—

*Overall risk of varicella embryopathy after maternal chickenpox in the first 27 weeks of gestation = 4/726 = 0.6% (0.2–1.4). Cases with embryopathy occurred after maternal infections at 12, 14, 16 and 19 weeks gestation.

infection. The low risk of fetal damage means that termination of pregnancy is not usually advised after maternal chickenpox.

The major problem with chickenpox in pregnancy relates to infection occurring just before or at the time of delivery. If the infection is transmitted to the fetus before substantial amounts of maternal antibody are produced and transferred across the placenta, the infant may develop severe, disseminated chickenpox—a condition with high mortality and morbidity (Gershon, 1975). To prevent or ameliorate disease, passive immunization with varicella-zoster immunoglobulin is recommended as soon as possible after birth for infants whose mothers develop the rash between 5 days before and two days after delivery.

Cytomegalovirus Infection

Cytomegalovirus (CMV) is a large DNA virus of the herpes family. The virus has the propensity to establish latent infection and may reactivate from time to time. In healthy individuals, infection is usually asymptomatic or mild and nonspecific and is rarely diagnosed. However, in immunosuppressed patients and very premature infants, CMV can be life threatening. CMV is the most common congenital infection and an established cause of handicap.

The different patterns of childhood acquisition of infection are reflected in adult seroprevalence. In developing countries, most women of child-bearing age are seropositive, having acquired CMV infection early in life. In contrast, in industrial countries about 50% of women of child-bearing age are still susceptible to infection and at risk of acquiring a primary infection in pregnancy. The birth prevalence of congenital CMV infection varies in different parts of the world—from 0.2% to 2.2% of live births—with no evidence of a seasonal variation (Stagno et al., 1983). As maternal infections are nearly always asymptomatic and over 90% of infected infants have no clinically recognizable signs of infection at birth, the majority of congenital infections pass unrecognized. The early studies, largely based on children admitted to a hospital, suggested that the prevalence of defects associated with congenital infection was high (McCracken et al., 1962; Pass et al., 1980; Weller & Hanshaw, 1964). Indeed, in the 1970s, CMV was described as a major cause of mental retardation, second only to Down syndrome. At that time repeat screening for infection in pregnancy was advocated so that women who acquired the infection could be identified and offered the option of termination, the assumption being that only primary infection early in pregnancy was likely to cause fetal damage. There was little scientific evidence available to support such a policy, and in the United Kingdom and elsewhere prospective studies were established to provide the epidemiologic information required for reaching decisions on the appropriateness of recommending screening in pregnancy. The results from these prospective studies, in which children were systematically screened for CMV at birth and those with congenital infection were followed up, demonstrated a lower incidence of adverse sequelae than was originally estimated (Ahlfors et al., 1979; Peckham et al., 1983; Saigal et al., 1982).

Fewer than 10% of congenitally infected infants have symptoms or signs of infections at births. The clinical manifestations include a rash, prolonged neonatal jaundice, hepatomegaly, splenomegaly, intrauterine growth retardation, microcephaly, pneumonitis, thrombocytopenia, and periventricular intracranial calcifications. The majority of this symptomatic group will have later complications, including permanent brain damage, which may include signs of cerebral palsy, mental retardation, or sensorineural hearing loss (Pass et al., 1980; Ramsey et al., 1991). Of the remaining children who are asymptomatic at birth, a small proportion will also develop long-term neurologic sequelae, with sensorineural hearing loss being the most frequent defect.

A large prospective study of CMV in pregnancy carried out in London revealed a congenital infection rate of 3 per 1000. In this study, 103 infants with congenital infection were identified; only 4 had neonatal symptoms or signs, and all 4 suffered serious permanent sequelae, including sensorineural hearing loss, cerebral palsy, mental retardation, and microcephaly. Of the remaining 99 asymptomatic children, 96 were followed to at least 3 years of age, and of these 6 were later found to have a bilateral or unilateral sensorineural hearing loss, which was associated with a motor handicap in 2 of the children. No statistically significant differences in IQ scores were found between the 90% of infected children with no discernible disabilities and matched controls—a finding consistent with other studies (Conboy et al., 1986; Pearl et al., 1986).

Unlike rubella, in which congenital infection is extremely rare after reinfection, intrauterine transmission of CMV infection commonly follows recurrent infection, even in the presence of substantial humoral immunity. Congenital infections resulting from a recurrence of CMV in pregnancy are considered less likely to result in fetal damage than primary infections (Stagno et al., 1982), although defects compatible with congenital CMV infection have been reported in children whose mothers were seropositive before their conception (Ahlfors et al., 1981; Rutter et al., 1985). Unlike rubella, CMV infection acquired in late pregnancy may cause fetal damage.

About 40% of women who acquire CMV infection during pregnancy will give birth to an infant with congenital infection. Based on this risk of transmission and on a risk of damage in a congenitally infected infant of 10%, a woman who acquires a primary CMV infection in pregnancy has a risk of approximately 1 in 25 of having a child with CMV-associated handicap. With about 780,000 births in England, Scotland, and Wales each year and a rate of congenital infection of 3 per 1000, an estimated 2,340 children would be born with congenital infection annually. Approximately 235 would have some CMV-related disability, and about half of these would have a unilateral or bilateral hearing loss but would be otherwise unaffected. It has also been estimated that about 12% of congenital sensorineural hearing loss in the United Kingdom is due to congenital CMV. The CMV etiology assumes a relatively greater importance with the decline in rubella hearing loss since the introduction of rubella vaccine. Based on a prevalence of cerebral palsy of 2.5 per 1000 live births, congenital CMV could also account for about 5% of cerebral palsy in the United Kingdom.

It must be emphasized that findings in one country cannot necessarily be extrapolated to another. Prospective studies in Sweden (Ahlfors et al., 1979) and Canada (Saigal et al., 1982) show similar results to those from the United Kingdom (Peckham et al., 1983), although studies from the United States show a much higher rate of damage in congenitally infected children (Fowler et al.,

1992). At present, antenatal screening is not considered to be appropriate in the United Kingdom. Such a program would neither be able to identify infections occurring in late pregnancy nor recurrent infections and would therefore fail to identify most pregnancies in which fetal damage had occurred. Because it is not possible to determine which infants will be damaged after maternal infection, approximately 24 normal fetuses would be terminated for each damaged fetus identified correctly.

Herpes Simplex Virus (HSV)

Although herpes simplex appears in the mnemonic traditionally used by physicians to remember the organisms causing congenital infections (TORCH), transplacental infection is probably rare. Reports of adverse effects following HSV infection in early pregnancy are few, and the evidence that transplacental HSV causes abnormalities is inconclusive. There have been only isolated case reports of primary maternal infection in the first 20 weeks of pregnancy resulting in congenital abnormality (Florman et al., 1973; Komorous et al., 1977; South et al., 1969). These infants suffered from microcephaly, microphthalmia, and cranial calcification and had cutaneous lesions at birth. No adequate estimation of risk is possible, but both type I and type II herpes infections are common in pregnancy and reports of damage rare. This suggests that the risk, if any, is extremely low. Early primary HSV infection is not therefore an indication for termination of pregnancy.

The acquisition of neonatal HSV infection during delivery is more common and is potentially devastating. There is good evidence that recurrent maternal genital HSV infection poses a low risk of transmission and that most cases of neonatal herpes result from a primary, often asymptomatic infection acquired in late pregnancy (Boucher et al., 1990; Brown et al., 1991; Prober et al., 1987).

Listeriosis

Listeria monocytogenes is a Gram-positive mobile bacterium. Its diagnosis depends on culture of the organism because serologic tests are not helpful. In the United Kingdom fewer than 300 cases per year are reported to the Public Health Laboratory Service on the basis of laboratory reports, although the organism can be isolated from the stools of up to 3% of normal individuals. Most reports of infection occur during pregnancy, in the neonatal period, in the elderly, or in immunocompromised individuals.

Listeria is found in many animal species, but direct spread to humans is not common. Food is implicated as a vehicle for transmission from animal to humans, and the organism has been isolated from raw poultry, raw vegetables, "cook-chill" meals, paté, milk, and soft cheese. Most cases are sporadic, but outbreaks have been reported. Direct "case-to-case" spread is rare (Jones, 1990).

Infection with *Listeria* in pregnancy may result in abortion, premature delivery, or fetal infection. Infection is most frequently documented in the third trimester of pregnancy, although cases have been confirmed much earlier. Unfortunately, no estimate of risk can be made on present evidence, and it is unclear whether it is a significant cause of fetal loss because bacterial cultures are not routinely performed on aborted fetuses. The fetus may acquire infection either transplacentally, by ascending infection from the genital tract, or at the time of delivery.

Infants infected prenatally may present soon after birth with a septicemic illness associated with a high mortality rate. The long-term morbidity among survivors is not known, but is thought to be low although hydrocephalus and neurodevelopmental handicap have been reported. Infants infected at the time of birth usually present with bacterial meningitis between 1 and 8 weeks of age (late-onset disease). With appropriate treatment the prognosis is good. If maternal infection is diagnosed during pregnancy, antibiotic treatment may reduce the risk of transmission.

HIV Infection

The World Health Organization (WHO) has estimated that ten million adults and one million children are infected with HIV worldwide. Most children acquire HIV infection through vertical transmission from their mother, and the increase in the number of women with HIV infection has been paralleled by an increase in the number of infected children.

Transmission of infection from mother to child can occur before, during, or shortly after birth. However, because of the difficulty of making an early diagnosis of infection in the child, the relative contribution of each of these routes is not known. Although there is clear evidence for intrauterine infection and HIV virus has been found in fetal tissue as early as 15 weeks gestation, increasingly it is being suggested that a substantial proportion of infection may occur around the time of delivery (Goedert et al., 1991; Fig. 6.4).

The diagnosis of an HIV infection even in an infant born to an HIV-positive mother is problematic. Children born to HIV antibody-positive mothers have no clinical manifestations of infection at birth, but possess maternal IgG antibodies and test HIV antibody positive. Maternal HIV antibodies persist in the child for a median of 10 months, but may remain for as long as 8 months (Fig. 6.4). Virologic tests, including virologic culture, P24 antigen, and the polymerase chain reaction, which detects and amplifies biogenetic material, are relatively insensitive in the first few months of life. Furthermore, these tests are costly, time consuming, and not routinely available.

Estimates of vertical transmission vary widely. The early studies are likely to have overestimated the risk of transmission because they were based on small, selected groups with bias toward women or children with symptoms or mothers who had already given birth to an infected child (Peckham et al., 1987b). Published estimates of vertical transmission derived from prospective studies, in which children born to HIV-seropositive women were identified before or at the time of birth and followed until their infection status could be determined, range from 7% to 39% (Newell, 1990). The estimate of vertical transmission from the European Collaborative Study (ECS, 1988, 1991) is about 15% and is markedly different from the rates reported from Africa. The reasons for this

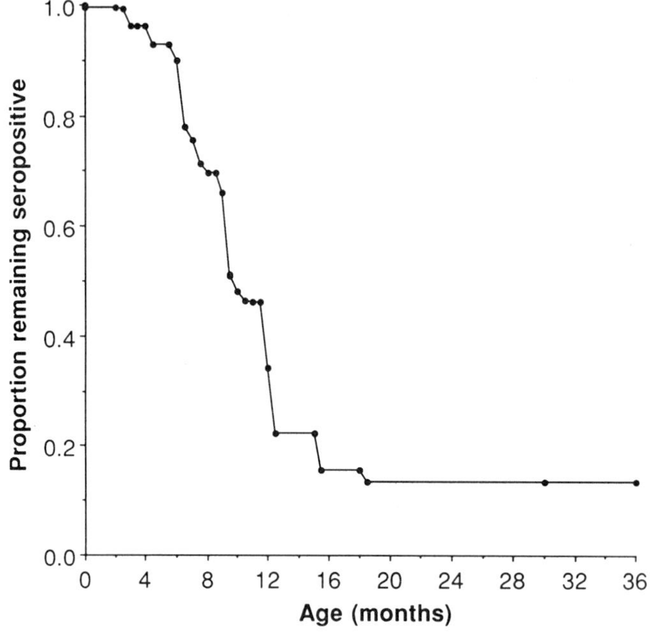

Fig. 6.4. Age at loss of HIV-1 antibody in a cohort of children born to infected mothers.

variance are unclear, and although methodologic differences, particularly loss to follow-up and early deaths, could account for some of it, it is likely that differences in maternal and environmental factors are also important. For example, infants born to mothers who have AIDS or low CD4 counts are at increased risk of infection (ECS, 1992).

The clinical presentation of infection is usually nonspecific and covers a wide spectrum of disease. The prognosis is variable and depends on the age of diagnosis and the presenting symptoms. Approximately one third of vertically infected children develop severe and rapidly progressing disease in the first year of life. The remainder have a more slowly progressive course, although nearly all show some manifestations of infection (clinical, immunologic, or both) by 1 year of age. However, the condition of these children may remain stable or even improve over the next few years, and much longer follow-up is required to establish the long-term outcome for this group.

Toxoplasma Gondii

When acquired in pregnancy, toxoplasmosis can cause fetal infection with potentially serious damage to the newborn. Although the life cycle of *Toxoplasma* is well described, little is known about its precise mode of transmission to humans. It is generally inferred from the life cycle that undercooked meat, resulting in the ingestion of *Toxoplasma* tissue cysts, or exposure to *Toxoplasma* oocysts in feline feces, either directly or through contaminated soil, are the major sources of infection.

Information on the current incidence of *Toxoplasma* infection in pregnancy is lacking. The prevalence of seropositivity varies markedly from country to country and between groups within a country. A review of studies conducted in several localities in the United Kingdom in the 1970s and 1980s suggests that the best estimate of incidence is around 2 per 1000 pregnancies, but the information on which this estimate is based is limited and may not apply in the United Kingdom in the 1990s nor to populations in other countries. Higher rates of infection have been reported from France, the United States, and other countries (Remington et al., 1990). There is some evidence from Europe that there may be a downward trend in the seroprevalence of toxoplasmosis (Forsgren et al., 1991; Walker et al., 1992).

Most healthy individuals with newly acquired infection are asymptomatic or present with nonspecific signs or symptoms that, as with CMV, can only be detected in pregnancy by repeated serologic testing. Transplacental infection occurs during the phase of parasitemia, and the risk of fetal infection following reactivated toxoplasmosis among women with previous evidence of infection is negligible.

Estimates of intrauterine transmission are based on studies carried out in Paris over 20 years ago (Remington et al., 1990). The transmission rate depends on the gestational age at the time of maternal infection: the rate is low (10%) in the first 2 weeks after conception, but rises to over 90% in the last 2 weeks of pregnancy. In contrast, the risk of damage to an infected fetus is much higher in those infected in early pregnancy.

Although congenital toxoplasmosis may present at birth with a spectrum of clinical effects ranging from the classic "triad" (hydrocephaly, chorioretinitis, and intracranial calcification) to nonspecific manifestations including intrauterine growth retardation, hepatosplenomegaly, jaundice, thrombocytopenia, and conclusions, 90% of congenitally infected infants are asymptomatic. Virtually all neonates with symptomatic congenital infection have long-term sequelae, the most common being neurologic impairment, epilepsy, and impaired vision due to bilateral or unilateral chorioretinitis (Desmonts et al., 1974).

There is a paucity of information on the long-term outcome of the 90% of congenitally infected neonates who are asymptomatic at birth. The few prospective studies of neonates with asymptomatic infections have only included small numbers of children. Because so few truly symptomless neonates were recruited and because of possible bias in ascertainment and the lack of controls, it is virtually impossible to derive generalizable information from these studies. In a Dutch study, six of nine asymptomatic congenitally infected neonates followed through 20 years developed chorioretinitis, one as late as 18 years; three had unilateral visual impairment, but no other neurologic defects were detected (Koppe et al., 1986). In another study from the United States, 13 neonates (10 asymptomatic and 3 with nonspecific problems at birth) were followed for an average of 8 years (Wilson et al., 1980). Eleven children subsequently developed chorioretinitis, three had unilateral blindness, and eight had normal vision. Five of the 13 had neurologic problems, but it is not clear which of these children with adverse outcomes had been symptomless neonates. One child had microcephaly, two children had mild and transient problems, and two had minor cerebellar signs. Without controls it is difficult to conclude that any of these conditions were due to toxoplasmosis.

Diagnosis is uncertain in asymptomatic infants and depends on the identification of specific IgM antibody in cord or neonatal blood or the demonstration of persistent IgG antibody. *Toxoplasma* IgM assays are relatively insensitive. Sequential measurements are therefore necessary for at least the first year to demonstrate changes in IgG antibody titer that differentiate passively acquired maternal antibody from fetal infection.

The incidence of congenital toxoplasmosis varies in different populations and most countries lack reliable information. The incidence in the United Kingdom is not known, but some evidence suggests that it is extremely low. Patients under 16 years with newly diagnosed symptomatic congenital infection were reported by pediatricians to the British Paediatric Surveillance Unit (BPSU), an active reporting scheme with 95% compliance (Hall & Glickham, 1990). Fourteen cases of symptomatic congenital toxoplasmosis, not all with CNS involvement, were observed in England and Wales in a 12-month period during 1989 to 1990 (Hall, 1992). However, with 680,000 births in England and Wales in 1989, and assuming a 2 per 1000 infection rate in pregnancy, there would be an estimated 1360 acute maternal *Toxoplasma* infections in that year. Assuming a 40% transmission rate and a proportion of 10% severely symptomatic, there should have been 544 fetal infections and about 54 neonates with serious clinically recognizable infection. The disparity between the estimated and observed figures for severely affected children reflects the need for further information on the incidence and natural history of toxoplasmosis in pregnancy. It is often argued that the incidence of chorioretinitis is high in children with congenital toxoplasmosis, but there is no evidence to support this assumption.

Conclusions

Epidemiology plays an important role in the study of congenital infections. Not only is it necessary for establishing the causal link between a microbe and clinical infection but it is also used for estimating the prevalence of specific infections in pregnancy in different geographical areas. It provides estimates of risk of maternal-child transmission of infection and serves to quantify the damage caused by congenital infection, both short and long term. This information is critical for the development of guidelines for the management of exposures to infection and for setting priorities for future research.

Not only is it necessary to follow up the congenitally infected child for prolonged periods after birth to assess the full impact of these congenital infections but also increasing emphasis is now being placed on the possible sequelae presenting in adult life. Such long-term effects of antenatal infection have proved difficult to investigate because of an absence of appropriate populations. There seems to be an increased risk of adult diabetes mellitus following exposure to congenital rubella (Forrest et al., 1971). There is also conflicting evidence linking antenatal viral infection and subsequent malignant disease (Adelstein & Donovan, 1976; Fine et al., 1985). Schizophrenia has been associated with prenatal exposure to the 1957 A2 influenza epidemic (O'Callaghan et al., 1991), and congenital HTLV-1 infection has been linked to adult T-cell leukemia (Yoshida et al., 1982) and to tropical spastic paraparesis (Rodgers-Johnson et al., 1988).

Finally, because the etiology of so many disabilities in childhood remains unknown, it is interesting to speculate how many more of these could be due to undiagnosed congenital infections.

References

Adelstein AM, Donovan JW, Leighton PC, Pike MC. Sequelae of virus infection in pregnancy. In: *Child Health: A Collection of Studies on Medical and Population Subjects*. London, OPCS, HMSO; 1976: No. 31.

Ahlfors K, Ivarsson S, Johnsson T, Svanberg L. A prospective study on congenital and acquired cytomegalovirus infections in infants. *Scand Infect Dis* 1979; 11:177–178.

Ahlfors K, Harris S, Ivarsson S, Svanberg L. Secondary material cytomegalovirus infection causing symptomatic congenital infection. *N Engl J Med* 1981; 305:284.

Boucher FD, Yasukawa L, Bronzan RN, Hensleigh PA, Arvin AM, Prober CG. A prospective evaluation of primary genital herpes simplex virus type 2 infections acquired during pregnancy. *Pediatr Infect Dis J* 1990; 9:499–504.

Bradford Hill A, Doll R, Galloway TM, Hughes JP. Virus diseases in pregnancy and congenital defects. *Br J Prev Soc Med* 1968; 12:1–7.

Brown ZA, Benedetti J, Ashley R et al. Neonatal herpes simplex virus infection in relation to asymptomatic maternal infection at the time of labor. *N Engl J Med* 1991; 324:1247–1252.

Centers for Disease Control. Parvovirus B19 Infection. *MMWR* 1989; 38:90–97.

Centers for Disease Control. Increase in rubella and congenital rubella syndrome—United States, 1988–1990. *MMWR* 1989; 38:90–97.

Centers for Disease Control. Cumulative totals for infectious diseases 1990–91 (table). *MMWR* 1992; 40:No 51 & 52.

Conboy T, Pass R, Stagno S, Britt W. Intellectual development in school-aged children with asymptomatic congenital cytomegalovirus infection. *Pediatrics* 1986; 77:801–806.

Cooper LZ. Congenital rubella in the United States. In: Krugman S, Gershon AA, eds. *Infections of the Fetus and the Newborn Infant*. New York: Alan R Liss Inc, 1975:1–22.

Desmonts G, Couvreur J. Congenital toxoplasmosis: a prospective study of 378 pregnancies. *N Engl J Med* 1974; 290:1110–1116.

Dudgeon JA. Congenital rubella. *Br Med Bull* 1976; 32:77–83.

Enders G. Varicella zoster virus infection in pregnancy. *Progr Med Virol* 1985; 29:166–96.

Enders G, Nickerl-Pacher U, Miller E, Cradock-Watson JE. Outcome of confirmed periconceptional maternal rubella. *Lancet* 1988; 1:1445–1447.

European Collaborative Study. Mother-to-child transmission of HIV infection. *Lancet* 1988; 2:1039–1042.

European Collaborative Study. Children born to women with HIV-1 infection: natural history and risk of transmission. *Lancet* 1991; 337:253–260.

European Collaborative Study. Risk factors for mother-to-child transmission of HIV-1. *Lancet* 1992; 339:1007–1012.

Fine PEM, Adelstein AM, Snowman J, Clarkson JA, Evans SM. Long term effects of exposure to viral infections in utero. *Br Med J* 1985; 90:509–511.

Florman AL, Gershon AA, Blackett PR, Nahmias AJ. Intrauterine infection with herpes simplex virus: resultant congenital malformations. *JAMA* 1973; 225:129–132.

Forrest JM, Menser MA, Burgess JA. High frequency of diabetes mellitus in young adults with congenital rubella. *Lancet* 1971; 2:332–334.

Forsgren M, Gille E, Ljungstrom I, Nokes DJ. *Toxoplasma gondii* antibodies in pregnant women in Stockholm in 1969, 1979, and 1987. *Lancet* 1991; 337:1413–1414.

Fowler KB, Stagno PHS, Pass RF, Britt WJ, Boll TJ, Alford CA. The outcome of congenital cytomegalovirus infection in relation to maternal antibody status. *N Engl J Med* 1992; 326:663–667.

Gershon AA. Varicella in mother and infant: problems old and new. In: Krugman S, Gershon AA eds. *Infections of the Fetus and the Newborn Infant*. New York: Alan R. Liss Inc; 1975:79–95.

Goedert JJ, Duliege A-M, Amos CI, Felton S, Biggar RJ. International Registry of HIV-Exposed Twins: The high risk of infection with human immunodeficiency virus type I for first-born, vaginally delivered twins. *Lancet* 1991; 338:1471–1475.

Gregg NM. Congenital cataract following German measles in the mother. *Trans Ophthalmol Soc Aust* 1941; 3:35–46.

Grilner L, Forsgren M, Barr B, Bottiger M, Danielsson L, de Verdier C. Outcome of rubella during pregnancy with special reference to the 17th–24th weeks of gestation. *Scand J Infect Dis* 1983; 15:321–325.

Hall SM. Congenital toxoplasmosis. *Br Med J* 1992; 305:291–297.

Hall S, Glickman M. Report from the British Paediatric Surveillance Unit. *Arch Dis Child* 1990; 65:807–809.

Haywood AM. Patterns of persistent viral infections. *N Engl J Med* 1986; 315:939–948.

Higa K, Kenjiro D, Haruchicko M. Varicella-zoster virus infection during pregnancy: hypothesis concerning the mechanisms of congenital malformations. *Obstet Gynecol* 1987; 68:214–222.

Jones D. Foodborne listeriosis. *Lancet* 1990; 336:1171–1174.

Komorous JM, Wheeler CE, Briggamann RA. Intrauterine herpes simplex infections. *Arch Dermatol* 1977; 113:918–922.

Koppe JG, Loewer-Sieger DH, de Roever-Bonnet H. Results of 20-year follow-up of congenital toxoplasmosis. *Lancet* 1986; 1:254–255.

Manson MM, Logan WPO, Loy RM. Rubella and other virus infections during pregnancy. *Rep Pub Health Medical Subj* 1960; 101.

Marshall WC. The clinical impact of intrauterine rubella. In: *Intrauterine Infections*. Ciba Foundation 10. Amsterdam: Associated Scientific Publishers; 1973; 3–22.

McCracken GH, Shinefield MR, Cobb K, Raunsen AR, Dische MR, Eichenwald MF. Congenital cytomegalic inclusion disease: a longitudinal study of 20 patients. *Am J Dis Child* 1969; 117:552–539.

Miller E. Rubella in the United Kingdom. *Epidemiol Infect* 1991; 107:31–42.

Miller E, Craddock-Watson JE, Pollock TM. Consequences of confirmed maternal rubella at successive stages of pregnancy. *Lancet* 1982; 2:781–784.

Newell ML, Peckham CS, Lepage P. HIV-1 infection in pregnancy: implications for women and children. *AIDS* 1990; 4:S111–S117.

O'Callaghan E, Sham P, Takei N, Glover G, Murray RM. Schizophrenia after prenatal exposure to 1957 A2 influenza epidemic. *Lancet* 1991; 337:1248–1250.

Pass RF, Stagno S, Myers GJ, Alford CA. Outcome of symptomatic congenital cytomegalovirus infection: results of long-term longitudinal follow-up. *J Pediatr* 1980; 66:758–762.

Pearl K, Preece P, Ades A, Peckham C. Neurodevelopmental assessment after congenital cytomegalovirus infection. *Arch Dis Child* 1986; 61:323–326.

Peckham CS, A clinical and laboratory study of children exposed in utero to maternal rubella. *Arch Dis Child* 1972; 47:571–577.

Peckham CS. Congenital rubella in the United Kingdom before 1970: the prevaccine era. *Rev Infect Dis* 1985; 7:S11–S16.

Peckham C, Coleman J, Hurley R, Chin K, Henderson K. Cytomegalovirus infection in pregnancy: preliminary findings from a prospective study. *Lancet* 1983; 1:1352–1356.

Peckham CS, Johnson C, Ades A, Pearl K, Chin KS. The early acquisition of cytomegalovirus infection. *Arch Dis Child* 1987a; 62:780–785.

Peckham CS, Senturia YD, Ades AE. Obstetric and perinatal consequences of human immunodeficiency virus (HIV) infection: a review. *Br J Obstet Gynaecol* 1987b; 94:403–407.

Prober CG, Sullender WM, Yasukawa LL, Av DS, Yeager A, Arvin AM. Low risk of herpes simplex virus infections in neonates exposed to the virus at the time of vaginal delivery to mothers with recurrent genital herpes simplex virus infection. *N Engl J Med* 1987; 316:240–244.

Public Health Laboratory Service (PHLS) Working Party on Fifth Disease. Prospective study of human parvovirus (B19) infection in pregnancy. *Br Med J* 1990; 300:1166–1170.

Ramsey MEB, Miller E, Peckham CS. Outcome of confirmed symptomatic congenital cytomegalovirus infection. *Arch Dis Child* 1991; 66:1068–1069.

Remington JS, Desmonts G. Toxoplasmosis. In: Remington JS, Klein JO, eds. *Infectious Diseases of the Fetus and Newborn Infant.* 3rd ed. Philadelphia: WB Saunders; 1990:89–195.

Rodgers-Johnson P, Morgan OC, Mora C, et al. The role of HTLV-1 in tropical spastic paraparesis in Jamaica. *Ann Neurol* 1988; 23:121–126.

Rutter D, Griffiths P, Trompeter R. Cytomegalic inclusion disease after recurrent maternal infection. *Lancet* 1985; 2:1182.

Saigal S, Lunyk O, Larke RPB, Chernesky MA. The outcome in children with congenital cytomegalovirus infection. *Am J Dis Child* 1982; 136:896–905.

Schwartz TF, Roggendorf M, Hottentrager B, et al. Human parvovirus B19 in pregnancy. *Lancet* 1988; 2:566–567.

Seigel M. Congenital malformations following chickenpox, measles, mumps and hepatitis. *JAMA* 1973; 226:1521–1524.

Sever J, White LR. Intrauterine viral infections. *Annu Rev Med* 1968; 19:471–486.

South MA, Tompkins WAF, Morris CR, Rawls ME. Congenital malformations of the central nervous system associated with genital type (type 2) herpes virus. *J Pediatr* 1969; 75:13–18.

Stagno S, Pass RF, Dworsky ME. Congenital cytomegalovirus infection: the relative importance of primary and recurrent maternal infection. *N Engl J Med* 1982; 306:945–949.

Stagno S, Pass RF, Dworsky ME, Alford CA. Congenital and perinatal cytomegalovirus infections. *Semin Perinatol* 1983; 7:31–42.

Torok TJ. Human parvovirus B19 infections in pregnancy. *Pediatr Infect Dis J* 1990; 9:772–776.

Walker J, Nokes DJ, Jennings R. Longitudinal study of toxoplasma seroprevalence in South Yorkshire. *Epidemiol Infect* 1992; 108:99–106.

Weller TH, Hanshaw JB. Virologic and clinical observations on cytomegalic inclusion disease. *N Engl J Med* 1964; 266:1233–1244.

Wilson CB, Remington JS, Stagno S, Reynolds DW. Development of adverse sequelae in children born with subclinical congenital toxoplasma infection. *Pediatrics* 1980; 66:767–774.

Yoshida M, Miyoshi I, Himuma Y. Isolation and characterization of human adult T-cell leukemia virus and its implication in disease. *Proc Natl Acad Sci USA* 1979; 79:2031–2035.

7

Respiratory Infections

NEIL M.H. GRAHAM

Although recognition of acute respiratory infections (ARI) as important causes of mortality (primarily among children in the developing world) and morbidity (in both developed and developing countries) has been slow in coming (Douglas, 1985; Monto, 1989), important advances have been made in understanding the epidemiology of these infections. Studies of risk factors for ARIs have been conducted predominantly in the developed world for reasons of funding availability, logistics, and the existence of an infrastructure capable of supporting large multidimensional studies. In general, results of epidemiologic studies conducted in the developed world have limited applicability in developing countries where risk factor exposures are often of a significantly greater magnitude or nature. The recent publication of the Board On Science and Technology for International Development (BOSTID) studies on ARI epidemiology in 12 developing countries has greatly broadened our knowledge outside the developed world (Bale, 1990). Thus, despite chronic underfunding of this type of research, several promising areas of epidemiologic investigation are being pursued, including nutritional risk factors and the effects of indoor and outdoor air pollution. Research on control strategies, including vaccines, case management, and risk factor modification, has also moved forward, albeit with varying success. In this chapter, the current state of knowledge on the magnitude, etiology, and risk factors for ARIs is reviewed, in addition to addressing several major methodologic problems and requirements for future research. Potential and existing control strategies at the public health level are also discussed.

Biologic Considerations

Viruses

Upper respiratory tract viral illnesses (URI) are caused by rhinoviruses (30% to 50%), coronaviruses (5% to 20%), influenza, parainfluenza, respiratory syncytial virus, adenoviruses, and certain enteroviruses (Berman & McIntosh, 1985; Reed, 1981). These illnesses are usually mild, self-limiting, and do not involve respiratory distress. Their importance in developed countries is largely social and economic through days lost from school and costs of treatment. However, in developing countries, they may herald the onset of pneumonia caused by secondary bacterial infection.

In children, lower respiratory viral illnesses are chiefly caused by respiratory syncytial virus; parainfluenza types 1, 2, and 3; influenza A and B; adenoviruses; and enteroviruses. These viruses can all cause bronchiolitis, croup, and pneumonia in children, but respiratory syncytial virus is most commonly associated with bronchiolitis and parainfluenza (especially type 1) with croup (Belshe et al., 1983; Foy et al., 1973; Mufson et al., 1970; Murphy et al., 1981). The extremely important role of respiratory syncytial virus in acute lower respiratory tract infections (LRI) has been emphasized in the BOSTID studies, where this virus was isolated in 65% to 80% of virus positive cases (Avila et al., 1990; Hortal et al., 1990a and b; Huq et al., 1990).

In developing countries the spectrum of viruses causing croup may be different, with measles playing a more important role (Berman et al., 1983; Wesley, 1975; see Chapter 9). Although often classified as a viral exanthem, the frequent association of measles with severe acute LRI in developing countries means it is often considered as an etiologic agent of acute respiratory illness (Escobar et al., 1976; Gonzaga et al., 1990). In the developed world it is not a serious cause of mortality in children (CDC, 1989). In general, however, virologic causes of acute infection of the lower respiratory tract in children seem to be similar in both developed and developing countries (Berman et al., 1981; Chanock et al., 1967; Escobar et al., 1976; Kloene et al., 1970; Monto & Johnson, 1968; Ogunbi, 1970; Olson et al., 1973; Shann et al., 1984a; Sobeslavsky et al., 1977; Spence & Barrat, 1968).

In most early epidemiologic studies, isolation of viral agents was limited by the laboratory techniques available. Isolation of virus from 20% to 25% of specimens was the maximum rate in several well-conducted studies (Denny & Clyde, 1986; Foy et al., 1973; Maletzky et al., 1971; Monto & Cavallaro, 1971; Monto et al., 1971). However, recent improvements in these techniques might make higher isolation rates more common. A recent study of LRI in infants reported a 66% positive isolation rate using combinations of viral culture and immunofluorescence techniques to identify viral antigens from throat and nasopharyngeal swabs (Wright et al., 1989b).

Bacteria

The major methodologic problem encountered in studying the bacterial causes of pneumonia is contamination of sputum specimens by nasopharyngeal and oropharyngeal organisms (Barrett-Connor, 1971). Thus, sputum cultures are of limited value. Because bronchoscopic and transtracheal aspirates are also at risk of contamination (Davidson et al., 1976; Halperin et al., 1982), most investigators now rely on percutaneous needle lung aspirates and blood culture for accurate diagnosis (Silverman et al., 1977). In the developed world, most cases of LRI in children are viral (Denny and Clyde, 1986; Glezen & Denny, 1973), but in developing countries mortality from bacterial pneumonia is a substantially larger problem. Studies of bacteria isolated from children in these areas, using lung aspiration techniques, have been reviewed by Berman and McIntosh (1985). The most important organisms identified in these studies were *Hemophilus influenzae* and *Streptococcus pneumoniae* (which together account for 54% of isolates) and *Staphylococcus aureus* (17%). Recent studies of children hospitalized with LRI in Argentina (Weissenbacher et al., 1990); Bangladesh (Rahman et al., 1990); Pakistan (Ghafoor et al., 1990), and the Philippines (Tupasi et al., 1990a) confirm that *S. pneumoniae* and *H. influenzae* (type B and untypable) were the most important bacterial causes of pneumonia. Other, less frequently encountered organisms were *Staph. aureus*, *K. pneumoniae*, and *H. parainfluenzae*. In otitis media, *S. pneumoniae* and *H. influenzae* are the most commonly isolated bacteria (Howie et al., 1970), but *Branhamella catarrhalis* has been isolated in 27% of cases in some series (Englehardt et al., 1989). *S. pneumoniae* and *H. influenzae* are also important causes of acute sinusitis in children (Wald et al., 1981). Bacteria cause pharyngitis and tonsillitis (*S. pyogenes*, *Corynebacterium diphtheriae*), acute epiglottitis (*H. influenzae* type B) and whooping cough (*Bordetella pertussis*); (Berman & McIntosh, 1985; Miller et al., 1982; Molleni, 1976).

Other Agents

The most important nonbacterial, nonviral respiratory pathogens are *Mycoplasma pneumoniae*, *Chlamydia* species, and *Pneumocystis carinii*. *M. pneumoniae* is most important as a cause of pneumonia and acute bronchitis (Denny & Clyde, 1986; Grayston et al., 1965; Jansson et al., 1964; Mufson et al., 1970). It may also cause upper respiratory illness (Grayston et al., 1965; Komaroff et al., 1983). *Chlamydia trachomatis* causes pneumonia in very young infants (Stagno et al., 1981; Suwanjutha et al., 1990), but *Chlamydia pneumoniae* (also called TWAR) seems to be more important as a cause of ARI (including pneumonia) in older children (Grayston, 1965; Marrie et al., 1987; Stagno et al., 1981). *Pneumocystis carinii*, a previously rare cause of pneumonia, has rapidly acquired major importance as a respiratory pathogen in individuals afflicted with the acquired immunodeficiency syndrome (AIDS). Before prophylaxis was widely used, approximately 60% to 80% of adult AIDS patients developed *P. carinii* pneumonia at some stage during the course of their illness (CDC, 1985; Murray et al., 1984). In developed countries, children with AIDS are also at significant risk for this organism, but at a lower rate than in adults. The importance of *P. carinii* secondary to HIV infection in children in the developing world, although apparently considerably less, has not been clearly defined (Quinn et al., 1986).

Classification of Acute Respiratory Infections

Although several classification systems have been proposed for ARIs, two basic systems are commonly used: the case-management classification system and the "traditional" clinical classification system.

Table 7.1. WHO Case-Management Classification System for ARI in Children Aged 2 Months to 5 Years in Developing Countries

Signs	Classification	Treatment
Central cyanosis Unable to drink	VERY SEVERE PNEUMONIA	ADMIT: O_2, antibiotic (Treat wheezing)
Chest in-drawing No central cyanosis Able to drink	SEVERE PNEUMONIA (Assess wheezing)	ADMIT: antibiotic (Treat wheezing)
No chest in-drawing Fast breathing	PNEUMONIA	HOME CARE: antibiotic (Treat wheezing)
No chest in-drawing No fast breathing	NO PNEUMONIA: COUGH OR COLD	HOME CARE: assess and treat chronic cough, otitis, sore throat (Treat wheezing)

Case-Management Classification

Given the importance of bacterial pneumonia as a cause of death in children in the developing world, WHO has developed a simple case-management approach designed to be used by village health care workers to reduce pneumonia mortality. Initial studies in India (McCord & Kielmann, 1978) and Papua New Guinea (Shann et al., 1984b) indicated that simplified case classifications could be successfully used by health workers to determine when children should be given antibiotics or referred to secondary- or tertiary-level care. These and several subsequent studies (Pandey et al., 1991; WHO, 1988) have also shown apparent reductions in pneumonia-related and overall mortality attributable to these interventions. In 1988, alterations were made to improve the specificity of these case-management guidelines (WHO, 1985a, 1988; 1989a and b). Although classification and management of syndromes causing stridor and wheezing are directly addressed and otitis media is classified separately, the primary focus remains on pneumonia. The major difference is in the group under 2 months of age. The facts that respiratory rate is often higher than 50 per minute and that some chest in-drawing can be normal in young infants make these signs less specific in this age group (WHO, 1989a). In addition, cough is often absent in neonates with pneumonia and is not sufficiently sensitive to be used as an indicator of severe disease. Thus, it has been recommended that signs of general sepsis should be sought (feeding problems, fever, hypothermia, drowsiness, convulsions, abdominal distention), as well as more specific signs of pneumonia (respiratory rate > 60, severe chest in-drawing, respiratory grunt) when deciding whether to give antibiotics and to admit to hospital (WHO, 1989a).

Clinical Classification

Although somewhat arbitrary, ARI syndromes have been often classified by the site of primary pathology. This system of classification creates some confusion because infections are not always limited to one part of the respiratory tract, and clinicians often disagree on what is "upper," "middle," and "lower." In addition, stridor-causing conditions have often been classified as upper respiratory tract infections, which is another source of confusion, because this classification is often held to be synonymous with mild disease. As these conditions can be fatal and may be inadvertently classified as acute LRI by primary health care workers (on the basis of respiratory distress), consideration has been given to classifying stridor-causing conditions within this category (WHO, 1985b). Nonetheless, classification by anatomic site remains the preferred system for most physicians and is compatible with the International Classification of Diseases (ICD) system. WHO has recommended using a simplified system that divides all respiratory conditions into upper and lower respiratory tract infections (Fig. 7.1).

Patterns of Occurrence

Developing Countries

The greatest health problem for developing countries is the mortality from ARIs in children aged younger than 5 years. Estimates of mortality associated with respiratory infection have been developed from the work of Bulla and Hitze (1978), Gwatkin (1980), and Leowski (1986). Gwatkin (1986) reckoned that each year during the late 1970s and early 1980s approximately 15 million children under the age of 5 years died. Based on the assumption that 25% to 33% of this mortality would have been due to ARIs, Leowski (1986) calculated that 2½ million infants and 1½ children aged 1 to 4 years would die from these infections each year. If developed countries are defined as those with infant mortality rates of 25 per 1000 births or less, 98% of those deaths in infants and 99% of those in children 1 to 4 years occur in less developed countries. Following the same reasoning, countries with infant mortalities of 100 per 1000 births or more contribute 58% of these deaths in infants and 66% in children 1 to 4 years. These figures may underestimate the magnitude of the problem because they are based on national mortality reporting systems of varying quality. Even the better systems may underreport total and specific mortality rates, whereas data from less established systems may be highly unreliable.

In addition to these estimates, other published data reflect large differences in mortality rates from respiratory infections between developed and developing countries. In 1977 infant deaths from pneumonia and influenza were five times higher in Costa Rica and 30 times higher in Paraguay than in the United States (Pio et al., 1985). For Filipino infants, pneumonia death rates have been reported to be 24 times higher than Australian infants, and 73 times higher in children 1 to 4 years (Douglas, 1979). Similarly, the Pan American Health Organization (PAHO) has reported pneumonia deaths in Peru as being 37 times higher in infants and 43 times higher in children 1 to 4 years compared to rates in North America (PAHO, 1980). Although the accuracy of these rates must be open to question since they rely on reporting mechanisms of variable fallibility, they illustrate the magnitude of the differences.

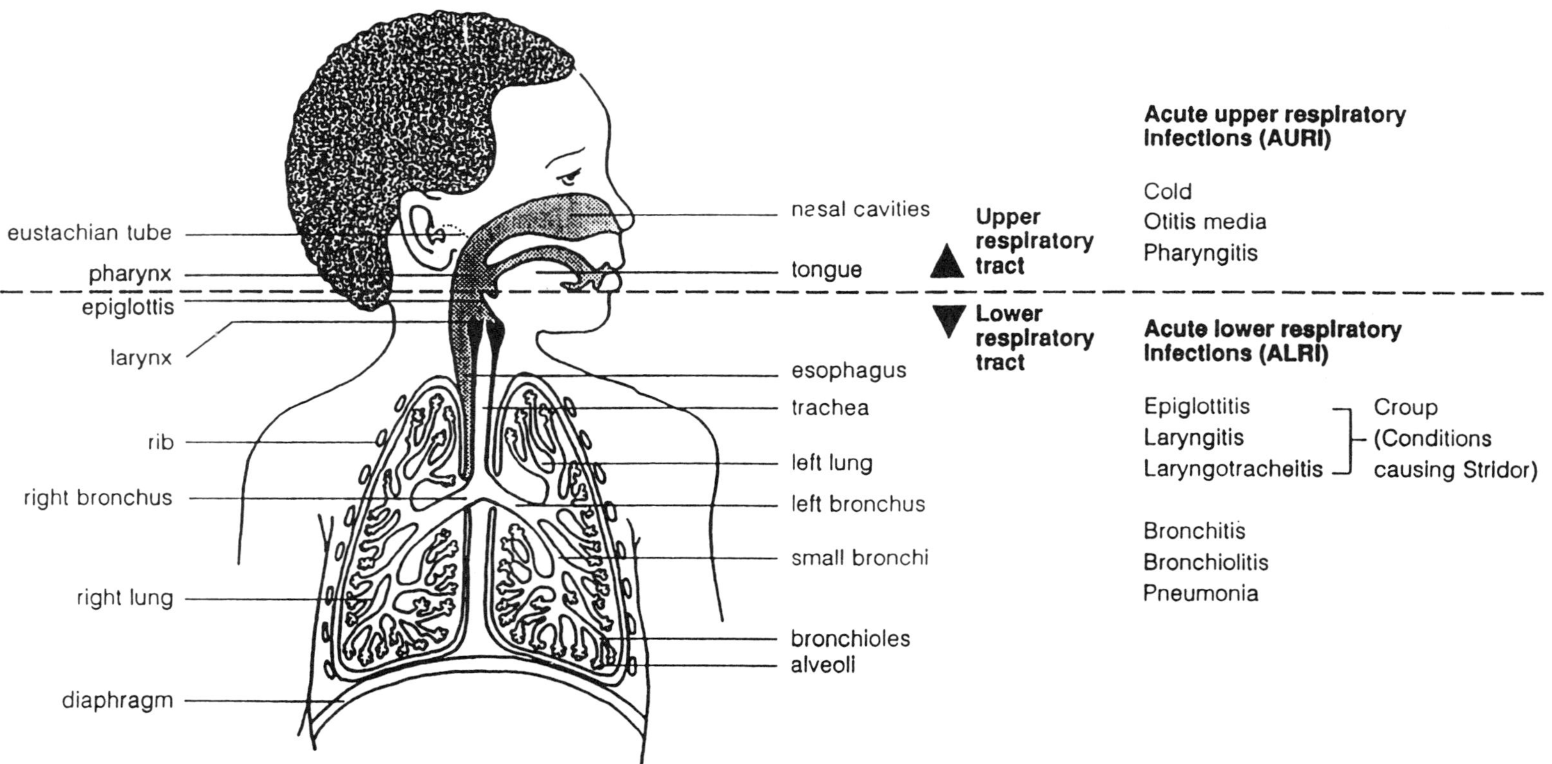

Fig. 7.1. Anatomically based classification system for upper and lower acute respiratory infections.

Despite these large variations in mortality, data from a number of studies suggest that morbidity rates from respiratory infections may be similar in developed and developing countries. In Tecumseh, Michigan, infants experienced a mean of 6.1 episodes of respiratory illness per year, and children 1 to 4 years had a mean of 5.2 episodes per year (Monto & Ullman, 1974). The Seattle Virus Watch from 1965 to 1969 reported that infants, on average, had 4.5 episodes per year (Fox et al., 1975). These rates are remarkably similar to those reported in urban settings in Costa Rica—4.9 and 5.7, respectively (James, 1972); in India—7.3 in children <2 years and 6.2 in children 3 to 5 years (Kamath et al., 1969); and in Ethiopia—7.9 and 6.6 for the same ages, respectively (Freij & Wall, 1977). More recent data from the carefully standardized BOSTID 12-country study confirm that six to eight episodes per child per year is the average throughout the world (McIntosh, 1990; Selwyn, 1990; Table 7.2).

These data suggest that severity, rather than incidence of ARI, explains the developed/developing world differentials in mortality. Nonetheless, morbidity in developing countries should not be ignored, because studies have shown that children have, on average, signs of ARI 20% to 40% (Selwyn, 1990) of the time. Indeed, one study reported rates as high as 60% in Bangladesh (Black et al., 1982), although in contrast to other studies, nasal discharge was included as a sign of ARI.

Developed Countries

The incidence rates of minor episodes of respiratory illness (chiefly upper respiratory tract infections) do not seem to have varied much over the past 60 years in the United States (Fox et al., 1972; Gwaltney et al., 1966; Monto & Ullman, 1974; van Volkenburg & Frost, 1933). Although studies have examined populations of differing compositions and have used differing study methods and definitions, the reported age-specific incidence rates have remained remarkably stable. In contrast, pneumonia mortality rates have fallen significantly in infants and young children, and moderate decreases have also been observed in older children and adolescents. Age-specific mortality rates from pneumonia and influenza in the United States from 1968 to 1986 are shown in Table 7.3.

Even though mortality rates for pneumonia and influenza have also fallen dramatically in young children and infants, LRI—croup, bronchitis, bronchiolitis, and pneumonia—is an important cause of morbidity affecting about 25% of children under 1 year and 18% of children 1 to 4 years annually (Denny & Clyde, 1986; Glezen & Denny, 1973; Henderson et al., 1979). A recent study reported the cumulative incidence of first episodes of LRI in infants to be 32.9% in children of families participating in a prepaid health plan (Wright et al., 1989a). This higher rate may be due in part to differing diagnostic criteria compared with previous studies or to increased physician attendance as a result of financial incentives in this health plan with an active, rather than passive, follow-up regimen.

In older children and adults in the United Kingdom, almost one quarter of all primary care health care visits and one third of days taken off work are attributable to acute respiratory illness (Cole & Wilson, 1989). In Australia,

Table 7.2. Incidence Rates per 100 Child-Weeks for ARI and LRI in BOSTID Community Studies

Region, Country of Study	ARI				LRI			
	Total No. of Child-Weeks at Risk	Total No. of New Episodes	Incidence Rate/100 Child-Weeks (95% CI)	Incidence Rate/100 Child-yrs*	Total No. of Child-Weeks at Risk	Total No. of New Episodes	Incidence Rate/100 Child-Weeks (95% CI)	Incidence Rate/100 Child-Years*
Africa								
Kenya	48,146	6,131	12.7(12.4, 13.0)	662	48,146	202	0.4(0.3, 0.5)	21
Nigeria	27,497	4,272	15.5(15.1, 16.0)	806	. . .	. . .	. . .	. . .
Oceania								
Papua New Guinea	. . .	. . .	. . .	. . .	6,543	168	2.6(2.2, 2.9)	135
Asia								
Philippines	65,108	8,643	13.3(13.0, 13.5)	692	65,108	747	1.1(1.1, 1.2)	57
Thailand	20,844	5,736	27.5(26.9, 28.1)	1,430	20,844	35	0.2(0.1, 0.2)	10
Latin America								
Colombia†	18,218	2,399	13.2(12.7, 13.6)	686	18,218	614	3.4(3.1, 3.6)	177
Uruguay†	4,014	620	15.4(14.3, 16.6)	562	4,014	327	8.1(7.3, 9.0)	296
Guatemala‡	15,280	2,572	16.8(16.2, 17.4)	874	15,280	92	0.6(0.5, 0.7)	31
Uruguay†§	6,332	829	13.1(12.3, 13.9)	478	6,332	399	6.3(5.7, 6.9)	230
Guatemala§	23,052	3,700	16.1(15.6, 16.5)	837	. . .	. . .	. . .	. . .

*Calculated by multiplying child-week rate by 52 (e.g., 0.4 × 52). For Uruguay 36.5 was used because visits were every 10 days.

†Cohort studies (birth to 36 months).

‡Index children only.

§Siblings, 0–4 years old, of index child.

Source: Selwyn, 1990.

Table 7.3. Age-Specific Mortality Rates from Pneumonia and Influenza in the United States, 1968–1986

		Age (years)		
Year	<1 year	1–4	5–14	15–24
1968	234.9	9.9	1.8	2.8
1970	180.8	7.6	1.6	2.4
1971	147.2	6.9	1.3	2.2
1973	115.7	5.9	1.4	2.0
1975	71.5	4.1	1.0	1.7
1977	53.2	3.1	0.9	1.3
1979	33.0	2.0	0.6	0.8
1981	22.6	1.8	0.5	0.8
1983	21.0	1.7	0.4	0.7
1986	17.6	1.4	0.4	0.7

Source: Data from National Center for Health Statistics. *Monthly Vital Statistics Report*, Hyattsville, MD: Public Health Service; 1968–1988.

1978 data from the Bureau of Statistics Health Survey show that 17% of participants 15 years or older consulted a physician for respiratory symptoms in the 2 weeks before the survey. Conversely, among children under 15 this figure rises to 43% (Australian Bureau of Statistics, 1977). Studies in Adelaide, Australia, suggest that each year children under age 5 experience a mean of seven episodes of respiratory illness, resulting in three doctor visits, the use of a pharmaceutical agent on 15 days, and 52 days of respiratory symptoms annually (Douglas, 1985). In the United States, upper and lower respiratory tract infections are estimated to be responsible for $15 billion in treatment costs per year in ambulatory and hospital settings (Dixon, 1985).

Risk Factors

Age

A large number of studies have shown that the incidence of acute viral respiratory illness peaks in infancy and early childhood and steadily declines with age (Fox et al., 1972, 1975; Gwaltney et al., 1966; Monto & Ullman, 1974; van Volkenburg, 1933; Table 7.4). This trend is generally attributed to changing patterns of exposure and the acquisition of specific immunity to an increasingly large array of virus types that occurs with age.

Infants are also at greater risk from bacterial pneumonia than older children, adolescents, and young adults (Tables 7.3 and 7.5). Similarly, in developing countries the incidence of ARI (particularly lower respiratory tract) peaks in the first year of life, remains elevated in the second year, and falls off rapidly thereafter.

Sex

Incidence rates of ARIs also vary by sex. van Volkenburg and Frost (1933) reported higher rates in boys under the age of 9 and the reverse pattern over

Table 7.4. Acute Respiratory Infection Morbidity Rates in Four U.S. Cohort Studies

			Mean Incidence/Year by Age Group					
Investigator	Years	Population	<1	1–2	3–4	5–9	10–14	15–19
Volkenburg & Frost	1924	Public Health Service families		3.0		2.7	1.9	
	1928–29	Baltimore families		4.5		3.5	3.5	2.4
	1929–30			4.5		3.8	2.8	2.3
Gwaltney	1963–66	Insurance co. employees						
Fox et al.	1965–69	Seattle families	5.1	5.8	5.8	3.8	2.3*	
Monto & Ullman	1969–71	Tecumseh families	6.1	5.7	4.7	3.5	2.7	2.4

*10–19 years

Table 7.5. Pneumonia Mortality Rates (per 100,000 Population) by Age and Sex in the United States, Costa Rica, and Cuba in 1987

		Age (years)			
Country	Sex	<1	1–4	5–14	15–24
United States	M	19.2	1.4	0.3	0.8
	F	15.7	1.2	0.3	0.6
Costa Rica	M	206.6	10.0	—	0.3
	F	127.6	5.2	0.3	—
Cuba	M	115.0	4.7	0.9	1.5
	F	102.9	4.3	0.6	1.7

Source: Data from World Health Organization. *World Health Statistics Annual.* Geneva, World Health Organization; 1989.

that age in Baltimore families in 1928 to 1930. However, no consistent pattern with gender was found in an earlier study in the same report. Monto and Ullman (1974) reported somewhat similar findings, with boys under 3 experiencing higher rates of illness and the opposite being true in older age groups. In contrast, a recent study of viral chest infections in infants found no differences in incidence by gender (Wright et al., 1989b). In developing countries the incidence of ARI is generally higher in boys than girls (an excess of 5% to 10%), although case fatality rates are commonly higher in girls (Selwyn, 1990). This paradoxical difference could be explained if girls are hospitalized or receive care at a later disease stage than boys.

Outdoor Air Pollution

In the earlier part of this century, episodes of acute, severe, particulate air pollution (in Meuse Valley, 1930; Donora, Pennsylvania, 1948; New York in 1953 and 1962; and Greater London in 1948, 1952, and 1956) resulted in rises in all-cause mortality due chiefly to increased deaths from pneumonia and cardiovascular disease in older adults (Ciocco and Thompson, 1961; Daley, 1959; Firket, 1931; Gore & Shaddick, 1958; Greenberg et al., 1962; Logan, 1952).

These studies have since stimulated research to examine the effects of much lower levels of air pollution on children for such outcomes as ARI, chronic respiratory disease, and changes in pulmonary function. This section focuses primarily on studies of respiratory infections. The components of air pollution most widely examined have been suspended respirable particulates, sulphur dioxide (SO_2), nitrogen dioxide, and ozone. Reports in the 1960s and 1970s were reviewed by Holland et al. (1979), but provided somewhat contradictory results. Nonetheless, a significant change occurred during this period: these studies began to focus on morbidity because it was likely to be a more sensitive outcome measure than mortality in studies of relatively low-level air pollution. Toyama (1964), in addition to reporting a correlation between bronchitis mortality and level of suspended particulates in children and older age groups, found that respiratory morbidity rates were higher in all ages and ventilatory function was poorer in children in air-polluted cities compared to relatively nonpolluted rural areas. Lunn and colleagues studied respiratory illness in Sheffield (United Kingdom) children (Lunn et al., 1967, 1970). In these studies, areas with relatively high and low levels of particulate matter (smoke) and SO_2 were compared. They found a relationship between exposure to high levels of particles and SO_2 in air, and repeated episodes of acute upper and lower respiratory tract illness, after adjusting for socioeconomic status. Conversely, Colley and Reid (1970) found a relationship between air pollution (urban:rural comparison) and acute lower, but not upper respiratory illness in children. This effect was most marked in the lower social classes. In these studies, adverse effects of air pollution were only apparent above moderately high threshold levels. Health effects in children have been estimated to occur above 180 $\mu g/m^3$ of SO_2 and 120 $\mu g/m^3$ of smoke, respectively (Levy et al., 1977).

In 1971, Collins, Kassap, and Holland reported that pneumonia and respiratory disease mortality in infants in England and Wales from 1958 to 1964 were most strongly associated with air pollution. A weaker but still significant relationship was also observed in children aged 1 to 4 years. In a study of Los Angeles college students, Durham (1974) found that upper respiratory symptoms reported by students presenting to campus health centers were significantly correlated with SO_2 and nitrogen dioxide levels, independent of the effects of age, weather, and smoking levels. Other investigators studied SO_2 and suspended sulphate levels in Salt Lake Basin, the Rocky Mountains, New York, and Chicago (French et al., 1973). In the Salt Lake Basin and the Rockies, high pollution levels were associated with excess reports of croup in children (age-sex-social class adjusted rates) who resided in a high pollution area for longer than 3 years. Similarly, in Chicago, acute upper and lower respiratory tract illness attack rates were reported to be higher in children, but in New York only the latter was significantly higher in residents of high pollution areas. Levy, Gent, and Newhouse (1977) found that high levels of SO_2 and particulate matter, but not nitrogen dioxide, carbon monoxide, or pollen, predicted hospital admission for acute respiratory disease, after adjusting for the effects of temperature. Penna and Duchiade (1991) also reported that particulate pollution levels in Rio de Janeiro were correlated with infant mortality from pneumonia, after adjusting for area of residence and income level. Particulate levels exceeded 240 $\mu g/m^3$ at 15 of the 22 stations where pollution levels were measured.

More recent studies have examined the effects of air pollution at much lower levels than earlier work and have endeavored to ascertain which components of air pollution are the most important causative factors. Study designs that allow concurrent comparison with similar demographic areas and adjustment for confounding factors (see Chapter 1), such as the Six Cities Study (Ware et al., 1986), have also been helpful in clarifying the role of outdoor air pollution in increasing susceptibility to acute respiratory illness in recent times. These investigators found that, between cities, annual mean differences in particulate and suspended sulphate concentrations as low as 80 $\mu g/m^3$ doubled the risk of acute cough and substantially increased the risk of bronchitis and other LRI in children. Associations with SO_2 were weaker, but significant. In another study, 24-hour fine particulate levels as low as 50 $\mu g/m^3$ were associated with significantly increased hospitalization rates in children for acute respiratory disease (Pope, 1989). The associations were stronger for bronchitis or asthma than for pneumonia or pleurisy and persisted when adjustments were made for meteorologic variables (see Chapter 15). Upper respiratory infections were twice as common in children residing in a more polluted city in Finland than in two less polluted cities (Jaakola et al., 1991). Sulphur dioxide, particulates, and nitrogen oxides at mean concentrations measuring 15–31 $\mu g/m^3$ were found in the more polluted city. These levels are relatively low, suggesting that there may be no lower threshold for health effects.

Other studies have confirmed the importance of the association between particulates, SO_2 and respiratory symptoms in children (Dales et al., 1989; Dockery et al., 1989), but the importance of ambient levels of nitrogen dioxide as a risk factor for respiratory illness is less certain (Dockery et al., 1989; Goings et al., 1989). Ozone exposures below the U.S. Ambient Air Quality Standard have been associated with acute changes in ventilatory function (Kinney et al., 1989) and with an increased risk of cough and LRI (Schwartz et al., 1989).

In sum, the evidence now clearly supports the hypothesis that suspended particulates, suspended sulphates, and SO_2 at levels currently being measured in ambient air significantly increase the risk of acute respiratory illness. However, since most studies do not include virologic sampling, it is unclear whether this morbidity is due chiefly to bronchial reactivity and respiratory tract irritation or to the effects of infection. Studies supported by virologic culture and serology are needed to answer this question. Data on nitrogen dioxide are somewhat less convincing, and it is too early to assess the importance of ozone as a risk factor for ARI.

Indoor Air Pollution

Passive smoking, nitrogen dioxide from gas cooking or heating, and smoke from biomass fuels are the three sources of indoor air pollution most often investigated in relation to ARIs. In children, many studies have focused on chronic lower respiratory symptoms or pulmonary function test abnormalities in relation to passive smoking (Schenker et al., 1983; Tager et al., 1979, 1983; Ware et al., 1984), but a substantial body of data also exist for risk of ARI with exposure to passive tobacco smoking (Colley et al., 1974; Fergusson & Horwood, 1985; Fergusson et al., 1980, 1981b; Harlap & Davies, 1974; Leeder et al., 1976;

Woodward et al., 1990). Exposure to passive smoking is associated with an increased risk of ARI in the first 2 years of life (Fergusson & Horwood, 1985), and maternal smoking seems more important than paternal smoking (Colley et al., 1974; Fergusson & Horwood, 1985; Woodward et al., 1990; Wright et al., 1991). Exposure to maternal cigarette smoke seems to approximately double the risk of lower respiratory tract illness in the first 2 years of life (Fergusson et al., 1981b; Ferris et al., 1985; Woodward et al., 1990). Negative studies have also been reported (Gardner et al., 1984; Lebowitz & Burrows, 1976; Love et al., 1981), but have been hampered by such factors as small numbers or did not report on smoking effects in children under 2 years of age. More recently, studies have focused on the effects of maternal smoking during pregnancy and the risk of respiratory infection in infants. Taylor and Wadsworth (1987) reported that prenatal smoking was a stronger risk factor for bronchitis in infants than postnatal smoking. Woodward et al. (1990) also examined this issue. Results were equivocal, but suggest that postnatal smoking was at least as important as prenatal smoking. The number of women who change smoking habits during or after pregnancy is small, and it may remain difficult to identify large enough comparison groups to fully settle this question in the future.

Natural gas cooking and heating stoves increase exposure of household members to nitrogen dioxide (Melia et al., 1978; Spangler et al., 1983), but at the relatively low levels attained in houses in developed countries it remains unclear whether these exposures significantly increase the risk of respiratory illness, despite numerous studies designed to test this question (Goings et al., 1989; Keller et al., 1979a and b; Melia et al., 1977, 1979; Ware et al., 1984). In studies of children in Adelaide, those who had gas heating in their homes were more likely to be prone to ARI than those with electric heating, but the level of significance was marginal (OR 1.6; 95% CI 1.0–2.6; Graham, 1987). Based on current data any effects attributable to nitrogen dioxide exposures are likely to be small (Samet et al., 1987). Of potentially far greater public health importance are the effects in children of smoke from the biomass fuels. In a study of Navajo children, cases of LRI were four times as likely to come from a home with a wood-burning stove than one without such a stove (Morris et al., 1990). This relationship persisted after multivariate analyses.

Children in many developing countries are exposed to peak and daily indoor concentrations of respirable particles from biomass fuels that are estimated to be about 20 times higher than the levels experienced in a developed country when two packs of cigarettes are smoked per day (Samet et al., 1987)—a level at which the risk of many respiratory symptoms approximately doubles (Ferris et al., 1985). In Zimbabwean huts, children exposed to wood-fire smoke from cooking have greatly raised carboxyhemoglobin (HbCO) concentrations (Martin, 1991). Concentration levels reached a mean of 6.45%, which are comparable to those found in smoking adults. Particulate exposures were also great, ranging from a mean of 546 $\mu g/m^3$ in children with URI to a mean of 1998 $\mu g/m^3$ in children with LRI. Reflecting this finding, in a study in Nepal, Pandey et al., (1989) found a relationship between hours per day spent near a stove and episodes of severe acute lower respiratory tract illness in children under age 2. However, in this study no adjustment was made for confounding factors, such as parental smoking (see Chapter 1). Campbell et al. (1989a) recently reported that children carried on their mother's back during cooking periods were at 2.8 times greater risk of an episode of "fast or difficult breathing" than children not so carried. Maternal reports of fast or difficult breathing were predictive of acute LRI in another study (Campbell et al., 1988). Armstrong and Campbell (1991) examined indoor air pollution and parental smoking in The Gambia. They found that paternal smoking increased the risk of LRI in children, but that regular carriage on a mother's back while cooking (a proxy for smoke exposure) was only predictive in girls. Kossove (1982) found that Zulu infants presenting to a medical clinic with acute LRI were more likely to be exposed to cooking smoke at home than children without respiratory illness, but the study was small and poorly controlled. These studies are difficult to conduct because in high ARI incidence areas exposure to indoor smoke is universally high and measurement of exposure dose is problematic. Intervention studies in high-incidence areas seem to be needed, but such interventions as building fluted stoves or providing smokeless fuel might not be economically feasible in many instances. Interestingly, in a U.S. study (Honicky et al., 1985; Osborne & Honicky, 1989), children from homes with wood-burning heating stoves also experienced more acute upper and lower respiratory tract illness than children from homes without stoves. Although the levels of the many gases, chemicals, and respirable particulates in wood smoke were not reported for either group, the relationship was not explained by social class, smoking, or other indoor sources of air pollution. Another study in the United States, which used a retrospective design, found no relationship between wood-smoke exposure and respiratory illness in school-aged children, suggesting that younger children may be those most at risk (Tuthill, 1984).

Social Factors: Crowding, Housing, Day Care, and Family Size

Because respiratory infections are contagious diseases, general conditions of crowding favor their propagation. Woods, as far back as 1927, reported a highly significant correlation between the proportion of overcrowded houses in a borough (two or more people per room) and pneumonia mortality in England and Wales. The strongest correlations were in the 0 to 5 age group, although an effect was also seen in adults. In 1945, Payling-Wright and Payling-Wright (1945) confirmed these findings by reporting strong correlations between crowding (persons per room and number of children per family) and mortality from bronchopneumonia in children under 2 years of age. Collins, Kassap, and Holland (1971) also reported significant correlations between crowding and death from bronchopneumonia in infancy, but pointed out that the relationship was confounded by indices of air pollution, social class, and educational status and the high intercorrelation of these factors. Holberg et al., (1991) found that in the first year of life sharing a bedroom with an older sibling increased the risk of RSV lower respiratory illness. More recent studies have focused on family size as a measure of crowding. The number and age of siblings in families predict the incidence of bronchitis and pneumonia in infants (Leeder et al., 1976), rates of acute respiratory illness in older children (Monto and Ross, 1977), and rates of acute LRI in infants (Gardner, et al., 1984). Aaby et al. (1988) reported that a decline in measles mortality in Guinea-Bissau after introduction of a vaccination program occurred despite increasing malnutrition and lower age at infection (see Chapter 9). Lower mortality was associated with low clustering of cases, i.e., isolated cases had a lower mortality than clustered cases. They argued that intensive exposure to measles virus through overcrowding and case clustering is a more important factor than malnutrition in predicting mortality from this disease. As support for this hypothesis, evidence is cited that mortality is high when a high proportion of measles patients have secondary cases. Given the extreme level of confounding between malnutrition and crowding as risk factors for ARI, it will require some considerable effort and care to tease out the separate effects of these factors. Nonetheless, this is not a trivial question and should be pursued further. Determining more precisely the attributable risks (see Chapter 1) for crowding or clustering and malnutrition in relation to acute LRI in developing countries would help focus interventions and improve their cost effectiveness.

In developed countries, the increasing use of day care centers for children, as mothers increasingly enter the workplace, has led to another illustration of the effects of crowding. Children attending group day care centers are at increased risk of acute upper and lower respiratory tract infections (Gardner et al., 1984; Strangert, 1976) and, in particular, increased risk of acute otitis media (Bell et al., 1989; Silipa et al., 1988; Strangert, 1977; Vinther et al., 1984), although not all studies have shown this relationship (Harsten et al., 1989). Harsten et al., (1990) found that up to 2.5 years of age children in group day care were at increased risk for ARI when compared to children at home or in family day care, who had similar rates. Group day care may also be associated with increased transmission of bacterial pathogens resulting in more severe invasive disease (Berg et al., 1991).

Nutrition

Despite the widely held belief that malnutrition increases the risk of severe, acute LRI, there are remarkably few epidemiologic data available that conclusively support this view. Because malnutrition is closely correlated with crowding, poverty, poor education, and poor housing in developing countries, it has proved difficult to identify an independent effect of this factor on risk for respiratory infection (Aaby, 1988; Aaby et al., 1988; Harsten et al., 1989). However, when taken together with studies of vitamin A and breast feeding, the picture regarding malnutrition and respiratory infection is becoming somewhat clearer.

Gomez et al. (1958) reported that mortality in hospitalized, underweight Mexican children was often associated with severe diarrhea and acute bronchopneumonia. In 1972, James published the results of a study from Costa Rica where the relationship of malnutrition (comparison of weight to standard measures) and respiratory illness was examined in poor children under the age of 5 years. Low-weight children experienced no more upper respiratory illness than normal-weight children, but episodes were of longer duration. However, in unadjusted analyses malnourished children experienced 2.7 times more bronchitis and 19 times more pneumonia and were far more likely to be hospitalized. Escobar et al., (1976) studied children hospitalized with LRI and found that mortality increased in relation to level of malnutrition (weight for age). Berman et al. (1983) found a significant relationship between malnutrition and pneumonia, but not with bronchitis or tracheobronchitis in children attending health centers in Cali, Columbia. Another report showed an increased relative risk of 27 for mortality from pneumonia in hospitalized children with third-degree malnutrition, with relative risks of 11.3 and 4.4 for second- and first-degree malnutrition, respectively (Tupasi et al., 1988). In the same report, malnutrition was not related to the incidence of respiratory morbidity in multivariate analyses, reportedly because of strong confounding from socioeconomic status (see Chapter 1). In another study the same investigators followed 1,978 children under 5 years and found that malnutrition increased the risk of LRI (RR = 1.9; 95% CI = 1.46–2.39) and substantially increased the risk of ARI mortality (two- to threefold; Tupasi, et al., 1990b). More recently, Smith et al., (1991) reported that in New Guinean children, low weight for age and low height for age (but not low weight for height) were associated with an increased incidence of LRI.

At the opposite end of the spectrum from malnutrition, obesity was reported to be associated with an increased incidence of respiratory illness in infants in one study (Tracey et al., 1971), but the normal-weight comparison group was breast-fed for longer and was of higher socioeconomic status so any effect of obesity may have been confounded by these factors (see Chapter 1).

Socioeconomic Status

Socioeconomic status has been measured in several different ways including rankings of occupational prestige, level of income, and educational status. Although these indices are intercorrelated, they do not all measure the same factors and tell little about the components of socioeconomic status that may act as risk factors for ARIs. Nonetheless, it has been clear for many years that socioeconomic status, no matter how it is measured, is associated with increased susceptibility to acute lower respiratory tract infections. Measures of occupational prestige and the proportion of families with incomes below the poverty line have been associated with increased mortality from bronchitis and pneumonia in children (Payling-Wright & Payling-Wright, 1945), as has educational status (Durham, 1974). Social class (as measured by occupational prestige) is also related to respiratory morbidity from predominantly lower respiratory tract conditions (Colley & Reid, 1970; Colley et al., 1973). However, the risk associated with lower socioeconomic status is not always consistent. Schenker et al., (1983), in a retrospective study, found relationships between low socioeconomic status (occupational status or educational level of parents) and severe chest illness and chronic respiratory symptoms in the first 2 years of life, but not with pneumonia or bronchitis. Gardner et al. (1984) used a combined measure of family income, insurance status, and parental educational level to measure socioeconomic status and found it is to be related to lower but not upper respiratory illness. Monto and co-workers (Monto & Ullman, 1974; Monto & Ross, 1977) found that lower-income families experienced more episodes of respiratory illness, but that lower-education level families experienced fewer episodes. This latter finding was unexpected and was attributed to differential symptom reporting rates by low and high educational groups. This finding illustrates how differently alternate measures of socioeconomic status can behave in predicting respiratory illness, but may also indicate that lower social class is a stronger risk factor for lower rather than upper respiratory illness, as was found in other studies (Gardner et al., 1984). The differentials in pneumonia and influenza mortality observed between economically developing and developed countries (Table 7.5) also reflect the association of low socioeconomic development with susceptibility to pneumonia in particular. However, the relatively similar levels of upper respiratory illness reported in developing and developed countries lends support to findings in developed countries that low socioeconomic status does not increase the risk of these conditions (see earlier section). Tupasi et al. (1988) confirmed that socioeconomic status *within* developing countries also strongly predicts the risk of ARI (they did not differentiate between upper and lower), but were unable to separate the effects of such factors as malnutrition, immunization status, and crowding.

These findings, of course, beg the key question: what is it about lower socioeconomic status that increases the risk of respiratory infection? Poverty and lower social status are associated with large family size, crowded living conditions, poorer access to health care, higher smoking rates, potential for nutritional deficit, lower breast-feeding rates, exposure to environmental pollutants (tobacco smoke, wood smoke, urban air pollution), and stressful living environments. These factors may contribute individually or perhaps interact to increase susceptibility to respiratory infections in these groups. In a study of young children in Adelaide who were prone and not prone to respiratory illness, lower parental occupational status was associated with having a prone child in bivariate analyses (Graham et al., 1990). However, after adjusting for such factors as maternal smoking, gender, number of siblings, parental history of respiratory illness, use of child care, maternal stress levels, and breast feeding, the relationship between social class and respiratory proneness disappeared. These data in young children help reflect the "grab-bag" nature of socioeconomic status as a risk factor and the importance of identifying the specific components that increase risk.

Meteorologic Factors

The seasonality of epidemics of ARIs has long been established, seeming to correlate best with low temperature, high humidity, and/or precipitation. These meteorologic conditions are generally associated with increased time spent indoors, either at home or at school, where many respiratory infections are transmitted (Beem, 1969; Dingle et al., 1964; Hendley et al., 1969). In these situations crowding allows more efficient viral transmission. Seasonality is most clear-cut in countries with temperate climates that have true seasons, but even in tropical countries case clustering tends to occur in the cool or wet season (Selwyn, 1990), although this is not absolutely universal. Whether meteorologic factors contribute to increased host susceptibility or enhanced viral integrity independently of this crowding effect has remained a matter of conjecture.

One factor that has been closely studied is the effect of low temperature or "chilling" on host susceptibility. Volunteers experimentally infected with rhinoviruses have been exposed to combinations of exposures of cold temperatures, wet clothes, and fatigue in studies in both the United States and the United Kingdom. In none of these studies were the volunteers who were exposed to chilling or cold more susceptible to infection (Christie, 1974; Douglas et al., 1968; Jackson et al., 1963). Other studies have found that low temperatures correlate with increases in mortality from pneumonia and bronchitis (Payling-Wright & Payling-Wright, 1945; Young 1924), but confounding from increased time spent indoors (leading to crowding) and higher levels of air pollution during winter makes these findings uninterpretable. This confounding is well illustrated in a recent study of air pollution and hospitalization for respiratory disease (Pope, 1989). Peak levels of respirable particulate air pollution occurred in mid-winter, presumably because condensation, cloud cover, and precipitation act to prevent dispersal of particulates and gases. In this study, low temperature was the meteorologic variable most closely correlated with hospitalization for respiratory disease and, together with mean fine particulate levels, explained 83% of the variance in total monthly hospital admissions for respiratory disease. Once again, it is impossible to disentangle the crowding effects of cold weather from any direct effects using these data.

Another meteorologic factor that might play a role is humidity. Gwaltney (1980) has pointed out that rhinoviruses may survive better at higher humidities. Thus, it might be postulated that higher humidity might favor transmission. However, in temperate or warm climates high humidity is often associated with the rainy season, so even in the absence of low temperatures, crowding from increased time spent indoors is likely to confound this relationship too.

Human Immunodeficiency Virus Infection

The newest risk factor for ARI is infection with the human immunodeficiency virus (HIV). The HIV epidemic has resulted in a dramatic increase in the incidence of *Pneumocystis carinii* pneumonia in the United States and other developed countries, particularly in adults (Hughes, 1987). Children with AIDS are also at risk from *Pneumocystis carinii*, but at a slightly lower rate than adults (Oleske et al., 1983; Rubinstein et al., 1983; Scott et al., 1984). Those with HIV are also at increased risk from bacterial pneumonia (Bernstein et al., 1985; Murray et al., 1984). *Streptococcus pneumoniae* and *Hemophilus influenzae* are the most commonly isolated organisms in community-acquired, HIV-associated bacterial pneumonia. The risk of pneumonia seems to be increased in HIV-infected patients with and without AIDS (Rolston et al., 1987; Schlamm & Yancowitz, 1989; Selwyn et al., 1988; White et al., 1985; Witt et al., 1987) and is believed to be due to a defect in humoral immune function seen in HIV infection (Ammann et al., 1984). The most common viral pulmonary infection found in children with AIDS is cytomegalovirus (Murray et al., 1984; Oleske et al., 1983; Scott et al., 1984). However, the pathogenicity of this virus in the lung is not always entirely clear, because it is sometimes isolated in the absence of histologic evidence of cytopathic change to lung parenchyma (Murray et al., 1987). The etiologic agents causing acute lower respiratory tract infections in HIV-infected children in Africa have not been completely elucidated at the present time. The most common pulmonary complication of HIV infection in Africa seems to be tuberculosis (Hira et al., 1990; Piot et al., 1990), although few studies have used appropriate microbiologic techniques to establish accurate estimates of risk in comparison with other organisms. It seems likely that HIV-infected children in Africa will also be at greatly increased risk from pneumonia caused by pyogenic bacteria, such as *S. pneumonia*, *H. influenzae*, and *Staph. aureus*, since these organisms are already important causes of pneumonia in that part of the world.

Whether HIV infection is associated with increased susceptibility to upper respiratory tract infections or to respiratory viruses in general is not known. It is also not known whether these less serious conditions can predispose to secondary bacterial invasion and pneumonia in AIDS patients.

Low Birthweight

Pio, Liowski, and Ten Dam (1985) have hypothesized that low birthweight may be an important risk factor for ARI (see Chapter 3). They cite the high incidence of low-weight births in developing countries and the higher mortality rates of these infants in the first year of life as support for this hypothesis. A recent study reporting on a 7-year birth cohort follow-up found that low birthweight (<2000 g) was associated with subsequent chronic cough, but not wheeze (Chan et al., 1989). No data were collected on acute respiratory symptoms in this study. Drillien (1959) in 1958 reported that low birthweight babies (<3 lbs, 1 oz) experienced higher rates of respiratory illness in the first 2 years of life than heavier babies. This relationship persisted when she stratified the infants by a "maternal care" index. Maternal care was poorly defined, but was reportedly closely correlated with the number of siblings in the family. However, after stratification by quality of housing and maternal care, low birthweight did not predict respiratory illness. Datta et al. (1987) studied low birthweight infants in India. These infants (<2500 g) experienced the same respiratory illness attack rate as normal-weight infants in the first year of life (4.65 versus 4.56 episodes), but had a much higher case fatality rate (24.6 versus 3.2 per 100 episodes of moderate or severe respiratory illness). Victora et al. (1989) also found that a birthweight of <2500 g was associated with increased mortality from respiratory infections, and this relationship persisted after adjustment for parental employment status, income, and education. However, in Uruguay, low birthweight was not associated with risk of ARI in children 1 to 4 years (Hortal et al., 1990b). Cerqueiro et al. (1990) found no relation between low birthweight and pneumonia treated as an outpatient, but for inpatients, low birthweight increased the risk of pneumonia twofold. These data suggest that low birthweight children do not experience higher rates of respiratory illness, but do experience more severe infections. Confounding from other factors associated with low birthweight—

crowding, poverty, poor nutrition—makes it difficult to ascertain whether the relationship is a causal one.

Lower Respiratory Tract Infection in Early Infancy

Several studies have now reported a relationship between acute lower respiratory tract infection in the first 2 years of life and chronic respiratory disease in later life (see Chapter 18). Childhood acute LRI has been related to chronic cough in young adults (Colley et al., 1973; Strachan et al., 1988), adult mortality from bronchitis (Barker & Osmond, 1986), and reduced ventilatory function and increased bronchial reactivity (Kattan et al., 1977; Mok & Simpson, 1948; Weiss et al., 1985; Woolcock et al., 1979). However, the relationship between early lower respiratory tract infection and subsequent ARI morbidity has not been studied as thoroughly. Data from two studies in Adelaide suggest that a similar relationship to that identified with chronic respiratory illness may exist. In a 3-year study of pneumococcal vaccine in young children, the strongest predictor of acute respiratory morbidity (recorded in respiratory symptom diaries by the mothers) in any 6-month period was the level of morbidity from the previous 6 months (Douglas & Miles, 1984; Pinnock et al., 1986). In a case-control study (Graham, 1987), young children who experienced high levels of respiratory illness morbidity (cases) were 11 times more likely to have experienced an episode of bronchitis, bronchiolitis, or pneumonia in the first year of life than children who had experienced low levels of morbidity (controls). After adjusting for the use of child care, number of siblings, breast feeding, maternal stress levels, parental occupational status, gender, exposure to gas heating, low birthweight, and parental history of respiratory illness, the relationship remained strong (OR = 9.5; 95% CI 5.5–16.6). These preliminary data, from both a prospective and a retrospective study, suggest that chest infections in infancy may predict subsequent levels of respiratory infection morbidity, at least in childhood. However, both of these analyses do not entirely disentangle acute from chronic morbidity nor did they address the etiology of symptoms i.e., whether it was infective or noninfective. Thus, further research is necessary to settle these questions.

Another key issue is whether LRI in early life acts as an early marker for genetically preprogrammed subsequent respiratory morbidity (chronic or acute) or whether it acts as a true risk factor by causing long-term damage to the lower respiratory tract. Until an effective intervention is available, such as a vaccine for respiratory syncytial virus, it may be difficult to determine which factor is more important. If previous respiratory morbidity predicts the level of subsequent morbidity from respiratory infections, there are also implications for statistical analyses of these types of data. Autocorrelation of this type suggests the need to control or adjust for repeated episodes of acute LRI. In prospective studies, the first episode can be used as the outcome for analysis, and Kaplan-Meier curves and Cox regression are then often used to estimate "survival time" (Wright et al., 1989b). For more frequent outcomes, such as upper respiratory tract infections, use of the first episode as an outcome would result in the loss of too much data. Although such techniques as autoregression (Rosner & Munoz,

1988) exist that allow adjustment for autocorrelated variables in multivariate models, they have not been widely used in studies of ARI. This is most likely due to the fact that the magnitude and nature of autocorrelation have not been clearly defined for respiratory infections in longitudinal studies.

Psychosocial Factors

Studies of relationships between psychosocial factors and respiratory infections have been conducted in experimental settings and using cross-sectional, retrospective, and prospective designs. All of the studies used upper respiratory infections or illnesses as the outcomes of interest, so data on LRI are lacking. Early cross-sectional studies conducted in college students reported relationships between anxiety and upper respiratory illness (Belfer et al., 1968), and between life changes, maladaptive coping, social isolation, unresolved role crisis, and illness behavior related to respiratory infection (Belfer et al., 1968; Jacobs et al., 1970). In the first report it was unclear how the outcome was measured, whereas in the other two studies illness behavior was addressed, but not the effects of psychosocial factors on the prevalence of respiratory infection. Boyce et al. (1977) undertook a longitudinal study of ARIs in children, but did not measure stress levels (or rigidity of family routines) until the end of the study. Nonetheless, they controlled for the effects of age, sex, race, income, and family size in the analyses and found that high life event scores and strict family routines were associated with increased duration and severity of respiratory illness. Other cross-sectional studies have found relationships between maternal stress and bronchitis in children (Hart et al., 1984), type A personality and respiratory illness in college students (Stout & Bloom, 1981), and poor family functioning and physician visits for ARIs in children (Foulke et al., 1988). None of these three studies could address the temporal relationship between psychosocial factors and respiratory illness, and none controlled for confounding factors.

However, there have also been several prospective studies showing that psychosocial factors may increase susceptibility to upper respiratory tract infections. In a series of studies involving experimentally induced colds at the Common Cold Unit in the United Kingdom, cognitive dissonance was associated with increased symptoms, introversion was associated with higher symptom and virus shedding scores, and certain life changes (resulting in decreased activity) predicted virus shedding (Broadbent et al., 1984; Totman et al., 1977, 1980). Although those subjects reporting higher stress or anxiety levels or who seem to be more introverted might be expected to report more symptoms, the finding that these factors were also associated with virus shedding in two of the studies is interesting. Most recently this group showed that rates of respiratory infection (confirmed by viral shedding) and clinical episodes significantly increase in relation to psychological stress in volunteers challenged with cold viruses (Cohen et al., 1991). These relationships persisted when confounding variables were taken into account and are strongly suggestive of a causal relationship. Meyer and Haggerty (1962), in a longitudinal study of 16 families (n = 100), reported that stressful life events in families were four times more likely to precede an episode of streptococcal pharyngitis than to follow it. High stress levels were also significantly associated with rises in ASO titer in this study. Although no adjustments were made for confounding factors, the objective outcome measures and prospective design lend strengths to their findings. In another prospective study, Kasl, Evans, and Niederman (1979) studied the relationship between a combination of high motivation and poor academic performance with clinical infectious mononucleosis in West Point cadets. During this 4-year survey, cadets who seroconverted against Epstein-Barr virus were monitored, and those with an "overachieving" father, high motivation, and a poor academic record were significantly more likely to have clinical infectious mononucleosis than a subclinical infection. High motivation and poor academic record interacted in this study to increase substantially the risk of clinical disease. Disease severity was confirmed by ascertaining the heterophile antibody titers in the clinical and subclinical cases.

We also studied the relationship between stress and upper respiratory tract infection in a prospective study in Adelaide (Graham et al., 1986). Episodes of illness were divided into definite, uncertain, and doubtful in a blinded fashion and confirmed, where possible, by a study nurse, virologic culture, or both. To improve the precision of stress measurement, a combination of three measures (major life events, minor life events, and psychological distress) was used in initial analyses. Prestudy stress variables predicted nurse-confirmed episodes and symptom days in "definite" episodes, even after adjusting for a range of confounding factors. A similar study was conducted examining the relationship between maternal stress levels and reported respiratory illness in children. We hypothesized that high maternal stress would reflect stress in the child, perhaps increasing the child's susceptibility to ARI in a manner similar to that seen in adults. Although the data were cross-sectional, a strong "dose-response" relationship was found between maternal stress levels and the risk of having a child who was highly prone to ARI (Graham et al., 1990). This relation persisted after adjusting for a wide range of potentially confounding factors and deserves further examination in a prospective study.

At present there are no data exclusively addressing the relationship between psychosocial factors and acute lower respiratory tract infection. Stress and anxiety might predispose to respiratory infection by two mechanisms. First, high stress levels may result in disruption of normal hygiene measures usually used to reduce transmission of respiratory viruses. Use of tissues and even handwashing (Dick et al., 1986; Gwaltney & Hendley, 1982; Gwaltney et al., 1978) may help reduce virus transmission, and high stress or anxiety levels may reduce adherence to these techniques.

This mechanism seems unlikely, however, first, because transmission factors were controlled in the experimental cold studies. Second, psychological stress and other psychological factors seem to suppress many components of immune function (Kiecolt-Glaser & Glaser, 1986), which may lead to increased susceptibility to respiratory infection. However, the immune function fluctuations observed to be associated with psychological factors may not have high clinical relevance, and until more data are available to address this issue their importance will remain uncertain.

Other Host Factors

In children, several host factors seem to influence susceptibility to LRI. Family history of asthma is associated with increased risk of bronchiolitis in infancy and seems to interact strongly with exposure factors, such as passive smoking and the presence of an older sibling in the home (McConnochie & Roghmann, 1986). This potential role of genetic factors seems to be supported by other studies reporting increased rates of wheeze-related respiratory illness in infants with small airway diameters (Martinez et al., 1988) and in those with higher virus-specific IgE responses to respiratory syncytial (Welliver et al., 1981) and parainfluenza viruses (Welliver et al., 1982). From a public health perspective, the most important host factor may be the observation that maternal antibodies in cord blood to respiratory syncytial and influenza viruses seem to be protective against subsequent infection in infants (Glezen et al., 1981; Puck et al., 1980). If maternal immunity can be passively transferred to infants, vaccination of pregnant women could be beneficial when appropriate vaccines become available.

Data Collection—Questionnaires

Although the optimal situation in any prospective study of ARI is to confirm the diagnosis through biologic means (Lim et al., 1989), in many situations there is a concurrent need for symptom data. Unfortunately, no standardized questionnaires exist for the collection of these ARI data (see Chapter 1). Measures developed by the American Thoracic Society (Speizer & Comstock, 1978) and the British Medical Research Council (Fletcher, 1960) were designed to measure chronic respiratory symptoms in adults. Their focus is so squarely set on symptoms of airway reactivity and allergy that they cannot be readily adapted for most studies of ARIs. Thus, many researchers have used either nonstandardized symptom diaries (Fig. 7.2) or recall questionnaires. Diaries have the advantage of minimizing recall bias and are useful in studies in which specific symptom complexes are important. Yet, they require daily recording by the study participant, usually the mother, and although this time commitment may not be a problem in studies of limited duration, it is likely to contribute to loss of follow-up in multiyear projects. An often-used alternative is to have research assistants call or visit parents on a weekly or fortnightly basis to inquire about symptom frequency and duration in the preceding period. This approach has all the problems associated with recall, but it is sustainable over long periods and the interviewer is able to define symptoms more clearly than would be otherwise possible using the diary approach. It is also likely to be easier to standardize a questionnaire than a symptom diary.

Gold et al. (1989) compared both approaches and found compliance greater with the questionnaire over the 2 years of the study. No differences in reporting of URIs were found, but an excess of LRI was reported in the questionnaires. The authors suggest that LRI symptoms (e.g., phlegm, wheezing, chest pain) may be easier to define by direct questioning. The diary method also recorded

CHILD's NAME ________ ID ________ RESPIRATORY EVENTS IN EARLY CHILDHOOD

DECEMBER 1988	1	2	3	4	5	6	7	8	9	10	11	12	13	14	15	16	17	18	19	20	21	22	23	24	25	26	27	28	29	30	31
Is he/she completely well ? Y=yes N=no																															
Do you think he/she has a cold? Y or N																															
Record each symptom he/she experiences each day. Mark with X.																															
Runny nose																															
Stopped-up nose																															
Hoarse throat																															
Wheezy/noisy breathing																															
Moist cough																															
Dry cough																															
Fever (feels hot)																															
Pulling at ears																															
Medication given (M)*																															
Doctor visits (D) *																															
Hospital visits(V)/ Hospital stays(S) * (*more details on back)																															
OTHER ILLNESSES (give brief details)																															

Fig. 7.2. Example of an acute respiratory illness symptom diary used in a 2-year cohort study of infants in Adelaide, Australia, 1988 to 1990.

a higher ratio of male to female LRI than the questionnaire method. Although the authors' interpretation may well be correct, both findings may equally reflect recall bias from the questionnaire. In Australian families respiratory diaries have been found to be superior to questionnaires and have been used successfully in long-term studies (Douglas & Miles, 1984). They are particularly useful when accurate determination of onset and duration of respiratory episodes is important. Ultimately, studies of both methods will be needed that utilize virologic culture and serologic methods to confirm episodes and to determine the best method of collecting these data.

The need for standardized questionnaires in developing countries is even greater (Miller, 1981). Not only are there considerable difficulties when standardizing measures of exposure between studies, but in many instances the clinical and laboratory expertise or facilities are not available to confirm diagnoses. A major attempt to standardize data collection protocols was undertaken in the recently completed National Research Council 12-countries project (Bale, 1990).

Most effort has focused on developing criteria for identifying acute LRIs from simple clinical signs. Studies now show that tachypnea and a history of fast breathing are highly sensitive and specific predictors of LRIs in both hospital and community settings (Cherian et al., 1988; Campbell et al., 1988; Leventhal, 1982; Shann et al., 1984a). If in-drawing is added, the sensitivity and specificity are improved (see Chapter 1). Debate has centered around whether to use different rates of tachypnea for children under 1 year and aged 1 to 4 years as the clinical cut-off for pneumonia. A recent paper by Harari et al. (1991) suggests that using 50 breaths per minute as a cut-off (± in-drawing) was equally useful above and below 1 year of age. Campbell et al. (1989b) recently reported that the best predictors of lobar pneumonia in infants were temperature >38.5° C and a respiratory rate >60 per minute. In studies of respiratory infection in developing countries, it may not be practical to aim for more specific diagnoses in every instance and may not always be within the resources of many studies. In areas where wheeze-related conditions are not highly prevalent, such specific diagnoses may not always be necessary.

Interventions

The case-management studies described earlier have been shown by several studies (Pandey et al., 1991; WHO, 1988) to result in reductions in pneumonia-related and overall mortality among infants treated with antibiotics in India and Papua New Guinea. In other areas where indoor air pollution from heating is prevalent, the obvious answer is to build fluted stoves or provide smokeless fuel, although doing so might not be economically feasible in many instances. Interestingly, in a U.S. study (Honicky et al., 1985; Osborne & Honicky, 1989) children from homes with wood-burning heating stoves also experienced more acute upper and lower respiratory tract illness than children from homes without stoves.

Interest in the relationship between vitamin A and respiratory infection began with the finding of Sommer and co-workers that vitamin A deficiency in children was associated with increased morbidity from respiratory infection and increased total mortality (Sommer et al., 1983, 1984). In a subsequent intervention study in Indonesia (Sommer et al., 1986; Tarwotjo et al., 1987), the same group reported a 34% reduction in all-cause mortality, but the reduction attributable to respiratory infections was not reported. Vitamin A supplementation has also been reported to reduce mortality from measles in a hospital-based study in Tanzania (Barclay et al., 1987). Subsequently, studies have confirmed these early reports of improved mortality (Rahmathullah et al., 1990; West et al., 1991), but whether vitamin A has any impact on ARI per se remains unclear (West et al., 1991).

In well-nourished Adelaide children, Pinnock and colleagues undertook two placebo-controlled vitamin A intervention studies (Pinnock et al., 1986, 1988). In the first study, respiratory morbidity in children with a history of frequent respiratory illness was reduced by 19% in those taking the supplement. However, this finding was not replicated in the second study in which children aged 2 to 7 who had an episode of bronchiolitis in the first year of life were followed for 12 months and no differences in respiratory morbidity were found. In Thailand, children with deficient serum retinol were four times more likely to experience respiratory morbidity than nondeficient children (Bloem et al., 1990). This study also found that supplementation with vitamin A offered some protection against respiratory illness, but it varied by age and length of follow-up, probably due to the study's small sample size. In a reanalysis of the original Indonesian vitamin A intervention study, no improvement in respiratory or enteric morbidity was seen in the children taking vitamin A (Abdeljaber et al., 1991). Clearly, further studies are needed to determine more conclusively what effects vitamin A supplementation has on morbidity and mortality from ARIs. It seems likely that beneficial effects will be limited to populations whose diets are significantly deficient in the vitamin and that any protective effects may only be seen for mortality, rather than morbidity.

Vitamin C has been advocated as a prophylaxis and treatment for upper respiratory tract infections. Several placebo-controlled trials have been undertaken, but generally, the results have been unimpressive in both treatment (Miller et al., 1977; Tyrell et al., 1977) and prophylactic situations (Pitt & Costrini, 1979).

In developed countries breast feeding seems to be clearly protective against the risk of acute otitis media (Saarinen, 1982; Teele et al., 1989), but perhaps not against other types of respiratory morbidity. Many studies have reported that breast-fed babies were at significantly lower risk of respiratory illness in bivariate analyses, only to have the relationship disappear after adjusting for confounding factors (Fergusson et al., 1978, 1985; Pullan et al., 19890; Taylor et al., 1982; Watkins et al., 1979; Woodward et al., 1990). However, two recent reports suggest the possibility of an interaction between breast feeding and other factors, such as passive smoking (Woodward et al., 1990), crowding, and minority status (Wright et al., 1989a). In addition, breast feeding has been found to be specifically protective for respiratory syncytial virus LRI in infants, even after adjusting for confounding factors (Holberg et al., 1991). These data suggest that breast feeding may reduce ARI morbidity in specific subgroups in developed countries. In developing countries, the weight of evidence also tends to support a protective effect of breast feeding. In Rwanda, mortality from acute LRI in hospitalized children under age 2 was lower in those who were breast fed (Lepage et al., 1981). In Brazil, in a community-based study breast feeding reduced respiratory infection mortality in children (Victora et al., 1987) and the incidence of upper respiratory morbidity, otitis media, and pneumonia in young infants (Forman et al., 1984). Whether the protective effect of breast milk is from its conferred anti-infective properties (Saarinen, 1982) improved hygiene, or nutritional factors per se is not entirely clear. Nonetheless, improved hygiene is more likely to protect against diarrheal diseases than respiratory infections (Victora et al., 1987), and nutritional factors are less likely to be important in developed countries than the anti-infective properties of breast milk.

Acknowledgments

The author would like to thank Dr. Antonio Pio of WHO, Dr. Robert M. Douglas of Australian National University, and Ms. Harriet Grossman for their assistance.

References

Aaby P. Malnutrition and overcrowding/intensive exposure in severe measles infection: review of community studies. *Rev Infect Dis* 1988; 10:478–491.

Aaby P, Bukh J, Lisse IM, et al. Decline in measles mortality: nutrition, age at infection or exposure. *Br Med J* 1988; 296:1226–1228.

Abdeljaber MH, Monto AS, Tilden RL, et al. The impact of vitamin A supplementation on morbidity: a randomized community intervention trial. *Am J Pub Health* 1991; 81:1654–1656.

Ammann AS, Schiffman G, Abrams D, et al. B-cell immunodeficiency in acquired immune deficiency syndrome. *JAMA* 1984; 251:1447–1449.

Armstrong JRM, Campbell H. Indoor air pollution exposure and lower respiratory infections in young Gambian children. *Int J Epidemiol* 1991; 20:424–429.

Australian Bureau of Statistics. *Australian Health Survey: Preliminary Bulletin No. 1.* Canberra: Australian Bureau of Statistics; 1977.

Avila M, Salomon H, Carballal G, et al. Isolation and identification of viral agents in Argentinian children with acute lower respiratory tract infection. *Rev Infect Dis* 1990; 12(suppl 8):S974–S981.

Bale S. Creation of a research program to determine the etiology and epidemiology of acute respiratory tract infection among children in developing countries. *Rev Infect Dis* 1990; 12(suppl 8):S861–S866.

Barclay AJG, Foster A, Sommer A. Vitamin A supplements and mortality related to measles: a randomized clinical trial. *Br Med J* 1987; 294:294–296.

Barker DJP, Osmond C. Childhood respiratory infection and adult chronic bronchitis in England and Wales. *Br Med J* 1986; 293:1271–1275.

Barrett–Connor E. The nonvalue of sputum culture in the diagnosis of pneumococcal pneumonia. *Am Rev Resp Dis* 1971; 103:845–848.

Beem MO. Acute respiratory illness in nursery school children: a longitudinal study of the occurrence of illness and respiratory viruses. *Am J Epidemol* 1969; 90:30–44.

Belfer ML, Shader RI, DiMascio A, et al. Stress and bronchitis. *Br Med J* 1968; 3:805–806.

Bell DM, Gleiber DW, Mercer AA, et al. Illness associated with child day care: a study of incidence and cost. *Am J Pub Health* 1989; 79:479–484.

Belshe RB, Van Voris LP, Mufson MA. Impact of viral respiratory diseases on infants and young children in a rural and urban area of southern West Virginia. *Am J Epidemiol* 1983; 117:467–474.

Berg AT, Shapiro ED, Capabianco LA, Group day care and the risk of serious infectious illnesses. *Am J Epidemiol* 1991; 133:154–163.

Berman S, Duenas A, Bedoya A, et al. Acute lower respiratory tract illnesses in Cali, Columbia: a two year ambulatory study. *Pediatrics* 1983; 71:210–218.

Berman S, McIntosh K. Selective primary health care: strategies for control of disease in the developing world XXI. Acute respiratory infections. *Rev Infect Dis* 1985; 7:674–691.

Bernstein LJ, Krieger BZ, Novick B, et al. Bacterial infection in the acquired immunodeficiency syndrome. *Pediatr Infect Dis* 1985; 4:472–475.

Black RE, Brown KH, Becker S, Yunus M. Longitudinal studies of infectious diseases and physical growth of children in rural Bangladesh. *Am J Epidemiol* 1982; 115:305–314.

Bloem MW, Wedel M, Egger RJ, et al. Mild vitamin A deficiency and risk of respiratory tract diseases and diarrhea in preschool and school children in Northeast Thailand. *Am J Epidemiol* 1990; 131:332–339.

Boyce WT, Jensen EW, Cassell JC, et al. Influence of life events and family routines on childhood respiratory tract illness. *Pediatrics* 1977; 60:609–615.

Broadbent DE, Broadbent MHP, Philpotts RJ, et al. Some further studies on the prediction of experimental colds in volunteers by psychological factors. *J Psychosom Res* 1984; 28:511–523.

Bulla A, Hitze KL. Acute respiratory infections: a review. *Bull WHO* 1978; 56:481–498.

Campbell H, Byass P, Greenwood BM. Simple clinical signs for the diagnosis of acute respiratory infections. *Lancet* 1988; 2:742–743.

Campbell H, Armstrong JRM, Byass P. Indoor air pollution in developing countries and acute respiratory infection in children. *Lancet* 1989a; 1:1012.

Campbell H, Byass P, Lamont AC, et al. Assessment of clinical criteria for identification of severe acute lower respiratory tract infections in children. *Lancet* 1989b; 1:297–299.

Centers of Disease Control. Update: acquired immunodeficiency syndrome—United States. *MMWR* 1985; 34:245–248.

Centers for Disease Control. Measles-United States, 1988. *MMWR* 1989; 38:601–605.

Cerqueiro CM, Murtagh P, Halac A, et al. Epidemiologic risk factors for children with lower respiratory tract infection in Buenos Aires, Argentina: A matched case-control study. *Rev Infect Dis* 1990; 12(suppl 8):995–997.

Chan KN, Elliman A, Bryan E, et al. Respiratory symptoms in children of low birth weight. *Arch Dis Child* 1989; 64:1294–1304.

Chanock R, Chambon L, Chang W, et al. WHO respiratory disease survey in children: a serological study. *Bull WHO* 1967; 37:363–369.

Cherian T, John TJ, Simoes E, et al. Evaluation of simple clinical signs for the diagnosis of acute lower respiratory tract infection. *Lancet* 1988; 2:125–128.

Christie AB. *Infectious Diseases: Epidemiology and Clinical Practice.* Edinburgh: Churchill Livingstone; 1974.

Ciocco A, Thompson DJ. A follow-up of Donora ten years after: methodology and findings. *Am J Pub Health* 1961; 51:155–164.

Cohen S, Tyrrell DAJ, Smith AP. Psychological stress and susceptibility to the common cold. *N Engl J Med* 1991; 325:606–612.

Cole P, Wilson R. Host-microbial interrelationships in respiratory infection. *Chest* 1989; 95(suppl):217s–221s.

Colley JRT, Reid DD. Urban and social origins of childhood bronchitis in England and Wales. *Br Med J* 1970; 2:213–217.

Colley JRT, Douglas JWB, Reid DD. Respiratory disease in young adults: influence of early childhood lower respiratory tract illness, social class, air pollution and smoking. *Br Med J* 1973; 3:195–198.

Colley JRT, Holland WW, Corkhill RT. Influence of passive smoking and parental phlegm on pneumonia and bronchitis in early childhood. *Lancet* 1974; 2:1031–1034.

Collins JJ, Kasap HS, Holland WW. Environmental factors in child mortality in England and Wales. *Am J Epidemiol* 1971; 93:10–22.

Dales RE, Spitzer WO, Suissa S, et al. Respiratory health of a population living downwind from natural gas refineries. *Am Rev Resp Dis* 1989; 139:595–600.

Daley C. Air pollution and causes of death. *Br J Prev Soc Med* 1959; 13:14–27.

Datta N, Kumar V, Kumar L, et al. Application of a case management approach to the control of acute respiratory infections in low birth weight infants: a feasibility study. *Bull WHO* 1987; 65:77–82.

Davidson M, Tempest B, Palmer DL. Bacteriologic diagnosis of acute pneumonia: comparison of sputum, transtracheal aspirates and lung aspirates. *JAMA* 1976; 235:158–163.

Denny FW, Clyde WA. Acute lower respiratory tract infections in non-hospitalized children. *J Pediatr* 1986; 108:635–646.

Dick EC, Houssain SV, Mink KA, et al. Interruption of transmission of rhinovirus colds among human volunteers using virucidal paper handkerchiefs. *J Infect Dis* 1986; 153:352–356.

Dingle JM, Badger GF, Jordan WS Jr. *Illness in the Home. A Study of 25,000 Illnesses in a Group of Cleveland Families.* Cleveland: Western Reserve University; 1964.

Dixon RE. Economic costs of respiratory tract infections in the United States. *Am J Med* 1985; 78(suppl 6B):45–51.

Dockery DW, Speizer FE, Stram DO, et al. Effects of inhalable particles on respiratory health of children. *Am Rev Resp Dis* 1989; 139:587–594.

Douglas RG Jr, Lindgram KM, Cough RB. Exposure to cold environment and rhinovirus cold. Failure to demonstrate an effect. *N Engl J Med* 1968; 279:742–747.

Douglas RM. *Acute Respiratory Infections.* Manila: World Health Organization, 1979.

Douglas RM. ARI—the Cinderella of communicable diseases. In: Douglas RM, Kerby-Eaton E, eds. *Acute Respiratory Infections in Children: Proceedings of an International Workshop.* Adelaide, SA: University of Adelaide; 1985:1–2.

Douglas RM, Miles HB. Vaccination against *Streptococcus pneumoniae* in childhood: lack of a demonstrable benefit in young Australia children. *J Infect Dis* 1984; 149:861–869.

Drillien CM. A longitudinal study of the growth and development of prematurely and maturely born children. Part IV. Morbidity. *Arch Dis Child* 1959; 34:210–217.

Durham WH. Air pollution and student health. *Arch Environ Health* 1974; 28:241–254.

Engelhardt D, Cohen D, Strauss N, et al. Randomized study of myringotomy, amoxycillin/clavulanate or both for acute otitis media in infants. *Lancet* 1989; 2:141–143.

Escobar JA, Dover AS, Duenas A, et al. Etiology of respiratory tract infections in children in Cali, Columbia. *Pediatrics* 1976; 57:123–130.

Fergusson DM, Horwood LJ. Parental smoking and respiratory illness during early childhood: a six year longitudinal study. *Pediatr Pulmonol* 1985; 1:99–106.

Fergusson DM, Horwood LJ, Shannon FT, et al. Infant health and breast feeding during the first 16 weeks of life. *Aust Pediatr J* 1978; 14:254–258.

Fergusson DM, Horwood LJ, Shannon FT. Parental smoking and respiratory illness in infancy. *Arch Dis Child* 1980; 55:358–361.

Fergusson DM, Horwood LJ, Shannon FT, et al. Breastfeeding, gastrointestinal and lower respiratory illness in the first two years. *Aust Pediatr J* 1981a; 17:191–195.

Fergusson DM, Horwood LJ, Taylor B. Parental smoking and lower respiratory illness in the first three years of life. *J Epidemiol Comm Health* 1981b; 1:99–106.

Ferris BG, Ware JH, Berkey CS, et al. Effects of passive smoking on health of children. *Environ Health Perspect* 1985; 62:289–295.

Firket J. The cause of the symptoms found in the Meuse Valley during the fog of December, 1930. *Bull Acad Roy Med Belg* 1931; 11:683–741.

Fletcher CM. Standardized questionnaire on respiratory symptoms. A statement prepared for and approved by the Medical Research Council's Committee on the etiology for chronic bronchitis. *Br Med J* 1960; 2:1665.

Forman MR, Gravbard BI, Hoffman HJ, et al. The Pima infant feeding study: breast-feeding and respiratory infections in the first year of life. *Int J Epidemol* 1984; 13:447–453.

Foulke FG, Reeb KG, Graham AV, et al. Family function, respiratory illness and otitis media in urban black infants. *Fam Med* 1988; 20:128–132.

Fox JP, Hall CE, Cooney MK, et al. The Seattle virus watch. II. Objectives, study population and its observation, data processing and summary of illnesses. *Am J Epidemiol* 1972; 96:270–285.

Fox JP, Cooney MK, Hall CE. The Seattle virus watch. V. Epidemiologic observations of rhinovirus infections, 1965–1969, in families with young children. *Am J Epidemiol* 1975; 101:122–143.

Fox JP, Cooney MK, Hall CE, et al. Rhinoviruses in Seattle families, 1975–1979. *Am J Epidemiol* 1985; 122:830–846.

Foy HM, Cooney MK, Maletsky AJ, et al. Incidence and etiology of pneumonia, croup and bronchiolitis in preschool children belonging to a prepaid medical care group over a four year period. *Am J Epidemiol* 1973; 97:80–92.

Freij L, Wall S. Exploring child health and its ecology. The Kirkos study in Addis Ababa. An evaluation of procedures in the measurement of acute morbidity and a search for causal structure. *Acta Paediatr Scand* 1977; 66(suppl):267.

French JG, Lowrimore G, Nelson WC, et al. The effect of sulphur dioxide and suspended sulphates on acute respiratory disease. *Arch Environ Health* 1973; 27:129–133.

Gardner G, Frank AL, Taber L. Effects of social and family factors on viral respiratory infection and illness in the first year of life. *J Epidemiol Comm Health* 1984; 38:42–48.

Ghafoor A, Nomani NK, Ishag Z, et al. Diagnoses of acute lower respiratory tract infections in Rwalpindi and Islamabad, Pakistan. *Rev Infect Dis* 1990; 12(suppl 8):S907–S914.

Glezen W, Denny FW. Epidemiology of acute lower respiratory disease in children. *N Engl J Med* 1973; 288:498–505.

Glezen WP, Paredes A, Allison JE, et al. Risk of respiratory syncytial virus infection for infants from low income families in relationship to age, sex, ethnic group and maternal antibody level. *J Pediatr* 1981; 98:708–715.

Goings SAJ, Kulle TJ, Bascom R, et al. Effect of nitrogen dioxide exposure on susceptibility to influenza. A virus infection in healthy adults. *Am Rev Resp Dis* 1989; 1075–1081.

Gold DR, Weiss ST, Tager IR, et al. Comparison of questionnaire and diary methods in acute childhood respiratory illness surveillance. *Am Rev Resp Dis* 1989; 139:847–849.

Gomez F, Glavan RR, Craviolo J, et al. Prevention and treatment of chronic severe infantile malnutrition (kwashiokor). *Ann NY Acad Sci* 1958; 69:969–981.

Gonzaga NC, Navarro EE, Lucero M, et al. Etiology of infection and morphologic changes in the lungs of Filipino children who die of pneumonia. *Rev Infect Dis* 1990; 12(suppl 8):S1055–S1064.

Gore AT, Shaddick CW. Atmosphere pollution and mortality in the county of London. *Br J Prev Soc Med* 1958; 12:104–113.

Graham NMH. *Psychosocial Factors in the Epidemiology of Acute Respiratory Infection*. Adelaide: University of Adelaide; 1987. Thesis.

Graham NMH, Douglas RM, Ryan P. Stress and acute respiratory infection. *Am J Epidemol* 1986; 124:389–401.

Graham NMH, Woodward AJ, Ryan P, Douglas RM. Acute respiratory illness in Adelaide children. II: The relationship of maternal stress, social supports and family functioning. *Int J Epidemiol* 1990; 19:937–944.

Grayston JT, Alexander E, Kenny G, et al. *Mycoplasma pneumoniae* infections. *JAMA* 1965; 19:369–374.

Grayston JT, Kuo CC, Wang SP, et al. A new *Chlamydia psittaci* strain, TWAR, isolated from acute respiratory tract infections. *N Engl J Med* 1986; 315:161–168.

Greenberg L, Jacobs MB, Droletti BM, et al. Report of an air pollution incident in New York City, November 1953. *Pub Health Rep* 1962; 77:7–16.

Greenberg L, Erhardt C, Field F, et al. Intermittent air pollution episodes in New York City 1962. *Pub Health Rep* 1963; 78:1061–1064.

Gwaltney JM. Epidemiology of the common cold. *Ann NY Acad Sci* 1980; 353:54–60.

Gwaltney JM, Hendley JO. Transmission of experimental rhinovirus infection by contaminated surfaces. *Am J Epidemiol* 1982; 116:828–833.

Gwaltney JM Jr, Hendley JO, Simon G, et al. Rhinovirus infections in an industrial population. I. The occurrence of illness. *N Engl J Med* 1966; 275:1261–1268.

Gwaltney JM, Moskolski PB, Hendley JO. Hand-to-hand transmission of rhinovirus colds. *Ann Intern Med* 1978; 88:463–467.

Gwatkin DR. How many will die? A set of demographic estimates of the annual number of infant and child deaths in the world. *Am J Pub Health* 1980; 70:1286–1289.

Halperin SA, Suratt PM, Gwaltney JM Jr, et al. Bacterial cultures of the lower respiratory tract in normal volunteers with and without experimental rhinovirus infection using a plugged double catheter system. *Am Rev Resp Dis* 1982; 125:678–680.

Harari M, Shann F, Spooner V, et al. Clinical signs of pneumonia in children. *Lancet* 1991; 338:928–930.

Harlap S, Davies AM. Infant admissions to hospital and maternal smoking. *Lancet* 1974; 2:529–532.

Harsten G, Prellner K, Heldrup J, et al. Recurrent otitis media: a prospective study of children during the first three years of life. *Acta Otolaryngol* 1989; 107:111–119.

Harsten G, Prellner K, Meldrup J, et al. Acute respiratory tract infections in children: a three year follow-up from birth. *Acta Paediatr Scand* 1990; 79:402–409.

Hart H, Bax M, Jenkins S. Health and behavior in preschool children. *Child Care Health Dev* 1984; 10:1–16.

Henderson FW, Clyde WA, Collier AM, et al. The etiologic and epidemiologic spectrum of bronchiolitis in pediatric practice. *J Pediatr* 1979; 95:183–190.

Hendley JO, Gwaltney JM, Jordan WS Jr. Rhinovirus infections in an industrial population. IV. Infections within two families of employees during two fall peaks of respiratory illness. *Am J Epidemiol* 1969; 89:184–196.

Hira SK, Ngandu N, Wadhawan D, et al. Clinical and epidemiological features of HIV infection at a referral clinic in Zambia. *J Acquir Immun Defic Syndr* 1990; 3:87–91.

Holberg CJ, Wright AL, Martinez FD, et al. Risk factors for respiratory syncytial virus-associated lower respiratory illnesses in the first year of life. *Am J Epidemiol* 1991; 133:1135–1151.

Holland WW, Bennett AE, Cameron IR, et al. Health effects of particulate air pollution: reappraising the evidence. *Am J Epidemiol* 1979; 110:533–659.

Honicky RE, Osborne JS, Akpom CA. Symptoms of respiratory illness in young children and the use of wood-burning stoves for indoor heating. *Pediatrics* 1985; 75:587–593.

Hortal M, Russi JC, Arbiza JR, et al. Identification of viruses in a study of acute respiratory tract infection in children from Uruguay. *Rev Infect Dis* 1990a; 12(suppl 8):S995–S997.

Hortal M, Benitex A, Contera M, et al. A community based study of acute respiratory tract infections in children in Uruguay. *Rev Infect Dis* 1990b; 12(suppl 8):S966–S973.

Howie VM, Ploussard JH, Lester RL Jr. Otitis media: a clinical and bacteriological correlation. *Pediatrics* 1970; 45:29–35.

Hughes WT. *Pneumocystis carinii* pneumonia. *N Engl J Med* 1987; 317:1021–1023.

Huq F, Rahman M, Nahar N, et al. Acute lower respiratory tract infection due to virus among hospitalized children in Dhaka, Bangladesh. *Rev Infect Dis* 1990; 12(suppl 8):S892–S897.

Jaakola JJK, Paunio M, Virtanen M, Heinonen OP. Low level air pollution and upper respiratory infections in children. *Am J Pub Health* 1991; 81:1060–1064.

Jackson GG, Muldoon RL, Johnson GC, Dowling HF. Contribution of volunteers to studies of the common cold. *Am Rev Resp Dis* 1963; 88(suppl):120–127.

Jacobs MA, Spilken AZ, Norman MM, et al. Life stress and respiratory illness. *Psychosom Med* 1970; 32:233–242.

James JW. Longitudinal study of the morbidity of diarrheal and respiratory infections in malnourished children. *Am J Clin Nutr* 1972; 25:690–694.

Jansson E, Wager O, Stenstrom R, et al. Studies on Eaton PPLO pneumonia. *Br Med J* 1964; 1:142–145.

Kamath KR, Feldman RA, Sundar Rao PSS, et al. Infection and disease in a group of South Indian families. II. General morbidity patterns in families and family members. *Am J Epidemiol* 1969; 89:375–383.

Kasl SV, Evans AS, Niederman JC. Psychosocial risk factors in the development of infectious mononucleosis. *Psychosom Med* 1979; 41:445–466.

Kattan M, Keens TG, Lapierre JG, et al. Pulmonary function abnormalities in symptom-free children after bronchiolitis. *Pediatrics* 1977; 59:683–688.

Keller MD, Lanese RR, Mitchell RI, et al. Respiratory illness in households using gas and electricity for cooking. I. Survey of incidence. *Environ Res* 1979a; 19:495–503.

Keller MD, Lanese RR, Mitchell RI, et al. Respiratory illness in households using gas and electricity for cooking. II. Symptoms and objective findings. *Environ Res* 1979b; 19:504–515.

Kiecolt-Glaser JK, Glaser R. Psychological influences on immunity. *Psychosomatics* 1986; 27:621–624.

Kinney PL, Ware JH, Spangler JD, et al. Short-term pulmonary function change in association with ozone levels. *Am Rev Respir Dis* 1989; 139:56–61.

Kloene W, Bang FB, Chakraborty SM, et al. A two-year respiratory virus survey in four villages in West Bengal, India. *Am J Epidemiol* 1970; 92:307–320.

Komaroff AL, Aronson MD, Pass TM, et al. Serologic evidence of chlamydia and mycoplasmal pharyngitis in adults. *Science* 1983; 222:927–929.

Kossove D. Smoke-filled rooms and lower respiratory disease in infants. *S Afr Med J* 1982; 61:622–624.

Lebowitz MD, Burrows B. Respiratory symptoms related to smoking habits of family adults. *Chest* 1976; 69:48–50.

Leeder S, Corkhill R, Irwig LM, et al. Influence of family factors on the incidence of lower respiratory illness during the first year of life. *Br J Prev Soc Med* 1976; 30:203–212.

Leowski J. Mortality from acute respiratory infections in children under 5 years of age: global estimates. *Rapp Trimest Statist Sanit Mond* 1986; 39:138–144.

Lepage P, Munyakazi C, Hennart P. Breastfeeding and hospital mortality in children in Rwanda. *Lancet* 1981; 2:409–411.

Leventhal JM. Clinical predictors of pneumonia as a guide to ordering chest roentgenograms. *Clin Pediatr* 1982; 21:730–734.

Levy D, Gent M, Newhouse MT. Relationship between acute respiratory illness and air pollution levels in an industrial city. *Am Rev Resp Dis* 1977; 116:167–173.

Lim I, Shaw DR, Stanley DP, et al. A prospective study of the aetiology of community acquired pneumonia. *Med J Aust* 1989; 151:87–91.

Logan WPD. Mortality in the London fog incident, 1952. *Lancet* 1953; 1:336–338.

Love GJ, Lan S, Shy CM, et al. The incidence and severity of acute respiratory illness in families exposed to different levels of air pollution, New York metropolitan area, 1971–2. *Arch Environ Health* 1981; 36:66–73.

Lunn JE, Knowelden J, Handyside AJ. Patterns of respiratory illness in Sheffield infant school children. *Br J Prev Soc Med* 1967; 21:7–16.

Lunn JE, Knowelden J, Roe JW. Patterns of respiratory illness in Sheffield infant school children. *Br J Prev Soc Med* 1970; 24:223–228.

Maletzky AJ, Cooney MK, Luce R, et al. Plan of study and observations on syndromes of acute respiratory disease. *Am J Epidemiol* 1971; 94:269–279.

Marrie TJ, Grayston JT, Wang SP, et al. Pneumonia associated with TWAR strain of *Chlamydia*. *Ann Intern Med* 1987; 106:507–511.

Martin KS. Indoor air pollution in developing countries. *Lancet* 1991; 337:358–359.

Martinez FD, Morgan WJ, Wright AL, et al. Diminished lung function as a predisposing factor for wheezing respiratory illness in children. *N Engl J Med* 1988; 319:1112–1117.

McConnochie KM, Roghmann KJ. Parental smoking, presence of older siblings and family history of asthma increase risk of bronchiolitis. *Am J Dis Child* 1986; 140:806–812.

McCord C, Kielmann AA. A successful programme for medical auxiliaries treating childhood diarrhea and pneumonia. *Trop Doctor* 1978; 8:220–225.

McIntosh K. Overview of the symposium. *Rev Infect Dis* 1990; 12(suppl 8):S867–S869.

Melia RJ, Florey C duV, Altman DG, et al. Association between gas cooking and respiratory disease in children. *Br Med J* 1977; 2:149–152.

Melia RJW, Florey C duV, Darby SC, et al. Differences in NO_2 levels in kitchens with gas or electric cookers. *Atmos Environ* 1978; 12:1379–1381.

Melia RJ, Florey C duV, Chinn S. The relation between respiratory illness in primary school children and the use of gas for cooking. I. Results from a national survey. *Int J Epidemiol* 1979; 8:333–338.

Meyer RJ, Haggerty RJ. Streptococcal infections in families: factors altering susceptibility. *Pediatrics* 1962; 29:539–549.

Miller DL. *Some Problems in the Classification of Acute Respiratory Infection in Young Children and Questionnaire Design*. Geneva: World Health Organization; 1981.

Miller DL, Alderslaide R, Ross EM. Whooping cough and whooping cough vaccine: the risks and benefits debate. *Epidemiol Rev* 1982; 4:1–24.

Miller JZ, Nance WE, Norton JA, et al. Therapeutic effect of vitamin C. A co-twin study. *JAMA* 1977; 237–251.

Mok JYQ, Simpson H. Outcome for acute bronchitis, bronchiolitis, and pneumonia in infancy. *Arch Dis Child* 1984; 59:306–309.

Molleni RA. Epiglottitis: incidence of extraepiglottic infection. Report of 72 cases and review of the literature. *Pediatrics* 1976; 58:526–531.

Monto AS. Acute respiratory infection in children in developing countries: challenge of the 1990s. *Rev Infect Dis* 1989; 11:498–505.

Monto AS, Cavallaro JJ. The Tecumseh study of respiratory illness. II. Patterns of occurrence of infection with respiratory pathogens 1965–1969. *Am J Epidemiol* 1971; 94:280–289.

Monto AJ, Johnson KM. Respiratory infections in the American tropics. *Am J Trop Med Hyg* 1968; 17:867–874.

Monto AS, Ross HW. Acute respiratory illness in the community; effect of family composition, smoking and chronic symptoms. *Br J Prev Soc Med* 1977; 31:101–108.

Monto AS, Ullman B. Acute respiratory illness in an American community. *JAMA* 1974; 227:164–169.

Monto AS, Napier JA, Metzner HL. The Tecumseh study of respiratory illness. I. Plan of study and observations on syndromes of acute respiratory disease. *Am J Epidemiol* 1971; 94:269–279.

Morris K, Morgenlander M, Covlehain JL, et al. Wood-burning stoves and lower respiratory tract infections in American Indian children. *Am J Dis Child* 1990; 144:105–108.

Mufson MA, Krause HE, Mocega HE, et al. Viruses, *Mycoplasma pneumoniae* and bacteria associated with lower respiratory tract disease among infants. *Am J Epidemiol* 1970; 91:192–202.

Murphy TF, Henderson FW, Clyde WA, et al. Pneumonia: an eleven-year study in a pediatric practice. *Am J Epidemiol* 1981; 113:12–21.

Murray JF, Felton CP, Garay SM, et al. Pulmonary complications of the acquired immunodeficiency syndrome. Report of a National Heart, Lung, and Blood Institute workshop. *N Engl J Med* 1984; 310:1682–1688.

Murray JF, Garay SM, Hopewell PC, et al. Pulmonary complications of the acquired immunodeficiency syndrome: an update. *Am Rev Resp Dis* 1987; 135:504–509.

Ogunbi O. Bacterial and viral etiology of bronchiolitis and bronchopneumonia in Lagos children. *J Trop Med Hyg* 1970; 73:138–140.

Oleske J, Minnefar AB, Cooper B, et al. Immune deficiency syndrome in children. *JAMA* 1983; 249:2345–2349.

Olson LC, Lexomboon U, Sithisarn P, et al. The etiology of respiratory tract infections in a tropical country. *Am J Epidemiol* 1973; 97:34–43.

Osborne JS, Honicky RE. Chest illness in young children and indoor heating with wood. *Am Rev Resp Dis* 1989; 139(suppl):A29.

Pan American Health Organization. Acute respiratory infections in the Americas. *Epidemiol Bull* 1980; 1:1–4.

Pandey MR, Boleij JSM, Smith KR, et al. Indoor air pollution in developing countries and acute respiratory infection in children. *Lancet* 1989; 1:427–429.

Pandey MR, Daulaire NMP, Starbuck ES, et al. Reduction in total under-five mortality in western Nepal through community-based antimicrobial treatment of pneumonia. *Lancet* 1991; 338:993–997.

Payling-Wright G, Payling-Wright H. Etiological factors in bronchopneumonia amongst infants in London. *J Hyg* (Camb) 1945; 44:15–30.

Penna MLF, Duchiade MP. Air pollution and infant mortality from pneumonia in the Rio de Janeriro metropolitan area. *Bull PAHO* 1991; 25:47–54.

Pinnock CB, Douglas RM, Badcock NR. Vitamin A status in children who are prone to respiratory tract infections. *Aust Pediatr J* 1986; 22:95–99.

Pinnock CB, Douglas RM, Martin AJ, et al. Vitamin A status of children with a history of respiratory syncytial virus infection in infancy. *Aust Pediatr J* 1988; 24:286–289.

Pio A, Leowski J, Ten Dam HG. The magnitude of the problem of acute respiratory infections. In: Douglas RM, Kerby-Eaton E, eds. *Acute Respiratory Infections: Proceedings of an International Workshop*. Adelaide, SA: University of Adelaide; 1985:3–16.

Piot P, Laga M, Ryder R, et al. The global epidemiology of HIV infection: continuity, heterogeneity, and change. *J Acq Immun Def Syn* 1990; 3:403–412.

Pitt HA, Costrini AM. Vitamin C prophylaxis in marine recruits. *JAMA* 1979; 241:908–911.

Pope CA. Respiratory disease associated with community air pollution and a steel mill, Utah Valley. *Am J Pub Health* 1989; 79:623–628.

Puck JM, Glezen WP, Frank AL, et al. Protection of infants from infection with influenza A virus by transplacentally acquired antibody. *J Infect Dis* 1980; 142:844–849.

Pullan CR, Toms GL, Martin AJ, et al. Breast feeding and respiratory syncytial virus infection. *Br Med J* 1980; 281:1034–1036.

Quinn TC, Mann JM, Curran JW, et al. AIDS in Africa: an epidemiologic paradigm. *Science* 1986; 234:955–963.

Rahman M, Huq F, Sack DA, et al. Acute lower respiratory tract infections in hospitalized patients with diarrhea in Dhaka, Bangladesh. *Rev Infect Dis* 1990; 12(suppl 8):S899–S906.

Rahmathullah L, Underwood BA, Thulasiraj RD, et al. Reduced mortality among children in Southern India receiving a small weekly dose of vitamin A. *N Engl J Med* 1990; 323:929–935.

Reed SE. The etiology and epidemiology of common colds and the possibilities of prevention. *Clin Otolaryngol* 1981; 6:379–387.

Rolston KVI, Uribe-Botero G, Mansell PWA. Bacterial infections in adult patients with the acquired immune deficiency syndrome (AIDS) and AIDS-related complex. *Am J Med* 1987; 83:604–605.

Rosner B, Munoz A. Autoregressive modelling for the analysis of longitudinal data with unequally spaced examinations. *Stat Med* 1988; 7:59–71.

Rubinstein A, Sicklick M, Gupta A, et al. Acquired immunodeficiency with reversed T4/T8 ratios in infants born to promiscuous and drug-addicted mothers. *JAMA* 1983; 249:2350–2356.

Saarinen UM. Prolonged breast feeding as a prophylaxis for recurrent otitis media. *Acta Pediatr Scand* 1982; 71:567–571.

Samet JM, Marbury MC, Spangler JD. Health effects and sources of indoor air pollution. Part 1. *Am Rev Resp Dis* 1987; 136:1486–1508.

Schenker MB, Samet JM, Spiezer FE. Risk factors for childhood respiratory disease. *Am Rev Resp Dis* 1983; 128:1038–1043.

Schlamm HT, Yancowitz SR. *Haemophilus influenzae* pneumonia in young adults with AIDS, ARC, or risk of AIDS. *Am J Med* 1989; 86:11–14.

Schwartz J, Dockery DW, Wypi D, et al. Acute effects of air pollution on respiratory symptom reporting in children. *Am Rev Resp Dis* 1989; 139(suppl):A27.

Scott GB, Buck BE, Leterman JG, Bloom FL, Parks WP. Acquired immunodeficiency syndrome in infants. *N Engl J Med* 1984; 310:76–81.

Selwyn BJ. The epidemiology of acute respiratory tract infection in young children: comparison of findings from several developing countries. *Rev Infect Dis* 1990; 12(suppl 8):S870–S888.

Selwyn PA, Feingold AR, Martel D, et al. Increased risk of bacterial pneumonia in HIV-infected intravenous drug users without AIDS. *AIDS* 1988; 2:267–272.

Shann FA, Hart K, Thomas D. Acute lower respiratory tract infections in children: possible criteria for selection of patients for antibiotic therapy and hospital admission. *Bull WHO* 1984a; 62:749–753.

Shann F, Graaten M, Germer S, et al. The etiology of pneumonia in children, Goroka Hospital, Papua New Guinea. *Lancet* 1984b; 2:537–541.

Silipa M, Karma P, Pukander J, et al. The Bayesian approach to the evaluation of risk factors in acute and recurrent otitis media. *Acta Otolaryngol* 1988; 106:94–101.

Silverman M, Stratton D, Diallo A, et al. Diagnosis of acute bacterial pneumonia in Nigerian children. Value of needle aspirations of lung and counter current electrophoresis. *Arch Dis Child* 1977; 52:925–931.

Smith TA, Lehmann D, Coakley C, et al. Relationships between growth and acute lower-respiratory infections in children aged < 5 y in a highland population of Papua New Guinea. *Am J Clin Nutr* 1991; 53:963–970.

Sobeslavsky O, Sebikari SRK, Harland PSEG, et al. The viral etiology of acute respiratory infections in children in Uganda. *Bull WHO* 1977; 55:625–631.

Sommer A, Tarwotjo I, Hussaini G, et al. Increased mortality in mild vitamin A deficiency. *Lancet* 1983; 2:585–588.

Sommer A, Katz J, Tarwotjo I. Increased risk of respiratory disease and diarrhea in children with pre-existing mild vitamin A deficiency. *Am J Clin Nutr* 1984; 40:1090–1095.

Sommer A, Tarwotjo I, Djunaedi E, et al. Impact of vitamin A supplementation on childhood mortality. A randomized controlled community trial. *Lancet* 1986; 1:1169–1173.

Spangler JD, Duffy CP, Letz R, et al. Nitrogen dioxide inside and outside 137 homes and implications for ambient air quality standards and health effects research. *Environ Sci Technol* 1983; 17:164–168.

Speizer F, Comstock G. Recommended respiratory disease questionnaires for use with adults and children in epidemiological research. *Am Rev Respir Dis* 1978; 118:7–53.

Spence L, Barrat N. Respiratory syncytial Virus associated with acute respiratory infection in Trinidadian patients. *Am J Epidemiol* 1968; 88:257–266.

Stagno S, Brasfield DM, Brown MB, et al. Infant pneumonitis associated with cytomegalovirus, chlamydia, pneumocystis and ureaplasma. *Pediatrics* 1981; 68:322–329.

Stout CW, Bloom LJ. Type A behavior and upper respiratory infections. *J Human Stress* 1981; 8:4–7.

Strachan DP, Anderson HR, Bland JM, et al. Asthma as a link between chest illness in childhood and chronic cough and phlegm in young adults. *Br Med J* 1988; 296:890–893.

Strangert K. Respiratory illness in preschool children with different forms of day care. *Pediatrics* 1976; 57:191–196.

Strangert K. Otitis media in young children in different types of day-care. *Scand J Infect Dis* 1977; 9:113–123.

Suwanjutha S, Chantarojanasiri T, Watthana-Kasetr S, et al. A study of non-bacterial agents of acute lower respiratory tract infection in Thai children. *Rev Infect Dis* 1990; 12(suppl 8):S923–S928.

Tager IB, Weiss ST, Rosner R, et al. Effect of parental cigarette smoking on the pulmonary function of children. *Am J Epidemiol* 1979; 110:15–26.

Tager IB, Weiss ST, Munoz A, et al. Longitudinal study of the effects of maternal smoking on pulmonary function in children. *N Engl J Med* 1983; 309:699–703.

Tarwotjo I, Sommer A, West KP, et al. Influence of participation on mortality in a randomized trial of vitamin A prophylaxis. *Am J Clin Nutr* 1987; 45:1466–1471.

Taylor B, Wadsworth J. Maternal smoking during pregnancy and lower respiratory tract illness early in life. *Arch Dis Child* 1987; 62:786–789.

Taylor B, Wadsworth J, Golding J, et al. Breast-feeding, bronchitis, and admissions for lower respiratory illness and gastroenteritis during the first five years. *Lancet* 1982; 1:1227–1229.

Teele DW, Klein JO, Rosner B, et al. Epidemiology of otitis media during the first seven years of life in children in greater Boston: A prospective cohort study. *J Infect Dis* 1989; 160:83–94.

Totman R, Reed SE, Craig JW. Cognitive dissonance, stress and virus-induced common colds. *J Psychosom Res* 1977; 21:51–61.

Totman R, Kiff J, Reed SE, et al. Predicting experimental colds in volunteers from different measures of life stress. *J Psychosom Res* 1980; 24:155–163.

Toyama T. Air pollution and its effects in Japan. *Arch Environ Health* 1964; 8:153–173.

Tracey VV, De NC, Harper JR. Obesity and respiratory infection in infants and young children. *Br Med J* 1971; 1:16–18.

Tupasi TE, Velmonte MA, Sanvictores MEG, et al. Determinants of morbidity and mortality due to acute respiratory infections: implications for intervention. *J Infect Dis* 1988; 157:615–623.

Tupasi TE, de Leon LE, Lupisan S, et al. Patterns of acute respiratory tract infection in children: a longitudinal study in a depressed community in Metro Manila. *Rev Infect Dis* 1990a; (suppl 8):S940–S949.

Tupasi TE, Mangubat NV, Sunico MES, et al. Malnutrition and acute respiratory tract infections in Filipino children. *Rev Infect Dis* 1990b; 12(suppl 8):S1047–S1054.

Tuthill RW. Woodstoves, formaldehyde and respiratory disease. *Am J Epidemiol* 1984; 120:952–955.

Tyrell DAJ, Wallace-Craig J, Meade TW, et al. A trial of ascorbic acid in the treatment of the common cold. *Br J Prev Soc Med* 1977; 31:189–191.

van Volkenburg VA, Frost WH. Acute minor respiratory diseases prevailing in a group of families residing in Baltimore, Maryland, 1928–1930. Prevalence, distribution and clinical description of observed cases. *Am J Hyg* 1933; 17:122–153.

Victora C, Smith PG, Vaughan JP, et al. Evidence of protection by breastfeeding against infant deaths from infectious diseases in Brazil. *Lancet* 1987; 2:319–322.

Victora CG, Smith PG, Barros FC, et al. Risk factors for deaths due to respiratory infections among Brazilian infants. *Int J Epidemiol* 1989; 18:918–925.

Vinther B, Pederson CB, Elbrond O. Otitis media in childhood. Sociomedical aspects with special reference to day care conditions. *Clin Otolaryngol* 1984; 9:3–8.

Wald ER, Milmoe GJ, Bowen A, et al. Acute maxillary sinusitis in children. *N Engl J Med* 1981; 304:749–754.

Ware JH, Dockery DW, Spiro A, et al. Passive smoking, gas cooking and respiratory health of children living in six cities. *Am Rev Resp Dis* 1984; 129:366–374.

Ware JH, Ferris BG, Dockery DW, et al. Effects of ambient sulphur oxides and suspended particles on respiratory health of preadolescent children. *Am Rev Resp Dis* 1986; 133:834–842.

Watkins CJ, Leeder SR, Corkhill RT. The relationship between breast and bottle feeding and respiratory illness in the first year of life. *J Epidemiol Comm Health* 1979; 33:180–182.

Weiss ST, Tager IB, Munoz A, et al. The relationship of respiratory infections in early childhood to the occurrence of increased levels of bronchial responsiveness and atropy. *Am Rev Resp Dis* 1985; 131:573–578.

Weissenbacher W, Carballal G, Avila M, et al. Etiologic and clinical evaluation of acute lower respiratory tract infections in young Argentinian children: an overview. *Rev Infect Dis* 1990; 12(suppl 8):S889–S898.

Welliver RC, Wong DT, Sun M, et al. The development of respiratory syncytial virus specific IgE and the release of histamine in nasopharyngeal secretions after infection. *N Engl J Med* 1981; 305:841–846.

Welliver RC, Wong DT, Middleton E, et al. Role of parainfluenza virus specific IgE in pathogenesis of croup and wheezing subsequent to infection. *J Pediatr* 1982; 101:889–896.

Wesley AG. Indications for intubation in laryngotracheobronchitis in black children. *S Afr Med J* 1975; 49:1126–1128.

West KP, Pokhrel RP, Katz, et al. Efficacy of vitamin A in reducing preschool child mortality in Nepal. *Lancet* 1991; 338:67–71.

White S, Tsou E, Waldhorn RE, et al. Life-threatening bacterial pneumonia in male homosexuals with laboratory features of the acquired immunodeficiency syndrome. *Chest* 1985; 87:486–488.

Witt DJ, Craven DE, McCabe WR. Bacterial infections in adult patients with the acquired immune deficiency syndrome (AIDS) and AIDS-related complex. *Am J Med* 1987; 82:900–906.

Woods HM. The influence of external factors on the mortality from pneumonia in childhood and later adult life. *J Hyg* (Camb) 1927; 26:36–43.

Woodward AJ, Douglas RM, Graham NMH, et al. Acute respiratory illness in Adelaide children: breast feeding modifies the effect of passive smoking. *J Epidemiol Comm Health* 1990; 44.

Woolcock AJ, Leeder SR, Pear JK, et al. The influence of lower respiratory illness in infancy and childhood and subsequent cigarette smoking on lung function in Sydney schoolchildren. *Am Rev Resp Dis* 1979; 120:5–14.

World Health Organization. *Proposal for the Classification of Acute Respiratory Infections and Tuberculosis for the Tenth Revision of the International Classification of Diseases.* Geneva: World Health Organization; 1985a.

World Health Organization. *Case Management of Acute Respiratory Infections in Children in Developing Countries.* Geneva: World Health Organization; 1985b.

World Health Organization. *Case Management of Acute Respiratory Infections in Children: Intervention Studies.* Geneva: World Health Organization; 1988.

World Health Organization. *Programme of Acute Respiratory Infections. Report of the Fourth Meeting of the Technical Advisory Group.* Geneva: World Health Organization; 1989a.

World Health Organization. *ARI Programme Report 1988.* Geneva: World Health Organization; 1989b.

Wright AL, Holberg CJ, Martinex FD, et al. Breastfeeding and lower respiratory tract illness in the first year of life. *Br Med J* 1989a; 229:946–949.

Wright AL, Taussig LM, Ray CG, et al. The Tucson children's respiratory study. II. Lower respiratory tract illness in the first year of life. *Am J Epidemiol* 1989b; 129:1232–1246.

Wright AL, Holberg LJ, Martinez FD, et al. The relationship of parental smoking to wheezing and non-wheezing lower respiratory illness in infancy. *J Pediatr* 1991; 118:207–214.

Young M. The influence of weather conditions on the mortality from bronchitis and pneumonia in children. *J Hyg* 1924; 23:151–175.

8

Gastroenteritis

ROGER I. GLASS AND CARYN BERN

Gastroenteritis is one of the most frequent illnesses affecting children, causing significant morbidity throughout the world and many deaths in developing countries. Although the term "gastroenteritis" implies inflammation of the stomach and intestines, the group of diseases involved can be caused by a wide variety of infectious agents. Many of these produce no inflammation and can be associated with a variety of conditions that are unrelated to the gastrointestinal tract. Consequently, the term now includes many enteric illnesses—acute and chronic diarrhea, dysentery, or vomiting regardless of whether inflammation is present or not. Throughout this chapter, the term "diarrhea" is often used interchangeably for gastroenteritis to emphasize the ambiguity.

Every child experiences diarrhea several times annually during the first 5 years of life, with the potential for severe disease, hospitalization, and death. Because the direct measurement of mortality from gastroenteritis requires surveillance of a large population for a prolonged period of time, estimates are generally based on survey data and extrapolation, resulting in substantial uncertainty (Bern et al., 1992a). However, diarrhea is undoubtedly one of the leading causes of death among children in developing countries, responsible for 25% to 30% of deaths among children younger than 5 years. In developed countries, diarrheal diseases also cause considerable morbidity and a substantial number of hospitalizations among children.

Biologic Considerations

Until recently, the cause of most episodes of gastroenteritis was unknown. It was attributed to a variety of childhood conditions—the introduction of weanling foods, malnutrition, gut allergies, enzyme deficiencies, changes in diet, and other conditions. Until 1970, an infectious agent could be identified in fewer than 30% of diarrheal episodes, thereby leaving ample opportunity for alternative explanations of disease etiology. Since then, many new infectious agents—viruses, bacteria, and parasites—have been discovered, and an etiology can be determined for a majority of cases when all diagnostic approaches are used. Consequently, infectious agents can now be identified for diarrhea previously attributed erroneously to weanling foods or malnutrition. The relative importance of each pathogen varies in developed and developing countries and by the age of the child.

Etiologic Agents

The diversity and peculiarities of these infectious agents have distinct implications for disease treatment, prevention, and control. Each agent has its own mode of transmission and requirements for control; specific drugs are required for some infectious diarrheas and not others; and some infections seem to be universal, causing disease in all children, whereas other infections are endemic among children in some developing countries but usually do not affect children in developed countries. The epidemiology of the newly identified agents has not been fully determined.

A large number of infectious agents—viruses, bacteria, and parasites—have been identified as causes of diarrhea in children (Table 8.1). Each agent has specific epidemiologic characteristics, including mode of transmission, reservoir, survival in the environment, and mechanism of disease production, such as toxins or tissue invasion. Agents, such as rotavirus, *Vibrio cholerae*, and enterotoxigenic *E. coli*, cause acute watery diarrhea, whereas such agents as *Shigella* and *E. histolytica* cause diarrhea with blood or mucus. Although the range of organisms associated with persistent diarrheal episodes is generally the same as those in acute episodes, enteroaggregative *E. coli* and *Cryptosporidium* have been identified more often (Bhan et al., 1988, 1989a and b), whereas multiple organisms are more commonly isolated in stools from persistent episodes (Bhan et al., 1989a; McAuliffe et al., 1986).

In general, bacterial pathogens are of greater importance in developing countries. Spread is generally by the fecal-oral route, and intensity of transmission is linked to poverty and poor sanitary conditions. By contrast, viral enteric agents, for which rotavirus is the prototype, are universal endemic pathogens of childhood, experienced by every child one or more times in the first few years of life (Kapikian & Chanock, 1990). This pattern has led researchers to speculate that rotavirus may have multiple routes of transmission, with contact or airborne

Table 8.1. Etiologic Agents of Gastroenteritis

Bacteria		Viruses	Parasites
Enterotoxigenic	Invasive		
Vibrio cholerae 0:1	*Shigella*	Rotaviruses	*Giardia lamblia*
V. cholerae non 0:1	*Salmonella*	Enteric adenovirus	*Cryptosporidium*
Escherichia coli histolytica	*Escherichia coli*	Norwalk virus	*Entamoeba*
C. perfringens fragilis	*Yersinia enterocolitica*	Astroviruses	*Dientamoeba*
Bacillus cereus	*Staphylococcus*	Caliciviruses	
Staphylococcus	*Campylobacter jejuni*	Coronaviruses	
C. difficile			
Other mechanisms			
V. parahemolyticus			
Aeromonas hydrophila			

Source: From Duggan et al., 1992.

droplet spread responsible for winter peaks of disease in developed countries and both contact/droplet and fecal-oral spread occurring in developing countries (Mahmoud & Feacham, 1987).

Finally, some etiologic agents require specific treatment. For example, depending on the clinical setting, antibiotics may be indicated for Shigellosis, cholera, or amebiasis. For all episodes of diarrhea, treatment should include rehydration and appropriate feeding.

The frequency of association of an etiologic agent with diarrheal episodes in a longitudinal study will be proportional to the overall incidence of diarrhea. For example, for an agent that causes diarrhea in every child once in the first 2 years of life, the proportion of episodes associated with the agent in a 2-year longitudinal study would be about 4% for a Bangladeshi child who has five to seven episodes per year, compared to 15% to 20% for a North American child with four to five episodes by age 2 (Table 8.2).

The total incidence of diarrhea due to an agent can be determined only through longitudinal studies, which are expensive and time consuming. However, the relative importance of agents causing moderately severe diarrhea can be estimated through outpatient studies and, for severe diarrhea, through inpatient studies. Thus, the rate of detection of an agent from longitudinal cohorts, outpatients, and inpatients with diarrhea, compared with that for controls, can be used to estimate the importance of that agent in causing mild, moderate, or severe disease and to confirm its pathogenicity.

Data compiled from 16 longitudinal studies in developing countries suggest that enterotoxigenic *E. coli* is the most commonly identified pathogen associated with mild endemic diarrhea; it was detected in a median of 23% of episodes (range, 1.9% to 38.1%). The next most common pathogens identified were *Campylobacter jejuni* (7.5%, range 1.5% to 12%), rotavirus (6.3%, range 2% to 22%), enteropathogenic *E. coli* (6%, range 3% to 9.7%), and *Shigella* species (5%, range 1.5 to 14.5%). Parasitic agents, in particular *E. histolytica* and *Giardia lamblia*, were detected more rarely (1% and 4%, respectively) and were found with equal frequency among asymptomatic children (Black et al., 1980, 1981, 1982, 1989; Cravioto et al., 1988; Cruz et al., 1988; Georges-Courbot et al., 1987; Giugliano et al., 1986; Guerrant et al., 1983; Rowland et al., 1988; Schorling et al., 1990; Sircar et al., 1984; Stanton et al., 1989; Varavithya et al., 1990; Zaki et al., 1986).

In longitudinal studies, researchers attempt to gain as complete a picture as

Table 8.2. Diarrheal Experience of Children in Bangladesh and the United States During the First 5 Years of Life

	Bangladeshi Child	American Child
Number of episodes per child per year	4–6	1.3–2.3
Total episodes	25	8
Number of episodes with:		
bacterial agent	4–6	0–1
viral agent	3–5	3–5
parasite	1–2	0–1
no agent identified	12	3
Risk of hospitalization	?	1/15 (6.5%)
Risk of death from diarrhea	1/20 (5%)	1/7000 (0.01%)

possible of the incidence and etiologic features of diarrheal episodes, no matter how mild. By contrast, outpatient and inpatient studies provide a measure of the relative importance of etiologic agents in causing disease severe enough to result in a clinic visit or health facility admission. In 14 outpatient studies, enterotoxigenic *E. coli* was found in a median of 14% (range 1% to 26%), whereas rotavirus was the most common agent detected (17%, range 1.3% to 24%); (Bhan et al., 1988; deMol et al., 1983; Echeverria et al., 1985, 1989; Hermann et al., 1988; Huilan et al., 1991; Linhares et al., 1983; MacKenjee et al., 1984; Mata et al., 1983, 1984; Mathewson et al., 1987; Mutanda, 1980; Osisanya et al., 1988; Rahman et al., 1990; Stoll et al., 1982). In all 11 inpatient studies, enterotoxigenic *E. coli* was found in a median of 9.3% (range 3.4% to 28%) and rotavirus in a median of 24% (range 14% to 41%) of episodes, confirming that rotavirus is the most important cause of severe dehydrating diarrhea (Bhan et al., 1988; deMol et al., 1983; Georges-Courbet et al., 1984; Mahmood et al., 1987; Mackenjee et al., 1984; Mata et al., 1983; Mutanda, 1980; Sethi & Khuffash, 1989; Sethi et al., 1989; Soenarto et al., 1983).

A similar body of longitudinal data is not available for developed countries, but a review of 12 inpatient and two outpatient studies yields median detection rates of enterotoxigenic *E. coli*, enteropathogenic *E. coli*, *C. jejuni*, *Shigella*, and *Salmonella* of 0.7% to 4%, whereas rotavirus was responsible for a median of 32% of episodes (range 11% to 68%) (Brandt et al., 1983; Donelli et al., 1988; Ellis et al., 1984; Gurwith & Williams, 1977; Kim et al., 1990; Kotloff et al., 1988; Riepenhoff-Talty et al., 1983; Uhnoo et al., 1986a and b; Vesikari et al., 1981; Wood et al., 1988). Enteric adenovirus, astrovirus, and other small round-structured viruses were detected in a median of 6% (range 0.9% to 10%), 3.6% (range 1% to 5%), and 3.9% (range 1.8% to 13%) of episodes of diarrhea, respectively. Thus, in developed countries, where the incidence of bacterial diarrhea is much lower, viral agents take on a proportionately greater role, although the absolute incidence of viral diarrhea is probably similar among children in developed and developing countries.

Agents associated with diarrhea are detected in the stools of asymptomatic individuals as well, with the ratio of symptomatic to inapparent infection varying by agent and with such host factors as age. For example, *C. jejuni* is detected in longitudinal studies at the same median rate in diarrheal stools (7.8%) as in control stools (7%). However, in a cohort of Mexican children, the ratio of symptomatic to asymptomatic infections fell with age, from 0.46 at 0 to 5 months of age, to 0.22 at 6 to 11 months, and to 0.17 at 12 to 23 months (Calva et al., 1988). For all established diarrheal agents, asymptomatic infections can occur. Hence, the mere finding of an enteric pathogen is not enough to determine with complete certainty that the agent was the specific cause of disease.

Patterns of Occurrence

Morbidity

The incidence of diarrhea among children has been measured in cohorts monitored for 1 or more years through active surveillance for diarrhea. Children in developing countries tend to have a higher incidence than those in developed countries (Table 8.2; Bern et al., 1992a; Glass et al., 1991). Most episodes are self-limited, but gastroenteritis always carries the potential for nutritional compromise, severe dehydration, and death.

In a recent review of 22 active surveillance studies in 12 developing countries, the median incidence of diarrhea for children younger than 5 years was 2.6 episodes per child per year, with a peak at age 6 to 11 months, corresponding to the introduction of weaning foods (Fig. 8.1; Bern et al., 1992a). In some studies, incidence rates as high as ten or more episodes per child per year have been observed among children younger than 2 years of age (Black et al., 1989; Lanata et al., 1989; Lopez de Romana et al., 1989; Schorling et al., 1990). Incidence varies widely even within the developing world. In one study in Brazil, children in poor rural and urban settings were compared with children from a more affluent area of the same city; poor children from rural and urban areas had incidence rates six and four times higher, respectively, than middle-class children (Guerrant et al., 1983).

Although most episodes are shorter than 7 days, from 3% to 20% of episodes in developing countries last longer than 14 days, meeting the definition for persistent diarrhea (WHO, 1988). In community-based studies from India, Bangladesh, and Brazil, several patterns emerge. Children who had persistent diarrhea at least once during the study period had more total days with diarrhea per year, as well as a higher incidence of diarrhea (Bhan et al., 1989a; Bhandari et al., 1992; Huttly et al., 1989; McAuliffe et al., 1986). In addition, persistent episodes carry a higher risk of mortality than acute cases (Bhandari et al., 1992). Thus, children with persistent diarrhea represent a group who are at increased risk of nutritional compromise and death.

The disease burden due to gastroenteritis is tremendous. On the basis of

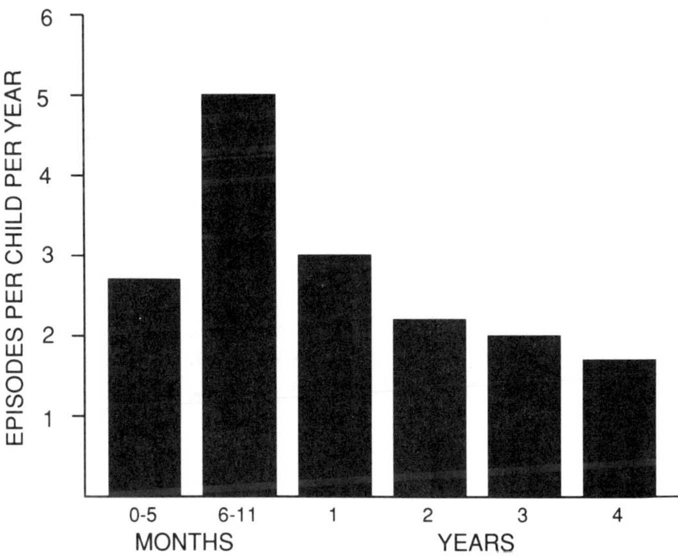

Fig. 8.1. Estimated median diarrheal morbidity for children younger than 5 years, based on results from 18 studies in developing countries. (From Bern et al., 1992a.)

three estimates of the median incidence in developing countries (Bern & Glass, 1992; Institute of Medicine, 1986; Snyder & Merson, 1982) and Institute of Medicine estimates for distribution of severity (Institute of Medicine, 1986), the world's 500 million children younger than 5 years have a calculated 1.1 to 1.7 billion episodes of diarrhea each year, of which 114 million are moderately severe and 29 million are severe (Bern & Glass, 1992). Thus, although the majority of episodes are mild enough to treat at home, a substantial proportion result in visits to health practitioners, expenditure on medicines, admission to health care facilities, or death.

Relatively few longitudinal studies have been performed in developed countries where diarrhea is generally believed to be a problem of lesser magnitude. However, a review of four such studies done in North America yields a summary rate of 1.3 to 2.3 episodes per child per year (Glass et al., 1991). In the same study, the authors, using national survey data, estimate that diarrhea results in 2.1 to 3.7 million physician visits and 220,000 hospitalizations per year in the United States, whereas another recent study estimates that 9% of all hospitalizations for children younger than 5 years are due to diarrhea (Gangarosa et al., 1992). Thus, diarrheal disease constitutes a significant public health burden in the developed world as well, carrying a high economic cost in physician visits, hospital admissions, and lost work time for parents.

Mortality

In Developing Countries

Although the incidence of diarrhea has been measured extensively in cohorts of children in developing countries, estimates of mortality from diarrhea are based on a composite of a few longitudinal studies and a larger number of surveys. Because these estimates carry important policy implications, it is important to bear in mind that the uncertainty in these figures is substantial.

In 1982, in a review of active surveillance data, Snyder and Merson estimated that 4.6 million children died of diarrhea each year, with 13.6 deaths per 1000 children younger than 5 years old. In a more recent report, based on a review of 15 studies in 10 developing countries, the median mortality from diarrhea was estimated to be 19.6 deaths per 1000 live births for infants (range 12.6 to 26.6) and 4.6 deaths per 1000 children 1 to 4 years of age (range 1.1 to 8.1; Bern et al., 1992a). On the basis of these estimates and the 1990 projected population for developing countries, excluding China, the authors calculated that 3.3 million children younger than 5 years die each year from diarrhea (range 1.5 to 5.1 million). The wide ranges of the estimates reflect their inherent uncertainty.

Estimates of diarrheal mortality have fallen substantially from 1982 to 1992 (Bern et al., 1992a). However, in all countries where a decline in mortality has been well documented, it began prior to the introduction of diarrheal control programs, and these decreases cannot be conclusively linked to public health interventions by the available data (El-Rafie et al., 1990; Pan American Health Organization, 1991). Better surveys are needed to substantiate the apparent decline (Bern et al., 1992a). Nonetheless, it seems plausible that increased global efforts to prevent diarrheal morbidity by improving access to oral rehydration therapy (ORT), emphasizing the importance of improved nutrition during and after diarrhea, and immunization against measles (see Chapter 9) may each have contributed to the global decline in mortality from diarrhea.

In the United States

Each year, about 350 children die from diarrhea in the United States, accounting for 0.5% to 3% of all deaths among children younger than 5 years, but 10% of preventable postneonatal infant mortality (Ho et al., 1988; Lew et al., 1991). No comparable data are available from other developed countries. Moreover, deaths from diarrhea that do occur in the United States primarily affect the most disadvantaged groups. The mother at greatest risk for having a child die of diarrhea is a black, unmarried mother in the South who is younger than 20 years of age, has not completed high school, and has not received prenatal care (Ho et al., 1988). These data imply that many diarrheal deaths in the United States are potentially avoidable by improvements in education, access to care, and earlier treatment.

Risk Factors

High-Risk Groups

Host factors are important determinants of risk of diarrheal disease. A group or individual may be at higher risk through increased susceptibility to pathogens, increased exposure to pathogens, being part of a concentration of susceptible individuals leading to outbreaks, or some combination of these factors (Table 8.3).

Table 8.3. Risk Factors for Diarrheal Disease Among Children

Increased susceptibility
Infancy
Congenital immunodeficiency, e.g., SCIDS
Acquired immunodeficiency, e.g., AIDS
Increased exposure
Low socioeconomic status
Non-breast-fed infants, weanlings
Travel to or residence in developing countries
Concentration of susceptible children
Day care centers
Hospital wards

Source: Adapted from Bern & Glass, 1992.

Age

Age may be the most important risk factor for gastroenteritis. Many diarrheal pathogens cause illness almost exclusively among children, although adults may be asymptomatically infected. The age of highest risk, and therefore of highest incidence of diarrheal episodes, is 6 to 11 months, when the infant is both more susceptible and subject to greater exposure to pathogens through the combination of waning maternal antibodies and the introduction of weanling foods (Bern et al., 1992a; Ho et al., 1988; Rowland et al., 1986; Snyder & Merson, 1982). Infection with rotavirus seems to cause more severe dehydration among children younger than 18 months than among older children (Bern et al., 1992b).

As a group, children in developing countries are at high risk because of increased exposure to pathogens in a contaminated environment. However, rates of diarrheal disease also vary by socioeconomic status within the same country (Guerrant et al., 1983), since more affluent members of the society have access to better sanitation and the means to limit contamination of food and water.

Breast Feeding

Breast feeding has long been known to protect children from enteric pathogens through decreasing exposure to contaminants (Gunn et al., 1979). For some pathogens, such as *Shigella* species and *V. cholerae*, even partial breast feeding confers protection from severe disease, either by transfer of maternal antibodies or toxin receptors in breast milk (Clemens et al., 1986, 1990a; Feachem & Koblinsky, 1984; Glass & Stoll, 1989; Mahmoud et al., 1989; Newburg et al., 1992). This protection appears to extend into the third year of life (Clemens et al., 1986). However, for rotavirus, the data are contradictory; some studies suggest that breast feeding is protective (Duffy et al., 1986) whereas others do not (Glass et al., 1986; Weinberg et al., 1984). There seems to be a dose-response relationship between number of breast feeds per day and the risk of death from diarrhea (Victora et al., 1989).

Malnutrition

In developing countries, malnutrition and diarrheal diseases are often linked in a cycle of declining health, with high attendant mortality. Although studies suggest that a malnourished child may not have an increased incidence of enteric infection, when that child is infected the illness tends to be of longer duration (Black et al., 1984) and may be of increased severity (Bern et al., 1992b; Mathur et al., 1985).

Immunodeficiency

Children with congenital or acquired immunodeficiency diseases are at particularly high risk for enteric infection from a wide variety of organisms (Chrystie et al., 1982; Yolken et al., 1982). In addition, immunosuppressed children may develop persistent infections with common agents, such as rotavirus, resulting in chronic diarrhea (Eiden et al., 1985; Pedley et al., 1984; Saulsbury et al., 1980).

Day Care

Day care centers contain a concentration of children in the susceptible age range and, as such, provide an opportunity for sporadic enteric infections to be amplified into outbreaks. Many outbreaks of diarrheal disease have been reported in day care centers, with the most common agents being rotavirus and *G. lamblia* (Bartlett et al., 1985, 1988; Grohmann et al., 1991; Pickering et al., 1986, 1988). Both of these organisms commonly result in a reservoir of asymptomatically infected children, which makes outbreak control difficult. Infants and toddlers cared for in day care centers have a higher incidence of endemic as well as epidemic gastroenteritis than children not in day care centers, and the effect is most marked for the youngest children (Bartlett et al., 1985; Sullivan et al., 1984). Contamination of surfaces and fomites, such as toys, may play a role in transmission, but covering diapers with a separate layer of clothing can decrease the rate of secondary spread (Van et al., 1991).

Pediatric Wards

Pediatric wards in hospitals contain another concentration of susceptible children, and gastroenteritis is one of the most common nosocomial infections. Rotavirus is the most frequent pathogen, but other agents, such as astrovirus, calicivirus, and small round-structured viruses, have been reported as well (Chiba et al., 1979; Cubitt et al., 1980; Esahli et al., 1991; Ford-Jones et al., 1990).

Interventions

Prevention

At the turn of the century, the United States and Europe had rates of diarrheal disease and diarrheal mortality comparable to those of developing countries today. Improvements in water and sanitation over the subsequent decades changed the patterns of disease from high incidence and summer peaks of bacterial diarrhea to the present low incidence rates, with winter peaks corresponding to rotavirus diarrhea among children. It is clear therefore that widespread improvements in water and sanitation would have an impact on diarrheal disease morbidity and mortality in developing countries. A review of 67 water and/or sanitation intervention studies suggests that in the short term, improved sanitary facilities have a greater impact than improvements in water quality and that a greater impact can be demonstrated for mortality or severe diarrhea than for milder disease (Esrey et al., 1985). However, such interventions are costly, and accordingly, diarrheal disease control programs have emphasized other preventive approaches judged to be more cost effective (Walsh & Warren, 1979).

On the basis of the demonstrated protective effect of breast feeding, diarrheal disease control programs in developing countries now include the promotion of exclusive breast feeding for the first 4 to 6 months of life and partial breast feeding for as long as 2 to 3 years (Feachem & Koblinsky, 1984). Even in developed countries, there is evidence that breast feeding may play a protective role (Duffy et al., 1986).

Measles immunization has been promoted as an intervention to avert diarrhea associated with acute measles (15% to 63% of measles cases) and postmeasles diarrhea (Feachem & Koblinksy, 1983, Koenig et al., 1990). Theoretical calculations suggest that measles coverage at 9 to 11 months of 45% to 90% could prevent 0.6% to 3.8% of diarrheal episodes and 6% to 26% of diarrheal deaths. However, because measles immunization is a part of national immunization programs in most countries, no additional costs would be involved for this intervention beyond those required to maintain high levels (see Chapter 9).

Rotavirus is responsible for an estimated 20% of all diarrheal deaths among children younger than 5 years, and an effective vaccine could decrease diarrheal morbidity by 2% to 3% and mortality by 6% to 10% in developing countries (de Zoysa & Feacham, 1985). Because rotavirus transmission is thought to occur by modes other than the fecal-oral routes, effective vaccines are the most promising intervention to decrease the morbidity associated with rotavirus in industrialized countries as well. To date, candidate rotavirus vaccines have varied widely in efficacy, and efficacy rates have generally been lower in developing than in developed countries (Clark, 1988; Flores et al., 1987; Georges-Courbet et al., 1991; Santosham et al., 1991; Vesikari et al., 1984).

Cholera vaccine has also been suggested as a selective intervention in areas with high incidence rates, such as Bangladesh (de Zoysa & Feacham, 1985). Unfortunately, the efficacy of the recent oral B subunit vaccine, although acceptable in adults, has been substantially lower among children (Clemens et al., 1990b).

Therapy

Interventions to prevent gastroenteritis include improved water and sanitation, exclusive breast feeding for young infants, and the timely administration of measles vaccine. Diarrheal episodes should be treated with appropriate rehydration and feeding; more widespread use of oral rehydration solutions (ORS) has the potential to prevent much of the morbidity and mortality associated with gastroenteritis.

The cornerstone of diarrheal case management is rehydration therapy (Table 8.4). Although a few bacterial and parasitic diarrheas may require treatment with antibiotics, most enteric infections are self-limited, and the resultant morbidity is largely due to dehydration and electrolyte imbalances. For severe dehydration, intravenous rehydration is required, but for the vast majority of diarrheal illnesses, oral rehydration therapy (ORT) can be administered successfully (Duggan et al., 1992). In addition to the appropriate use of ORT, it

Table 8.4. Diarrhea Treatment Chart

Degree of Dehydration	Signs*	Rehydration Therapy (within 4 hr)	Replacement of Stool Losses	Dietary Therapy†
Mild	Slightly dry buccal mucous membranes, increased thirst	ORS 50 mL/kg	10 mL/kg or 1/2 to 1 cup of ORS for each diarrheal stool	Human milk feeding, half- or full-strength lactose-containing milk or undiluted lactose-free formula
Moderate	Sunken eyes, sunken fontanelle, loss of skin turgor, dry buccal mucous membranes	ORS 100 mL/kg	Same as above	Same as above
Severe	Signs of moderate dehydration plus one of the following: rapid thready pulse, cyanosis, rapid breathing, lethargy, coma	Intravenous fluids (Ringer lactate), 40 mL/kg/hr until pulse and state of consciousness return to normal; then 50 to 100 mL/kg of ORS	Same as above	Same as above

*If no signs of dehydration are present, rehydration therapy is not required. Proceed with maintenance therapy and replacement of stool losses.

†Infants and children who receive solid food may continue their usual diet.

Source: Adapted from Duggan et al., 1992.

is important to continue feeding the child with diarrhea (Table 8-4). Although ORT is now widely accepted as the mainstay of treatment in the developing world, it is still underutilized in the United States (Avery & Snyder, 1990).

ORT has been demonstrated to be as effective as intravenous therapy in the treatment of hospitalized children with acute gastroenteritis, resulting in equally prompt resolution of diarrhea and electrolyte abnormalities (Santosham et al., 1982). The wider use of ORT could prevent or shorten many pediatric admissions for diarrhea, resulting in substantial savings. It would also help limit the use of other liquids (e.g., fruit drinks, soda, soups) that do not contain the appropriate concentration of electrolytes.

Conclusions

Gastroenteritis is one of the most common illnesses of children, and although evidence suggests that diarrheal mortality has declined over the past decade in many areas, diarrhea remains one of the major causes of death among children younger than 5 years in developing countries. Morbidity associated with diarrhea is substantial. Children throughout the world experience one to ten episodes per year, with attendant nutritional impairment, costs of health facility visits and medications, and a large number of costly hospital admissions.

A diverse array of microbiologic agents are responsible for diarrhea, but the bacterial agents are relatively more important in developing countries, whereas viral agents are more prominent in industrialized nations. Rotavirus is the most important agent causing severe dehydrating diarrhea in both settings.

Individuals may be at increased risk of diarrheal disease by virtue of increased susceptibility (e.g., immunodeficiency disorders), increased exposure, such as infants at the time of introduction of weaning foods, or being part of a concentration of susceptible individuals, e.g., the day care setting.

Interventions to prevent diarrhea require improvements in water supply, sanitary facilities, and domestic hygiene, promotion of breast feeding, and improved measles immunization coverage (Feacham & Koblinsky, 1983, 1984). Rotavirus vaccines hold promise for the future and, if effective, would represent an intervention equally important for preventing morbidity in developed countries as for preventing morbidity and mortality in the developing world. A cholera vaccine that would be effective in children would be an important adjunct in areas of high incidence. Therapy for gastroenteritis, regardless of etiology, should include appropriate rehydration therapy and continued feeding. Only a few bacterial and parasitic pathogens require antimicrobial therapy.

In summary, gastroenteritis remains an important cause of morbidity and mortality among children throughout the world. In future control efforts, both general interventions, such as ORT, and specific preventive measures, such as vaccines, will play important roles.

References

Avery ME, Snyder JD. Oral therapy for acute diarrhea: the underutilized simple solution. *N Engl J Med* 1990; 323:891–894.

Bartlett AV, Moore M, Gary GW, Starko KM, Erben JJ, Meredith BA. Diarrheal illness among infants and toddlers in day care centers. II. Comparison with day care homes and households. *J Pediatr* 1985; 107:503–509.

Bartlett AV, Reves RR, Pickering LK. Rotavirus in infant-toddler day care centers: epidemiology relevant to disease control strategies. *J Pediatr* 1988; 113:435–441.

Bern C, Glass RI. Impact of diarrheal diseases worldwide. In: Kapikian AZ, eds. *Viral Infections of the Gastrointestinal Tract*. New York: Marcel Dekker; 1993, pp. 1–26.

Bern C, Martines J, de Zoysa I, Glass RI. The magnitude of the global problem of diarrhoeal disease: a ten-year update. *Bull WHO* 1992a; 70(6): 705–714.

Bern C, Unicomb L, Gentsch J, Banul N, Sack RB, Glass RI. Rotavirus diarrhea in Bangladeshi children: correlation of disease severity with serotypes. *J Clin Microbiol*. 1992b; 30(12); 3234–3238.

Bhan MK, Raj P, Bhandari N, Svensson L, Stintzing G, Prasad AK, Jayashree S, Srivastava R. Role of enteric adenoviruses and rotaviruses in mild and severe acute enteritis. *Pediatr Infect Dis J* 1988; 7:320–323.

Bhan MK, Bhandari N, Sazawai S, Clemens J, Raj P, Levine MM, Kaper JB. Descriptive epidemiology of persistent diarrhoea among young children in rural northern India. *Bull WHO* 1989a; 67:281–288.

Bhan MK, Raj P, Levine MM, Kaper JB, Bhandari N, Srivastava R, Kumar R, Sazawal S. Enteroaggregative *Escherichia Coli* associated with persistent diarrhea in a cohort of rural children in India. *J Infect Dis* 1989b; 159:1061–1064.

Bhandari N, Bhan MK, Sazawal S. Mortality associated with acute watery diarrhea, dysentery, and persistent diarrhea in rural north India. *Acta Paediatr Scand* 1992; 81(suppl 381):3–6.

Black RE, Merson MH, Rahman ASMM, Yunus M, Alim ARMA, Huq I, Yolken RH, Curlin GT. A two-year study of bacterial, viral, and parasitic agents associated with diarrhea in rural Bangladesh. *J Infect Dis* 1980; 142:660–664.

Black RE, Merson MH, Huq I, Alim ARMA, Yunus M. Incidence and severity of rotavirus and *Escherichia Coli* diarrhoea in rural Bangladesh: implications for vaccine development. *Lancet* 1981; 1:141–143.

Black RE, Brown KH, Becker S, Alim ARMA, Huq I. Longitudinal studies of infectious diseases and physical growth of children in rural Bangladesh. II. Incidence of diarrhea and association with known pathogens. *Am J Epidemiol* 1982; 115:315–324.

Black RE, Brown KH, Becker S. Malnutrition is a determining factor in diarrheal duration, but not incidence, among young children in a longitudinal study in rural Bangladesh. *Am J Clin Nutr* 1984; 37:87–94.

Black RE, Lopez de Romana G, Brown KH, Bravo N, Grados Bazalar O, Kanashiro HC. Incidence and etiology of infantile diarrhea and major routes of transmission in Huascar, Peru. *Am J Epidemol* 1989; 129:785–799.

Brandt CD, Kim HW, Rodriguez WJ, Arrobio JO, Jeffries BC, Stallings EP, Lewis C, Miles AJ, Chanock RM, Kapikian AZ, Parrott RH. Pediatric viral gastroenteritis during eight years of study. *J Clin Microbiol* 1983; 18:71–78.

Calva JJ, Ruiz-Palacios GM, Lopez-Vidal AB, Ramos A, Bojalil R. Cohort study of intestinal infection with *Campylobacter* in Mexican children. *Lancet* 1988; 1:503–506.

Chiba S, Sakuma Y, Kogasaka R, Akihara M, Horino K, Nakao T, Fukui S. An outbreak of gastroenteritis associated with calicivirus in an infant home. *J Med Virol* 1979; 4:249–254.

Chrystie IL, Booth IW, Kidd AH, Marshall WC, Banatvala JE. Multiple faecal virus excretion in immunodeficiency (letter). *Lancet* 1982; 1:282.

Clark HF. Rotavirus vaccines. In: Plotkin SA, Mortimer EA, eds. *Vaccines*. Philadelphia: WB Saunders; 1988, pp. 517–525.

Clemens JD, Stanton B, Stoll B, Shahid NS, Banu H, Chowdhury AKMA. Breast feeding as a determinant of severity in shigellosis: evidence for protection throughout the first three years of life in Bangladeshi children. *Am J Epidemiol* 1986; 123:710–720.

Clemens JD, Sack DA, Harris JR, Khan MR, Chakraborty J, Chowdhury S, Rao MR, van Loon FP, Stanton B, Yunus M. Breast feeding and the risk of severe cholera in rural Bangladeshi children. *Am J Epidemiol* 1990a; 131:400–411.

Clemens JD, Sack DA, Harris JR, van Loon FP, Chakraborty J, Ahmed F, Rao MR, Khan MR, Yunus M, Huda N. Field trial of oral cholera vaccines in Bangladesh: results from three-year follow-up. *Lancet* 1990b; 2:270–273.

Cravioto A, Reyes RE, Ortega R, Fernandez G, Hernandez R, Lopez D. Prospective study of diarrhoeal disease in a cohort of rural Mexican children: incidence and isolated pathogens during the first two years of life. *Epidemiol Infect* 1988; 101:123–134.

Cruz JR, Cano F, Caceres P, Chew F, Pareja G. Infection and diarrhea caused by *Cryptosporidum sp.* among Guatemalan infants. *J Clin Microbiol* 1988; 26:88–91.

Cubitt WD, McSwiggan DA, Artstall S. An outbreak of calicivirus infection in a mother and a baby unit. *J Clin Pathol* 1980; 3:1095–1098.

deMol P, Hemelhof W, Butzler JP, Brasseur D, Kalala T, Vis HL. Enteropathogenic agents in children with diarrhoea in rural Zaire. *Lancet* 1983; 1:516–518.

de Zoysa I, Feachem RG. Interventions for the control of diarrhoeal diseases among young children: rotavirus and cholera immunization. *Bull WHO* 1985; 63:569–583.

Donelli G, Ruggieri FM, Tinari A, Marziano ML, Menichella D, Caione D, Concato C, Rocchi G, Vella S. A three-year diagnostic and epidemiologic study on viral infantile diarrhoea in Rome. *Epidemiol Infect* 1988; 100:311–320.

Duffy LC, Byers TE, Riepenhoff-Talty M, La Scolea LJ, Zielezny M, Ogra PL. The effects of infant feeding on rotavirus-induced gastroenteritis: a prospective study. *Am J Pub Health* 1986; 76:259–263.

Duggan C, Santosham M, Glass RI. The management of acute diarrhea in children: oral therapy—rehydration, maintenance, and nutrition. *MMWR* 1992; 41:(suppl 16): 1–20.

Echeverria P, Seriwatana J, Taylor DN, Yanggratoke S, Tirapat C. A comparative study of enterotoxigenic *Escherichia Coli*, *Shigella*, *Aeromonas*, and *Vibrio* as etiologies of diarrhea in northeastern Thailand. *Am J Trop Med Hyg* 1985; 34:547–554.

Echeverria P, Taylor DN, Lexsomboon U, Bhaibulaya M, Blacklow NR, Tamura K, Sakazaki R. Case-control study of endemic diarrheal disease in Thai children. *J Infect Dis* 1989; 159:543–548.

Eiden J, Losonsky GA, Johnson J, Yolken RH. Rotavirus RNA variation during chronic infection of immunocompromised children. *Pediatr Infect Dis J* 1985; 4:632–637.

Ellis ME, Watson B, Mandal BK, Dunbar EM, Craske J, Curry A, Roberts J, Lomax J. Micro-organisms in gastroenteritis. *Arch Dis Child* 1984; 59:848–855.

El-Rafie M, Hassouna WA, Hirschhorn N, Loza S, Miller P, Nagaty A, Nasser S, Riyad S. Effect of diarrhoeal disease control on infant and childhood mortality in Egypt. *Lancet* 1990; 335:334–338.

Esahli H, Breback K, Bennet R, Ehrnst A, Eriksson M, Hedlund K-O. Astroviruses as a cause of nosocomial outbreaks of infant diarrhea. *Pediatr Infect Dis J* 10:511–5.

Esrey SA, Feachem RG, Hughes JM. Interventions for the control of diarrhoeal diseases among young children: improving water supplies and excreta disposal facilities. *Bull WHO* 1985; 63:757–772.

Feachem RG, Koblinsky MA. Interventions for the control of diarrhoeal diseases among young children: measles immunization. *Bull WHO* 1983; 61:641–652.

Feachem RG, Koblinksy MA. Interventions for the control of diarrhoeal diseases among young children: promotion of breast feeding. *Bull WHO* 1984; 62:271–291.

Flores J, Perez-Schael I, Gonzalez M, Garcia D, Perez M, Daoud N, Cunto W, Chanock

RM, Kapikian AZ. Protection against severe rotavirus diarrhoea by rhesus rotavirus vaccine in Venezuelan infants. *Lancet* 1987; 1:1882–1882.

Ford-Jones EL, Mindorff CM, Gold R, Petric M. The incidence of viral-associated diarrhea after admission to a pediatric hospital. *Am J Epidemiol* 1990; 131:711–718.

Gangarosa RE, Glass RI, Lew JF, Boring JR. Hospitalizations with gastroenteritis in the United States, 1985: the special burden of disease among the elderly. *Am J Epidemiol* 1992; 135:281–290.

Georges-Courbet MC, Wachsmuth IK, Meunier DMV, Nebout N, Didier F, Siopathis MR, Georges AJ. Parasitic, bacterial, and viral enteric pathogens associated with diarrhea in the Central African Republic. *J Clin Microbiol* 1984; 19:571–575.

Georges-Courbot MC, Beraud-Cassel AM, Gouandjika I, Georges AJ. Prospective study of enteric *Campylobacter* infections in children from birth to 6 months in the Central African Republic. *J Clin Microbiol* 1987; 25:836–839.

Georges-Courbet MC, Monges J, Siopathis MR, Roungou JB, Gresenguet G, Bellec L, Bouquety JC, Lanckriet C, Cadoz M, Hessel L. Evaluation of the efficacy of a low-passage bovine rotavirus (strain WC3) vaccine in children in Central Africa. *Res Virol* 1991; 142:405–411.

Giugliano LG, Bernardi MGP, Vasconcelos JC, Costa CA, Giugliano R. Longitudinal study of diarrhoeal disease in a peri-urban community in Manaus (Amazon-Brazil). *Ann Trop Med Parasitol* 1986; 80:443–450.

Glass RI, Stoll BJ. The protective effect of human breast milk against diarrhea: a review of studies from Bangladesh. *Acta Paediatr Scand* 1989; 351(suppl):131–136.

Glass RI, Stoll BJ, Wyatt RG, Hoshino Y, Banu H, Kapikian AZ. Observations questioning a protective role for breastfeeding in severe rotavirus diarrhea. *Acta Paediatr Scand* 1986; 75:713–718.

Glass RI, Lew JF, Gangarosa RE, LeBaron CW, Ho Mei-S. Estimates of morbidity and mortality rates for diarrheal diseases in American children. *J Pediatr* 1991; 118:27–33.

Grohmann G, Glass RI, Gold J, James M, Edwards P, Borg T, Stine S, Goldsmith C, Monroe SS. An outbreak of human calicivirus gastroenteritis in a day-care center in Sydney, Australia. *J Infect Dis* 1991; 29:544–550.

Guerrant RL, Kirchhoff LV, Shields DS, Nations MK, Leslie J, de Sousa MA, Araujo JG, Correia LL, Sauer KT, McClelland KE, Trowbridge FL, Hughes JM. Prospective study of diarrheal illnesses in northeastern Brazil: patterns of disease, nutritional impact, etiologies, and risk factors. *J Infect Dis* 1982; 148:986–997.

Gunn RA, Kimball AM, Pollard RA, Feeley JC, Feldman RA, Dutta SR, Matthew PP, Mahmoud RA, Levine MM. Bottle feeding as a risk factor for cholera in infants. *Lancet* 1979; 2:730–732.

Gurwith MJ, Williams TW. Gastroenteritis in children: a two-year review in Manitoba. I. Etiology. *J Infect Dis* 1977; 136:239–247.

Hermann JE, Blacklow NR, Perron-Henry DM, Clements E, Taylor DN, Echeverria P. Incidence of enteric adenoviruses among children in Thailand and the significance of these viruses in gastroenteritis. *J Clin Microbiol* 1988; 26:1783–1786.

Herrmann JE, Nowak NA, Perron-Henry DM, Hudson RW, Cubitt WD, Blacklow NR. Diagnosis of astrovirus gastroenteritis by antigen detection with monoclonal antibodies. *J Infect Dis* 1990; 161:226–229.

Ho Mei-S, Glass RI, Pinsky PF, Young-Okoh NaC, Sappenfield WM, Buehler JW, Gunter N, Anderson LJ. Diarrheal deaths in American children: are they preventable? *JAMA* 1988;260:3281–3285.

Huilan S, Zhen LG, Mathan MM, Mathew MM, Olarte J, Espejo R, Ghafoor MA, Khan MA, Sami Z, Sutton RG. Etiology of acute diarrhea among children in developing countries: a multicentre study in five countries. *Bull WHO* 1991; 69:549–555.

Huttly SRA, Hoque BA, Aziz KMA, Hasan KZ, Patwary MY, Rahaman MM, Feachem RG. Persistent diarrhea in a rural area of Bangladesh: a community based longitudinal study. *Int J Epidemiol* 1989; 18:964–969.

Institute of Medicine. *New Vaccine Development: Establishing Priorities. Vol. II: Diseases of Importance in Developing Countries.* Washington, DC: National Academy Press; 1989.

Kapikian AZ, Chanock RM. Rotaviruses. In: Fields BN, Knipe DM, eds. *Virology*. New York: Raven Press; 1990.

Kim Kyung-H, Yang Jai-M, Joo Se-I, Cho Young-G, Glass RI, Cho Yang-J. Importance of rotavirus and adenovirus types 40 and 41 in acute gastroenteritis in Korean children. *J Clin Microbiol* 1990; 28:2279–2284.

Koenig MA, Khan MA, Wojtyniak B, Clemens JD, et al. Impact of measles vaccination on childhood mortality in rural Bangladesh. *Bull WHO* 1990; 68:441–447.

Kotloff KL, Wasserman SS, Steciak JY, Tall BD, Losonsky GA, Nair P, Morris JG, Levine MM. Acute diarrhea in Baltimore children attending an outpatient clinic. *Pediatr Infect Dis J* 1988; 7:753–759.

Lanata CF, Black RE, del Aguila R, Gil A, Verastegui H, Gerna G, Flores J, Kapikian AZ, Andre FE. Protection of Peruvian children against rotavirus diarrhea of specific serotypes by one, two, or three doses of the RIT 4237 attenuated bovine rotavirus vaccine. *J Infect Dis* 1989; 159:452–459.

Lew JF, Glass RI, Gangarosa RE, Cohen IP, Bern C, Moe CL. Diarrheal deaths in the United States, 1979 through 1987: a special problem for the elderly. *JAMA* 1991; 265:3280–3284.

Linhares AC, Moncao HC, Gabbay YB, de Araujo VLC, Serruya AC, Loureiro ECB. Acute diarrhoea associated with rotavirus among children living in Belem, Brazil. *Trans Roy Soc Trop Med Hyg* 1983; 77:384–390.

Lopez de Romana G, Brown KH, Black RE, Kanashiro HC. Longitudinal studies of infectious diseases and physical growth of infants in Huascar, an underprivileged peri-urban community in Lima, Peru. *Am J Epidemiol* 1989; 129:769–784.

Mackenjee MKR, Coovadia YM, Coovadia HM, Hewitt J, Robins-Browne RM. Aetiology of diarrhoea in adequately nourished young African children in Durban, South Africa. *Ann Trop Paediatr* 1984; 4:183–187.

Mahmood DA, Feacham RG. Clinical and epidemiological characteristics of rotavirus- and EPEC-associated hospitalized infantile diarrhoea in Basrah, Iraq. *J Trop Pediatr* 1987; 33:319–325.

Mahmood DA, Feachem RG, Huttly SRA. Infant feeding and risk of severe diarrhoea in Basrah city, Iraq: a case-control study. *Bull Who* 1989; 67:701–706.

Mata L, Simhon A, Padilla R, del Mar Gamboa M, Vargas G, Hernandez F, Mohs E, Lizano C. Diarrhea associated with rotaviruses, enterotoxigenic *Escherichia coli*, *Campylobacter*, and other agents in Costa Rican children, 1976-1981. *Am J Trop Med Hyg* 1983; 32:146–153.

Mata L, Bolanos H, Pizarro D, Vives M. Cryptosporidiosis in children from some highland Costa Rican rural and urban areas. *Am J Trop Med Hyg* 1984; 33:24–29.

Mathewson JJ, Oberhelman RA, Dupont HL, de la Cabada FJ, Garibay EV. Enteroadherent *Escherichia coli* as a cause of diarrhea among children in Mexico. *J Clin Microbiol* 1987; 25:1917–1919.

Mathur R, Reddy V, Naidu AN, Ravikumar Krishnamachari KAVR. Nutritional status and diarrhoeal morbidity: a longitudinal study in rural Indian preschool children. *Hum Nutr Clin Nutr* 1985; 39C:447–454.

McAuliffe JF, Shields DS, de Sousa MA, Sakell J, Schorling J, Guerrant RL. Prolonged and recurring diarrhea in the northeast of Brazil: examination of cases from a community-based study. *J Pediatr Gastroenterol Nutr* 1986; 5:902–906.

Mutanda LN. Epidemiology of acute gastroenteritis in early childhood in Kenya. III. Distribution of aetiological pathogens. *East Afr Med J* 1980; 57:317–326.

Newburg DS, Ashkenazi S, Cleary T. Human milk contains the Shiga toxin receptor glycolipid Gb3. *J Infect Dis* 1992; 166:832–836.

Osisanya JOS, Daniel SO, Sehgal SC, Afigbo A, Iyanda A, Okoro FI, Mbelu N. Acute diarrhoeal disease in Nigeria: detection of enteropathogens in a rural sub-Saharan population. *Trans Roy Soc Trop Med Hyg* 1988; 82:773–777.

Pan American Health Organization. Mortality due to intestinal infectious diseases in Latin America and the Caribbean, 1965–1990. *Epidemiol Bull PAHO* 1991; 12:1–10.

Pedley S, Hundley F, Chrystie I, McCrae MA, Desselberger U. The genomes of rotaviruses isolated from chronically infected immunodeficient children. *J Gen Virol* 1984; 65:1141–1150.

Pickering LK, Bartlett AV, Woodward WE. Acute infectious diarrhea among children in day care: epidemiology and control. *Rev Infect Dis* 1986; 8:539–547.

Pickering LK, Bartlett AV, Reves RR, Morrow A. Asymptomatic excretion of rotavirus before and after rotavirus diarrhea in children in day care centers. *J Pediatr* 1988; 112:361–365.

Rahman M, Shahid NS, Rahman H, Sack DA, Rahman N, Hossain S. Cryptosporidiosis: a cause of diarrhea in Bangladesh. *Am J Trop Med Hyg* 1990; 42:127–130.

Riepenhoff-Talty M, Saif LJ, Barrett HJ, Suzuki H, Ogra PL. Potential spectrum of etiological agents of viral enteritis in hospitalized infants. *J Clin Microbiol* 1983; 17:352–356.

Rowland MGM, Goh-Rowland SGJ, Dunn DT. The relation between weaning practices and patterns of morbidity from diarrhoea: an urban Gambian case study. In: Walker-Smith JA, McNeish AS, eds. *Diarrhea and Malnutrition in Childhood.* London: Butterworths; 1986.

Rowland MGM, Rowland SGJ, Cole TJ. Impact of infection on the growth of children from 0 to 2 years in an urban West African community. *Am J Clin Nutr* 1988; 47:134–138.

Santosham M, Daum RS, Dillman L. Oral rehydration therapy of infantile diarrhea: a controlled study of well-nourished children hospitalized in the United States and Panama. *N Engl J Med* 1982; 306:1070–1076.

Santosham M, Letson GW, Wolff M, Reid R, Gahagan S, Adams R, Callahan C, Sack RB, Kapikian AZ. A field study of the safety and efficacy of two candidate rotavirus vaccines in a Native American population. *J Infect Dis* 1991; 163:483–487.

Saulsbury FT, Winkelstein JA, Yolken RH. Chronic rotavirus infection in immunodeficiency. *J Pediatr* 1980; 97:61–65.

Schorling JB, Wanke CA, Schorling SK, McAuliffe JF, de Souza MA, Guerrant RL. A prospective study of persistent diarrhea among children in an urban Brazilian slum. *Am J Epidemiol* 1990; 132:144–156.

Sethi SK, Khuffash F. Bacterial and viral causes of acute diarrhoea in children in Kuwait. *J Diarr Dis Res* 1989; 7:85–88.

Sethi SK, Khuffash FA, Al-Nakib W. Microbial etiology of acute gastroenteritis in hospitalized children in Kuwait. *Pediatr Infect Dis J* 1989; 8:593–597.

Sircar BK, Deb BC, Sengupta PG, Mondal S, De SP, Sen D, Saha MR, Ghosh S, Sikdar SN, Pal SC. A longitudinal study of diarrhoea among children in Calcutta communities. *Ind J Med Res* 1984; 80:546–550.

Snyder JD, Merson MH. The magnitude of the global problem of acute diarrhoeal disease: a review of the active surveillance data. Bull *WHO* 1982; 60:605–613.

Soenarto Y, Sebodo T, Suryantoro P, Krisnomurti, Haksohusodo S, Ristanto IK, Romas MA, Noerhajati Muswiroh S, Rohde JE, Ryan NJ, Luke RKJ, Barnes GL, Bishop RF. Bacterial, parasitic agents and rotaviruses associated with acute diarrhoea in hospital in-patient Indonesian children. *Trans Roy Soc Trop Med Hyg* 1983; 77:724–730.

Stanton B, Silimperi DR, Khatun K, Kay B, Ahmed S, Khatun J, Alam K. Parasitic, bacterial and viral pathogens isolated from diarrhoeal and routine stool specimens of urban Bangladeshi children. *J Trop Med Hyg* 1989; 92:46–55.

Stoll BJ, Glass RI, Huq MI, Khan MU, Holt JE, Banu H. Surveillance of patients attending a diarrhoeal disease hospital in Bangladesh. *Br Med J* 1982; 285:1185–1188.

Sullivan P, Woodward WE, Pickering LK, DuPont HL. Longitudinal study of occurrence of diarrheal disease in day care centers. *Am J Pub Health* 1984; 74:987–991.

Uhnoo I, Olding-Stenkvist E, Kreuger A. Clinical features of acute gastroenteritis associated with rotavirus, enteric adenoviruses, and bacteria. *Arch Dis Child* 1986a; 61:732–738.

Uhnoo I, Wadell G, Svensson L, Olding-Stenkvist E, Ekwall E, Molby R. Aetiology and epidemiology of acute gastroenteritis in Swedish children. *J Infect* 1986b; 13:73–89.

Van R, Wun CC, Morrow AL, Pickering LK. The effect of diaper type and/or clothing on fecal contamination in day-care centers. *JAMA* 1991; 265:1840–1844.

Varavithya W, Vathanophas K, Bodhidatta L, Punyaratabandhu P, Sangchai R, Athipanyakom S, Wasi C, Echeverria P. Importance of *Salmonellae* and *Campylobacter jejuni* in the etiology of diarrheal disease among children less than 5 years of age in a community in Bangkok, Thailand. *J Clin Microbiol* 1990; 28:2507–2510.

Vesikari T, Maki M, Sarkkinen HK, Arstila PP, Halonen PE. Rotavirus, adenovirus, and non-viral enteropathogens in diarrhoea. *Arch Dis Child* 1981; 56:264–270.

Vesikari T, Isolauri E, D'Hondt E. Protection of infants against rotavirus diarrhoea by RIT 4237 attenuated bovine rotavirus strain vaccine. *Lancet* 1984; 1: 977–981.

Victora CG, Smith PG, Vaughan JP, Nobre LC, Lombardi C, Teixeira AM, Fuchs SC, Moreira LB, Gigante LP, Barros FC. Infant feeding and deaths due to diarrhea: a case-control study. *Am J Epidemiol* 1989; 129:1032–1041.

Walsh JA, Warren KS. Selective primary health care: an interim strategy for disease control in developing countries. *N Engl J Med* 1979; 301:967–974.

Weinberg RJ, Tipton G, Klish WJ, Brown MR. Effect of breast-feeding on morbidity in rotavirus gastroenteritis. *Pediatrics* 1984; 74:250–253.

Wood DJ, Longhurst D, Killough RI, David TJ. One-year prospective cross-sectional study to assess the importance of Group F adenovirus infections in children under 2 years admitted to hospital. *J Med Virol* 1988; 26:429–435.

World Health Organization. Persistent diarrhoea in children in developing countries: Memorandum from a WHO meeting. Bull *WHO* 1988; 66:709–717.

Yolken RH, Bishop CA, Townsend TR, Bolyard EA, Bartlett J, Santos GW, Saral R. Infectious gastroenteritis in bone-marrow transplant recipients. *N Engl J Med* 1982; 306:1009–1012.

Zaki AM, Dupont HL, El Alamy MA, Arafat RR, Amin K, Awad MM, Bassiouni L, Imam IZ, El Malih GS, El Marsafie A, Mohieldin MS, Naguib T, Rakha MA, Sidaros M, Wasef N, Wright CE, Wyatt RG. The detection of enteropathogens in acute diarrhea in a family cohort population in rural Egypt. *Am J Trop Med Hyg* 1986; 35:1013–1022.

9

Communicable Diseases

EDWARD A. MORTIMER, JR.

The epidemiology of the common contagious diseases of childhood (which sometimes occur in adults) depends on interactions among four variables: the infecting organism, the mechanism(s) of transmission, host defenses, and environmental factors. These variables affect not only the likelihood that an individual will acquire an infection but also population epidemiology.

Biologic Considerations

Features of **the organism** that influence disease epidemiology include its infectivity, which is usually measured by the number of organisms required for colonization; its pathogenicity (i.e., the production of disease once infection has occurred); its immunogenicity and antigenic stability; its ability to survive outside the host; whether it can persist in the host (the carrier state); the production of exotoxins, which may vary among strains of the same organism; and, in the case of bacteria, whether resistance to antibiotics develops.

The second variable is the **mode of transmission**, which for most of the contagious diseases of childhood is via aerosols from the respiratory tract, either by direct or indirect mechanisms. Direct transmission requires close contact between the infected individual and the susceptible person; it may be actual physical contact or close proximity, usually within 5 to 8 feet. Most organisms that require hundreds or thousands of infectious units to colonize, such as group A streptococci, are transmitted by the direct route in large aerosolized droplets. Indirect transmission, in contrast, includes the airborne route, as well as by organisms from a variety of inanimate sources, such as fomites and other objects in the environment, or in dust, water, and food. These inanimate sources seem to be of little importance in the transmission of the common contagious diseases of childhood. However, tiny aerosolized particles (airborne droplet nuclei), containing one or at most very few organisms, may be wafted at considerable distances through the air and constitute an important mechanism of transmission for many infections, including some of the common contagious diseases.

The third component of this quartet of interacting factors that determine the likelihood of infection is **the host**. For the common contagious diseases the most important host determinant is the immune status of the exposed individual. The underlying health status of the exposed, susceptible person usually has little to do with whether infection occurs, but the presence of malnutrition, other infections, and the like strongly influences morbidity and mortality from the various contagious diseases of childhood.

The fourth factor is **the environment**, which affects the likelihood that the susceptible individual will be exposed to the organism under conditions conducive to transmission. This likelihood in turn, depends on several other factors—not only the physical environment, such as season, but also patterns of social intermingling and the prevalence of infection in those with whom the susceptible individual comes in contact.

The four interacting factors that determine infection in the individual also govern the epidemiology of these diseases in communities and larger populations. Whether these contagious diseases are endemic in a population, occur in epidemics, or both is dependent on these factors, which collectively contribute to the phenomenon known as **herd immunity**. It may be defined as the circumstances in a population in which the proportion of the population immune to the disease in question is sufficiently large to prevent propagation of the disease by limiting the opportunities for susceptible persons to come into effective contact with those who are infected. Herd immunity is sometimes interpreted as the simple total proportion of the population that is immune; for example, the often-quoted belief that, if diphtheria is introduced into a population, an outbreak will not occur if 60% to 65% of the individuals in that population are immune. Of course, if a very high proportion of the total population is immune to a given contagious disease, the infection cannot maintain itself in that population (Anderson & May, 1990). However, the issue of herd immunity is usually far more complex and cannot be reduced to a single proportion that fails to take into account a number of factors (Fox et al., 1971). Among these is the fact that mixing (the frequency of contact among individuals) is not random in communities, which comprise many subgroups—the smallest being the family and extending to school populations, social groups, workplaces, and the like. The frequency of contacts within and between such groups obviously varies, which affects the likelihood of disease transmission. Further, among such groups the proportions of individuals who are immune vary markedly, most commonly because of age. These proportions may also be influenced by disparate past experiences with disease outbreaks or with immunization. Thus, whether minor or major epidemics of contagious diseases occur depends on the extent of intermingling within populations and subpopulations and on the immune status of individuals in various groups. An example is the near absence of diphtheria in the developed world, in spite of the fact that approximately half of adults, middle-aged and older, have been shown serologically to be susceptible (Karzon & Edwards, 1988). There can be little doubt that this is a consequence of remarkably high levels of vaccine-induced immunity in the childhood population.

How these various factors affect the epidemiologic characteristics of the several contagious diseases is discussed in the section on each disease. Additionally, because most are vaccine-preventable, the epidemiology before and after widespread use of immunization is considered. Certain characteristics of each disease are included when uniquely relevant to its epidemiology. This chapter covers the five common contagious diseases of childhood: pertussis, measles, rubella, mumps, and varicella. For consideration of other infections, the reader is referred to the general references.

PERTUSSIS

Clinical Features

Pertussis (whooping cough) is a highly contagious bacterial respiratory disease with a protracted course. After an incubation period of 7 to 13 days, the initial symptoms are indistinguishable from those of a nonspecific respiratory infection with a dry cough, but progress over the next 2 weeks to the appearance of paroxysms. As the frequency of paroxysms increases, the characteristic respiratory whoop appears at the end of a paroxysm, often associated with vomiting. The paroxysms persist for 2 to 6 weeks, after which the cough gradually subsides over a period of several weeks. Important complications include atelectasis and bronchopneumonia, which are responsible for the vast majority of deaths; encephalopathy (probably anoxic) in approximately 1 in 10,000 cases; and, in the past, inanition due to repeated vomiting.

Biologic Considerations

Pertussis is caused by a Gram-negative bacillus, *Bordetella pertussis*. Humans are the only natural host. It is a somewhat fastidious organism, requiring special culture media. The frequency with which *B. pertussis* is recovered from clinical specimens is directly related to the experience of the laboratory, and accordingly, the number of reported cases of pertussis proven by culture (the gold standard for diagnosis) is undoubtedly far less than the number that actually occur (Onorato & Wassilak, 1987). Identification by direct fluorescent antibody is frequently used, but its specificity is relatively unsatisfactory because of large numbers of false-positive tests. Serologic testing has been quite satisfactory for investigational purposes, but is not available for routine use (Onorato & Wassilak, 1987). Less satisfactory, but nonetheless helpful diagnostically, are a history of exposure to pertussis and the well-known lymphocytosis. Thus, from an epidemiologic standpoint, difficulties in establishing a precise bacteriologic diagnosis compromise estimates of the true incidence of the disease.

Another feature of the organism that has had an indirect effect on whooping cough epidemiology has been less than optimal understanding of the antigens of the organism that are responsible for clinical immunity, whether induced by disease or by the whole-cell vaccine. Recent advancements in knowledge (Wardlaw & Parton, 1988) have made it possible in recent years to produce a vaccine limited to the components probably responsible for clinical immunity and largely free of those believed to cause the well-known reactivity of the whole-cell preparation (Cody et al., 1981). This reactivity led to the belief, now shown to be largely fallacious (Howson & Fineberg, 1992), that the vaccine not infrequently caused permanently disabling neurologic reactions or death, resulting in poor acceptance of the vaccine in several countries and the consequent return of epidemic pertussis (Cherry, 1984; Kimura & Kuno-Sakai, 1990; Romanus et al., 1987; Stuart-Harris, 1979) and, in the United States, extensive personal injury litigation and increased vaccine costs (Hinman, 1986; Koplan & Hinman, 1987).

B. pertussis infects by attaching to respiratory cilia, and, by damaging the ciliated cells, it compromises the normal tracheobronchial toilet. Cultures are most likely to be positive during the catarrhal stage (a week or two before the onset of paroxysms), but organisms usually cannot be isolated by 2 weeks after the onset of paroxysms (Onorato & Wassilak, 1987).

Transmission

Pertussis seems to be transmitted invariably via the respiratory route by direct, close contact. It is most contagious during the catarrhal and early paroxysmal stages and becomes noninfectious as the paroxysms begin to disappear. Indirect transmission via fomites or airborne droplet nuclei has not been demonstrated. The disease is highly contagious; up to 90% of susceptible household contacts acquire the disease (Clark et al., 1946; Cockburn, 1955; Fine et al., 1988; Kendrick, 1940; Sako, 1947). There is no animal reservoir, nor has a carrier state been demonstrated.

Transmission in school settings also occurs at a high rate, although data are sparse. An elegant example of shoeleather epidemiology is a little-known report of a 1940 outbreak of pertussis in an elementary school in Rochester, New York (Clark et al., 1946). Among the 205 pupils, kindergarten through the eighth grade, 93 (45%) had a prior history of pertussis. Of the 112 susceptible by history, 57 (51%) developed pertussis, but 17 of these were believed to have acquired the disease at home. Forty of the susceptible children exposed only at school became ill. However, the rate of infection in the older susceptibles (grades 5 through 8) was only 10% compared to 58% in the younger grades. This difference suggests that a considerable number of children who were said not to have had prior pertussis had indeed experienced it in the past. The school included some children who had received the crude pertussis vaccines of that era; removal of these children from the analysis gave an attack rate of 54% among susceptibles. Of considerable interest is that there were three successive waves of infection over a 6-week period in this outbreak.

Immunity

It has always been assumed that clinical pertussis induces lifelong immunity, although anecdotal reports of second attacks, which have not been laboratory proven, exist, e.g., the grandmother who acquired pertussis from her ill grandchild. Whether these represent true second attacks, parapertussis, or some other illness is unknown. Effective transplacental immunity does not exist, thus placing young infants in jeopardy.

Patterns of Occurrence

Incidence

In the past in the absence of immunization nearly everyone experienced pertussis, almost always in childhood. The small proportion of individuals without a record or history of pertussis is probably largely explained by missed diagnoses; atypical clinical manifestations, which are often characteristic of the disease in very young infants; and milder illnesses. Before World War I in New York City 50% of reported cases occurred in children of elementary school age; this group was the major reservoir for pertussis (Luttinger, 1916). Twenty percent of cases occurred in infants, who accounted for more than half of the mortality from pertussis, and a similar proportion occurred in preschool children (1 to 4 years), whereas very few cases were reported in adolescents and adults. In the United States from 1980 to 1989, nearly three-quarters of reported cases occurred in infants and preschool children, the majority of whom were either too young to be immunized or had failed to be properly immunized according to the current U.S. recommended schedule (Farizo et al., 1992).

Temporal Trends

A noteworthy phenomenon in the epidemiology of pertussis is that a distinct decline in pertussis mortality occurred in the United States, United Kingdom, and Sweden (and presumably in other developed countries) during the first half of this century before the implementation of any effective preventive or therapeutic measures (Cherry, 1984; Dauer, 1943; Kimura & Kuno-Sakai, 1990; Mortimer & Jones, 1979; Romanus et al., 1987). Indeed, in the United States, infant mortality from pertussis declined 80% from the period of 1900–1904 to the period of 1940 to 1944 (Mortimer & Jones, 1979; Fig. 9.1). Similarly, infant mortality from pertussis in the United Kingdom declined approximately 90% from 1915 to 1955 before the widespread use of the vaccine (Cherry, 1984). In Sweden, annual deaths from pertussis decreased from about 1000 in 1916 to approximately 200 in the early 1930s (Romanus et al., 1987).

Two unproved and probably unprovable hypotheses may explain this decline in mortality in the absence of effective prevention and treatment, even though nearly everyone experienced pertussis. The first hypothesis relates to a 42% decline in the U.S. birth rate to women aged 15 to 44 years between 1900 and 1935 to 1939 (U.S. Bureau of the Census, 1975). It is assumed that such a decline, with consequent smaller families, resulted in less frequent exposure of infants, who are at highest risk of death from pertussis. The other hypothesis is that case-fatality rates in infants and young children who acquired pertussis declined as infant nutrition improved and the incidence of debilitating disorders, such as recurrent enteric infections, decreased. However, data that show a decline in case-fatality rates in infants during the prevaccine years are unavailable.

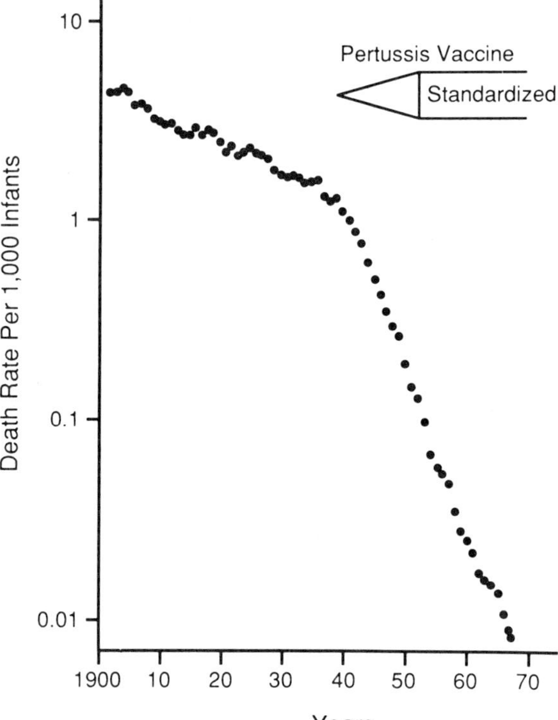

Fig. 9.1. Infant mortality rate from pertussis. United States, 1900 to 1974, expressed as a 5-year moving average (Mortimer & Jones, 1979).

Temporal Variations in Morbidity

Examination of year-to-year variations in the incidence of pertussis indicates that peaks in reported cases usually occur every 2 to 4 years; rarely is the interval a year or two longer (Cherry, 1984; Farizo et al., 1992; Gordon & Hood, 1951; Miller et al., 1974). Curiously, this pattern has not been influenced by immunization, although fewer cases occur. Presumably this periodicity represents replenishment of the population of susceptibles by annual birth cohorts.

Seasonality

Examination of seasonal variations has yielded inconsistent results. Lapin found none of consequence (Lapin, 1943), whereas in 1951 Gordon and Hood (1951) observed that the highest incidence occurred during winter and spring, although these variations were not striking. In a review in 1975 Olson concluded that there was no seasonality of the disease. This seeming inconsistency may be explained by the fact that some of the earlier data were based on mortality figures, which would reflect the coexistence of other diseases, such as gastroenteritis, that in turn may have compromised survival in infants and young children with pertussis. More recently, reported cases of pertussis in the United States from 1980 to 1989 were examined (Farizo et al., 1992). In the southern states a peak incidence was observed during the early summer, whereas in the northern states the highest rates extended from June through October. Although pertussis was observed yearround, peak rates were two- to threefold those observed at other times of the year.

Sex

Pertussis displays a curious, unexplained sex distribution. It was and still is more often reported in females than in males; case-fatality rates are also higher in females (Farizo et al., 1992; Gordon & Hood, 1951; Olson, 1975). It is difficult to believe that male children would be more likely to escape the disease than females; whether, for some unknown reason, the disease is more severe in females, which would make it more easily recognized and also result in higher mortality, is unknown.

Race

In the past mortality from pertussis was higher in blacks than in whites, undoubtedly as a consequence of socioeconomic status, including age distribution (Gordon & Hood, 1951).

Socioeconomic Status

Low socioeconomic status (SES) affects pertussis epidemiology in two ways. Age-specific incidence rates in very young children are highest in low socioeconomic groups, presumably because of crowding and perhaps, currently, because of lower rates of immunization in preschool children in these groups. Mortality rates from pertussis are also inversely related to SES, probably largely due to the higher incidence of the disease in the very young but also in part due to higher case-fatality rates attributable to other factors, such as low birthweight and underlying problems including other infections and nutritional deficits.

International Comparisons

Although pertussis morbidity and mortality have declined remarkably in the industrialized world, the situation has been very different in developing countries. Indeed, in the 1980s mortality rates in infants and young children in these nations continued to be similar to, or exceeded, those in the United States at the turn of the century. It was estimated by the World Health Organization (WHO) that, among the approximately 110 million children born annually in developing countries in the early 1980s, nearly 850,000 succumbed to pertussis, the majority before their fifth birthdays, for a mortality rate of 7.7 per 1000 (Grant, 1985). Underlying or recurrent disorders, such as low birthweight, malnutrition, and debilitation by recurrent respiratory and intestinal infections, undoubtedly play major roles in these high mortality rates. An additional reason for high pertussis mortality in these countries is the high proportion of cases that occur in very young children, including infants (Mahieu et al., 1978, Morley et al., 1966). It is to be anticipated that the continuing success of the Expanded Programme on Immunization (EPI) of WHO will achieve important reductions in pertussis mortality in these countries (Fig. 9.2); (EPI, 1992).

Interventions

Treatment

The treatment of pertussis is largely symptomatic. Although *B. pertussis* is susceptible to several antibiotics, particularly erythromycin, therapy has little or no effect on established disease (Sprauer et al., 1992). There is evidence that erythromycin administered in the catarrhal stage may ameliorate or shorten the course of the disease. Additionally, if administered to exposed susceptibles before the onset of symptoms, it may avert or modify subsequent illness. Because erythromycin hastens the disappearance of *B. pertussis* from the respiratory tract, as judged by recovery on culture even in individuals with full-blown disease, it should be prescribed for all individuals with pertussis in the hope that it will minimize disease transmission to others. Unfortunately, the use of erythromycin and other antibiotics in an effort to control pertussis and prevent its transmission has little or no public health value, primarily because they are effective only in the early stages of the illness before it is recognized as pertussis. Accordingly, the only effective approach to controlling pertussis at the present time is wide-

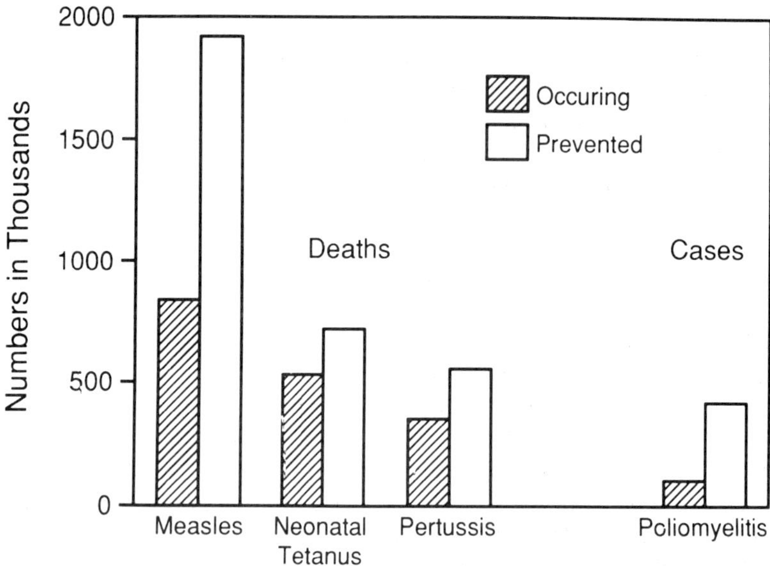

Fig. 9.2. Estimated deaths from measles, neonatal tetanus, and pertussis and cases of poliomyelitis occurring and prevented by immunization in developing countries, 1990 (Expanded Programme on Immunization, 1992).

spread immunization. Quarantine is also of negligible benefit because the disease is highly contagious before characteristic symptoms occur.

Prevention: Immunization

Remarkable changes in the epidemiology of pertussis have occurred in the last four decades as a result of the development and widespread use of pertussis vaccine. However, these effects have been largely limited to those countries of the industrialized world in which pertussis vaccine (almost always in combination with diphtheria and tetanus toxoids, the familiar DTP) has been widely used beginning 30 or 40 years ago. Only in the last decade has the impact of increasing immunization of children on pertussis epidemiology been observed in the developing world as a result of the EPI (Expanded Programme on Immunization, 1992).

The demonstration that *B. pertussis* could be propagated on culture in the laboratory in 1906 prompted attempts to produce inactivated whole-cell vaccines and even a few acellular vaccines prepared from the supernatant fluids of broth cultures. In an effort to enhance efficacy, the whole-cell vaccines were manipulated in several ways, including the use of fresh cultures, quantification of the numbers of bacteria per dose, the addition of other respiratory flora, and experimenting with subcutaneous versus intramuscular administration. The composition of these vaccines, produced by several manufacturers in different countries, can only be speculated. In the United States, vaccines were licensed by the Public Health Service only for interstate or foreign commerce; at least some states licensed these vaccines for intrastate use as early as 1914. Beginning about the time of World War I and for some years thereafter, the medical literature contained several reports of case series of children who received these vaccines, both for treatment and prophylaxis, published by well-known physicians of that era (Friedlander, 1925; Luttinger, 1917). The results presented in these reports, usually characterized by a maximum of enthusiasm and a minimum of controls, cannot be assessed.

Attempts to develop effective pertussis vaccines, which were largely hit or miss, continued, and by the beginning of the 1940s it was evident that preexposure use of pertussis vaccines effectively prevented the disease in many or most recipients (Lapin, 1943). Continued improvements were made; in the United States the current whole-cell preparation was licensed in 1945, and production requirements were standardized by Federal Regulation in 1954.

By the mid-1950s most industrialized countries recommended pertussis vaccine, usually as DTP, as a routine preventive measure for all children. Increasing acceptance of this recommendation by physicians and the public in ensuing years altered the epidemiology of pertussis remarkably. In some instances, school entry requirements mandating immunization in the absence of contraindications have further augmented the prevalence of full immunization against pertussis.

Striking reductions in the morbidity and mortality rates from pertussis have occurred, despite the fact that whole-cell pertussis vaccine is less effective as an immunizing agent against clinical disease in the exposed individual than are most other vaccines used in childhood, notably oral polio virus vaccine, tetanus toxoid, and measles vaccine. This less-than-optimal efficacy of pertussis vaccine has led to challenges of the policy of routine pertussis immunization in the past two decades in the public media and by some scientists. These challenges have also, in part, been based on reports of pertussis in immunized individuals and the fact that mortality from pertussis declined before advent of the vaccine (Dauer, 1943; Mortimer & Jones, 1979; Stuart-Harris, 1979). However, there is ample evidence of the efficacy of whole-cell pertussis vaccine (Cherry, 1984).

In relation to protection afforded to the individual subject, the most stringent test is the **household contact study**, which assesses the proportion of immunized individuals who fail to acquire the disease in question after household exposure compared to those who are unimmunized. An additional merit of the household contact study is that it provides optimal comparability of exposure for all subjects. Two early reports from 1947 (Sako, 1947) and 1959 (Medical Research Council, 1959) showed protective efficacy of 79% and up to 90%, respectively. The most recent, carefully conducted household contact study in the United States also showed high efficacy (Onorato et al., 1992). In this study several definitions of pertussis were employed, as well as confirmation by culture and/or serology in many instances. Vaccine efficacy for fully immunized preschool children was estimated to be 95%, 81%, and 64% for severe, typical, and mild pertussis, respectively. Additionally, there was evidence of partial protection afforded by incomplete immunization, perhaps even following a single dose. Thus, there is little question that pertussis vaccine offers high, but not absolute, protection against clinical pertussis on exposure; the best point estimate is probably 80% to 90%.

From the public health standpoint, pertussis vaccine is much more efficacious than this estimate. The decline in reported cases of pertussis in the United States since the advent of the vaccine has been too great to be accounted for by the known underreporting of the disease. The crude rates of reported cases of pertussis in the early 1940s would suggest that in 1988 to 1991 approximately 400,000 cases of pertussis should have been reported annually in the United States; instead, an average of only about 3700 cases were reported each year (CDC, 1991d). These results suggest that, on a population basis, pertussis vaccine efficacy approaches 99%, presumably because of herd immunity.

Nonetheless, there is no question that, at least in the United States, pertussis is vastly underreported and that this underreporting may extend to hospitalizations and mortality as well. A recent study estimated the extent of this problem, and, hence, the true incidence of pertussis morbidity and mortality by taking advantage of the existence of several surveillance systems (Sutter & Cochi, 1992). Simply stated, by examining the overlap (or lack of overlap) in pertussis cases reported to two different systems, it was possible to estimate the numbers of events that were missed by both systems. As a hypothetical example, if 100 events are reported to both reporting systems serving the same population, but one system identified a total of 400 cases (four times as many) and the other 300 cases (three times as many), it may be estimated that the total number of events was actually $3 \times 4 \times 100$, or 1200. On this basis, this study estimated that more than 13,000 individuals were hospitalized for pertussis during the 4 years 1985 to 1988, a figure that is three- to fourfold greater than the number reported by either system alone. Using other sources for prediction, it was estimated that the total number of cases of pertussis in the United States for those 4 years was actually between 30,000 and 100,000, rather than the 14,057 cases reported to the CDC.

Although it is clear that pertussis mortality in the industrialized world declined before widespread use of the vaccine, there is a great deal of information (too vast to review in detail here) that shows that the vaccine has resulted in striking decreases in morbidity, as well as mortality, with or without underreporting. Evidence other than the accelerated decline in incidence rates with the advent of pertussis vaccine includes the recurrence of major outbreaks of pertussis in the United Kingdom, Japan, and Sweden when vaccine acceptance rates declined beginning in the 1970s, chiefly because of fears of vaccine reactions (Cherry, 1984; Kimura & Kuno-Sakai, 1990; Romanus et al., 1987). Further, it has been shown that there is an inverse relationship between vaccine acceptance rates and disease incidence in different communities in the same country (Pollard, 1980). Finally, in communities with pertussis outbreaks, much higher disease rates occur in unimmunized children compared to those who have received pertussis vaccine (Church, 1979). However, there is no question that protection afforded by the vaccine is not perfect; in well-exposed individuals efficacy is probably only between 80% and 90%. Unfortunately, the fact that pertussis does occur in some immunized individuals has led some to draw the fallacious conclusion that the vaccine is of no merit for the reason that, in a highly immunized population with a local outbreak of pertussis, vaccine failures will represent a high proportion of cases. Indeed, in the unlikely situation that 100% of the population was immunized, 100% of cases would occur in immunized individuals!

In the developing world, pertussis is not yet under control (Fig. 9.2). At the time WHO initiated EPI in 1974, 5% or fewer children in developing countries had received three doses of pertussis vaccine as DTP (Expanded Programme on Immunization, 1992). Although precise figures are unavailable, as recently as the early 1980s it was estimated that up to 850,000 children succumbed annually to pertussis in the developing world. During the decade of the 1980s childhood immunization coverage expanded remarkably to the point that, by 1990, more than 80% of children had received three doses of DTP and the estimate of deaths was 350,000 or less (Expanded Programme on Immunization, 1992). Of course, underlying or concomitant disorders, such as malnutrition, recurrent enteritis, low birthweight, and the like, contribute to high case-fatality rates from pertussis and other contagious diseases, such as measles, in the developing world. Accordingly, full immunization is only part of the solution to high mortality from these infections in these nations.

In the past decade or so two other changes, which are possibly interrelated, have occurred in the epidemiology of pertussis in the United States. One change is the disproportionate number of cases of pertussis that are being recognized in adolescents and adults (Mortimer, 1990). Indeed, for the years 1980 to 1989, approximately 12% of all cases were reported in individuals 15 years and older, and about 40% of these occurred in individuals 30 years and older (Farizo et al., 1992). The second change is the increasing recognition that mild, atypical cases of pertussis may occur in previously immunized persons (Etkind et al., 1992; Steketee et al., 1988). There has also been a two- to threefold increase in the overall incidence of reported cases of pertussis in the past 15 years; this increase has affected all age groups, but the greatest increment is in individuals

15 years and older (Farizo et al., 1992). Nonetheless, it is important to note that approximately half of all cases of pertussis continue to occur in infants less than 1 year of age, more than three-quarters of whom are too young to have completed primary immunization (Farizo et al., 1992).

These two changes in the epidemiology of pertussis in the United States—the recent increase in reported cases and the high proportion of cases in older individuals—have not been entirely explained. Because it is well known that pertussis is incompletely reported, it may be that there has been enhanced recognition and reporting of the disease subsequent to publicity about alleged reactions to the vaccine. Although there has been an apparent increase in refusals to permit inoculation of children with pertussis vaccine among some sectarian and other groups, with resultant small localized outbreaks of whooping cough, these outbreaks are insufficient to explain the recent increment in reported cases (Etkind et al., 1992).

A possible explanation for the higher rates observed in older individuals is that of waning immunity following immunization or even the disease itself. There is at least some evidence of waning clinical protection with years elapsed since completion of immunization; half or more individuals become susceptible 5 to 10 years later (Jenkinson, 1988; Lambert, 1965; Lautrop & Mikkelson, 1969). Additionally, in an outbreak of pertussis in a Wisconsin institution among individuals, almost all of whom had been immunized against pertussis, there was also evidence of waning immunity related to years since last immunized (Steketee et al., 1988). Furthermore, serologic evidence of pertussis was identified in 26% of 130 university students with a cough of 6 days duration or more but without classical symptoms of pertussis (Mink et al., 1992). Finally, it has been shown that subclinical cases of pertussis frequently occur in families along with clinical cases (Long et al., 1990).

Whether pertussis in the adult is a new phenomenon that is only now recognized because of a greater index of suspicion and better diagnostic methods or whether it existed in the past can only be speculated. It is, however, tempting to hypothesize that the reduced incidence of pertussis with the advent of widespread immunization has resulted in less opportunity for casual exposure to the disease and consequent reinforcement of immunity. This question cannot be answered. It is also unclear whether milder or subclinical cases in adolescents and adults play a role in transmission of the disease, for example, to unimmunized young infants, because those persons with milder infections may be less likely to transmit the organism to others than are those with full-blown disease. Nonetheless, in the future it may become advisable to administer reinforcing doses of pertussis vaccine to adults if it can be shown that this age group serves as a source of infection for others. Such adult immunization would very likely be facilitated by the recently developed, less reactive, acellular pertussis vaccines (Shapiro, 1992).

Measles (Rubeola)

Clinical Features

Measles is a highly contagious, severe, systemic viral infection, the most prominent manifestations of which are fever, respiratory symptoms, and a characteristic rash. The illness runs a course of about 7 days. It is initiated by gradually increasing fever, coryza, conjunctivitis, and cough. In about 3 days the pathognomonic Koplik spots on the buccal mucosa appear and persist for about 24 hours, at about which time the characteristic rash begins on the head, neck, and face. Over the next few days the rash gradually spreads over the trunk and extremities. About 2 or 3 days after the initial appearance of the rash, fever subsides, and over a period of a week or so the rash and the respiratory symptoms disappear. Measles is expected to provide clinical immunity for life.

Measles is important for two reasons. First, even the uncomplicated acute illness is exhaustingly severe; it is often said that children with measles are "really sick." Second, respiratory complications, such as otitis media and pneumonia, occur, the latter being the most common cause of death. In approximately 1 in 1000 cases measles encephalitis occurs, which may result in permanent brain damage or death. A rare but devastating degenerative central nervous system disorder, subacute sclerosing panencephalitis (SSPE), occurs with an incidence of approximately 1 to 2 per 100,000 cases of measles. SSPE is best characterized as a slow virus measles infection of the brain, with symptoms appearing after an interval of 3 to 10 years.

Biologic Considerations

The measles virus is highly infective in humans, who seem to be the only natural host, although under some circumstances monkeys can be affected. The virus contains several antigens that are quite immunogenic. Serologic responses to these antigens are of diagnostic utility, and their presence in serum correlates well with clinical immunity. Clinically significant antigenic variation among strains from different locales or over time has not been demonstrated. The organism is relatively fragile, being readily inactivated by heat, cold, ultraviolet light, and a variety of substances.

Transmission

Measles is highly contagious; at least 90% of nonimmune household contacts of an individual with active disease will be infected. Rates of transmission in classrooms and other places where children gather are lower, but vary considerably depending on the intimacy and duration of exposure. Although other routes are possible, in the vast majority of instances the disease is communicated by air. Effective transmission occurs not only by the direct respiratory route via large aerosolized droplets but also by smaller aerosols (indirect airborne transmission). As with the common cold, physical contact may result in transmission via contaminated secretions. Measles is most contagious during the catarrhal stage; once the rash appears the individual becomes noninfectious within 1 to 3 days. An occasional source of infection is the urine, from which virus can be recovered during the height of the illness and throughout the period of eruption of the rash.

The interval from exposure to the onset of symptoms is estimated to be 10 days and from exposure to rash about 14 days with little variation. There is no effective animal reservoir, although primates in contact with humans often develop measles antibody and can be infected in the laboratory. It has been demonstrated that previously immune individuals may show serum antibody increases in the absence of symptoms after exposure, but there is no evidence to suggest that they are infectious (Markowitz et al., 1990a; Preblud & Katz, 1988).

Patterns of Occurrence

As with most of the "usual" contagious diseases of childhood, the epidemiology of measles has been remarkably altered by the advent of effective immunization, particularly in the industrialized world. Accordingly, it is useful to consider not only the current epidemiology of measles in developed countries but also its behavior in these countries in the past and in less fortunate parts of the world at present.

Incidence

In the past, nearly everyone experienced measles, usually in childhood. Before widespread immunization, however, the age incidence was strongly influenced by population characteristics that determined the likelihood of exposure to the disease. Black (1989) reviewed data from sparsely populated communities with little outside communication where measles did not maintain itself, and many years or rarely even a generation or two might elapse before the disease was introduced from the outside. Under such circumstances the importation of measles would result in infection of most or all of the children (and sometimes adults) who had not had prior experience with the disease, and mortality was high, if only due to lack of care. However, in this century, with the growth of large cities of sufficient size to maintain measles transmission and with the increasing volume and speed of national and international travel, the epidemiology of measles became less dependent on the probability of disease introduction and related more to the proportions of susceptibles in the population, particularly in large cities. In these situations outbreaks occurred every 2 to 5 years—the interval required to develop a large susceptible population through birth cohorts. In the industrialized world the interval was usually shorter in large, crowded cities and longer in more sparsely populated areas. However, measles occurred every year. Examination of the numbers of cases reported annually in the United States in the prevaccine era—1942 to 1963—(CDC, 1991d) and in New York City, 1912 to 1917 (Herrman, 1925), indicate that differences between peak years of incidence and intervening years were usually not very striking. The numbers of reported cases during epidemic years was usually less than twice the number in nonepidemic years.

Population densities also affected the age distribution of measles. Although the age incidence was usually highest in children of elementary school age, in large cities where the disease was endemic the highest rates were often observed in children of preschool age (Herrman, 1925). Usually spared were children under 1 year due to transplacental immunity. Mortality was also apt to be greater in crowded inner cities due to the higher disease incidence in the very young.

A remarkable account of epidemic measles in an urban area six decades ago is provided by the Medical Officer of Health and the School Medical Officer in a report to the London County Council (Central Public Health Committee, 1933). In the 1920s London experienced epidemics of measles biennially; this report describes an outbreak that began in October 1931, peaked in May of 1932, and finally subsided in the summer, perhaps in part due to the summer holiday. More than 55,000 children with measles were identified, of whom more than 11,000 (20%) were admitted to infectious disease hospitals. The most common reason for admission was severe measles, deemed to be unsuitable for home care. However, the diagnosis of bronchopneumonia was made in 1362 (12%) of those admitted, and more than one third (460) of those patients died. The age distributions of cases and deaths, as reported from 24 of London's 28 boroughs, was characteristic of urban outbreaks in unimmunized populations. As Table 9.1 indicates, attack rates were highest in 3- to 4-year-olds, many of whom attended what would currently be called preschool. Attack rates were considerably lower in children under 1 year, presumably largely attributable to maternal antibody, but also possibly to less exposure. However, case-fatality rates were highest in infants and toddlers less than 2 years old. Attack rates in children 3 to 5 years who attended school were much higher than in those who did not.

Temporal Trends

This type of epidemic behavior was characteristic of measles in the first half of this century, particularly in large urban populations. However, it is noteworthy that in the United States crude mortality rates from measles gradually declined nearly 90% in the first 40 years of this century *before* the development of an effective preventive measure. This decline also occurred in the absence of specific therapy, such as antibiotics, that might reduce mortality from complications. Although these are crude rates, the magnitude of the decline in mortality, as with pertussis, cannot be discounted as an artifact caused by the data not being adjusted for changes in population age distribution. Instead, it seems reasonable that the declining birthrate reduced the likelihood of exposure of infants at highest risk of death, and in addition, better nutrition and reductions in the prevalence of underlying or concomitant disorders, such as enteric infections,

Table 9.1. Age Distributions of Measles Cases, Deaths, Case-Fatality Rates, and Mortality Rates, London, 1931–1932

Age (Yrs)	Cases	Cases/ 100,000	Deaths	Deaths/ 100,000*	Case-Fatality Rates (%)
<1	1,793	1,437	155	145	8.6
1	4,280	3,627	360	364	8.4
2	4,319	3,717	121	130	2.8
3	6,088	5,248	48	58	0.8
4	8.569	7,262	37	39	0.4
5–13	23,155	N.A.	52	N.A.	0.2
>13	616	N.A.	3	N.A.	0.5
All ages	48,820	556	776	10.7	1.6

*Calculated from Central Public Health Committee, 1933.

played major roles in this decline. Thus, because nearly every child experienced measles, the decline in mortality resulted from decreases in case-fatality rates, not in overall disease incidence.

Seasonal Variations

In the past, in temperate zones measles displayed striking seasonal variations. The incidence consistently began to increase in November, approximately doubling every month until March when it began to level off, with the incidence usually reaching a peak in May (Central Public Health Committee, 1933; Herrman, 1925). Beginning in June there was a sharp decline each month so that by September and October the incidence was 5% or less of that observed in peak months. Since the development of widespread immunization, the same seasonality has occurred, although with blunted variations (CDC, 1991d). It is presumed, but not proven, that the seasonal changes relate to closer contact of individuals who are indoors in colder months, such as in schools. In tropical and other warmer areas there is little effect of season.

Sex

Because measles is a highly contagious disease experienced by nearly everyone in the absence of immunization, there is no sex difference in incidence. In the above-described London outbreak, mortality was approximately 20% higher in males than in females (Central Public Health Committee, 1933). Whether this disparity reflects differing age distributions of measles between the two sexes, with males acquiring the disease younger when mortality is higher, or whether it reflects a difference in age-specific case-fatality rates is unclear.

Race

There is no evidence that race per se has any influence on measles epidemiology. Any racial differences are a consequence of socioeconomic factors.

Socioeconomic Status (SES)

Mortality rates from measles are higher in crowded, inner-city areas, presumably because of enhanced exposure of infants and very young children who are at highest risk of death. Other factors may be the presence of underlying disease, less than optimal nutrition, or other factors related to lower SES, including lack of immunization.

International Comparisons

Until very recently the situation in the developing world remained similar to that in industrialized countries during the early part of this century. Indeed, as recently as the early 1980s WHO estimated that 2.6 million or more children died annually in the developing world from measles, a figure approaching 2.5%

of the annual birth cohort (Grant, 1985). In these countries the highest incidence and mortality rates were in infants and children younger than 5 years of age.

Interventions

Prevention: Immunization

The isolation and propagation of measles virus in 1954 provided opportunities not only for better understanding of measles pathogenesis and immunity but also for the development of active immunization (CDC, 1989c; Preblud & Katz, 1988). By 1963 both inactivated and live, attenuated measles vaccines were available. The inactivated vaccine was usually given as two or three doses 4 weeks apart, sometimes with a subsequent dose of the live attenuated vaccine. It soon became apparent that the immunity after the inactivated vaccine not only waned within a very few years but was also defective. Consequently, exposed individuals often developed an atypical form of measles, which was often severe, with a variety of systemic and cutaneous phenomena not ordinarily associated with measles. For this reason the inactivated vaccine was abandoned and is no longer available.

Most individuals who receive live, attenuated measles vaccine are expected to display some symptoms 6 to 9 days after its administration—the so-called mild measles. However, from 1963 to 1975 in the United States the live vaccine comprised the Edmonston B strain, which was much more reactive than current strains in the sense of producing more pronounced symptoms. For this reason immune serum globulin was commonly administered at the time of immunization to ameliorate the subsequent vaccine-related illness.

Other attenuated vaccines (the Schwarz and Moraten strains) were introduced in the late 1960s, and by 1975 the Edmonston B vaccine was no longer available (Markowitz et al., 1990b). At the present time the Schwarz strain is used primarily in Europe and the Moraten strain in the United States. Both are associated with far less reactivity and with excellent immunogenicity and clinical protection. In most of the industrialized world, live measles vaccine is combined with live, attenuated mumps and rubella vaccines—usually referred to as MMR. Immune serum globulin is not employed with either of these two vaccine strains.

Measles vaccine, now recommended or mandated for all children in most developed countries, has had remarkable effects on the epidemiology of measles, although the eradication of measles, which was hoped for or anticipated in some countries, has not been achieved. In the United States live measles vaccine was originally recommended for administration at 9 months of age; because of vaccine failures attributed to persistent maternal antibody, the recommended age was raised to 1 year in 1965. However, it subsequently became apparent that vaccine failures attributable to persistent maternal antibody occurred in up to 5% of children when it was given at 1 year, and in 1976 the recommended age was changed to 15 months (Preblud & Katz, 1988).

Figure 9.3 shows the numbers of cases of measles reported annually in the United States from 1950 to 1991 (CDC, 1991d). Undoubtedly, the figures before use of the vaccine are underestimates, because the average number of cases

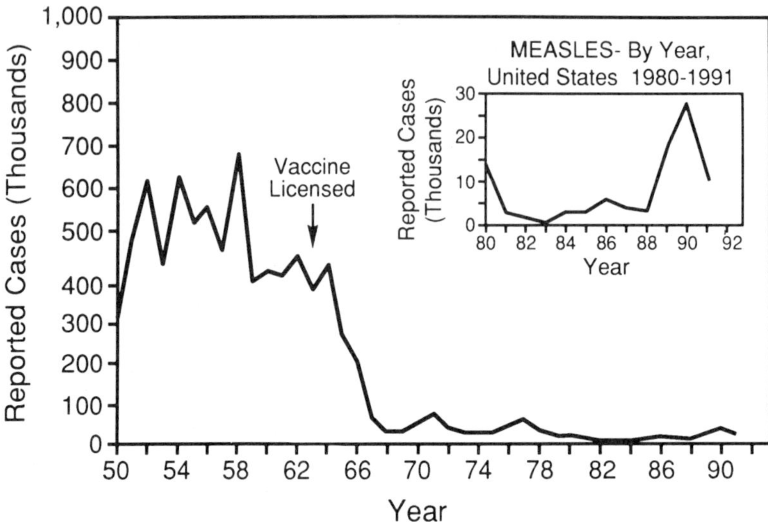

Fig. 9.3. Reported cases of measles, United States, 1950 to 1991 (CDC, 1991d).

annually had to have approximated the birth cohort inasmuch as very few individuals escaped measles. It is likely, however, that in the last decade, reported cases more closely reflected actual cases because of enhanced surveillance and increased interest in measles.

The striking reductions following the widespread use of measles vaccine stimulated efforts in industrialized nations to eliminate indigenous measles (Preblud & Katz, 1988). In the United States in 1978 an attempt to accomplish this goal within 4 years was initiated. Although this ambitious goal was not achieved, that effort did achieve a reduction of 90% or more from an average of 40,000 or more reported cases annually from 1971 to 1977 by the early 1980s (CDC, 1991d). Indeed, the total number of cases reported for the 2 years, 1982 to 1983, was only 3,211. For the 10 years from 1979 to 1988, an average of less than four deaths from measles occurred annually. However, this salutary situation did not continue; from the nadir in 1983 the number of reported cases approximately doubled in the next 5 years, and in 1989 to 1990 the United States experienced the worst epidemic of measles in nearly two decades, with nearly 46,000 cases and 130 deaths (Gindler et al., 1992). Although there was approximately a 50% decline in cases by 1991, and fewer cases reported in the first half of 1992, the incidence of measles in the United States in the 1990s continued to exceed that of the early 1980s. It should be noted that this increase in cases of measles in 1989 to 1990 was not limited to the United States; many other Western Hemisphere nations were affected, including Canada, the Caribbean, and Central America (Gindler et al., 1992; McLean et al., 1990).

A careful examination of the epidemiologic characteristics of this two-year outbreak in the United States explains its occurrence (Gindler et al., 1992). Of particular importance are the age and ethnic distributions of those affected. Table 9.2 compares the age distributions for measles in the United States before vaccine use (1960 to 1964), during years of low incidence in the vaccine era

Table 9.2. Proportions of Cases and Incidence of Measles by Age, United States, 1960–1964, 1984–1985 and 1989–1990

	Percent of Cases			Cases per 100,000		
Age	1960–1964*	1984–1985	1989–1990	1960–1964*	1984–1985	1989–1990
0–4	37.2	26.8	43.7	766.0	4.1	53.8
5–9	52.8	9.9	9.6	1,236.9	1.6	21.4
10–14	6.5	21.8	9.8	169.1	3.3	13.3
15+	3.4	41.5	36.8	10.0	0.6	29.1
Total cases	2,190,391	5,409	45,979			

*Estimates from a sample of the U.S. population.

Source: Adapted and recalculated from CDC (1990b, 1991c) and Preblud & Katz (1988).

(1984 to 1985), and during the 1989 to 1990 outbreak. From 1960–1964 to 1984–1985 there was a marked decline in the incidence in all age groups. Indeed, the magnitude of the decline in incidence in children was such that more than 40% of cases occurred in persons 15 years and older. However, by 1989–1990 all age groups were affected by recurrent epidemic measles, although the greatest effect was in children younger than 4 years and in persons 15 years and older—these two groups accounted for 80% of cases. Indeed, the incidence in this older group in 1989–1990 actually increased nearly threefold from 1960–1964. From the standpoint of race and ethnicity, rates were highest among Hispanics, intermediate in blacks, and lowest in non-Hispanic whites, being 29.5, 12.3, and 5.2 per 100,000, respectively. Geographically, the outbreak was also remarkable in that most of the cases occurred in regional or local outbreaks, primarily in urban areas. Indeed, five urban areas—Los Angeles, Dallas, New York City, San Diego, and Bakersfield, California—accounted for nearly half of all cases. These outbreaks largely affected children under age 5. However, some large urban areas, such as Atlanta, Boston, and New Orleans, were in the main spared.

Of considerable importance for the prevention of such outbreaks in the future and the ultimate control of measles are data regarding the immunization status of those who acquired the disease. Table 9.3 classifies the cases of measles that occurred in 1989–1990 in the United States according to whether they had been appropriately vaccinated and, if unvaccinated, the reasons why they had not been (CDC, 1990b, 1991c). About 27% of cases occurred in individuals who had been properly vaccinated. The majority of cases (73%) occurred in unimmunized persons, for more than half of whom the vaccine had been indicated but simply was not received. However, about 27% of all cases occurred in individuals for whom immunization was not routinely recommended; most of these were in infants and young children younger than the recommended age for immunization (15 months). Nearly 4% of cases occurred in adults born before 1957 for whom measles vaccine had not been routinely advised because most had experienced measles. It is distressing to note that more than 2,200 cases (5%) occurred in individuals who were not immunized because of religious or philosophic objections.

The epidemiologic data derived from this U.S. epidemic of measles, which had approximately 46,000 cases in a 2-year period, highlight several problems that need to be addressed. First, it is clear that U.S. immunization programs do

Table 9.3. Vaccination Status of Measles Cases, United States, 1989 to 1990*

Vaccine Status	Number	% of Total
Unvaccinated	33,186	73.0
Vaccine indicated	18,341	40.4
Vaccine not indicated	12,397	27.3
Age <16 months	10,460	23.0
Born before 1957	1,586	3.5
Immune by serology or physician diagnosis	36	0.1
Medical exemption	315	0.7
Other reasons	2,488	5.5
Non-U.S citizen	243	0.5
Religious or philosophic exemption	2,205	4.9
Appropriately vaccinated	12,249	27.0

*Combined for the 2 years from Centers for Disease Control (1990b, 1991c).

not adequately reach children before entry into elementary school at which time immunization requirements, mandated in most states, take effect. This deficit most often occurs in large urban areas among lower-income groups. Indeed, a retrospective survey of children entering school in 1990 showed that, among eight large cities, the proportions of children who had received measles vaccine by 2 years of age ranged between 51% and 81% (CDC, 1991a). This is a failure of the health care system, and recommendations for correction have been made (National Vaccine Advisory Committee, 1991).

The second problem is that in 1989–1990 23% of measles cases occurred in children younger than the age recommended for the administration of vaccine. This may be in part a consequence of the fact that at present most pregnant women have acquired measles immunity from immunization, not from natural disease. Serum antibody levels after immunization are lower than those after natural disease (Lennon & Black, 1986). Because acquired antibody (but not necessarily clinical protection) declines gradually over years, the amount of transplacental antibody received from an immunized mother may well be considerably less than that acquired from a mother who experienced the disease, thus shortening the duration of protection. Although such levels are unpredictable in individual infants, consideration is being given to lowering the age of routine immunization to 1 year for routine immunization and to 9 months (as already recommended) or earlier in outbreak situations. Any vaccine failures that occur in the few infants whose mothers have higher levels of serum antibody to measles should be corrected by a second dose of measles vaccine as MMR, which has been recommended in the United States since 1989 (CDC, 1989c).

An additional concern is that 12,249 cases (27% of the total) occurred in 1989–1990 in individuals who had previously been immunized. This is three times the total of all cases, immunized and unimmunized, that occurred in 1983. Because most individuals immunized as early as 12 months were considered to be immune, some of these may represent vaccine failures due to persistent maternal antibody, as noted above. Others may have resulted from improper vaccine storage or similar problems. Some may have occurred because of the simultaneous administration of immune serum globulin in the past, particularly if it was given with one of the more attenuated vaccines contrary to recommendations. Finally, it is also likely that a proportion of unknown magnitude comprises individuals who responded appropriately to measles vaccine but whose immunity waned to nonprotective levels over a period of some years. Because it is known that immune individuals exposed to measles often acquire anamnestic serologic responses that may assist in maintaining immunity (Markowitz et al., 1990a; Preblud and Katz, 1988) it is possible that waning immunity in some was facilitated by the near-disappearance of measles by the mid-1980s. Nonetheless, whatever the reasons for the occurrence of measles in satisfactorily immunized persons, the problems should be controlled by a second dose of measles vaccine.

Measles Vaccine in the Developing World

Major contributing factors to high measles mortality in developing countries have been the high incidence in the very young and the prevalence of debilitating underlying or associated disorders, including low birthweight, malnutrition, prior or subsequent diarrhea, and a variety of lower respiratory tract infections. All contribute to higher case-fatality rates (Assad, 1983; Koster et al., 1981; Loening & Coovadia, 1983; Morley, 1969). However, by 1990 WHO estimated that 80% of children in developing countries had received measles vaccine, recommended at 9 months of age (EPI, 1992). Estimates indicate that measles mortality in these nations had declined to approximately 600,000 annually compared to 2.5 million 10 years ago (Fig. 9.2); this decrease is largely attributable to measles vaccine, but undoubtedly in part to other factors, such as better nutrition and oral rehydration therapy (ORT) for diarrheal diseases.

In these developing nations, particularly in urban areas (Loening & Coovadia, 1983), a considerable proportion of cases of measles with high mortality occur in infants younger than 9 months of age and are associated with loss of transplacental protection for reasons that are not clear (Halsey et al., 1985). Additionally, levels of immunization of children 9 months and older achieved in urban areas did not affect transmission to infants satisfactorily (Taylor et al., 1988). Accordingly, measles vaccines of higher potency have been developed, which are designed to overcome the unpredictable levels of transplacental antibody and thus to be effective in infants 6 months of age or younger. Three such vaccines were developed: the Edmonston-Zagreb (EZ) strain developed in Yugoslavia, the AIK-C strain from Japan, and the higher titer Schwarz strain. These strains proved to be immunogenic in infants as young as 4 months of age (Aaby et al., 1988; Markowitz et al., 1990b; Tidjani et al., 1989), and accordingly, in 1989 WHO and EPI recommended the use of the EZ measles vaccine in infants under age 6 months in nations with high infant mortality from measles (Expanded Programme on Immunization, 1991).

However, in late 1991 a report appeared indicating that children in Africa who had received the high-titer EZ vaccine at 4 to 6 months in the original clinical trials showed excess mortality during the ensuing 2 or 3 years compared to infants who received the Schwarz vaccine at 9 months (EPI, 1991; Garenne et al., 1991). After careful review by EPI and outside consultants, it was concluded that these data were valid, and the recommendation for the use of EZ vaccine at 6 months of age was withdrawn (Weiss, 1992). Several epidemiologic features of this unexpected delayed mortality are of interest. First, the excess mortality seemed to continue for at least 2 years, the longest period of observation. Second, it was not attributable to measles, but instead to a variety of infections known to be problems in these particular populations, including malaria, pneumonia, and diarrheal diseases. Third, the excess mortality seemed to be multiplicative, rather than additive, increasing the expected mortality by approximately 25%, and not associated with a specific death rate. In this regard it should be noted that the excess mortality was not evident in areas with very low death rates in infants and young children. Fourth, and perhaps most remarkable, is that the excess mortality seemed to affect only female children. Fifth, the excess mortality seemed to be associated with the high titer of the vaccine, rather than the age at which it was administered. A biologic explanation for these phenomena is unknown. Because both measles and the vaccine produce changes in the immune system, it is tempting to hypothesize an immunologic mechanism, but this is unproven. In the absence of an explanation that would lead to a corrective modification of the vaccine, further studies of high-titer measles vaccines in young infants are not planned.

Nutrition

Another approach to reducing measles mortality in developing nations is based on the observations that serum vitamin A levels are depressed during measles and that this depression is associated with increased morbidity and mortality (Frieden et al., 1991). Clinical trials of vitamin A supplementation during measles have shown a clear reduction in disease severity, including mortality (Coutsoudis et al., 1991; Hussey & Klein, 1990). Accordingly, WHO has recommended such supplementation during the illness. Remarkably in the 1931–1932 outbreak of measles in London a controlled clinical trial of fish-liver oil concentrate administered to hospitalized children with measles was associated with reduced mortality but not morbidity (Central Public Health Committee, 1933).

Nonetheless, the worldwide goal of reducing measles mortality by 95% from pre-EPI levels by 1995 continues (Expanded Programme on Immunization, 1992). With 80% of the population served by EPI immunized against measles by 1990, an estimated 70% reduction in mortality occurred. To achieve this 95% goal, at least 90% of 1-year-old children (and more in some areas) will need to be immunized against measles. This goal will not be easily achieved, but the success of EPI programs to date suggests that it is possible.

Rubella (German Measles)

Clinical Features

Rubella is an acute exanthematous viral disease experienced by most persons during their lifetimes, most often in childhood. It is usually a mild disease with low-grade fever and minimal or no systemic symptoms; in children the first manifestation is usually the rash. It is rather fine and maculopapular in appearance, sometimes confluent on the trunk, and usually lasts 3 or 4 days. Serologic studies have demonstrated that rubella sometimes occurs without a rash. Quite characteristic is enlargement of posterior cervical and postauricular nodes. In contrast to measles, the diagnosis can be somewhat difficult to make clinically, and there is often confusion with other rash-producing infections, including mild scarlet fever. Isolation of the rubella virus (Parkman et al., 1962; Weller & Neva, 1962) and the subsequent development of serologic methods for diagnosis have facilitated better definition of the clinical manifestations and epidemiology of the disease.

The importance of rubella in pediatrics lies in the congenital rubella syndrome (CRS), a devastating infection of the fetus that frequently occurs when a pregnant woman experiences the disease in the first trimester. CRS is variably associated with a wide spectrum of manifestations. Cherry (1992) reviews these manifestations in detail and includes estimates of their frequency. In brief, infants with the syndrome are born with a chronic or subacute rubella virus infection that may persist up to a year after birth. There is a high rate of spontaneous abortions and stillbirths. Many infants are born with symptoms of active infection, including meningoencephalitis, pneumonitis, bone involvement, hepatitis, and thrombocytopenia. Such cases fall into the TORCH syndrome—defects caused by toxoplasmosis, rubella, cytomegalovirus, as well as herpes simplex. Other manifestations of CRS include intrauterine and postnatal growth retardation, sensorineural deafness, cataracts and other ophthalmic disorders, and congenital heart disease. Some of these manifestations, such as developmental retardation, deafness, and some forms of congenital heart disease, are not recognized for several months or a few years after birth. The affected infants often shed virus from the respiratory tract and in the urine for up to a year after birth. The diagnosis is best made by virus isolation or serologically by high levels of rubella-specific IgM.

Acquired rubella is frequently associated with arthritis or arthralgia, which may affect large and small joints (Chantler et al., 1982; Judelsohn & Wyll, 1971). It usually begins about the time the rash is disappearing. It often resembles the arthritis associated with rheumatoid arthritis and in some instances is sufficiently acute and severe to mimic acute rheumatic fever. It is usually transient, disappearing within a few weeks. The incidence of arthritis is directly related to age; it is quite uncommon in children and occurs far more often in females than in males. Rates as high as 50% have been described in adult females, although these joint disorders are usually, if not always, transient. In some instances rubella virus has been identified in synovial fluid (Grahame et al., 1981). Occasional instances of apparent progression to rheumatoid arthritis have been described, but, given the frequency of rheumatoid arthritis, such cases may well represent simple coincidence (Howson & Fineberg, 1992).

Rarely, rubella encephalitis has been described, sometimes with death and permanent disability; the incidence is probably no more than 1 per 5,000 cases. In approximately 1 in 3,000 cases of rubella, transient acute thrombocytopenia occurs (Cherry, 1992).

Biologic Considerations

Transmission

It is generally accepted that rubella is usually transmitted by the respiratory route. The virus is readily recovered from nasal pharyngeal secretions; shedding may begin as early as a week before onset of the rash and may persist for 10 days or longer after the eruption appears. However, maximum shedding occurs during the period from 4 to 5 days before rash onset and for about a week thereafter. Because rates of infection in exposed susceptibles are lower than those of some other contagious diseases, such as measles, it is assumed that transmission is primarily by large aerosolized droplets containing many organisms (the direct respiratory route), rather than by smaller droplets containing very few organisms (indirect airborne transmission). It is possible that transmission occasionally occurs by direct physical contact, such as from contaminated hands. Curiously, during rubella outbreaks a small proportion of affected individuals seem to transmit the disease at unusually high rates; these "spreaders" shed large amounts of virus (Hattis et al., 1973). A potentially important source of transmission is the infant with congenital rubella who may shed the virus for many months.

Immunity

Both serologic and cell-mediated immune responses occur with rubella. Clinical immunity is generally assumed to be lifelong; the majority of alleged second attacks most likely represent erroneous diagnoses, given the ease with which rubella can be confused with other rashes. However, there are isolated instances of laboratory-proven second attacks. Transplacental immunity in infants born to mothers who were immune before conception provides clinical protection for about 6 months and perhaps longer, though not as long as with measles. Additionally, as with some other contagious diseases, evidence of subclinical infection after exposure occurs in some individuals (Plotkin, 1988).

Patterns of Occurrence

For several reasons, data regarding the incidence of rubella are less precise than those for many other infectious diseases, both in industrialized and developing nations. First, the disease if often sufficiently mild that it may not come to the attention of a physician. It is not an easy diagnosis to make and is frequently missed. Second, except for its pregnancy-related effects, it is not considered an important disease. In the United States it was not nationally reportable until 1966; data before that year come from localized areas where it was reportable or from special studies. In the developing world rubella is of low priority compared to other more devastating, vaccine-preventable diseases, and few data, even regarding CRS, are available. Additionally, because rubella is rarely fatal, mortality data are of no value.

An approach that has proven valuable in determining the true incidence of rubella is to determine the prevalence of serum antibody at various ages. Such information regarding the incidence of rubella in the absence of immunization is limited, however, because serologic testing for rubella antibodies did not become available until the late 1960s, immediately following which widespread rubella immunization was initiated in many industrialized countries. Somewhat surprisingly, data from the United States indicate that up to 20% of adults have not experienced rubella. There seems to be considerable variation, however, among nations, at least in the Western Hemisphere. Serologic studies conducted in the prevaccine era suggested that 90% or more of adults in industrialized nations were immune to rubella, with the curious exception of Japan (Cockburn, 1969). In some Caribbean islands and some remote areas, the prevalence of adult immunity was much lower, indicating the absence of endemic disease.

Temporal Variations

Data from several states and communities in the United States where the disease was reportable indicate that, before widespread immunization, outbreaks of rubella occurred every 6 to 9 years (Witte et al., 1969). Although rubella was probably endemic during the intervening years, the incidence was extremely low.

In 1964 to 1965 in the United States, a major outbreak occurred with nearly 550,000 reported cases—a considerable underestimate because rubella was not reportable in 15 states containing about 45% of the U.S. population, including large urban centers (Orenstein et al., 1984). Up to about 30,000 pregnancies were affected; approximately 20,000 infants with CRS were born, most with residual handicaps. Approximately half again as many pregnancies were lost, either due to stillbirths or spontaneous or induced abortion.

Seasonality

In the temperate zones the peak incidence of rubella is in the spring, March through June, although the disease seems to be endemic yearround, except in isolated areas.

Age

Some age-specific incidence data are available from reported cases for the prevaccine era. These data indicate that, in the United States, the highest incidence was in children aged 5 to 14, in whom about two thirds of all cases occurred (Witte et al., 1969). Less than 15% of cases were reported in preschool children, and another 20% occurred after the age of 14.

Sex

There are no effects of sex on rubella epidemiology, other than the higher rate of rubella arthritis in females.

Race

Presumably all races are equally susceptible. It is of interest, however, that in the United States in 1991 there were only 15 cases reported in blacks compared to 980 in non-Hispanic whites (CDC, 1991d). This is surprising, given the fact that the incidence of measles is disproportionately higher in blacks, presumably due to delayed immunization in inner cities. It is likely that this apparent disparity in the racial incidence of rubella reflects the difficulty in diagnosis caused by a less readily recognized rash in blacks.

Socioeconomic Status (SES)

There is no recognized effect of SES on rubella, although it is logical that the disease might occur earlier in life in crowded inner cities.

Interventions

Prevention: Immunization

The recovery of rubella virus on tissue culture in 1962 and its subsequent propagation facilitated the development of live, attenuated rubella vaccines; this effort was accelerated in anticipation of the next epidemic cycle, which was expected in the early 1970s. By 1970 in the United States and at about the same time in Europe, several such vaccines were licensed after clinical trials demonstrated their safety and efficacy. In some countries these earlier vaccines have been replaced by products that are at least as effective and somewhat less reactive; in the United States, for example, the currently used RA/27, licensed in 1979, is universally employed. In the United States, as in many countries, rubella vaccine is combined with live, attenuated measles and mumps vaccine as MMR.

The initial immunization strategy used in the United States was designed to avert or ameliorate the incidence of CRS when and if epidemic disease returned in the early 1970s as expected. To this end the group initially targeted for intense immunization efforts comprised young school-aged children for three reasons. First, elementary schools were a major site of propagation of rubella in previous epidemic years. Second, most children in the early elementary school grades were born after the 1964 to 1965 epidemic and were expected to be susceptible. Third, the younger the elementary school child, the more likely was the mother to be pregnant. Yet, the anticipated epidemic did not occur in the United States. Whether it was prevented by this unique application of the principles of herd immunity or whether it would have failed to appear for other reasons is a matter for conjecture. Since that initial immunization effort, rubella vaccine has been recommended at 15 months of age as part of the MMR, this age being selected to provide maximum protection against measles. Since 1989 in the United States a second dose of MMR has been recommended in early adolescence, primarily to achieve maximum population immunity against measles, but secondarily against rubella and mumps (CDC, 1990a). In the United Kingdom a different approach was taken, which was to immunize in early adolescence (Clarke et al., 1979).

Rubella vaccine is the only vaccine given to humans for which the primary justification is the prevention of disease in others. Thus, the measure of success of widespread rubella immunization is the incidence of CRS. Figure 9.4 shows the incidence of reported rubella and CRS in the United States from 1966 to 1988 (CDC, 1989a). Beginning in 1990 in the United States a slight increase in cases occurred; many of these were in Amish or other religious populations that

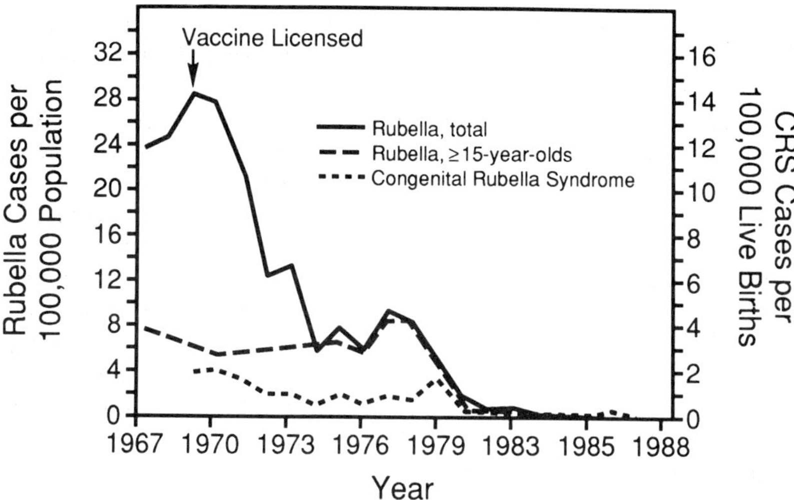

Fig. 9.4. Incidence of rubella and the rubella syndrome, United States, 1967 to 1988 (CDC, 1989a).

do not accept routine immunization, whereas others occurred in underimmunized inner-city areas (CDC, 1992a; Lee et al., 1992). During the years 1986 through 1991, 86 cases of the syndrome were reported in the United States, the majority in the last 2½ years (CDC, 1991d). One half or more of these could have been prevented if women had been screened for rubella immunity during a prior pregnancy and immunized after delivery if they were susceptible.

An interesting epidemiologic phenomenon of herd immunity is a consequence of the interaction between age at rubella immunization and the proportion of persons immunized to achieve the goal of preventing rubella in women of child-bearing age (Anderson & May, 1990). If immunization is optional for preschool children, less than full acceptance (such as 50%) may be sufficient to reduce the transmission of rubella disease in childhood, but will still leave the unimmunized children susceptible to rubella on reaching adulthood. Under such circumstances the result might be a larger proportion of women of child-bearing age being nonimmune, with a consequent increase in CRS. Indeed, this situation occurred in Finland. Therefore, when acceptance of rubella vaccine among young children is low but sufficient to reduce transmission in schools, a better approach is to immunize in early adolescence as is done in the United Kingdom, which allows many or most children to experience the disease and subsequently immunizes those who did not.

Rubella Vaccine Reactivity

There have been three concerns about rubella vaccine. First is the question whether the vaccine could produce the CRS if given to a woman early in pregnancy. Assuming that it has the potential for producing the syndrome, the second question is whether a recently immunized child could transmit the vaccine virus to others, particularly the child's pregnant mother. The third concern is whether the vaccine produces a chronic rheumatoid arthritis-like disorder in some recipients. Answers to the first two of these concerns are available; the third is under continuing study.

Although studies of an earlier, less attenuated rubella vaccine indicated that the virus could be recovered from approximately 20% of aborted fetuses of recently immunized susceptible mothers (albeit, significantly less often if the mother had received the RA 27/3 vaccine), vaccine-related teratogenicity does not seem to occur. The U.S. Public Health Service monitored the outcomes of 321 term pregnancies of women who had received rubella vaccine between 3 months before and 3 months after the estimated date of conception (CDC, 1990a). Of these, 226 (70%) had received the RA 27/3 vaccine; 97 (30%) had received the earlier, less attenuated vaccine, and in one the vaccine was unknown. Five of these infants displayed serologic evidence of intrauterine infection without clinical manifestations. For the RA 27/3 vaccine the 95% confidence interval of the risk of CRS to the infant under these circumstances is 0% to 1.2%. Because this risk is negligible, the U.S. Public Health Service discontinued further surveillance of rubella vaccine and pregnancy outcomes in 1989. Furthermore, there seems to be little or no risk of transmission of vaccine virus from an inoculated child (Plotkin, 1988).

There is no question that acute arthritic symptoms frequently occur after rubella vaccine, although the rate is considerably lower than that after natural disease, but with the same sex and age predilections (Plotkin, 1988). Anecdotal reports, including one case series, suggest that chronic joint manifestations follow both the disease and rubella immunization in a few individuals. From previously immunized, affected persons, rubella virus has been recovered from peripheral blood and synovial fluid leukocytes some months later (Chantler et al., 1982; Grahame et al., 1981). These results suggest but do not prove that both rubella disease and rubella immunization are occasionally followed by chronic or recurrent arthritis (Howson & Fineberg, 1992). A more definitive resolution of this question should be provided by well-designed clinical, laboratory, and epidemiologic studies currently in progress.

Mumps

Clinical Features

Mumps is a systemic viral disease, usually occurring in childhood, that primarily affects both exocrine and endocrine glands and, less commonly, the neurologic system. It is a nuisance disease that can be quite unpleasant, but sequelae are extremely rare.

After initial infection, viremia occurs with subsequent localization of the virus in various glandular tissues or in nervous tissue or both. The incubation period is usually 16 to 18 days, but often seems to be several days longer or shorter because of variations in the onset of clinical symptoms. As a rule, mumps is associated with slight to moderate fever and a short prodrome before the onset of parotid swelling. Characteristically, the salivary glands, most often the parotid, exhibit varying degrees of pain and swelling for up to 10 days. Other glands that may be affected include the pancreas, the ovaries, the thyroid and, rather frequently, the testes. Orchitis is usually unilateral, and the concern that bilateral orchitis produces sterility is probably a myth. Serologic studies have shown that one third or more of all cases of mumps are asymptomatic.

Mumps meningoencephalitis begins a few days to a week after onset of symptoms and is usually mild, but may be a severe illness with high fever, vomiting, nuchal rigidity, some encephalitic signs, and, occasionally, convulsions. Usually this complication is self-limited, and sequelae are rare. Severe hearing impairment, occurring with or without meningoencephalitis, is an extremely rare, permanent complication; fortunately, it is usually unilateral.

Except during epidemics, clinical accuracy in the diagnosis of mumps is far from satisfactory. Many cases are asymptomatic, and mild cases are often not recognized. Diagnostic confusion with cervical adenitis is a frequent problem. Additionally, there are other causes of parotitis, some recurrent and some due to other viruses. Serologic tests are widely available for clinical use and are of particular value in the differential diagnosis of meningoencephalitis in the absence of parotitis.

Biologic Considerations

Transmission

It is generally agreed that mumps is transmitted by the respiratory route. Because it is less readily transmitted than some other contagious diseases, such as measles, pertussis, and varicella, it may be that a larger inoculum as contained in heavy droplets requires close respiratory contact. One reason for lower transmission rates than those of measles and pertussis is the absence of respiratory manifestations, such as cough. Acquisition of clinical mumps by susceptible contacts exposed in households seems to be between 30% to 40% (Dingle et al., 1964; Harris et al., 1968; Hope-Simpson, 1952; Meyer, 1962) and varies with age, being highest in children ages 2 to 9 with a range of about 40% to 60%.

Immunity

Immunity after the natural disease is assumed to be lifelong, although antibodies decline after infection (Philip et al., 1959). The severity of the clinical disease has no effect on immunity. Although data are less precise than those for measles, infants of immune mothers are protected by transplacental antibodies for at least 6 months. In immune persons exposure to mumps frequently results in an anamnestic serologic response (Dingle et al., 1964).

Patterns of Occurrence

Incidence

Relatively few data are available on the incidence and age distribution of mumps before the advent of immunization or even today in nations where mumps vaccine is not routinely employed. To a large extent this lack of information is because mumps is generally considered to be a nuisance disease of relatively little consequence compared to other contagious diseases of childhood. Indeed, in the United States mumps was reportable nationally beginning in 1922, but not from 1950 until 1968 when mumps vaccine was first marketed. However, many states continued to maintain data in the interim (Witte & Karchmer, 1968). Additionally, physicians frequently fail to report mumps, and parents often did not contact a physician when mumps occurred in their children (Levitt et al., 1970).

Most of the data regarding the incidence of mumps, including its age distribution, come from prevaccine serologic studies, epidemics, and some communities or states where it was reportable. Because death from mumps is extremely rare and even when reported may be misdiagnosed, mortality data have no value.

It is reasonable to assume that few individuals escape mumps infection in their lifetimes, as with the other contagious diseases, except those who reside in remote areas. Although this assumption is likely to be true, it is difficult to substantiate. Personal recollections of past contagious diseases are quite unreliable and are particularly so with mumps, if only because up to a third of serologically proven infections are asymptomatic. Survey data from the United States in the prevaccine era indicate that, at most, only about 60% of adolescents give a history of mumps.

Geographic Variations

Mumps occurs worldwide. However, data regarding its incidence and age distribution in developing countries are not available, in part because the disease is of minor importance compared to many other infections.

As with other contagious diseases, outbreaks occasionally occur in isolated areas where there has been no experience with the disease for several generations. In 1957 one such outbreak occurred in an Eskimo population on an Alaskan island where there had been no mumps for at least 50 years (Philip et al., 1959). Of 561 residents, 363 (65%) experienced clinical mumps; after serologic testing it was shown that 494 (88%) were infected. Among the small proportion who escaped mumps, some who were elderly may have experienced it in the past, and others might not have been exposed on this sparsely populated island.

Temporal Variations

Mumps is both an endemic and epidemic disease. Peaks in incidence are said to occur about every 7 years (Gordon & Kilham, 1949). However, data from U.S. urban areas before the use of mumps vaccine suggest that the interepidemic interval was 3 to 4 years (Bader, 1977; Dingle et al., 1964; Witte & Karchmer, 1968).

Seasonality

In urban areas mumps is endemic the yearround, but peaks with a two- or threefold increase occur during the spring months (Witte & Karchmer, 1968).

Age

Serologic studies, reviewed by Feldman (1989), have showed wide variations in the presence of antibody depending on age, geography, and the characteristics of the populations studied. Although these studies are difficult to interpret, in part because some were conducted in the United States after vaccine licensure and in others there are considerable variations in the populations studied, it seems that the majority of individuals acquired mumps antibody in childhood. Data on the age incidence of reported mumps from four urban areas in the United States, 1960 to 1964, indicated that about 25% of cases occurred in children younger than 5 years of age, 56% from 5 to 9 years, 13% from 10 to 19 years, and 6% in persons 20 years and older (Witte & Karchmer, 1968). For meningoencephalitis, reported cases indicate that the rate of this complication is likely higher (or more apt to be recognized) in older individuals; 16% of cases were reported in persons 20 years and older.

Unpublished data that suggest that most individuals experience mumps during their lifetimes are derived from serologic studies conducted in Cleveland in 1980. Sera were available from 340 women up to 90 years of age, all but 9 of whom were 25 years or older and thus would not have received mumps vaccine. Indeed, 52% were 45 to 64 years of age, and 25% were 65 or older. A positive hemagglutination antibody titer of 1:10 or greater was found in 321 (91.5%) of this group. However, only 61% reported a past history of mumps, 26% denied having had mumps, and 13% stated that they did not know whether they had had it or not (Hodder et al., unpublished data).

The data cited above that indicate that up to 80% of U.S. children in the prevaccine era experienced mumps by 10 years of age are derived from urban areas. Circumstantial evidence indicates that the age distribution is older in rural areas, presumably because of lack of contact with the disease. This evidence is derived from British, French, and U.S. military experiences (Gordon & Heeren, 1940). In the U.S. Army in World War I more than 230,000 cases of mumps resulting in hospitalization or restricted duty occurred, for an annual rate of 56 per 1000 troops (Stokes, 1958). This incidence rate exceeded those for all other infectious diseases, with the exceptions of influenza and gonorrhea. Additionally, nearly four million man-days were lost from duty in World War I, for a rate of 2.6 per 2000 days, also ranking third among infectious diseases. In World War II mumps epidemics again occurred in the military, although at rates one tenth or less those of World War I. However, among the common contagious diseases, the incidence of mumps exceeded those of all others and was threefold that of measles, which ranked second. In these military outbreaks, mumps was most likely to occur in recent recruits on large bases and particularly affected those from rural areas. It is generally believed that recruits from rural areas had been less likely to be exposed to mumps in childhood simply because of lack of contact.

Rates in the military are presumed to have been lower in World War II than in World War I because of greater urbanization and increased contacts among different populations due to improved transportation, all of which resulted in fewer susceptible recruits.

Sex

Both sexes seem equally susceptible, but there is a predilection for meningoencephalitis in males (Witte & Karchmer, 1968).

Race

All races are equally susceptible. However, among U.S. military recruits in the two world wars, rates were much higher in blacks than in whites, presumably because a large proportion of black recruits came from rural areas, especially in the South (Stokes, 1958).

Socioeconomic Status (SES)

The effects of SES on the epidemiology of mumps have not been defined. Presumably the poor in inner cities would acquire mumps at younger ages, whereas the rural poor might incur infection later, as noted above.

Interventions

Prevention: Immunization

In the United States, live, attenuated monovalent mumps vaccine was licensed in 1967. In the next few years bivalent combinations with measles vaccine or rubella vaccine were licensed, but these are no longer used. In 1971 the current trivalent preparation containing live, attenuated measles, mumps, and rubella vaccines (MMR) was licensed in the United States and in Canada shortly thereafter. However, because of its cost, the U.S. Public Health Service did not recommend mumps vaccine for all children until 1977 (CDC, 1989b). For a number of years other industrialized nations eschewed mumps vaccine, often employing monovalent or bivalent measles and rubella vaccines. MMR was introduced in Scandinavia in the early 1980s, in the Netherlands in 1987, and in the United Kingdom in 1988 (Isaacs & Menser, 1990). In clinical trials mumps vaccine produced seroconversion and clinical protection in about 95% of recipients. In most vaccinees protection is long lived, probably for life. Studies of efficacy under outbreak conditions since licensure have suggested slightly lower efficacy between 80% and 85% (Cochi et al., 1988; Hersh et al., 1991).

Because of the usually benign nature of mumps and the added expense of the vaccine, whether in monovalent or combined form, its widespread acceptance developed somewhat slowly. However, at present in the United States MMR is required for school entry in 42 of the 50 states and in the District of Columbia. In developing nations mumps vaccine has been used rarely or not at all, and mumps is not a vaccine-preventable disease targeted in EPI programs because of costs and the higher priority of other vaccine-preventable diseases with far greater morbidity and mortality.

Figure 9.5 shows the incidence rate of reported mumps, 1968 to 1991, and the numbers of reported cases, 1980 to 1991, in the United States (CDC, 1991d). The incidence declined about 90% in the 10 years after introduction of the vaccine—a decrease that was somewhat less precipitous than that for measles. This decline continued through 1985, following which outbreaks of mumps recurred with nearly a fourfold increase in incidence by 1987. Comparison of the reported age distribution of mumps in 1985 to 1987 provides a reasonable explanation for its recurrence when considered in the light of mumps vaccine utilization since licensure and the decline in reported cases of mumps during this period (CDC, 1985, 1987b, 1991d; Cochi et al., 1988). Although there was an increased incidence of mumps in all age groups, the most striking increase occurred in those 10 to 19 years. Indeed, in 1985 53% of reported cases occurred in individuals 10 years and older, whereas in 1987 the proportion was 75%. This shift in the age distribution of mumps was reflected by a number of outbreaks in schools and colleges (Sosin et al., 1989), and even in the workplace (CDC, 1987a; Kaplan et al., 1988).

An explanation for this recrudescence of mumps, including its age distribution, has been offered by Cochi, Preblud, and Orenstein (1988). During the 9 years between licensure of mumps vaccine in 1968 and U.S. Public Health Service recommendation that it be used for all children in 1977, it received only gradual acceptance. The number of doses of vaccine during that interval was only about half those of measles and rubella vaccines, the latter being used first in 1970. However, apparently enough mumps vaccine was employed to reduce the incidence and consequent transmission of the disease to the extent that a

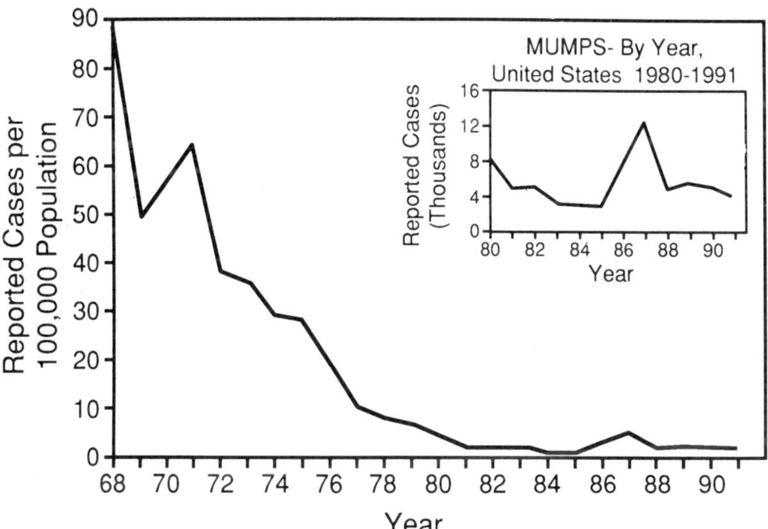

Fig. 9.5. Incidence rates of mumps, 1968 to 1991, and numbers of reported cases, 1980 to 1991, United States (CDC, 1991d).

considerable proportion of unimmunized elementary school children escaped and entered adolescence susceptible to infection. Because the 1977 recommendation for universal immunization of children resulted in an increasing number of states with school entry immunization laws, succeeding birth cohorts were protected, but many unimmunized children progressed to adolescence and young adult life unprotected. The proportion of individuals in this susceptible cohort, most of whom are now in their twenties, who are still vulnerable to mumps is unknown. However, only about 6,000 cases of mumps were reported in the United States during 1991 and 1992 (CDC, 1991d, 1992b). In 1991 nearly two thirds of cases occurred in persons 10 years and older, nearly 75% of whom were 10 to 19 years. Although precise data for these years are not available, other experience suggests that the majority occurred in persons who had never been vaccinated, rather than representing vaccine failures (Kaplan et al., 1988; Wharton et al., 1988).

An unexpected complication associated with vaccines containing one strain of attenuated virus was observed initially in 1987 and subsequently confirmed (Mumps meningitis, 1989; Furesz & Hockin, 1990). Self-limited mumps meningoencephalitis without sequelae occurred rarely (about 1 per 100,000 cases) after receipt of vaccine prepared with the URABE vaccine strain, but not with the Jeryl Lynn strain. Use of the implicated vaccine strains was subsequently discontinued in Canada and the United Kingdom (Furesz & Hockin, 1990; Two MMR vaccines withdrawn, 1992).

Varicella

Clinical Features

Varicella, or chickenpox, is a usually benign infection that nearly everyone experiences, most frequently in childhood. Colonization of the respiratory tract by the varicella zoster (VZ) virus is followed by viremia, viral multiplication in various organs, and secondary viremia with invasion of the skin. The incubation period may range from 10 to 21 days, but usually it is 14 to 17 days from exposure to the first appearance of vesicles. There may be a very mild flu-like prodrome of no more than a day, followed by the characteristic vesicular eruption, usually appearing in three or four "crops" 24 to 36 hours apart. Initially, the vesicles are described as a "dew drop on a rose petal" because of the small red areola around the vesicle. The vesicular fluid contains large amounts of virus. The vesicles rupture or desiccate within a day or two, with the formation of small, noninfectious scabs that disappear in 7 to 10 days. During the course of the illness, systemic symptoms, including fever, are usually mild; the fever is said to rise slightly just before each new crop of vesicles.

The importance of varicella is measured by frequent minor but sometimes major acute complications, severe disease in the immunocompromised person, and herpes zoster, an unpleasant late sequela. The most common acute complication of varicella is secondary infection of the lesions, which is usually superficial and mild but is occasionally invasive with cellulitis, lymphadenitis, abscess formation, or, rarely, gangrene (Bullowa & Wishik, 1935; Wishik & Bullowa,

1935). The frequency of secondary cutaneous infection is uncertain; the rate was 3% among hospitalized children with varicella, but this was obviously a group selected for more severe disease. The most frequent infecting organism in the past was hemolytic streptococcus, presumably group A. Otitis media and pneumonia were reported to occur at rates of 1.5% and 0.8%, respectively, but it is not clear whether these represent complications or simply intercurrent disease. Population-based data regarding complications of varicella are limited. Guess et al. (1986) provided estimates for the United States for 1979 to 1982 from federal surveys and for Olmstead County, Minnesota, based on a prospective population-based system of collecting data from providers. For children younger than age 5, the most common cause of hospital admission was bacterial skin infection (206 per 10,000 cases of varicella). From age 5 to 14, varicella encephalitis (usually manifested as self-limited acute cerebellar ataxia) and Reye's syndrome were most frequent (about 1.5 hospitalizations per 10,000 cases of varicella each). In adults the incidence of encephalitis was about double that in children, and the incidence of varicella pneumonia was nearly 27 per 10,000 cases. Mortality in symptomatic pneumonia is estimated to be 10% to 30% and is highest in pregnant women and immunocompromised persons (Triebwasser et al., 1967). Overall, it was estimated that nearly 4,000 hospital admissions occur annually in the United States for varicella and its complications (Guess et al., 1986). The disease also can be very severe in the neonate, and a congenital varicella syndrome, primarily affecting the nervous system, occurs in infants of mothers who experienced the disease in the first trimester (Brunell, 1992; see Chapter 6).

Herpes zoster (shingles) is a late sequela of chickenpox, ascribed to latent virus in sensory nerve roots, which may reactivate spontaneously or as a result of debilitating illness or therapeutic immunosuppression. Although often little more than an uncomfortable nuisance, zoster can be disabling, particularly if it involves the trigeminal or facial nerve. Hope-Simpson (1965) estimated that 50% of individuals who survive to 85 years of age will have at least one episode of zoster.

Biologic Considerations

Transmission

Varicella is highly contagious. Hope-Simpson (1952) found that 61% of children and adolescents under 15 years without known histories of varicella acquired the disease on initial household exposure. In a large series Ross (1962) found that 87% of susceptible children acquired chickenpox on initial household exposure. In those households in which two or more siblings were exposed to the index child who brought it home and at least one escaped the disease on initial exposure, 71% were infected by the secondary cases.

The major mode of spread of chickenpox is transmission of virus from the cutaneous lesions to the respiratory tract of the susceptible host. Humans are the only reservoir. Transmission usually occurs via the air, either from intimate contact or by airborne droplet nuclei, which may be wafted long distances, particularly in indoor settings, such as schools and hospitals. Transmission can also occur by direct physical contact and via contaminated fomites. Transmission from the respiratory tract of an infected individual seems to occur rarely, probably because the amount of virus present in respiratory secretions during the course of the illness is small. The cutaneous lesions are infective for only 3 to 5 days after onset of the eruption, whereas scabbed lesions are not infectious. The eruption of herpes zoster is infectious, but considerably less so than that of chickenpox, if only because the vesicles are fewer in number (Weller, 1992).

Immunity

Varicella induces both humoral and cellular immunity that is usually lifelong, although rare second attacks of chickenpox occur (Weller, 1983). Infants born to varicella-immune mothers are usually protected against clinical disease for several weeks. However, detectable serum transplacental antibody fades rapidly and in at least half of all infants is lost by 6 months (Gershon et al., 1976). Varicella may occur in infants younger than 6 months in spite of detectable antibody, although before 2 months the disease is milder (Baba et al., 1982). The immunology of herpes zoster is a complex issue (Weller, 1983, 1992).

Patterns of Occurrence

Incidence

Because everyone is expected to experience chickenpox, over time reported cases should equal the annual birth cohort. This is difficult to confirm, however, because in many nations data are not tabulated, and in industrialized countries this common disease is vastly underreported. For example, in the United States the average number of cases notified annually over the past 20 years is equal to only about 5% of each year's birth cohort.

Age

In industrialized nations within temperate zones, almost all chickenpox occurs in children, approximately 95% of whom have experienced the disease by their 15th birthdays. Nearly two thirds of all cases occur in the elementary school age group (age 5 to 9 years). Less than 2% of cases occur before 1 year of age and less than 3% beyond the age of 20 years. In Massachusetts during the years 1952 to 1961 about 29% of reported cases occurred in children under age 5 (Gordon, 1962) compared to less than 20% in the United States during the years 1989 to 1991 (CDC, 1989d, 1990c, 1991d). Yet, the high proportion in those earlier years probably reflects the post-World War II baby boom in the United States. It has been known for some years that the age distribution of varicella differs in warmer climates, with a much higher proportion of cases occurring in adults (Weller, 1992) with the potential for pregnancy-related problems. Weller (1989) has suggested three possible explanations for this variance, including diminished transmission in sparsely populated areas, viral interference due to the presence of other viruses, and limited survival of VZ virus outside the host because of higher ambient temperatures.

An interesting phenomenon that may relate at least in part to the older age distribution of varicella in warmer climates is a recently observed increase in chickenpox in U.S. military personnel, particularly among young recruits (Gray et al., 1990). In the U.S. Army there was more than a fourfold increase from 1980 to 1988 from a rate of approximately 3 to 13 per 10,000 annually. For the U.S. Navy, the increase during those same years was ninefold (from 3 to 27 per 10,000 annually). Risk factors for acquiring chickenpox in this military population were primarily ethnicity and age. The risks were highest for blacks and Hispanics and for personnel whose homes of record were in the Caribbean, these two factors undoubtedly being interrelated. Between 85% and 95% of cases occurred in persons under 26, with very high odds ratios compared to other personnel. Although clearly military personnel from warmer climates (the Caribbean) were at much higher risk for chickenpox, the increase is far greater than could be explained by changes in the geographic or ethnic origin of personnel. Additionally, the increase cannot be explained by a disproportionate number of young recruits because the annual incidence of varicella in the U.S. Army did not change in World War II. Indeed, for 1940 to 1942, when the strength of the U.S. Army increased 11-fold with many draftees, the annual rates of chickenpox per 10,000 were 3.3, 4.2, and 3.7 for those 3 years, respectively (Stokes 1958). This striking increase in varicella in the U.S. Army and Navy in the last decade indicates the need to consider varicella vaccine for all recruits (Gray et al., 1990).

The major risks of death from varicella are in adults and infants under 10 days, the latter mostly due to varicella acquired from a mother who contracted the disease in the last week or two of pregnancy. Death is usually due to pneumonia. Varicella after 10 days of age does not seem to be associated with excessive mortality (Brunell, 1992). The higher mortality in adults is usually due to varicella pneumonia.

Temporal Variations

Varicella is an endemic disease in all but the most isolated areas of the world. Year-to-year variations are far from striking, although there is a suggestion from U.S. data that peaks with 25% to 30% increase in incidence occur every 4 or 5 years. In contrast, seasonal variations are remarkable, with 10- to 20-fold variations between low and high incidence months throughout the year. In the United States rates are lowest in the summer and early fall, begin to rise in December, and are highest during March, April, and May. It has been suggested that one continuing reservoir for the maintenance of endemic varicella is latent infections that may later be manifested as herpes zoster (Gordon, 1962).

Sex

There are no epidemiologic differences by sex.

Race

All races are equally susceptible to varicella, and there is no evidence of excessive morbidity or mortality attributable to race per se. Therefore, differences that might be observed in morbidity or mortality associated with race must be attributable to geographic effects on age distribution of the disease, underlying disorders, and, possibly, socioeconomic factors, including the availability of care for complications.

Socioeconomic Status (SES)

There is no evidence that SES affects the incidence of varicella, although it is reasonable to suspect that infants in crowded inner cities and in large families might acquire the disease at earlier ages.

Epidemiology of Reye's Syndrome

Reye's syndrome is an acute disorder clinically characterized by encephalopathy that varies in severity, but is associated with death in up to one third of reported cases and with permanent neurologic disability in another third. It is primarily a disease of children. During the years 1977 to 1985 in the United States 2,546 cases were reported to the CDC; 549 (22%) were associated with chickenpox and the majority of the remainder with influenza (CDC, 1991b). Beginning in 1980 a series of studies demonstrated a consistently strong relationship with the administration of salicylates during the acute viral illness (Forsyth et al., 1989; Hurwitz et al., 1987). In the United States there was widespread publicity about the potential risk of aspirin in these two viral diseases. Hence, in 1986, after considerable disagreement and delay (Mortimer, 1987), a label warning was implemented and resulted in the near disappearance of the syndrome. Indeed, during the 4 years, of 1986 to 1989, only 19 cases of Reye's syndrome associated with varicella were reported (CDC, 1991b).

Interventions

Control of Varicella

Interest in pharmacologic and immunologic control of varicella has been stimulated for four reasons. First, it can be a severe disease with high mortality in newborns, pregnant women and other adults, and immunocompromised persons. Second, nosocomial outbreaks pose considerable problems, particularly because of increasing numbers of immunocompromised children and adults who are hospitalized (Weber et al., 1988). Third, varicella is a potential problem in the military. Fourth, the health care costs associated with its complications are not inconsequential (Preblud, 1986).

Pharmacotherapy

The effects of acyclovir and vidarabine on varicella zoster infections have recently been reviewed by Whitley (1992) and may be summarized as follows. The administration of acyclovir to children and adults within 24 hours of onset of chickenpox ameliorates the disease course by reducing the number of subsequent lesions and shortening the duration of new crops, apparently without compromising the immune response. However, its value in normal children has been questioned, in part because of its cost (Controversy about chickenpox, 1992), but it may be of therapeutic utility for adolescents and adults. However, evidence that it will reduce transmission or is of prophylactic value after exposure does not exist. In immunocompromised hosts with varicella, both acyclovir and vidarabine effectively reduce severe complications. Somewhat similar results were obtained in immunocompromised hosts with herpes zoster, although acyclovir seemed to be more effective. A major drawback to vidarabine is that it requires hospitalization for parenteral administration.

Passive Immunotherapy

Interferon has been shown to reduce complications of varicella in immunosuppressed children with malignancies, but limited information to date does not indicate any benefit for immunosuppressed adults with herpes zoster (Whitley, 1992).

In part because of the study by Ross (1962) that showed modification of varicella by immune serum globulin, high-titer varicella zoster immune globulin (VZIG) has been employed for prophylaxis in seronegative adults and others at high risk with some apparent effect (Brunell, 1992). Presumably, VZIG should also have some modifying effect in infants whose mothers develop varicella in the few days before or after delivery, but this has been difficult to demonstrate (Brunell, 1992).

Active Immunization

Because the above modalities offer only modest benefit to exposed or infected individuals and are of no value from the public health standpoint, and in part because an increasing proportion of hospitalized patients are at risk from varicella due to immunosuppression, a live, attenuated vaccine was developed and evaluated, originally in Japan where it has been increasingly used since the 1970s (Takahashi, 1986). The vaccine has also been studied extensively in the United States (Gershon, 1992; Gershon et al., 1992), and licensure is expected in 1993. Efficacy seems to be high in normal children and adults and even in leukemic children. Concerns about the vaccine have included transmission to others because the vaccine is often associated with a rash, particularly in leukemic children, waning immunity with consequent susceptibility to varicella in adult life when risks are greater, and the possibility of an increase in herpes zoster in later years. These concerns have largely been answered. There is a low risk of transmission from leukemic children, but the infections in contacts are very mild. To date protection in healthy and leukemic children has persisted for as long as a decade, and the few breakthrough infections have been mild. Finally, the risk of herpes zoster after the vaccine seems to be less than that after the disease (Controversy about chickenpox, 1992; Gershon, 1992, Gershon et al., 1992). Thus, the vaccine seems to be safe and effective in healthy children and adults and in leukemic children, although questions remain including the need for a second dose.

Conclusions

There are, of course, many other communicable diseases of childhood. Among those of traditional concern, one important omission is poliomyelitis, another is diphtheria, and the third is tetanus. In large part the success of vaccines has led to their virtual disappearance in Western nations, although they are still of concern in many parts of the developing world. The diseases reviewed in this chapter are a window into the fascinating history of pediatric epidemiology of the classical, big E, variety. They also illustrate, often in a dramatic manner, the effectiveness of vaccines and other preventive and control measures and the role played by epidemiology in the assessment of these measures.

References

Aaby P, Jensen TG, Hansen HL, Kristiansen H, Tharup J, Poulsen A, Sodemann M, Jakobsen M, Knudsen K, daSilva ML, Whittle H. Trial of high-dose Edmonston-Zagreb measles vaccine in Guinea-Bissau: protective efficacy. *Lancet* 1988; 2:809–811.

Anderson RM, May RM. Immunisation and herd immunity. *Lancet* 1990; 335:641–645.

Assaad F. Measles: summary of worldwide impact. *Rev Infect Dis* 1983; 5:452–459.

Baba K, Yabuuchi H, Takahashi M, Ogra P. Immunologic and epidemiologic aspects of varicella infection acquired during infancy and early childhood. *J Pediatr* 1982; 100:881–885.

Bader M. Mumps in Seattle-King County, Washington 1920-1976. *Am J Pub Health* 1977; 67:1089–1091.

Black FL. Measles. In: Evans AS, ed. *Viral Infections of Humans: Epidemiology and Control.* 3rd ed. New York: Plenum Medical Book Company, 1989; 451–469.

Brunell PA. Varicella in pregnancy, the fetus, and the newborn: problems in management. *J Infect Dis* 1992; 166(suppl 1):S42–47.

Bullowa JGM, Wishik SM. Complications of varicella. I. Their occurrence among 2,534 patients. *Am J Dis Child* 1935; 49:923–926.

Centers for Disease Control. Summary of notifiable diseases, United States, 1985. *MMWR* 1985; 34(54).

Centers for Disease Control: Mumps outbreaks on university campuses—Illinois, Wisconsin, South Dakota. *MMWR* 1987a; 36:496–498, 503–505.

Centers for Disease Control. Summary of notifiable diseases, United States, 1987. *MMWR* 1987b; 36(54).

Centers for Disease Control. Rubella and congenital rubella syndrome, United States, 1985-1988. *MMWR* 1989a; 38:173–178.

Centers for Disease Control. Mumps prevention: recommendations of the Immunization Practices Advisory Committee (ACIP). *MMWR* 1989b; 38:388–392; 397–400.

Centers for Disease Control. Measles prevention: recommendations of the Immunization Practices Advisory Committee (ACIP). *MMWR* 1989c; 38 (S9):1–18.

Centers for Disease Control. Summary of notifiable diseases, United States, 1989. *MMWR* 1989d; 38(54).

Centers for Disease Control. Measles—United States, 1989 and first 26 weeks, 1990. *MMWR* 1990a; 39:353–355; 361–363.

Centers for Disease Control. Rubella prevention: recommendations of the Immunization Practices Advisory Committee (ACIP) *MMWR* 1990b; 39(RR-15):1–18.

Centers for Disease Control. Summary of notifiable diseases, United States, 1990 *MMWR* 1990c; 39(53).

Centers for Disease Control. Measles vaccination levels among select groups of preschool-aged children: United States. *MMWR* 1991a; 40:36–39.

Centers for Disease Control. Reye syndrome surveillance—United States, 1989 *MMWR* 1991b; 40:88–90.

Centers for Disease Control. Measles—United States, 1990. *MMWR* 1991c; 40:369–372.

Centers for Disease Control. Summary of notifiable diseases, United States, 1991. *MMWR* 1991d; 40(53).

Centers for Disease Control. Congenital rubella syndrome among the Amish—Pennsylvania, 1991-1992. *MMWR* 1992a; 41:468–469, 475–476.

Centers for Disease Control. Table II. Cases of selected notifiable diseases, United States, weeks ending November 21, 1992 and November 23, 1991 (47th week). *MMWR* 1992b; 4:886.

Central Public Health Committee. *Measles. Report of the Medical Officer of Health and School Medical Officer on the Measles Epidemic, 1931–32*. London: London County Council; 1933.

Chantler JK, Ford DK, Tingle AJ. Persistent rubella infection and rubella-associated arthritis. *Lancet* 1982; 1:1323–1325.

Cherry JD. The epidemiology of pertussis and pertussis vaccine in the United Kingdom and the United States: a comparative study. In: Lockhart JD, ed. *Current Problems in Pediatrics*. Chicago: Year Book Medical Publishers, 1984; Vol. 14, No 2.

Cherry JD. Rubella In: Feigin RD, Cherry JD, eds. *Textbook of Pediatric Infectious Diseases*. 3rd ed. Philadelphia: WB Saunders CO, 1992; Vol 2:1792–1817.

Church MA. Evidence of whooping cough vaccine efficacy from 1978 whooping cough epidemic in Hertfordshire. *Lancet* 1979; 2:188–190.

Clark AC, Bradford WL, Berry GP. An epidemiological study of an outbreak of pertussis in a public school. *Am J Pub Health* 1946; 36:1156–1162.

Clarke M, Schild GC, Boustred J, Seagroatt V. Effect of rubella vaccination programme on serological status of young adults in United Kingdom. *Lancet* 1979; 1:1224–1226.

Cochi SL, Preblud SR, Orenstein WA. Perspectives on the relative resurgence of mumps in the United States. *Am J Dis Child* 1988; 142:499–507.

Cockburn WC. Large-scale field trials of active immunizing agents. *Bull WHO* 1955; 13:395–407.

Cockburn CW. World aspects of the epidemiology of rubella. *Am J Dis Child* 1969; 118:112–122.

Cody CL, Baraff LJ, Cherry JD, Marcy SM, Manclark CR. Nature and rates of adverse reactions associated with DTP and DT immunizations in infants and children. *Pediatrics* 1981; 68:650–660.

Controversy about chickenpox. *Lancet* 1992; 340:639–640.

Coutsoudis A, Broughton M, Coovadia HM. Vitamin A supplementation reduces measles morbidity in young African children: a randomized, placebo-controlled double-blind trial. *Am J Clin Nutr* 1991; 54:890–895.

Dauer CC. Reported whooping cough morbidity and mortality in the United States. *Pub Health Rep* 1943; 58:661–676.

Dingle JH, Badger GF, Jordan WS Jr. *Illness in the Home. A Study of 25,000 Illnesses in a Group of Cleveland Families*. Cleveland: The Press of Western Reserve University; 1964: 260–265.

Etkind P, Lett SM, MacDonald PD, et al. Pertussis outbreaks in groups claiming religious exemptions to vaccinations. *Am J Dis Child* 1992; 146:173–176.

Expanded Programme on Immunization. Safety and efficacy of high titre measles vaccine at 6 months of age. *Weekly Epidemiol Rec* 1991; 66:249–251.

Expanded Programme on Immunization. *EPI for the 1990s*. World Health Organization; Geneva: 1992:15.

Farizo KM, Cochi SL, Zell ER, Brink ED, Wassilak SG, Patriarca PA. Epidemiological features of pertussis in the United States, 1980–1989. *Clin Infect Dis* 1992; 14:708–719.

Feldman HA. Mumps. In: Evans AS, ed. *Viral Infections of Humans: Epidemiology and Control*. 3rd ed. New York: Plenum Medical Book Co; 1989:471–491.

Fine PEM, Clarkson JA, Miller E. The efficacy of pertussis vaccines under conditions of household exposure. Further analysis of the 1978–80 PHLS/ERL study in 21 Area Health Authorities in England. *Int J Epidemiol* 1988; 17:635–642.

Forsyth BW, Horwitz RI, Acampora D, Shapiro ED, Viscoli CM, Feinstein AR, Henner R, Holabird NB, Jones BA, Karabelas ADE, Kramer MS, Miclette M, Wells JA. New epidemiologic evidence that bias does not explain the aspirin/Reye's syndrome association. *JAMA* 1989; 261:2517–2524.

Fox JP, Elveback L, Scott S, et al. Commentary. Herd immunity: basic concept and relevance to public health immunization practices. *Am J Epidemiol* 1971; 94:179–189.

Frieden TR, Sowell AL, Henning KJ, Huff, DL, Gunn RA. Vitamin A levels and severity of measles: New York City. *Am J Dis Child* 1992; 146:182–186.

Friedlander A. Whooping cough. In: Abt IA, ed. *Pediatrics*. Philadelphia: WB Saunders Co 1925: 6:128–147.

Furesz J, Hockin JC. Vaccine-related mumps meningitis—Canada. *Can Dis Weekly Rep* 1990; 16:253–254.

Garenne M, Leroy O, Beau JP, Sene I. Child mortality after high-titre measles vaccines: prospective study in Senegal. *Lancet* 1991; 338:903–907.

Gershon AA. Varicella vaccine: still at the crossroads. *Pediatrics* 1992; 90(suppl):144–148.

Gershon A, Raker R, Steinberg S, Topf-Olstein B, Drusin LM. Antibody to varicella-zoster virus in parturient women and their offspring during the first year of life. *Pediatrics* 1976; 58:692–696.

Gershon AA, LaRussa P, Hardy I, Steinberg S, Silverstein S. Varicella vaccine: the American experience. *J Infect Dis* 1992; 166(suppl):S63–68.

Gindler JS, Atkinson WL, Markowitz LE, Hutchins SS. Epidemiology of measles in the United States in 1989 and 1990. *Pediatr Infect Dis J* 1992; 11:841–846.

Gordon JE. Chickenpox: an epidemiological review. *Am J Med Sci* 1962; 244:362–389.

Gordon JE, Heeren RH. The epidemiology of mumps. *Am J Med Sci* 1940; 200:412–428.

Gordon JE, Hood RI. Whooping cough and its epidemiological anomalies. *Am J Med Sci* 1951; 222:333–361.

Gordon JE, Kilham L. Ten years in the epidemiology of mumps. *Am J Med Sci* 1949; 218:338–359.

Grahame R, Armstrong R, Simmons NA, Mims CA, Wilton JMA, Laurent R. Isolation of rubella virus from synovial fluid in five cases of seronegative arthritis. *Lancet* 1981; 2:649–651.

Grant JP. *The State of the World's Children 1985. UNICEF.* New York: Oxford University Press; 1985:36.

Gray CG, Palinkas LA, Kelley PW. Increasing incidence of varicella hospitalizations in United States Army and Navy personnel: are today's teenagers more susceptible? Should recruits be vaccinated? *Pediatrics* 1990; 86:867–873.

Guess HA, Broughton DD, Melton LJ III, Kurland LT. Population-based studies of varicella complications. *Pediatrics* 1986; 78(suppl):723–727.

Halsey NA, Boulos R, Mode F, Andre J, Bowman L, Yaeger RG, Toureau S, Rohde J, Boulos C. Response to measles vaccine in Haitian infants 6 to 12 months old. Influence of maternal antibodies, malnutrition, and concurrent illnesses. *N Engl J Med* 1985; 313:544–549.

Harris RW, Turnbull CD, Isacson P, Karzon DT, Winkelstein W Jr. Mumps in a northeast metropolitan community. I. Epidemiology of clinical mumps. *Am J Epidemiol* 1968; 88:224–233.

Hattis RP, Halstead SB, Herrmann KL, Witte JJ. Rubella in an immunized island population. *JAMA* 1973; 223:1019–1021.

Herrman C. Measles. In: ABT IA, ed. *Pediatrics*. Philadelphia: WB Saunders Co; 1925: 6:363–407.

Hersh BS, Fine PEM, Kent WK, Cochi SL, Kahn LH, Zell ER, Hays PL, Wood CL. Mumps outbreak in a highly vaccinated population. *J Pediatr* 1991; 119:187–193.

Hinman AR. DTP vaccine litigation. *Am J Dis Child* 1986; 140:528–530.

Hope-Simpson RE. Infectiousness of communicable diseases in the household (measles, chickenpox and mumps). *Lancet* 1952; 2:549–554.

Hope-Simpson RE. The nature of herpes zoster: a long term study and a new hypothesis. *Proc Roy Soc Med* 1965; 58:1–20.

Howson CP, Fineberg HV. Adverse events following pertussis and rubella vaccines. Summary of a report of the Institute of Medicine. *JAMA* 1992; 267:392–396.

Hurwitz ES, Barrett MJ, Bregman D, Gunn WJ, Pinsky P, Schonberger LB, Drage JS, Kaslow RA, Burlington DB, Quinnan GV, LaMontagne JR, Fairweather WR, Dayton D, Dowdle WR. Public Health Service Study of Reye's syndrome and medications: report of the main study. *JAMA* 1987; 257:1905–1911.

Hussey GD, Klein M. A randomized, controlled trial of vitamin A in children with severe measles. *N Engl J Med* 1990; 323:160–164.

Isaacs D, Menser M. Modern vaccines. Measles, mumps, rubella, and varicella. *Lancet* 1990; 335:1384–1387.

Jenkinson D. Duration and effectiveness of pertussis vaccine: evidence from a 10 year community study. *Br Med J* 1988; 296:612–614.

Judelsohn RG, Wyll SA. Rubella in Bermuda. Termination of an epidemic by mass vaccination. *JAMA* 1971; 223:401–406.

Kaplan KM, Marder DC, Cochi SL, Preblud SR. Mumps in the workplace. Further evidence of changing epidemiology of a childhood vaccine-preventable disease. *JAMA* 1988; 260:1434–1438.

Karzon DT, Edwards KM. Editorial. Diphtheria outbreaks in immunized populations. *N Engl J Med* 1988; 318:41–43.

Kendrick PL. Secondary attack rates from pertussis in vaccinated and unvaccinated children. *Am J Hyg* 1940; 32:89–91.

Kimura M, Kuno-Sakai H. Developments in pertussis immunisation in Japan. *Lancet* 1990; 336:30–32.

Koplan JP, Hinman AR. Editorial. Decision analysis, public policy, and pertussis: are they compatible? *Med Decis Making* 1987; 7:71–73.

Koster FT, Curlin GC, Aziz KMA, Haque A. Synergistic impact of measles and diarrhoea on nutrition and mortality in Bangladesh. *Bull WHO* 1981; 59:901–908.

Lambert HJ. Epidemiology of a small pertussis outbreak in Kent County, Michigan. *Pub Health Rep* 1965; 80:365–369.

Lapin LH. *Whooping Cough*. Springfield, IL: Charles C Thomas; 1943: 1–237.

Lautrop H, Mikkelson OS. The effect of prophylactic whooping-cough vaccination. An attempt at an evaluation based on experiences in Denmark. *Ugeskr Laeg* 1969; 131:735–741.

Lee SH, Ewert DP, Frederick PD, Mascola L. Resurgence of congenital rubella syndrome in the 1990s. Report on missed opportunities and failed prevention policies among women of childbearing age. *JAMA* 1992; 267:2616–2620.

Lennon JL, Black FL. Maternally derived measles immunity in era of vaccine-protected mothers. *J Pediatr* 1986; 108:671–676.

Levitt LP, Mahoney DH Jr, Casey HL, Bond JO. Mumps in a general population. A sero-epidemiologic study. *Am J Dis Child* 1970; 120:134–138.

Loening WEK, Coovadia HM. Age-specific occurrence rates of measles in urban, peri-urban, and rural environments: implications for time of vaccination. *Lancet* 1983; 2:324–326.

Long SS, Welkon C, Clark JL. Widespread silent transmission of pertussis in families: antibody correlates of infection and symtomatology. *J Infect Dis* 1990; 161:480–486.

Luttinger P. The epidemiology of pertussis. *Am J Dis Child* 1916; 12:290–315.

Luttinger P. Pertussis vaccine. Its value as a curative and prophylactic agent in whooping cough. *JAMA* 1917; 68:1461–1464.

Mahieu JM, Muller AS, Voorhoeve AM, Dikken H. Pertussis in a rural area of Kenya: epidemiology and a preliminary report on a vaccine trial. *Bull WHO* 1978; 56:773–780.

Markowitz LE, Preblud SR, Fine PEM, Orenstein WA. Duration of live measles vaccine-induced immunity. *Pediatr Infect Dis J* 1990a; 9:101–110.

Markowitz LE, Sepulveda J, Diaz-Ortega JL, Valdespino JL, Albrecht P, Zell ER, Stewart J, Zarate ML, Bernier RH. Immunization of six-month old infants with different doses of Edmonston-Zagreb and Schwarz measles vaccines. *N Engl J Med* 1990b; 322:580–587.

McLean ME, Walsh PJ, Carter AO, Lavigne PM. Measles in Canada—1989. *CDWR* 1990; 16:213–218.

Medical Research Council. Vaccination against whooping-cough. The final report to the Immunization Committee of the Medical Research Council and to the medical officers of health for Battersea and Wandsworth, Bradford, Liverpool and Newcastle. *Br Med J* 1959; 1:994–1000.

Meyer MB. An epidemiologic study of mumps; its spread in schools and families. *Am J Hyg* 1962; 75:259–281.

Miller CL, Pollock TM, Clewer ADE. Whooping cough vaccination. An assessment. *Lancet* 1974; 2:510–513.

Mink CAM, Cherry JD, Christenson P, Lewis K, Pineda E, Shlian D, Dawson JA, Blumberg DA. A search for *Bordetella pertussis* infection in university students. *Clin Infect Dis* 1992; 14:464–471.

Morley D. Current practice. Medicine in the tropics. Severe measles in the tropics. *Br Med J* 1969; 1:297–300.

Morley D, Woodland M, Martin WJ. Whooping cough in Nigerian children. *Trop Geogh Med* 1966; 18:169–182.

Mortimer EA Jr. Reye's syndrome, salicylates, epidemiology and public policy. *JAMA* 1987; 257:1941.

Mortimer EA Jr. Perspective. Pertussis and its prevention: a family affair. *J Infect Dis* 1990; 161:473–479.

Mortimer EA Jr, Jones PK. An evaluation of pertussis vaccine. *Rev Infect Dis* 1979; 1:927–932.

Mumps meningitis and MMR vaccine. *Lancet* 1989; 2:1015–1016.

National Vaccine Advisory Committee. *The Measles Epidemic. The Problems, Barriers, and Recommendations*. Washington, DC: US Dept of Health and Human Services; 1991.

Olson LC. Pertussis. *Medicine* 1975; 54:427–469.

Onorato IM, Wassilak SGF. Laboratory diagnosis of pertussis: the state of the art. *Pediatr Infect Dis J* 1987; 6:145–151.

Onorato IM, Wassilak SG, Meade B. Efficacy of whole-cell pertussis vaccine in preschool children in the United States. *JAMA* 1992; 267:2745–2749.

Orenstein WA, Bart KJ, Hinman AR, Preblud SR, Greaves WL, Doster SW, Stetler HC, Sirotkin B. The opportunity and obligation to eliminate rubella from the United States. *JAMA* 1984; 251:1988–1994.

Parkman PO, Beuscher EL, Artenstein MS. Recovery of rubella virus from army recruits. *Proc Soc Exp Biol Med* 1962; 111:225–230.

Philip RN, Reinhard KR, Lackman DB. Observations on a mumps epidemic in a "virgin" population. *Am J Hyg* 1959; 69:91–111.

Plotkin SA. Rubella vaccine. In: Plotkin SA, Mortimer EA Jr, eds. *Vaccines*. Philadelphia: WB Saunders Co; 1988:235–262.

Pollard R. Relation between vaccination and notification rates for whooping cough in England and Wales. *Lancet* 1980; 1:1180–1182.

Preblud SR. Varicella: complications and costs. *Pediatrics* 1986; 78(suppl):728–735.

Preblud SR, Katz SL. Measles vaccine. In: Plotkin SA, Mortimer EA Jr, eds. *Vaccines*. Philadelphia: WB Saunders Co; 1988:182–222.

Romanus V, Jonsell R, Bergquist S-O. Pertussis in Sweden after the cessation of general immunization in 1979. *Pediatr Infect Dis J* 1987; 6:664–671.

Ross AH. Modification of chickenpox in family contacts by administration of gamma globulin. *N Engl J Med* 1962; 267:369–376.

Sako W. Studies on pertussis immunization. *J Pediatr* 1947; 30:29–40.

Shapiro ED. Editorial. Pertussis vaccines. Seeking a better mousetrap. *JAMA* 1992; 267:2788–2790.

Sosin DM, Cochi SL, Guinn RA, Jennings CE, Preblud SR. Changing epidemiology of mumps and its impact on university campuses. *Pediatrics* 1989; 84:779–784.

Sprauer MA, Cochi SL, Zell ER, et al. Prevention of secondary transmission of pertussis in households with early use of erythromycin. *Am J Dis Child* 1992; 146:177–181.

Starr SE. Status of varicella vaccine for healthy children. *Pediatrics* 1989; 84:1097–1099.

Steketee RW, Burstyn DG, Wassilak SGF, Adkins WN Jr, Polyak MB, Davis JP, Manclark CR. A comparison of laboratory and clinical methods for diagnosing pertussis in an outbreak in a facility for the developmentally disabled. *J Infect Dis* 1988; 157:441–449.

Stokes JC Jr. Mumps. In: Coates JB Jr, Hoff EC, Hoff PM, eds. *Preventive Medicine in World War II. Communicable Diseases Transmitted Chiefly Through Respiratory and Alimentary Tracts*. Washington, DC: Office of the Surgeon General, Department of the Army; 1958: Vol. IV:135–140.

Stuart-Harris CH. Experiences of pertussis in the United Kingdom. In: Manclark CR, Hill JC, eds. *International Symposium on Pertussis*. Washington DC: US Government Printing Office; 1979: 256–261.

Sutter RW, Cochi SL. Pertussis hospitalizations and mortality. 1985-1988. Evaluation of the completeness of national reporting. *JAMA* 1992; 267:386–391.

Takahashi M. Clinical overview of varicella vaccine: development and early studies. *Pediatrics* 1986; 78(suppl):736–741.

Taylor WR, Ruti-Kalisa, ma-Disu M, Weinman JM. Measles control efforts in urban Africa complicated by high incidence in the first year of life. *Am J Epidemiol* 1988; 127:788–794.

Tidjani O, Grunitsky B, Guerin N, Levy-Bruhl D, Lecam N, Xuereff C, Tatagan K. Serological effects of Edmonston-Zagreb, Schwarz, and AIK-C measles vaccine strains given at ages 4-5 or 8-10 months. *Lancet* 1989; 2:1357–1360.

Triebwasser JH, Harris RE, Bryant RE, Rhoades ER. Varicella pneumonia in adults. Report of seven cases and a review of literature. *Medicine* 1967; 46:409–423.

Two MMR vaccines withdrawn. *Lancet* 1992; 340:722.

U.S. Bureau of the Census. *Historical Statistics of the United States, Colonial Times to 1970*. Bicentennial Edition, Part 1, Table B 5-10 p. 49. Washington, DC: US Government Printing Office; 1975.

Wardlaw AC, Parton R, eds. *Pathogenesis and Immunity in Pertussis*. New York: John Wiley and Sons, Ltd; 1988.

Weber DJ, Rutala WA, Parham C. Impact and costs of varicella prevention in a university hospital. *Am J Pub Health* 1988; 78:19–23.

Weiss R. Measles battle loses potent weapon. *Science* 1992; 258:546–547.

Weller TH. Varicella and herpes zoster. Changing concepts of the natural history, control and importance of a not-so-benign virus. *N Engl J Med* 1983; 309:1362–1368; 1434–1440.

Weller TH. Varicella-herpes zoster virus. In: Evans As, ed. *Viral Infections of Humans: Epidemiology and Control*. 3rd ed. New York: Plenum Medical Book Company; 1989: 659–683.

Weller TH. Varicella and herpes zoster: a perspective and overview. *J Infect Dis* 1992; 166 (suppl 1):S1–6.

Weller TH, Neva FA. Propagation in tissue culture of cytopathic agents from patients with rubella-like illness. *Proc Soc Exp Biol Med* 1962; 111:211–215.

Wharton M, Cochi SL, Hutcheson RH, Bistowish JM, Schaffner W. A large outbreak of mumps in the postvaccine era. *J Infect Dis* 1988; 158:1253–1260.

Whitley RJ. Therapeutic approaches to varicella-zoster virus infections. *J Infect Dis* 1992; 166(suppl):S51–57.

Wishik SM, Bullowa JGM. Complications of varicella. II. Surface complications. *Am J Dis Child* 1935; 49:927–932.

Witte JJ, Karchmer AW, Case C, Herrmann KL, Abrutyn E, Kassanoff I, Neill JS. Epidemiology of rubella. *Am J Dis Child* 1969; 118:107–111.

Witte JJ, Karchmer AW. Surveillance of mumps in the United States as background for use of vaccine. *Pub Health Rep* 1968; 83:95–100.

Suggested Readings

Evans AS, ed. *Viral Infections of Humans: Epidemiology and Control*. 3rd ed. New York: Plenum Medical Book Company; 1989.

Feigin RD, Cherry JD, eds. *Textbook of Pediatric Infectious Diseases*. 3rd ed. Philadelphia: WB Saunders Co; 1992: Vol. II:1205–2395.

Krugman S, Katz, SL, Gershon AA, Wilfert CM, eds. *Infectious Diseases of Children*. 9th ed. St. Louis: Mosby Year Book; 1992.

Plotkin SA, Mortimer EA Jr, eds. *Vaccines*. Philadelphia: WB Saunders Co; 1988.

PART III

MENTAL AND BEHAVIORAL DISORDERS

10

Mental Retardation

STEPHEN A. RICHARDSON AND HELENE KOLLER

The term "mental retardation" (MR) covers the range of severity of intellectual impairment, from mild to profound. The criteria for the diagnosis have traditionally been based primarily on tests of intelligence, and this continues despite frequent challenges to the underlying assumptions. MR and corresponding terms—mental subnormality and mental deficiency—refer to a heterogeneous group of conditions, most of which are genetic or chromosomal or reflect the consequences of intrauterine infection or iso-immunization. Other biologic causes include anoxia at birth, other obstetric difficulties, as well as a relatively few postnatal events, such as sequelae of central nervous system infection or injury, anoxia from repeated or prolonged convulsions, and a variety of other causes including degenerative diseases (such as Tay-Sachs) and toxic encephalopathies (such as lead poisoning). A large proportion of cases of MR have, however, no known origin.

Therefore, it is not surprising that epidemiologic studies have varied widely in the rate of mental retardation found among children. The prevalence in different studies ranges from 6.7 to over 30 per 1,000. However, studies frequently report the prevalence of severe retardation separately from that of mild retardation. This traditional dichotomization has been found useful in distinguishing those who are likely to need lifelong support and supervision (severe mental retardation, or SMR) from those who may be able to function as adults without special services (mild mental retardation, or MMR). The following sections review studies of the epidemiology of SMR and MMR, including factors that may account for differences found between them. Variability in prevalence is found mainly in the studies of MMR. This chapter also examines how mental retardation is distributed in the general population and its main etiologic and risk factors.

Defining Mental Retardation

As in any epidemiologic enquiry, the investigator needs to define the entity under study to minimize misclassification. This task is particularly difficult around the upper border of MR, i.e., where mental retardation shades into normal levels of intelligence. It is an example of a disorder defined, in part, by an arbitrary cut-off point on a continuous scale—never a satisfactory situation from either a clinical or an epidemiologic perspective.

In the current definition, three conditions must be present (Grossman, 1983).

1. significantly subaverage intellectual functioning
2. deficits in adaptive behavior
3. retardation manifest during the developmental period, the end point of which is around the age of leaving school

How the first two criteria may be defined to distinguish between cases that do and do not fit the criteria has been the subject of much debate over many years.

Significantly Subaverage Intellectual Functioning

Intellectual functioning is determined by tests that provide an intelligence test score or IQ. These tests are standardized with a mean of 100, and an IQ below 70 is now accepted as defining subaverage intellectual functioning. This score is two standard deviations below the mean on the Wechsler Intelligence Scale for Children (WISC). Rutter et al. (1970) using the WISC, ascertained IQ scores for all 10- to 12-year-old children on the Isle of Wight in England and found that 25.3 per 1000 children scored two standard deviations or more below the mean. Because the same intelligence test is not always used, the American Association on Mental Deficiency classification states: "This upper limit (70) is intended as a guideline; it could be extended upward through IQ 75 or more, depending on the reliability of the intelligence test used (Grossman, 1983)."

Intelligence testing is valuable because it provides a more objective measure than a personal judgment of a teacher or of any other person who knows a child well. The intelligence test was originally developed by Simon and Binet "to furnish to the teacher a *first* means by which he may single out mentally backward children, who, upon further examination may also be found to have some mental deficit, or peculiarity which prevents them from fully profiting by the education of the ordinary school and who would probably benefit more by being educated in a special school or special class" (Darroch, 1914).

Several surveys have used cut-off points above 70, e.g., Holland—80 (Sorel, 1974) and Scotland—75 (Birch et al., 1970). Others have used lower cut-off points, e.g., Germany—60 (Cooper, 1990). For studies that distinguish those with MR into mild (IQ 50 and above) and severe MR (IQ below 50), there is always some point where an IQ point or two around 50 differentiates between those with mild and severe MR. Accordingly, any slight differences in test usage or in test differences may alter the prevalence of both MMR and SMR.

Another difficulty in comparing prevalence studies of mental retardation is that, over time, there has been an upward drift in test performance, i.e., children have been scoring higher on IQ tests. In the United States, the Stanford-Binet was restandardized in the mid-1970s (Terman & Merrill, 1973) because of this upward drift. Age-specific means before restandardization for those of school age ranged from 109.7 at age 5 to 101.9 at age 10 (Gallagher, 1985).

Sonnander (1990) in Sweden administered the WISC to a representative school population aged 6 to 12 years using norms standardized for the test in the 1960s. The results showed a clear upward shift, although the distribution of scores was normal, with a mean of 107.94. Sonnander concluded that the use of the old norms in current testing makes the assessment unreliable.

It is not clear what factors are responsible for this upward drift. One possibility is that the general level of intellectual functioning of children is rising. Another is that the shift is only an artifact of the test. Assuming that children are gradually becoming brighter, if test scores are not again restandardized, the number of children with IQ scores below 70 will decrease because fewer children will score around the upper end of the MMR range. If the test is restandardized, more children will have IQ scores below 70, and over time the intellectual ability of some children with IQs below 70 will be greater. Assuming the second possibility, that the drift of test scores is an artifact of the test, restandardizing will increase the prevalence of psychometrically defined mental retardation.

Deficits in Adaptive Behavior

This criterion relates to the ability of children to meet societal standards for behavior and functioning in the various activities expected for others of their age and sex. The earliest indicators of poor adaptive behavior may be delayed developmental milestones in infancy. Behavior of children in the school setting has also been widely used in the assessment of adaptive behavior. Where there is compulsory education and children of similar ages are placed in the same classes, the school is a valuable setting for teachers to compare behavior and school performance. In addition, formal tests have been developed to assess adaptive behavior, the most recent of which are the Adaptive Behavior Scales (ABS) developed for the American Association on Mental Retardation (Nihira, et al., 1974). These scales deal with sensorimotor development, self-sufficiency, language, and socialization. However, these scales have not been used in any community prevalence studies of MR.

For purposes of administrative classification of MR by educational authorities, a judgment on adaptive behavior is generally based on observations of the child at school, together with information from parents and others who see the child in other settings.

Manifestation During the Developmental Period

This criterion excludes from the definition of mental retardation any intellectual impairment that has its onset during adulthood for whatever cause. Within the developmental period, prevalence rates do not remain stable, however. As is discussed later, some causes of mental retardation occur prenatally, such as various genetic disorders (see Chapter 5). There are also peri- and postnatal causes, such as brain damage due to asphyxia, viral infections, toxicities, and trauma (see Chapters 3, 4 and 6). Reductions in prevalence arise from deaths, which occur more often among children with SMR and multiple disabilities than among children with MMR. During the developmental period, only a few children with MMR improve in their functioning to a level where they are no longer considered to have MR.

Prevalence rates during the developmental period depend on the age at which the diagnosis is made. SMR is usually recognized in the preschool period, whereas milder forms of MR are not generally identified until the school years when demands for abstract thought increase. Studies using age-specific rates generally show increases in prevalence up to ages 10 to 12. It is important then, when comparing prevalence rates in different studies to take age into account.

Combinations of the Three Criteria

All studies of MR must comply with the third criterion: restricting cases to those manifest during the developmental period. To identify MMR, both intellectual impairment and adaptive behavior need to be taken into account, especially at the upper end of the range of MMR. Mittler (1979) points out that "based on school experience . . . it is obvious that many people with IQs lower than 70 manage reasonably well and do not require special help, whereas many others with IQs considerably higher than this experience serious difficulties in learning and living."

To identify children with SMR, the criterion of intellectual impairment may be sufficient. Fryers (1987) has proposed that "*all* people with an IQ below 50, at all ages, in all societies and in all services, will be considered retarded, and no other feature is *necessary* for this category. Therefore, IQ is actually the sole criterion for definition, and Severe Mental Retardation/Handicap (SMR) is coterminus with Severe Intellectual Handicap." Because all cases of SMR during childhood are readily identifiable, it is unlikely that cases will be missed.

Definitions Used in Prevalence Studies

The criteria for mental retardation described in the previous section were intended primarily for use in the clinical evaluation of individual children. There are no epidemiologic studies in which an IQ test *and* the ABS are used to assess all children known to have, or at risk of having, mental retardation. The definitions actually used may usefully be considered in relation to history of services for children with mental retardation.

Prevalence Studies

Early Studies: Before Special MR Services for Children

The methods used by Lewis (1929) in an early study are described in some detail because of that study's pivotal place in the history of MR services. It was designed to provide estimates of the number of MR children for whom special school provisions should be made by local authorities. At the time, there were few established programs to meet the needs of these children. The study provides an elegant example of the work of a pioneer in the epidemiology of mental retardation.

In 1913, the Mental Deficiency Act in England required education authorities to identify all mentally deficient children aged 14 to 16 years of age, and the Elementary Education Act in 1914 required these authorities to develop specific educational opportunities for all children who were considered able to follow some form of education. The implementation of the Act was delayed by World War I, but in the 1920s the need for accurate prevalence information about mental retardation was evident. Lewis carried out a survey of three urban and three rural areas in England and Wales and published his report in 1929 (Lewis, 1929). He visited every school in each of the areas under study. Each teacher provided a list of the 15% to 16% of the children in the class who were judged the most backward in school performance. Lewis then personally tested each of these children using the Otis group intelligence test and removed those who were clearly not retarded. The remaining children were tested individually, using a form of the Binet-Simon test and several performance and school tests. He also obtained information from teachers or others who knew the child and tested children excluded from the schools and in institutions. In urban areas he found 18.21 per 1000 who were "feebleminded" (IQ 50+) and 4.39 per 1000 who were classified as "imbeciles" or "idiots" (IQ<50).

Gruenberg (1955), as did Lewis, carried out a prevalence study because "for the purpose of planning community services, facts about the amount and kinds of mental retardation in the general population are necessary" (Goodman et al., 1956). Onondaga County in New York State was chosen because at that time it had no comprehensive services for children with MR.

> Responsible child-care agencies were requested to report all children under 18 years of age and residents of Onondaga County on March 1, 1953 identified as definitely mentally retarded, or suspected of mental retardation on the basis of developmental history, poor academic performance, IQ score, or social adaption when contrasted with the performance of their peers (p. 87).

It was recognized that it was questionable whether all the children reported actually had MR, and it was expected that any reporting error would be on the side of overinclusiveness. Based only on the cases reported, the prevalence of suspected cases rose with age to a maximum of 77.3 per 1000 for ages 10 to 14 and then dropped to 44.6 per 1000 for ages 15 to 17. Fifty-eight percent of all school-aged cases had intelligence test quotients available. For these children, the prevalence was 3.6 per 1000 for IQs below 50 (SMR) and 18.3 per 1000 for IQs 50 to 74 (Gruenberg, 1955). These results are in close agreement with Lewis's rates of 4.39 and 18.21, respectively.

Later Studies: Different Approaches After World War II

After World War II a large number of schools established mental retardation services along with procedures for identifying children who might benefit from these programs. Placing children with MR in special classes or schools was common practice, as was the use of residential institutions for severely retarded children. Those with other forms of disability, such as physical disabilities, epilepsy, blindness, and deafness, were also segregated. Parents had little say in decisions about these placements. IQ testing was widely used to evaluate whether a child had MR and was sometimes used for screening. Several epidemiologic studies were carried out, using as a definition of MR those children in the community who were classified as MR by the education and health authorities. The selection of a community for study was based on an assessment of the thoroughness of the local authorities' screening and evaluation procedures and the existence of enough special facilities to meet the needs of all thought to require them.

Birch et al. (1970) began with an administrative classification in their definition of MR in a study of 8- to 10-year-old children. In addition, however, they independently tested all children so defined to confirm that the classification was correct. Every child in the community had been given a group intelligence test at age 7, so those who remained in regular classes and were not administratively classified as MR but who had IQ scores on the group tests in the MMR range were known.

Using the same study population of Birch et al. (1970), different prevalence rates may be obtained for MMR depending on the definition used, as seen in Table 10.1, below.

Use of Health Registers

Some investigators have used registers of people with mental retardation compiled by health authorities. These registers were intended for children with MR who also had health problems that the educational authorities could not deal with and who were therefore referred to the health authorities. Because these are a subset of all children with MR, the prevalence rates obtained from health registers are invariably lower than the other rates shown, e.g., for Salford, England, ages 10 to 14, SMR 2.54:1000, MMR 0.29 (Susser & Kushlick, 1961); for Wessex, England, SMR 2.57, MMR 0.48 (Kushlick & Blunden, 1974); and for British Columbia, Canada, ages 15 to 29, SMR 2.37, MMR 1.7 (Baird & Sadovnick, 1985).

Table 10.1. Prevalence Rates as a Function of Definitions Used

Definitions	Mildly Mentally Retarded	Severely Mentally Retarded	Total
Children administratively classified as MR, with IQ below 70	5.7	3.7	9.4
Children administratively classified as MR, including those with IQ of 70 and above	8.9	3.7	12.6
Children in regular classes with IQ below 75 + administratively classified	23.7	3.7	27.4

Source: Based on data from Birch et al. (1970).

Social Factors Affecting Prevalence

In the 1960s and 1970s, there was still widespread acceptance of the segregation of children with MR in special schools or residential institutions, and school systems continued to use intelligence tests for both administrative and research purposes.

During the last quarter century, however, several social changes have occurred that have had a major influence on epidemiologic studies of MR. The earlier practice of segregating children with disabilities (including MR) has slowly given way to mainstreaming, integration, and normalization. Much of the impetus for these changes came from the Scandinavian countries, based on a growing concern for the stigmatizing consequences of classifying children as MR. The term "labeling" was introduced, which intentionally has a more pejorative connotation than "classifying." There was concern that the segregated environments of special schools, classes, and institutions deprived children of experiences essential for effective socialization. It was also recognized that the widespread use of IQ testing could have stigmatizing consequences. Thus, such testing in schools is now greatly restricted, and in any case, attitudes toward the test influence how the test is scored. For example, it has been reported that in Scandinavia, psychologists, sympathetic to the concepts of normalization and mainstreaming, have in testing children become more lenient in interpreting answers. This practice results in higher scores. In addition, whereas earlier, teachers willingly cooperated in helping to identify children they thought might have MR, they have since become increasingly reluctant to assist in such identification for fear of contributing to stigmatization.

It is difficult to assess accurately the consequences of these social changes, together with the upward drift in intelligence test scores. It would be reasonable to expect that they would lower the prevalence rates of MMR found in recent studies. Kebbon (1987) reviewed six prevalence studies that were conducted in Scandinavia between 1981 and 1986. The prevalence ranged from 3.7 to 7.5 per 1000 for MMR. (In these studies the definition of MMR was an IQ between 50 and 69.) The results are, as expected, lower than those obtained from studies done before the social changes described.

A review of community studies of SMR in children of school age shows that the range of prevalence is from 2.6 to 6.3 per 1000. However, few reports are at the extremes of the range, and most cluster around 4 per 1000. There is no evidence of any steady increase or decline over the past 50 years since the study of Lewis (1929), who found a prevalence of 3.7 per 1000 for urban children. In a review of studies of SMR carried out in the 1950s and 1960s, Abramowicz and Richardson (1975) selected 27 studies judged to be of reasonable reliability and arrived at a best estimate of 3.7 per 1000. In Scandinavia in the 1980s, the median prevalence for SMR was 3.85 per 1000, with a range of 3.0 to 6.3 per 1000 (Kebbon, 1987). Fryers (1984) calculated the annual prevalence of SMR for children in Salford, England from 1961 to 1980. During this period the rate rose slowly from a low of 2.62 in 1961 to a high of 5.71 in 1976 and then showed a slow decline until 1980.

From these figures, a reasonable estimate of the prevalence of SMR in industrialized societies seems to be from 3 to 5 per 1000. In more impoverished societies, where there are high child mortality rates, the prevalence may be lower because of the greater risk of death for children with severe disabilities.

In summary, the prevalence of SMR has remained relatively constant for over half a century, with a range of about 3 to 5 per 1000. However, the rate of MMR has varied widely, depending on the definition used and the social circumstances. For children 10 to 14 years of age, the best estimate at present is between 5 and 12 per 1000, using as the criterion an IQ of less than 70. It may be expected that the prevalence of MMR will be higher than for SMR.

An Alternative Definition

Perhaps one reason for the tradition of using an IQ of 50 as the cut-off point between mild and severe MR was the distinction made by Lewis (1929) between "organic" and "subcultural" retardation. His view was that those with scores below IQ 50 had some form of brain dysfunction (organic), whereas those with IQs of 50 and above did not. However, later research has shown that brain dysfunction is also present among those with MMR. Birch et al. (1970) found that approximately 30% of children with MMR had evidence of CNS damage. In a study based on an expansion of the Scottish population originally studied by Birch et al. (1970), Goulden et al. (1988) assigned, on clinical grounds, degrees of probability of a biologic etiology of MR. For those with an IQ of 50+ (MMR), 20% had a high probability, 5% a medium probability, and 6% a low probability of a biologic etiology. In recent epidemiologic studies of Swedish schoolchildren, Hagberg and Kyllerman (1983) estimated that 43% of those with MMR had an established or highly probable biologic basis for their mental retardation. (This high percentage is probably due to the lower prevalence of MMR found in Sweden than in the Scottish study.) These results suggest that the long-established dichotomy of MR into MMR and SMR needs to be reconsidered. The dichotomy ignores the adaptive behavior component of the definition of MR and places undue faith in IQ scores. This faith is questioned by Mittler (1979):

> Most psychologists are now well aware of the limitations of placing too much emphasis on an IQ score in judging the presence or extent of mental handicap. It is important to stress that the IQ is in no sense a "magic" number. Unfortunately, it has been credited with a degree of psychological significance out of all proportion either to its scientific status or its relevance to the practical problems of normal or handicapped persons (p. 23).

The IQ score alone largely determined whether those with scores around 50 were MMR or SMR, and accordingly any slight error influenced the prevalence of SMR. The cut-off point at the upper end of the MMR range was frequently used to decide whether to include or exclude a child as MMR.

An alternative to using an IQ score alone to dichotomize those with MR is to distinguish between those who will and will not require continuous services and supervision as adults. To make such an identification requires that a population of children with MR be followed into adulthood to identify those who continue to need services after leaving school. In a follow-up study to age 22 of a representative population of children with MR, we found that 45% of those with IQ scores below 70 continued receiving mental retardation services in the 6 years after leaving school (Richardson, et al., 1984a and b). The use of services during this period varied by IQ level. All those with IQs below 50 were receiving MR services, in contrast to only 18% of those with IQ scores between 50 and 69. In population terms, the follow-up showed that 77 per 13,842 or 5.6 per 1000 of all children had MR and needed continuous care. If this finding can be generalized, it suggests that in the Hagberg and the Blomquist studies in Sweden (Kebbon, 1987), which report a prevalence for all children with mental retardation of 6.7 and 8.1 per 1000, respectively, a large majority of these children will require MR services continuing into adulthood.

To predict which children with MMR will require continuing services in the postschool years requires an examination of the factors that best identify this subgroup. Clearly, an IQ score above 50 alone is a poor predictor, and other factors, such as other forms of disability, personal characteristics, and childhood experiences, need to be included in a predictive model.

Multiple Disabilities (Co-Morbidity)

In much of the epidemiologic research on mental retardation, the focus is on intellectual level, and other disabilities are disregarded. In some cases, biologic factors that cause mental retardation also cause other disabilities, such as cerebral palsy and epilepsy. To ascertain all the needs of a child with MR, it is essential therefore to know which other disorders are also present. Increasingly, epidemiologic studies include information on multiple disabilities, or co-morbidity. Some use medical diagnostic categories, whereas others use terms descriptive of functional impairment, such as nonambulatory or incontinent. For service purposes, classifications of the degree and kinds of functional impairments are more useful because diagnostic terms, such as cerebral palsy and epilepsy, do not indicate the severity of the disorders nor how much they interfere with everyday living. Further, knowing the patterns of associated disabilities of each child in a population with MR is more useful than knowing what proportion of children with MR have various disabilities.

Several studies report the frequency of various disabilities found in populations of children with SMR. Two of the most common disabilities are epilepsy and cerebral palsy. For all those with SMR, the percentage with epilepsy ranges from 19% to 36%: 19% (Corbett et al., 1975); 22% (Wald et al., 1977); 27% (Gillberg et al., 1986); 35% (Goulden et al., 1991); and 36% (Gustavson et al., 1977). Among children with SMR, Fryers (1984) in a review, estimated a range for cerebral palsy of 20% to 40%. Specific studies report 18% (Gustavson et al., 1977); 41% (Blomquist, 1982); and 40% (Richardson et al., unpublished result from the Aberdeen study).

A few studies have examined how various disabilities combine for each child in a population of children with MR (Hagberg & Kyllerman, 1983; Kushlick & Blunden, 1974; Richardson et al., 1984b; Rutter et al., 1981). These studies show that multiple disabilities in addition to MR are far more frequent among those with severe than mild mental retardation. Among those with SMR, the presence of three or more disabilities in addition to MR was found in 22% in a Danish study by Bernsen (1976) and 23% in a Scottish study by Richardson et al. (1984b).

For children with severe sensory disabilities, evaluating the presence and severity of MR may be very difficult, and it is among these children that misdiagnoses of MR are most likely.

Age

SMR is identified at an earlier age than MMR. For genetic disorders that have objective diagnostic markers, prenatal diagnosis is possible in some cases. Generally, all cases of severe MR are identified before the school years. Gruenberg (1964), in a review, showed that the overall prevalence of MR increased with age until the late school years and after leaving school dropped by approximately half. This is illustrated in a follow-up study of a population of children with MR up to age 22 (Richardson et al., 1984a). Figure 10.1 shows the variation in prevalence rates by age. The decline at ages 16 to 17 is accounted for by those

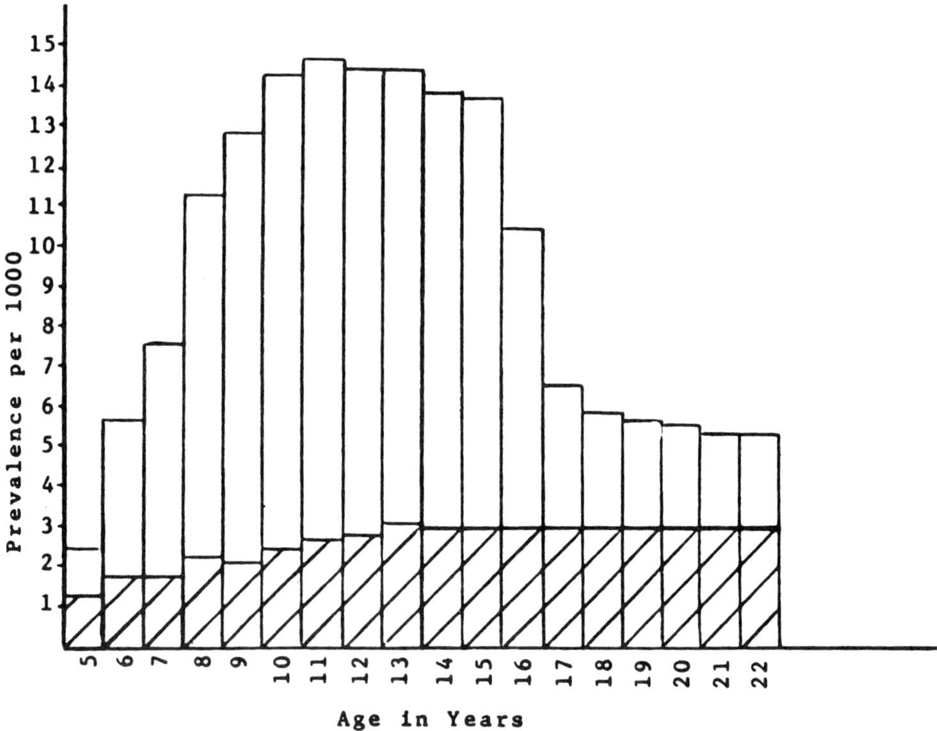

Fig. 10.1. Level of functioning during school years based on placement. White areas = educable mentally retarded. Cross-hatched areas = trainable mentally retarded or lower (postschool level of functioning based on final school age placement).
Source: Richardson et al. (1984a).

attending the special classes who are able to manage without services after leaving school.

In recent studies (where the prevalence rate for MMR is lower than in the earlier studies), there is less variation in age-specific rates than that shown in Figure 10.1.

Sex

Studies of SMR, with few exceptions, show that there is a somewhat higher rate for boys than girls (Abramowicz & Richardson, 1975). For MMR a somewhat higher prevalence for boys than girls has also been found consistently (Richardson et al., 1986a and b). The ratio of boys to girls seems to depend on the upper IQ cut-off point used in the definition of MR because the excess of boys is found at the upper end of the range of MMR. The excess is higher in the IQ range of 70 and above, which is included in many of the prevalence studies. In our follow-up, we found no gender difference in the IQ range of 50 to 69, but from 70 upward the excess of boys became marked.

Family Background

The most commonly used measure of family background is social class. In Britain this measure is based on the Registrar General's classification of occupations on a five-point scale from I (Professional) to V (Unskilled Manual). The classification of the head of the household provides a general indicator of the lifestyle of the family. Other indicators that have been used in assessing socioeconomic status are family income and parent education. One of the most consistent findings in the literature on MR is the stepwise increase in the prevalence of MR as the social class moves from I to V. In the study of Birch et al. (1970), the range in prevalence across social class was 3.7 per 1000 for social classes I–IIIa, nonmanual, to 32.6 per 1000 for social class V, nonskilled-manual, for children with MR aged 8 to 10. When retardation is subdivided into MMR and SMR, this gradient is found to be largely or wholly accounted for by the MMR.

It was expected, based on the generally poorer health of poor people, that those at the lower end of the social class scale would have a higher prevalence of SMR than those at the upper end. Rather surprisingly, several prevalence studies show that SMR was randomly distributed across social classes (Birch et al., 1970; Lewis, 1929; Stein & Susser, 1963). However, some studies show that SMR is overrepresented in lower social class families (Bayley, 1973; Cooper & Lackus, 1984; Drillien et al., 1966). Whether SMR is randomly distributed across social class must remain an open question pending new studies, but it is clear that the difference in prevalence between upper and lower social class families is far more marked for children with MMR than with SMR.

The measure of social class assumes a traditional family with an employed head of household. A study in Norway by Skaarbrevik (1971) calls this assumption into question. In a follow-up of educable mentally retarded children, he found that 32% of those studied had a deviant family background; hence, for this group, social class was often impossible to identify. In our follow-up, we found that 45% of the children with MMR came from unstable families, and for 6%, it was impossible to assign a social class (Richardson et al., 1985).

Urban-Rural Differences

Several studies have found higher prevalence rates for mental retardation in rural than urban areas: Lewis (1929) in England and Wales; Akesson (1961) in Sweden; Mulcahy and Reynolds (1984) in Ireland; Dupont (1989) in Denmark, and Diaz-Fernandez (1987) in Spain. On the basis of a school survey in Maine, Levinson (1962) concluded that a higher proportion of children scored below IQ 75 in rural than urban areas. In the Diaz-Fernandez study, largely involving SMR, the highest prevalence rates were found in the most isolated, mountainous areas, far from the coast of Spain, which were mostly depressed and disadvantaged. Reasons suggested for the higher rural rates included inbreeding and selective migration, with the more competent people leaving.

However, other studies do not find significant urban-rural differences. Innes et al. (1978) found no differences in the Northeast of Scotland nor did Kushlick and Cox (1973) in Wessex, England. The differences between urban and rural prevalence may be lessened or may even disappear when national health and educational services of uniform quality are present in all parts and when the availability of transportation and improved communication systems change the circumstances and conditions for people in rural areas.

Risk Factors

The problems of defining a "case" (i.e., who should be counted as having mental retardation) discussed in the previous section are related to attribution of cause. Some children are classified based on the presence of organic abnormalities known to be associated with mental retardation. Other children are classified based only on a below-average IQ score. Still others reflect some combination of an organic abnormality associated with brain dysfunction, a subaverage IQ score, and a problem with school performance or behavior. Once a child has been classified, if no clear organic basis has been identified, cause is frequently attributed to what is more correctly considered a "risk factor," such as low birthweight or a deprived social environment (see Chapter 1). The biosocial interaction that has been shown to occur, perhaps most clearly between the two risk factors just mentioned, is not usually considered. However, many biologic and social factors are inseparably intertwined in a dynamic process that occurs throughout growth and development. Even in cases where a clear biologic insult has occurred, the outcome may be mediated through the social environment. This biosocial interaction is addressed later, but first causal factors that are clearly biologic need to be considered.

Biologic Risk Factors

Biologic determinants are most frequently identified in children with the more severe grades of mental retardation (Birch et al., 1970; Grossman, 1983). For these children, when a biologic cause cannot be assigned, it is generally assumed. In contrast, among those with mild mental retardation, when a biologic cause is not found, a familial, social, or cultural attribution is often made. Although the etiology of most MMR remains unclear, new technology has uncovered biologic causes not expected a generation ago. Sometimes, however, assignment of cause is based on associations between a risk factor and mental retardation. The problem is the direction of these associations; they show that a large proportion of children with mental retardation may have a history of a particular risk factor (when studied retrospectively), but most children with a history of that risk factor (studied prospectively) do not become mentally retarded, i.e., in epidemiologic terms, their relative risk is low. In the reports that follow, therefore, it is necessary to bear in mind that many investigators consider risk factors as "causes."

In a study in Israel, Costeff et al. (1983) found abnormal medical histories, particularly maternal "reproductive insufficiency," in more than a quarter of the study population with MMR. In another population-based study of mild mental handicap in Wales (Rao, 1990), adverse obstetric factors were found in 69% of children with MMR, and an additional 3% had chromosomal anomalies. Investigators in two epidemiologic studies of MMR in Swedish schoolchildren, both with low prevalence rates of about 4 per 1000, found a biologic cause in almost half the children (Blomquist et al., 1981; Hagberg et al., 1981). In the study carried out by Hagberg et al. (1981), the authors state they were unable "to find any convincing evidence that a materially deficient environment alone could have been decisive" for any of the children studied. Similarly, Blomquist et al. (1981) found only three children of 171 for whom the retardation was considered to be a consequence of neglect or understimulation. They expected that some of the cases assigned to the unknown group had an unidentified biologic etiology and suggested that their finding of a large male excess ratio (1.6 to 1) could at least partly be due to unidentified X-linked genetic disorders.

For many years, the theory prevailed, expounded particularly by the eugenics movement, that MMR was in large part due to the pooling of genes of constitutionally inferior individuals who pass on low intelligence from one generation to the next. Akesson (1987), reviewing certain epidemiologic observations published since 1970, reassessed the long-standing belief that polygenic inheritance is the primary cause of MMR. Citing the study by Blomquist et al. (1981) in which 10% of the MMR population was found to have a chromosomal defect and a further 8% had a well-defined disease due to a major gene, Akesson suggested that these and other findings "are not easily accommodated" to theories assuming polygenic inheritance.

The remaining biolog determinants may reasonably be subdivided as follows: (1) genetic factors, (2) infections and intoxications, and (3) other factors.

Genetic Factors

Genetic factors known to cause mental retardation are of four different types: chromosomal anomalies, single-gene disorders, X-linked patterns of inheritance, and sex chromosome disorders (see Chapters 4 and 5).

Chromosomal anomalies are estimated to cause at least one third of cases of SMR and a smaller, but as yet not clearly delineated, proportion of MMR cases (Baraitser, 1984). Most of the chromosomal anomalies causing mental retardation are trisomies or translocations. The most common and most readily recognized is Down syndrome, which can be caused by a translocation, but is usually due to a trisomy on chromosome 21. Children with Down syndrome have a wide range of IQs, from below 20 to 100 (in a few cases), even though most fall within a narrower band (Mittler, 1984). There is some evidence that, among children with Down syndrome, IQ is related to upbringing and socialization, with children raised from infancy in institutions showing lower IQs than children raised in families providing intellectual stimulation (Evans & Hamerton, 1985). According to Mittler (1984), however, some children with Down syndrome function at very low levels despite heroic efforts, whereas others reach a high level of functioning without special measures. A review of prevalence studies of SMR between 1925 and 1969—the period when institutionalization of children with Down syndrome was common—showed that Down syndrome comprised between one sixth and one third of cases of SMR in children (Abramowicz & Richardson, 1975).

Epidemiologic studies have long shown an increasing risk of bearing a child with Down syndrome with advancing maternal age, especially after age 34 (Lilienfeld & Benesch, 1969). Changes in child-bearing practices and availability of amniocentesis and, more recently, chorionic villi sampling were expected to decrease the prevalence of Down syndrome, which had occurred with a frequency of 1.25 per 1000 live births in most populations (Hook & Hamerton, 1977). Dolk et al. (1990) surveyed the prevalence of Down syndrome births between 1980 and 1986 in 19 European regions and found that live birth prevalence rates ranged from 0.58 per 1000 in Odense, Denmark, to 1.98 per 1000 in Galway, Ireland. The percentages of mothers over ages 34 and 40 in these two populations are instructive and may account for this difference. In Odense, mothers over 34 comprised 15.8% of the study population, and there were none over 40. In Galway, the figures were 57.9% and 28.9%, respectively. Dolk et al. (1990) reasonably attributed the rate differences to differential use of prenatal diagnosis resulting in the termination of pregnancy. To compare the rates in these 19 European regions with Hook and Hamerton's 1977 rate of 1.25 per 1000 noted above, we examined the frequencies of regions with rates below 1.2 per 1000, rates between 1.2 and 1.3 per 1000, and rates above 1.3 per 1000. There were nine regions with lower rates, three between 1.2 and 1.3 per 1000, and seven with higher rates. Thus, more than half the regions reported rates that showed a decline from 1.25 per 1000. Recently, significantly reduced levels of serum alphafetoprotein between the 16th and 18th week of pregnancy in women of all ages has been found to be associated with carrying a Down syndrome fetus, thus identifying another high-risk group for whom prenatal diagnosis is warranted (Cuckle et al., 1984). This indicator is further expected to decrease the incidence of Down syndrome births in populations that avail themselves of prenatal diagnosis and pregnancy termination.

Single-gene disorders are most frequently inborn errors of metabolism. They may or may not be X-linked (see Table 10.2). Single-gene and X-linked inborn errors of metabolism are together responsible for approximately 5% of SMR cases. In many of these cases, the metabolic defect has already been defined, and methods exist for carrier detection and hence can be used in prenatal and postnatal diagnosis. Some of those conditions that can be detected by mass screening of newborns, such as phenylketonuria (PKU) can be treated before symptoms develop. For other conditions that remain untreatable, such as Tay-Sachs disease, carrier identification and counseling are useful in prevention. Finally, specific treatment is becoming available for a small but growing number of inborn errors of metabolism. In the near future, it may be feasible to transfer normal genes into mutant cell lines, which would revolutionize the entire approach to inborn errors of metabolism (Moser, 1985).

X-linked disorders as already mentioned, include some inborn errors of metabolism, but vastly outnumbering all other X-linked diagnoses at present is the fragile-X syndrome. In a review, Brown et al. (1987) calculated that approximately 1 per 981 males carry the fragile-X chromosome, 1 per 1226 are affected by the syndrome, and more than 75% of those affected are moderately to severely retarded. For females, they calculated that approximately 1 per 677 carry the chromosome, 1 per 2033 are affected, and about 90% of those affected are moderately to severely retarded. Brown et al. (1987) estimated that, in populations of individuals with all grades of mental retardation, between 5% and 10% have the fragile-X syndrome.

Two studies from the United Kingdom and one from Finland are illustrative. In a study of boys with SMR in the West Midlands, Bundey et al., (1985) found the fragile-X chromosome in 7% of those whose mental retardation was otherwise unexplained. The same investigators, studying children with MMR in Coventry (Thake et al., 1987), found the fragile-X chromosome in 7% of boys and 10% of girls whose mental retardation was otherwise unexplained. In Finland, Kahkonen et al. (1987) found the fragile-X syndrome in 5% of children with all grades of mental retardation.

Other forms of X-linked mental retardation have also recently been identified, and Partington et al. (1984) suggest that X-linked mental retardation, including the fragile-X syndrome, may be found to make a far larger contribution to mental retardation than had been suspected previously. Strategies to prevent

Table 10.2. Inborn Errors of Metabolism Associated with Mental Retardation

Autosomal (Not Sex Linked)	Sex Linked
Galactosemia	Lesch-Nyhan syndrome
Tay-Sachs disease	Hunter's syndrome
Homocystinuria	Glucose-6-phosphate dehydrogenase (G6PD) variants
Hurler's syndrome	
Phenylketonuria (PKU)	Glycogen storage disease with phosphorylase kinase deficiency
Porphyria	
Wilson's disease	Pseudohypoparathyroidism

X-linked mental retardation now center around genetic screening and family counseling, although mass screening and prenatal diagnosis of female carriers are not generally feasible.

The sex chromosome disorders that are associated with mental retardation rarely cause severe retardation and make only a small contribution to the prevalence of mild retardation. These disorders include Klinefelter's syndrome (37,XXY), triple-X females, (47,XXX) and other X polysomies. They are all identifiable prenatally from amniotic fluid, but again, routine screening is not presently feasible. Turner's syndrome (45,X), although associated with some learning disabilities, is not generally associated with mental retardation.

Infections and Intoxications

When such infections as rubella, syphilis, cytomegalovirus (CMV), and toxoplasmosis occur in pregnant women, the infants may have a congenital condition that includes mental retardation (see Chapter 6). In addition, many other maternal infections, particularly viral, may affect the embryo (Grossman, 1983). Syphilis, which is treatable with antibiotics, and rubella, for which a vaccine is available (see Chapter 9), should now be within our control, and fetal damage from these causes no longer need occur. However, in the United States, the recent increase in syphilis in some segments of the population is a growing cause for concern. The Centers for Disease Control reported a rise from 6392 cases in 1956 to 40,275 cases in 1988, resulting in a marked increase in congenital syphilis (Kandall, 1991). Congenital CMV infections resulting in neurologic sequelae were found to occur in Sweden at a rate of approximately 6 per 10,000, whereas the rates for toxoplasmosis were lower. Useful prevention and intervention measures for these conditions are not yet available (Hagberg & Hagberg, 1984).

In the infant, such infections as meningitis and encephalitis following measles and pertussis can also result in mental retardation (see Chapter 9). However, vaccination for measles can prevent the disease and its sequelae. The risk of postinfectious encephalitis due to pertussis versus the risk of encephalitis following vaccination for the disease has been hotly debated. Most investigators have concluded that the estimated risk of residual defects from encephalitis under conditions of widespread vaccination is much lower than the estimated increase in mortality if pertussis again becomes widespread and thus recommend vaccination (Dudgeon, 1984).

It has been known for some time that such maternal disorders as toxemia of pregnancy or diabetes are frequently associated with insult to the unborn child (Grossman, 1983). Maternal diabetes can now be better controlled, resulting in a marked decrease in problems for the newborn (Fuhrmann et al., 1983). The effects of toxemia of pregnancy on the fetus are difficult to sort out, because toxemia is often associated with other obstetric complications. In the study carried out by Birch et al. (1970) in Aberdeen, Scotland, moderate and severe degrees of preeclamptic toxemia were found with significantly greater frequency in mothers of mentally subnormal children than in a comparison population. However, of the seven cases of severe toxemia that occurred in the mentally subnormal population, five occurred in combination with other potentially damaging complications and circumstances, such as twinning and low birthweight. Moreover, in the twin pregnancies in which severe toxemia occurred, the second twin was unaffected. Other researchers have also found it difficult to isolate the role of toxemia as a cause of mental retardation because of the confounding effects of other complications (Stein & Susser, 1974).

Maternal PKU is another potential threat to the developing fetus. The limiting of dietary treatment of PKU to childhood has been questioned for some time (Barabas et al., 1984), but in the past, treatment was frequently stopped after the first few years of life. The high blood levels of phenylalanine that are toxic to infants were not considered damaging to the mature brain, and women successfully treated for PKU in childhood no longer were given a special diet for their own protection. However, their high blood levels of phenylalanine can be damaging to their unborn children. Reinstitution of the special dietary regimen to reduce phenylalanine levels immediately before and throughout pregnancy seems to lessen the risk for fetal damage (Lenke & Levy, 1980), but vigilant surveillance of young women treated for PKU in childhood may prove difficult (Kirkman, 1982).

Hyperbilirubinemia, when severe, produces kernicterus, a neurotoxicity that has been a principal cause of neurologic abnormalities (Grossman, 1983). There are several causes for this disorder, the most common being maternal-fetal blood group incompatibility. The ability to immunize Rh-negative mothers against Rh sensitization by Rh-positive fetuses has sharply limited kernicterus from this cause. In addition, phenobarbital, phototherapy, and exchange transfusions have been successful in reducing hyperbilirubinemia before kernicterus occurs.

Women taking anticonvulsant drugs during pregnancy are also at increased risk of bearing a child with developmental disabilities, including mental retardation. There is, however, an increased risk to children born to epileptic mothers, irrespective of whether they receive anticonvulsant therapy. At present, there seems to be a consensus that "the need to maintain seizure control during pregnancy outweighs the increased incidence of fetal malformations when these medications are administered during the first trimester" (Moser, 1985, p. 144).

Excessive alcohol intake during pregnancy can result in the fetal alcohol syndrome, which is characterized by a cluster of abnormalities including mental retardation. The full syndrome has been found mainly in children born to chronically alcoholic women, although it may also be associated with lesser total alcohol consumption, e.g., binge drinking at critical stages of gestation (Landesman-Dwyer, 1982). Olegard et al. (1987) report that in Gothenburg, Sweden, in 1976 to 1977, the incidence of the full-blown fetal alcohol syndrome was 1.7 per 1000. It declined to 0.4 per 1000 in 1983 to 1984. The authors attributed the drop to educational prevention programs. They report, however, that the decline seems to have been replaced by an increasing incidence of a similar, but not identical syndrome caused by high doses of benzodiazapines during pregnancy.

The recent increase in cocaine use among the child-bearing population has resulted in growing numbers of infants affected by cocaine exposure in the perinatal period. In an extensive review, Neuspiel and Hamel (1991) concluded that, "thus far, independent effects of cocaine have not been conclusively demonstrated in human infants, and studies beyond infancy have not been reported." One reason it is difficult to isolate the effects of perinatal drug exposure is that these infants are exposed to multiple risk factors of biologic, social, and cultural origin (Kandall, 1991). HIV infections in the newborn also place a child at risk for mental retardation; however, as with cocaine exposure, reliable information is scant, inconclusive, and confounded by many other risk factors.

Other Biologic Factors

The last category of biologic determinants includes a wide array of factors. The course of events after birth clearly influences the later development of the child, and there is evidence that pre-existing congenital conditions may contribute to that course (Drillien et al., 1980; Stein & Susser, 1974).

There are many conditions of unknown prenatal influence for which no definite etiology has been established. This partial list is from the AAMD Medical Etiological Classification (Grossman, 1983):

cerebral malformation, e.g., anencephaly, microencephaly
craniofacial anomaly, e.g., holoprosencephaly, Cornelia de Lange syndrome, microcephalus, macroencephaly, Crouzon's syndrome, Apert's syndrome, craniostenosis, Laurence-Moon-Biedl syndrome
status dysraphicus, e.g., meningoencephalocele, meningomyelocele
congenital hydrocephalus.
hydroencephaly.
single umbilical artery

Hazards in the immediate perinatal period have long been known to place the newborn at risk for disabilities, including mental retardation. However, "by the beginning of the 1970s, obstetric practices had changed to the degree that physical traumas during labor and delivery were becoming uncommon . . . (and) intrapartum asphyxia, characterized by biochemical events leading to tissue ischemia and/or hemorrhage, was far more apparent as a cause for severe brain damage" (Rosen, 1985). However, there are a wide array of prenatal and perinatal factors, as well as chromosomal abnormalities and nongenetic congenital anomalies, that outweigh intrapartum asphyxia as contributors to brain damage.

Low birthweight (LBW), defined as <2500 g, is associated with developmental disabilities, including mental retardation. This association is due to the extensive complications that can occur in the LBW neonate, the incidence and severity of which are inversely related to gestational age and birthweight (Hack, 1990). LBW may be due to preterm birth (<37 weeks) or intrauterine growth failure. These causes of LBW can result in different outcomes, but few studies make the distinction. Social factors, including maternal smoking and diet, have been associated mainly with preterm birth (Avery, 1985).

Medical advances over the past quarter of a century have dramatically increased the survival of very low birthweight (VLBW) infants. VLBW is defined as <1500 g, although the lower limit for survival has continued to drop and now seems to be holding at about 600 g (24 weeks gestation). The extent to which these VLBW infants survive relatively intact has not yet been answered fully. In a review, Hack (1990, p. 9) concluded that improved survival is tempered by "enormous neonatal morbidity . . . and less than optimal later development. Although the impairment rate of these survivors has not changed during the last

10 to 20 years, the absolute number of impaired children has increased due to the overall increase in survival." Survival rates remained relatively constant over the 3 years before the review, indicating that the survival limit had been reached, at least for the present.

Studies that have examined the intellectual functioning of survivors followed to school age necessarily lag behind studies of survival rates. In a recent study in Montreal, Lefebvre et al. (1988) followed the 46 survivors of 241 VLBW (501 g to 1000 g) infants born between 1976 and 1979. The mean age at follow-up was 6.8 years, and only two children were lost to follow-up. Among the remainder, morbidity was extremely high; 4.5% had severe mental retardation and 27% had mild retardation. Only 36% had no significant educational problems.

By way of balancing this pessimistic picture, Fryers (1990) notes that "the proportion of (low birthweight) children with significant disabilities seems to have diminished as obstetric and pediatric techniques have improved, and the same interventions which save the lives of very small babies, some damaged, are likely to prevent damage in larger babies previously at high risk. The end product of this dynamic equation in any population is impossible to estimate." Hack (1990) suggests that new therapeutic measures, such as the use of surfactants to prevent or ameliorate respiratory distress syndrome, indomethacin to prevent intraventricular bleeds, and immunoglobulin to prevent infection, may eventually increase survival rates even higher.

Endocrine disorders also cause mental retardation. The most common is hypothyroidism, which may be either congenital or acquired. The latter form has largely disappeared in developed countries (Stern, 1985). The congenital form (cretinism) comprises the majority of cases and has multiple causes, which include "maldevelopment or maldescent of the thyroid, inborn errors of the metabolism of the thyroid hormone, iodine deficiency, pituitary or hypothalamic disorder, the ingestion of goitrogens" (Stern, 1985). The incidence of congenital hypothyroidism is between 1 per 4000 to 1 per 7000 births, making it the most common endocrine disorder in infants. However, early detection and rigorous replacement therapy should dramatically reduce the prevalence of mental retardation due to this disorder (Stern, 1985).

Finally, many prenatal and postnatal environmental hazards may cause mental retardation. These dangers include irradiation during pregnancy in clinical settings and through nuclear explosion and lead and mercury poisoning, acquired prenatally and postnatally. In the postnatal period, causal factors include severe head trauma and anoxia. It is within our power, through public health and welfare measures, to eliminate these potential hazards and effectively reduce the incidence of mental retardation associated with them.

Social and Environmental Risk Factors

Social deprivation, when severe, can cause mental retardation. Clarke and Clarke (1976) point to individual case studies describing extreme deprivation, including deplorable institutional treatment, that resulted in very poor intellectual functioning, which was then reversed in a facilitating social environment. The proportion of cases for whom social deprivation is the sole determinant, however, is probably very small. Increasingly, researchers in a variety of areas have pointed to the interactive effects of the social environment with biologic factors.

Begab (1981) suggests that the particular factors in the social environment that influence intellectual development are those that relate most particularly to the mother and her child-rearing practices. Important elements in the environment are sensory, verbal, and intellectual stimulation. When children are denied this stimulation, it is frequently because their parents are intellectually limited themselves, and they lack the ability to stimulate the child properly in language and analytical skills. The genetic contribution to the poor intellectual development of these children may, however, limit the influence of the social environment.

Intervention programs designed to preclude or interrupt the sequence of disadvantage emanating from poor home environments have had inconclusive results. Preschool remedial programs generally showed benefits that tended to diminish with time (Bronfenbrenner, 1975). More intensive prevention-oriented programs were then tried. The Milwaukee Project typifies and is the most well known of these programs. Begun in 1966, the final report was only recently published (Garber, 1988). This study was designed to test whether an experimental intervention could prevent the declines in IQ expected for children being raised by a retarded mother. An experimental group of children born to mothers with IQs of 75 or lower was given supplemental educational experiences outside the home, and the rate of intellectual development for these children was compared to that for an untreated control group of children who remained at home with similarly retarded mothers (Garber et al., 1991). A second control group consisted of children of mothers living in the same disadvantaged area of the city who had full-scale WAIS IQs over 100. The study report has been subjected to intense peer review, partly because of some controversy surrounding the project and partly because the implications of the findings are so important and yet so equivocal (*American Journal on Mental Retardation*, 1991, Special Book Review Section.)

The reviews indicate that this program of intensive intervention with both child and mother resulted in higher test scores for children of mothers with MMR than for children in the no-intervention control groups. These higher scores did not, however, translate to similar increments in achievement. The response to the reviewers by Garber et al. (1991) included what the researchers judged to be the important findings coming from the project. They considered that the need to distinguish between two groups of children is not fully appreciated, i.e., those who experience declines in intellectual development and those who consistently demonstrate a low IQ level. The Milwaukee Project found that the risk for declining IQs was highest for and almost totally limited to children of intellectually limited mothers. For these children, Garber et al. (1991) considered the risk to be familial, rather than social or cultural. They concluded, "the specific etiology for the majority of cases of mild intellectual retardation remains unknown and *should not* (authors' italics) be attributed to 'presumed' psychosocial influences" (Garber et al., 1991).

Biosocial Interactions

A biosocial interaction (or multifactorial cause) may be involved in the incidence of neural tube defects. The most common neural tube defects are anencephaly, which is lethal, and spina bifida, which often results in severe disability and mental retardation. Although a genetic component is clearly suggested by the magnitude of the recurrence risk of neural tube defects for relatives, the genetic contribution has not been clarified as well as it has been for other disorders. Further, the recurrence risk is social-class-related, with an incidence two to four times greater in lower than higher socioeconomic groups. This socioeconomic distribution led to the suspicion that diet might be a contributory factor, and recent evidence points to a possible therapeutic effect of multivitamin supplementation instituted before conception and continued into the first trimester of pregnancy. Neural tube defects can be detected by measuring alphafetoprotein levels in amniotic fluid and by ultrasound examination. Accordingly, maternal serum alphafetoprotein levels, if properly timed, can be useful in identifying at-risk pregnancies (Moser, 1985; see Chapter 4).

Several other biologic insults seem to place a child at risk for mental retardation, and they are frequently associated with social or environmental risk factors. They include low birthweight, prenatal infections, and malnutrition. When they occur together, that risk increases. This phenomenon makes it difficult to sort out potential causal mechanisms.

It has been well established that the developmental outcome for many low birthweight infants is mediated through the social environment (see Sameroff, 1981, for a review). In another review, Escalona (1984) concluded that "child-rearing conditions that support and enrich early development make it possible for young children to overcome or compensate for early deficits."

Berg (1985) summarized the complex nature of the phenomenon:

> Small, underweight babies are more likely than better-developed newborns to show mental and physical handicaps at various ages. The reasons for this association are manifold and include preconceptual genetic influences and environmental factors of both physical and psychosocial kinds. In that sense, it is very difficult to envisage smallness at birth as such as a cause of mental defect; the association is much more likely to exist because preceding circumstances were responsible for both manifestations and/or because small infants are more vulnerable (and in some instances more exposed) to peri- and postnatal environmental hazards of various kinds.

Similar interactive effects have been suggested by researchers examining the impact of the social environment on children with subclinical prenatal infections in general (Alford, 1977) and congenital cytomegalovirus infections in particular (Scheiner et al., 1977). These researchers have concluded that intellectual outcomes for these children were clearly social-class-related.

Researchers examining the effects of malnutrition on intellectual development have concluded either that there are interactive effects between malnutrition and the social environment or that an unfavorable social environment is the common cause of both the malnutrition and the retarded mental development. In one study, Jamaican boys who had been severely malnourished in infancy were found to have significantly lower IQs than a comparison population at school age (Hertzig et al., 1972). Subsequent analyses of these children also examined height at follow-up (as an indicator of nutrition subsequent to the episode of severe malnutrition) and social background. The social background score turned out to be by far the best predictor of IQ. Further, when social background and height were held constant for the previously malnourished and comparison children, only a 2-point difference in IQ was found between the two groups under the most favorable conditions of tall stature and advantageous social background. Under the least favorable conditions, the difference was 9 points (Richardson, 1976).

Whether considering low birthweight, prenatal infections, malnutrition, or other insults to the newborn, it is important to remember that their associations with mental retardation do not usually demonstrate cause. "Indeed, it is often more likely that each was due to the same preceding causal factors, whether recognizable or not" (Berg, 1985, p. 123).

Conclusions

The causes of mental retardation are numerous and varied, and research findings related to one cause may have little bearing on other causes. There are still a great many gaps in our understanding of causal mechanisms, and we still lack some basic scientific knowledge about how the brain develops. Down syndrome is an example of the limits of our understanding. Although the genetic anomaly and its relationship to mental retardation are clear, we do not understand the causes of the nondisjunction responsible for the trisomy or the physiology of how the genetic anomaly relates to mental retardation. Nevertheless, it is hard not to be impressed with the pace at which new knowledge is developing.

Public health and welfare measures can decrease the incidence of mental retardation from some causes, but these measures must approach the problems in a comprehensive manner. Otherwise, one damaging factor may replace another, as seems to have occurred in Sweden, where a public education campaign resulted in a lowered incidence of fetal alcohol syndrome, which was then replaced by another syndrome due to benzodiazapine use. Further, prepregnancy planning and prenatal care must be made more widely available in those places where it is not yet universal, and improvements in the social conditions in which children are raised must be made a priority.

References

Abramowicz HK, Richardson SA. Epidemiology of severe mental retardation in children: community studies. *Am J Ment Defic* 1975; 80:18–39.

Akesson HO. *Epidemiology and Genetics of Mental Deficiency in a Southern Swedish Population*. Uppsala, Sweden: Institute for Medical Genetics of the University of Uppsala; 1961.

Akesson HO. Traditional views and new perspectives on the genetics of mild mental retardation. *Upsalla J Med Sci* 1987; 44(suppl):30–33.

Alford CA. Prenatal infections and psychosocial development in children born into lower socioeconomic settings. In: Mittler P, (ed.), *Research to Practice in Mental Retardation*. Vol III. Baltimore: University Park Press, 1977.

American Journal on Mental Retardation. Special Book Review Section. 1991; 95:447–493.

Avery G. Effects of social, cultural and economic factors on brain development. In: Freeman JM, ed. *Prenatal and Perinatal Factors Associated with Brain Disorders*. Bethesda, MD: NIH Publication No. 85-1149; 1985:162–176.

Baird PA, Sadovnick AD. Mental retardation in over half a million consecutive livebirths. An epidemiological study. *Am J Ment Defic* 1985; 89:p 323–330.

Barabas G, Matthews WS, Koch D, Taft LT. Diet reinstitution in phenylketonuria. In Berg JM, ed. *Perspectives and Progress in Mental Retardation*. Vol II. Baltimore: University Park Press; 1984.

Baraitser M. Chromosomal aspects of mental retardation. In Dobbing J, Clarke ADB, Corbett JA, Hogg J, Robinson RO, eds. *Scientific Studies in Mental Retardation*. London: Royal Society of Medicine; 1984.

Bayley M. *Mental Handicap and Community Care. A Study of Mentally Handicapped People in Sheffield*. London: Routledge and Kegan Paul; 1973.

Begab MJ. Issues in the prevention of psychosocial retardation. In: Begab MJ, Haywood HC, Garber HL, eds. *Psychosocial Influences in Retarded Development*. Vol I. Baltimore: University Park Press; 1981.

Berg JM. Physical determinants of environmental origin. In: Clarke AM, Clarke ADB, Berg JM, eds. *Mental Deficiency. The Changing Outlook*. 4th ed. London: Methuen and Co, Ltd; 1985.

Bernsen AH. Severe mental retardation among children in the County of Arhus, Denmark. *Acta Psychiat Scand* 1976; 54:43–66.

Birch H, Richardson SA, Baird D, Horobin G, Illsley R. *Mental Subnormality in the Community: A Clinical and Epidemiologic Study*. Baltimore: Williams & Wilkins; 1970.

Blomquist HK, Gustavson K-H, Holmgren G. Mild mental retardation in children in a Northern Swedish community. *J Ment Defic Res* 1981; 25:169–186.

Bronfenbrenner U. Is early intervention effective? In: Guttentag G, Struening E, eds. *Handbook of Evaluation Research*. Vol 2. Beverly Hills, CA: Sage; 1975:279–303.

Brown TW, Jenkins EC, Gross AC, et al. Genetics and expression of the fragile-X syndrome. *Uppsala J Med Sci* 1987; 44(suppl):137–154.

Bundy S, Webb TP, Thake A, Todd J. A community study of severe mental retardation in the West Midlands and the importance of the fragile X chromosome in its aetiology. *J Med Genetics* 1985; 22:258–266.

Clarke AM, Clarke ADB, eds. *Early Experience: Myth and Evidence*. London: Open Books; 1976.

Cooper B, Lackus B. The social-class background of mentally retarded children. A study in Mannheim. *Soc Psychiatry* 19:3–12.

Cooper B. 1990. Mental handicap in school age children of Mannheim. An epidemiologic contribution. *Nervenarzt* 61:550–560.

Corbett JA, Harris R, Robinson RA. Epilepsy. In: Wortis J, ed. *Mental Retardation*. Vol 7. New York: Brunner/Mazel; 1985.

Costeff H, Cohen BE, Weller LE. Biological factors in mild mental retardation. *Dev Med Child Neurol* 1983; 25:580–587.

Cuckle HS, Wald NJ, Lindenbaum RH. Maternal serum alpha-fetoprotein measurement: A screening test for Down syndrome. *Lancet* 1984; 1:926–929.

Darroch A. Introduction. In: Binet A, Simon TH, eds. *Mentally Defective Children*. Trans. WB Drummond. London: Edward Arnold; 1914.

Diaz-Fernandez F. Descriptive epidemiology of registered mentally retarded persons in Galicia (Northwest Spain). *Am J Ment Retard* 1988; 92:385–392.

Dolk H, DeWals P, Gillerot Y, et al. The prevalence at birth of Down syndrome in 19 regions of Europe, 1980-86. In: Fraser WI, ed. *Key Issues in Mental Retardation Research*. London: Routledge, 1990.

Drillien CM, Jameson S, Wilkinson EM. Studies in mental handicap, Part 1. Prevalence and distribution by clinical type and severity of defect. *Arch Dis Child Health* 1966; 41:528.

Drillien CM, Thomson AJM, Burgoyne K. Low birthweight children at early school age: a longitudinal study. *Dev Med Child Neurol* 1980; 22:26–47.

Dudgeon JA. Infectious agents in the aetiology of mental retardation. In: Dobbing J, Clarke ADB, Corbett JA, Hogg J, Robinson RO, eds. *Scientific Studies in Mental Retardation*. London: Royal Society of Medicine; 1984.

Dupont A. 140 years of Danish studies on the prevalence of mental retardation. *Acta Psychiatr Scand* 1989:79(suppl 348):105–112.

Escalona SK. Social and other environmental influences on the cognitive and personality development of low birthweight infants. *Am J Ment Defic* 1984; 87:505.

Evans JA, Hamerton JL. Chromosomal anomalies. In: Clark AM, Clarke ADB, Berg JM, eds. *Mental Deficiency—The Changing Outlook*. 4th ed. London: Methuen and Co, Ltd; 1985.

Fryers T. *The Epidemiology of Severe Intellectual Impairment*. London: Academic Press; 1984.

Fryers T. Epidemiological issues in mental retardation. *J Ment Defic Res* 1987; 31:365–384.

Fryers T. Epidemiology of severe mental retardation. In: Evans PLC, Clarke ADB, eds. *Combatting Mental Handicap*. Oxon: AB Academic Publishers; 1990.

Fuhrmann K, Reiher H, Semmler K, et al. Prevention of congenital malformations in infants of insulin-dependent diabetic mothers. *Diab Care* 1983; 6:219–223.

Gallagher JJ. The prevalences of mental retardation: cross-cultural considerations from Sweden and the United States. *Intelligence* 1985; 9:97–108.

Garber HL. *The Milwaukee Project: Preventing Mental Retardation in Children at Risk*. Washington DC: American Association on Mental Retardation; 1988.

Garber HL, Hodge JD, Rynders J, Dever R, Velu R. The Milwaukee Project: setting the record straight. *Am J Ment Retard* 1991; 95:493–525.

Gillberg C, Persson E, Grofmann M, Themner U. Psychiatric disorders in mildly and severely mentally retarded urban children and adolescents: epidemiological aspects. *Br J Psychiatr* 149:68–74.

Goodman MB, Gruenberg EM, Downing JJ, Rogot EA. Prevalence study of mental retardation in a metropolitan area. *Am J Pub Health* 1956; 46: no. 6.

Goulden KJ, Richardson SA, Shinnar S. Factors suggesting biological etiology of mental retardation from the Aberdeen cohort (abstr). *Dev Med Child Neurol* 1988; 30(suppl 52).

Goulden KJ, Shinnar S, Koller H, Katz M, Richardson SA. Epilepsy in children with mental retardation: a cohort study. *Epilepsia* 1991; 32:690–697.

Grossman HJ. *Classification in Mental Retardation*. Washington, DC. American Association on Mental Deficiency; 1983.

Gruenberg EM. *Technical Report of the Mental Health Research Unit, New York State Department of Mental Hygiene*. New York: Milbank Memorial Fund; 1955.

Gruenberg EM. Epidemiology. In: Stevens HA, Heber R, eds. Chicago: University of Chicago Press; 1964.

Gustavson KH, Holmgren A, Jonsell R, Blomquist HK. Severe mental retardation in children in a northern Swedish county. *J Ment Defic Res* 1977; 21:161.

Hack M. *Changing Outcome of the Tiny Infant. The Tiny Baby*. Ithaca, NY: Perinatology Press; 1990.

Hagberg B, Hagberg G. Aspects of prevention of pre-, peri- and postnatal brain pathology in severe and mild mental retardation. In: Dobbing J, Clarke ADB, Corbett JA, Hogg J, Robinson RO, eds. *Scientific Studies in Mental Retardation*. London: Royal Society of Medicine; 1984.

Hagberg B, Kyllerman M. Epidemiology of mental retardation—a Swedish survey. *Brain Dev* 1983; 5:No. 5.

Hagberg B, Hagberg G, Lewerth A, Lindberg U. Mild mental retardation in Swedish school children. *Acta Paediatr Scand* 1981; 70:441–444.

Hertzig ME, Birch HG, Richardson SA, Tizard J. Intellectual levels of school children severely malnourished during the first two years of life. *Pediatrics* 1972; 49: 814–824.

Hook EB, Hamerton JL. The frequency of chromosomal abnormalities detected in consecutive newborn studies—differences between studies—results by sex and by severity of phenotypic involvement. In: Hook EB, Porter IH, eds. *Population Cytogenetics*. New York: Academic Press, 1977.

Innes G, Johnston AW, Millar WM. Mental subnormality in northeast Scotland—a multidisciplinary study of total population. *Scot Health Serv Stud* 1978; No. 38.

Kahkonen M, Alitalo T, Airaksinen E, Matilainen R, Launiala K, Autio S, Leisti J. Prevalence of the fragile-X syndrome in four birth cohorts of children of school age. *Hum Genet* 1987; 77:85–87.

Kandall SR. Perinatal effects of cocaine and amphetamine use. Pregnancy and substance abuse: perspectives and directions. *Bull NY Acad Med* 1991; 67:240–255.

Kebbon L. Relation between criteria: case-finding method and prevalence. *Uppsala J Med Sci* 1987; 44:19–23.

Kirkman HN. Projections of a rebound in frequency of mental retardation from phenylketonuria. *Appl Res Ment Retard* 1983; 3:319–328.

Kushlick A, Cox AR. The epidemiology of mental handicap. *Dev Med Child Neurol* 1973; 15:748–759.

Kushlick A, Blunden R. The epidemiology of mental subnormality. In: Clarke AM, Clarke ADB, eds. *Mental Deficiency—The Changing Outlook*. 3rd ed. London: Methuen and Co, Ltd; 1974:31–81.

Landesman-Dwyer S. Maternal drinking and pregnancy outcome. *Appl Res Ment Retard* 1982; 3:241–263.

Lefebvre F, Bard H, Veilleux A, Martel C. Outcome at school age of children with birthweights of 1000 grams or less. *Dev Med Child Neurol* 1988; 30:170–180.

Lenke RR, Levy HL. Maternal phenylketonuria and hyperphenylalaninemia. *N Engl J Med* 1980; 303:1202–1208.

Levinson EJ. *Retarded Children in Maine*. Second series, No. 77. Orono: University of Maine Press, 1962.

Lewis EO. *Report of the Mental Deficiency Committee*. Part II. London; HMSO; 1929.

Lilienfeld AM, Benesch CH. *Epidemiology of Mongolism*. Baltimore: Johns Hopkins Press; 1969.

Mittler P. *People, Not Patients*. London: Methuen and Co, Ltd; 1979.

Mittler P. Comment on chromosomal aspects of mental retardation. In: Dobbing J, et al., eds. *Scientific Studies in Mental Retardation*. London: Royal Society of Medicine; 1984:87.

Moser HW. Biologic factors of development. In: Freeman JM, ed. *Prenatal and Perinatal*

Factors Associated with Brain Disorders. Bethesda, MD: NIH Publication No. 85-1149; 1985:121–162.

Mulcahy H, Reynolds A. *Census of Mental Handicap In The Republic of Ireland, 1981*. Dublin: The Medico-Social Research Board; 1984.

Neuspiel DR, Hamel SC. Cocaine and infant behavior. *J Dev Behav Pediatr* 1991; 12:55–64.

Nihira K, Foster R, Shellhaas M, Leland H. *Adaptive Behavior Scales*. Washington, DC: American Association on Mental Deficiency; 1974.

Olegard R, Laegreid L, Wahlstrom J. Prenatal environmental factors including fetal alcohol syndrome. *Uppsala J Med Sci* 1987; 44(suppl):169–172.

Partington MW, Hunter PE, Lockhart KA, Maidment B, Sears EVP. Simple X-linked mental retardation: clinical diagnosis and impact on the family. In: Berg JM, ed. *Perspectives and Progress in Mental Retardation*. Vol II. Baltimore: University Park Press; 1984.

Rao JM. A population-based study of mild mental handicap in children: preliminary analysis of obstetric associations. *J Ment Defic Res* 1990; 34:59–65.

Richardson SA. The relation of severe malnutrition in infancy to the intelligence of school children with differing life histories. *Pediatr Res* 1976; 10:57–61.

Richardson SA, Koller H. Epidemiology. In: Clarke AM, Clarke ADB, Berg J, eds. *Mental Deficiency—The Changing Outlook*. 4th ed. London: Methuen and Co, Ltd; 1985.

Richardson SA, Koller H, Katz M, McLaren J. Career paths through mental retardation services: an epidemiological perspective. *Appl Res Ment Retard* 1984a; 5:53–67.

Richardson SA, Koller H, Katz M, McLaren J. Patterns of disability in a mentally retarded population between ages 16 and 22 years. In: Berg JM, ed. *Perspectives and Progress in Mental Retardation*. Vol II: *Biomedical Aspects*. Baltimore: University Park Press; 1984b.

Richardson SA, Koller H, Katz M. Relationship of upbringing to later behavior disturbance of mildly retarded young people. *Am J Ment Defic* 1985; 90:1–8.

Richardson SA, Katz M, Koller H. Sex differences in the numbers of children administratively classified as mildly menatlly retarded: an epidemiological review. *Am J Ment Defic* 1986a; 91:250–256.

Richardson SA, Koller H, Katz M. A longitudinal study of numbers of males and females in mental retardation services by age, I.Q. and placement. *Am J Ment Defic* 1986b; 30:291–300.

Rosen MG. Factors during labor and delivery that influence brain disorders. In: Freemen JM, ed. *Prenatal and Perinatal Factors Associated with Brain Disorders*. Bethesda, MD: NIH Publication No. 85-1149; 1985:237–262.

Rutter M, Tizard J, Whitmore K. *Education, Health and Behavior*. London: Longman Group, Ltd; 1970.

Sameroff AJ. Longitudinal studies of preterm infants. In: Friedman SL, Sigman M, eds. *Preterm Birth and Psychological Development*. New York: Academic Press; 1981.

Scheiner AP, Hansaw JB, Simeonsson RJ, Scheiner B. The study of children with congenital cytomegalovirus infection. In: Mittler P, ed. *Research to Practice in Mental Retardation*. Vol III. Baltimore: University Park Press; 1977.

Skaarbrevik KJ. A follow-up study of educable mentally retarded in Norway. *Am J Ment Defic* 1971; 75:560–565.

Sonnander K. Prevalence of mental retardation: an empirical study of an unselected school population. In: Fraser WI, ed. *Key Issues in Mental Retardation Research*. London: Routledge; 1990.

Sorel FM. *Prevalences of Mental Retardation*. The Netherlands: Tilburg University Press; 1974.

Stein ZA, Susser M. The Social Distribution of Mental Retardation. *Am J Ment Defic* 1963; 67:811–821.

Stein ZA, Susser M. The epidemiology of mental retardation. In: Caplan G, ed. *American Handbook of Psychiatry*. 2nd ed. *Child and Adolescent Psychiatry, Socio-cultural and Community Psychiatry*. New York: Basic Books; 1974.

Stern J. Biochemical aspects. In: Clarke AM, Clarke ADB, Berg J, eds. *Mental Deficiency. The Changing Outlook*. 4th ed. London: Methuen and Co, Ltd; 1985.

Susser MW, Kushlick A. *Report on the Mental Health Services of the City of Salford for the Year 1960*. Salford City: Salford City Health Dept; 1961.

Terman L, Merrill N. *Stanford Binet Intelligence Scale: Manual for the third revision, Form L-N*. Boston: Houghton Mifflin; 1973.

Thake A, Todd J, Webb T, Bundy S. Children with the fragile-X syndrome at schools for the mildly mentally retarded. *Dev Med Child Neurol* 1987; 29:711–719.

Wald I, Zdzienieka E, Bartnik M, Kalinska A, Mrugalska K. *The Ten Years' Follow-Up Study of Representative Samples of the Low-Grade Mentally Retarded in Poland*. Warsaw, Poland: Psychoneurological Institute; 1977.

Webb TP, Thake AI, Bundy SE, Todd J. A cytogenetic survey of a mentally retarded school-age population with special reference to fragile sites. *J Ment Defic Res* 1987; 31:61–71.

11

Emotional and Behavioral Problems

JESSIE ANDERSON AND JOHN SCOTT WERRY

The identification of children with emotional and behavioral problems in the community setting has important implications for the children themselves and for the community, both in terms of current disability and future disorder (Robins, 1966, 1983; Rutter, 1984). Although the roots of adult disorders in childhood experiences have long been recognized in psychiatry, the existence of emotional and behavioral problems among children, requiring attention in their own right and not just as precursors of adult disorder and disability, has gained recognition only in the past few decades (Achenbach, 1981; Quay, 1979; Rutter, 1965; Skinner, 1981). Although much research has focused on individual disorders, such as hyperactivity, depression, and delinquency, using both clinical and general population samples, the investigation of the epidemiologic aspects of childhood psychopathology in general has received less attention.

The extent of the suffering for children and their families arising from disordered behavior and emotional dysfunction is evident: epidemiologic surveys of unselected populations give prevalences ranging from 7% to 22% (Costello, 1989; Graham, 1979; Links, 1983; Rutter, 1989; Vikan, 1985).

This chapter examines both early and more recent population studies of child and adolescent psychopathology. Classification systems and how they affect prevalence rates, are discussed, along with some areas of special interest, including cross-cultural studies, studies of pediatric practice populations, and studies across different age groups.

Definitions

Because of the looseness with which certain terms are used by nonpsychiatrists, these terms are defined at the outset. In psychiatry, *emotional* or *internalizing* disorder has a specific meaning; as the name suggests, it is one characterized by emotional symptoms of anxiety, misery, or depression. *Behavior* or *externalizing* disorders are characterized by annoyance or disruption of others, such as parents, teachers or peers. *Conduct* disorder is one in which the behavior deliberately violates the rights of others (aggression, stealing, etc.).

Although clinicians have debated the usefulness of diagnosis in child and adolescent psychiatry and many prefer to use more analytically oriented formulations of children's perceived conflicts as a basis for treatment, the value of diagnosis or case identification in epidemiology is undeniable (Werry, 1990). The ability to identify homogeneous groups of disturbed children whose symptoms, correlates of disorder, and precursors of disorder are similar permits risk factors or causes to be studied and distinctive treatments to be evaluated. Case identification depends on reliable and valid classification systems (Blashfield & Draguns, 1976; Cantwell, 1980; Wing, 1981).

Because of the critical nature of "caseness" to sound epidemiologic studies and the skeptical and poorly understood view of psychiatric diagnosis outside psychiatry itself, considerable attention must be devoted to this issue.

Systems of Classification

A common division of systems of classification is the "category versus dimension" distinction, that is, whether the syndromes describe distinct illnesses or describe severity on a continuum or dimension of behavior or mood, analogous to physical dimensions, such as weight or height (Kendell, 1975; Maxwell, 1971, 1972; Quay, 1986). Most emotional and behavioral states in childhood and adolescence are normally distributed, making the dimensional approach more appropriate. Yet, the issue of "category or dimension" is not a simple either-or choice because they are not mutually exclusive or incompatible, and many true clinical categories represent extreme ends of normally distributed attributes, e.g., gigantism or mental retardation. There are, however, some disorders that are clearly categorical, the major psychoses (insanity) being a good example.

Because child psychiatry lacks a sound etiologic base, with a few exceptions the major classification systems have been clinically derived, descriptive, and based on symptom clusters that form syndromes. Some recent studies have also used multivariate analytic methods to derive dimensional syndromes from empiric data (Achenbach, 1981). Yet, in independent reviews, Achenbach and Edelbrock (1978) and Quay (1979, 1986) found considerable convergence between empiric and clinical systems, in that several robust categories could be identified by factor analysis—conduct disorders, anxiety, attention deficit, socialized aggressive, and, more rarely, psychotic disorders (see La Greca & Quay, 1984). The present lack of precise knowledge of etiology in child psychiatry supports an empiric rather than an a priori medical approach to defining reliable and valid syndromes. These classifications should then be validated by tests of predictive power and treatment response and can be then used to detect etiologic differences. Of course, there are limitations to this empiric approach, and solid theory is still needed.

Diagnostic Classification

The history of official taxonomies of childhood disorders is a relatively brief one. Widespread dissatisfaction with the use of adult categories had resulted in the nondiagnosis of many children seen in clinics (Achenbach & Edelbrock, 1978; Rosen et al., 1964). For example, the American Psychiatric Association's first version of the *Diagnostic and Statistical Manual* (DSM-I) in 1952 had only two categories for child psychopathology. By 1968, its successor, DSM-II, had added six behavioral disturbances of childhood—hyperkinetic reaction, withdrawing reaction, overanxious reaction, runaway reaction, unsocialized-aggressive reaction, and group delinquent reaction. These classifications were based on the pioneering factor analyses by Hewitt and Jenkins (1946) and Jenkins (1966) of symptoms reported by children attending child guidance clinics.

Acceptance of DSM-II was neither widespread in the United States nor elsewhere. The WHO International Classification of Diseases (ICD) was the most widely used system, although this changed dramatically in 1980 with the publication of DSM-III. The ninth edition (ICD 9) and its accompanying multiaxial system are described in detail in the next sections, along with the American system (DSM-III), and other systems based on multivariate statistical analyses.

ICD 9. The child section of ICD 9 was developed from earlier versions primarily by Rutter and colleagues. The categories are symptomatologic and are only intended to be used if no adult category is suitable. There is a wide range of specificity of the syndromes, they are relatively easy to apply, and broad groupings of "emotional" or "conduct" disorders can be used, avoiding more refined, less reliable diagnostic categories (Yule, 1981). However, the disorders are not age specific, nor are clear rules given for applying the categories. The ICD 9 system incorporates conditions widely regarded as describing abnormal psychological function but not necessarily psychiatric conditions, thus creating potential territory disputes between practitioners of different professions (Yule, 1981). In addition to categories, the system was made multiaxial to include areas also felt to be important—intellectual level, delays in development, medical conditions, and abnormal psychosocial situations (Rutter et al., 1975b). A multiaxial system was thought to provide a more comprehensive picture of the child and the psychosocial situation than traditional medical uniaxial systems (Achenbach, 1981).

DSM-III. DSM-III is quite radical and innovative, being the only medical system of classification that sets out necessary and sufficient criteria for the diagnosis of each disorder. The structure is multiaxial and somewhat similar to ICD 9, in that many of the categories are the same and it is both descriptive and empirical. Accordingly, both systems are relatively compatible.

The disorders in DSM-III—four times as many as in DSM-II—are grouped into five major areas: (1) Intellectual (Mental Retardation), (2) Behavioral (Attention Deficit and Conduct Disorders), (3) Emotional (Anxiety Disorders and Others), (4) Physical (Eating, Movement Disorders) and (5) Developmental Disorders (which replace adult personality disorders on axis II). Subcategories for each group give a total of 49 disorders in the section of DSM-III devoted to Disorders Arising in Childhood and Adolescence, without including all the adult disorders—most of which can also occur in children.

The major claims for the system are in the "operationalized" criteria, which provide increasing reliability, good coverage, and high acceptability to clinicians. DSM-III also provides guidance to and decision trees for differential diagnosis (Cantwell, 1980) and a manual of attributes of each disorder. Although still controversial, DSM-III as it relates to childhood disorders is now widely used, is clinically acceptable, and remains the most structured and only operationalized classification system available.

The major criticisms center on DSM-III's low reliability for some newer categories, such as Oppositional Disorder, and for most subcategories (Achenbach, 1980; Quay, 1986; Werry et al., 1983). Resistance to using DSM-III may stem from the subjectivity of some criteria. These criteria require frequent recourse to the manual, which, if not used, increases its complexity, error, and unreliability (Werry, 1985). Nevertheless, epidemiologic studies using DSM-III generally provide good information on the common disorders and shed light on their natural history and possible etiology.

DSM-III-R. This revision of DSM-III appeared in 1987. There have been significant changes in the disorders of childhood and adolescence, and as a result the 1987 revision created considerable confusion in both clinicians and researchers, who were just becoming familiar with DSM-III.

Changes have included: (1) placing Attention Deficit Disorder, Conduct Disorders, and Oppositional Disorder in a group of "Disruptive behaviour disorders," (2) raising the threshold for the unreliable Oppositional Defiant Disorders to five symptoms, (3) putting hyperactivity back into Attention Deficit-Hyperactivity Disorder (ADHD) and requiring of its symptoms some degree of pervasiveness, (4) reducing the unreliable subtypes of Conduct Disorder to two, and (5) moving autism to Axis II (developmental disorders).

Mood disorders and anxiety disorders remain similar to DSM-III, as do eating disorders, gender identity disorder, and developmental disorders. Evidence of the impact of these changes is found in Lahey et al. (1990), who diagnosed both DSM-III and DSM-III-R disorders concurrently in 177 outpatients. Compared to DSM-III, DSM-III-R diagnoses for Oppositional Disorder were 26% less prevalent, Dysthymia 38% less, and Conduct Disorder 44% less, and the only disorder that was more prevalent was Attention Deficit-Hyperactivity Disorder (14%). Comparisons of the family, social, and legal characteristics of children with DSM-III and DSM-III-R Conduct disorders indicated that DSM-III-R Conduct disorders were more strongly associated with police contacts, school suspensions, and parental personality disorders. Together, this suggests an increase in their severity (Lahey et al., 1990). The changes in prevalence rates indicate quite major differences in threshold for the major DSM disorders and play havoc with epidemiologic studies, which rely so heavily on stability of diagnosis across time.

Dimensional Systems

Although there are other classification systems (Quay, 1986), the major competitor to the categorical (medical) approach is the dimensional system, best exemplified by the Child Behavior Checklist (CBCL; Achenbach & Edelbrock, 1983, 1986, 1987), which includes Parent, Teacher and Youth Self-Report versions. In a recent review of empirically derived syndromes, the authors of several different dimensional systems (see Quay, 1986) joined forces to analyze results using the CBCL and a modified version, the ACQ behavior checklist (Achenbach et al., 1983) in American and Dutch samples referred to mental health services. Using principal components analysis to identify syndromes, their replicability across gender, age group, and location of the sample was examined and compared to other classifications, notably DSM-III-R. The results showed that six syndromes, labeled Aggressive, Anxious/Depressed, Attention Problems, Delinquent, Somatic Complaints, and Withdrawn, were generally replicable. In addition, boys had a replicable Socially Inept syndrome and girls a "Mean" (or unkind and unpleasant) syndrome.

The core syndromes were strongly replicable in other empiric studies, particularly those reviewed by Quay (1986). In comparison to DSM-III-R, the empiric data made a clearer distinction between aggressive and delinquent (i.e., law breaking) types of conduct disorders and were more explicit in the distinctions of subtypes of Conduct Disorder. The empiric data did not find a group corresponding to Oppositional-Defiant Disorder in DSM-III-R, and the authors regarded the symptoms from DSM-III-R as a mild form of Conduct Disorder, a finding similar to others (Anderson et al., 1987; Werry et al., 1983). The empiric syndrome combining inattention and overactivity corresponds with DSM-III-R ADHD, the category of somatic complaints corresponds with Somatization Disorder, and the anxious-depressed syndrome combines Overanxious Disorder and Dysthymia. No empiric syndromes were found that corresponded to DSM-III-R Major Depression, Separation Anxiety, or Phobias (Achenbach et al., 1989).

Because the empirically derived syndromes were based only on parent reports, the next step would seem to be to include child or adolescent and teacher data into the analyses to refine and strengthen the syndromes. The findings offer some support for DSM-III-R categories, and it is expected they will influence future taxonomic revisions (DSM-IV and ICD 10).

Validity

The ultimate test lies in the predictive power of each system for such issues as correlates, etiology, treatment, and outcome. It will come as no surprise to find that some disorders are more valid than others, when using various measures of validity. There is also a problem of observer perception of disorder.

Patterns of Occurrence

Early Studies

Early studies of behavior and emotional problems of children have been well summarized by Achenbach and Edelbrock (1978), Graham (1977, 1979), and Links (1983). The major population studies of preadolescent children carried out by Rutter, Graham, and colleagues 20 years ago were the most influential of the earlier studies. Using a multistage design, Rutter, Tizard, and Whitmore (1970) screened the entire 10- and 11-year-old population of the Isle of Wight and then interviewed those children with likely disorders, as well as randomly chosen controls. They produced prevalence rates of 2.5% and 4% for emotional and conduct disorders, respectively, and a total prevalence of 6.8% (corrected for cases likely to have been missed). The same methods were used in Inner London (Rutter et al., 1975a), giving rates of 24.5% for boys and 13.2% for girls, more than twice the rates in the Isle of Wight.

Other studies have yielded prevalence rates ranging from 19.4% of children in Newcastle (Miller et al., 1974) to 18% in urban Queensland, 10% in rural Queensland (Connell et al., 1982), 14% of children "in need of mental health services" in Hawaii (Werner & Smith, 1977, 1979), 8% to 11% of Danish children (Kastrup, 1976), and 8% of girls and 16% of boys in the National Child Development Study (Pringle et al., 1966). In general, urban children have higher rates of disorder than rural children, although this was not so for the Danish study.

A review of 25 American studies by Schwartz-Gould et al. (1981) showed that most reported only global estimates of disorder, giving prevalences from 6.6% to 37%, with teacher-informant studies consistently yielding lower prevalences than parent-informant studies. They noted the lack of interviews with children in these studies and the difficulties in making corrections for missed cases. In their review of epidemiologic studies of childhood psychopathology, La Greca and Quay (1984) concluded that estimates are likely to be 10% for all disorders, 6.0% for conduct disorders, 5.0% for attention deficit disorders, and 3.0% for anxious-withdrawn disorders (which may co-occur).

In summary, although there is some disagreement in these early estimates of prevalence rates there is also an encouraging element of consistency in broad diagnostic categories.

Difficulties with Early Studies

The basic unit in epidemiology is the "identified case," which is often poorly defined in prevalence studies (Graham, 1979). Variations in prevalence in the early studies may therefore be due to different methods of assessing disorder and a lack of uniform diagnostic criteria. Methods of eliciting information also varied, from questioning randomly selected households to surveying teachers in local schools by questionnaire or having parents respond to mailed questionnaires. The samples were clinical, nonclinical, and mixed, with variations in age group and sex distribution. The nature of the disorders described, their symptom structure, defining characteristics, and the reliability and validity of their identification were equally disparate, with similar names defining several different constellations of signs and symptoms, e.g., Minimal Brain Dysfunction—see Ross & Ross, 1982; Rutter, 1982. Recent advances in both classification systems and structured interview/diagnostic instruments have resulted in improvements in epidemiologic studies. Instruments now available for assessing disorder in childhood and adolescence include parent, teacher, and child questionnaires; structured and semistructured interview schedules; and checklists. Any description of these instruments is beyond the scope of this chapter, but good reviews include Boyle and Jones (1985); Edelbrock and Costello (1988); the special section on "Structured Diagnostic Interviews" of the *Journal of the American*

Academy of Child and Adolescent Psychiatry (1987); Orvaschel et al. (1983); Orvaschel and Walsh (1984); and Rutter et al. (1988).

Recent Studies

The prevalence of all common disorders (as defined by DSM-III criteria, ICD 9, or by dimensional systems) and the extent to which disorders coexist have been studied recently in several general population samples (Costello, 1989). Although in the past children had rarely been used as a source of information, despite the evidence that they can be reliable reporters of their own symptoms (Herjanic & Reich, 1982; Herjanic et al., 1975; Reich et al., 1982), the more recent studies are notable both for their use of child interviews and for multi-source information gathering. For the purposes of this chapter, only studies published in 1985 or later and those with randomly selected, population-based samples of adequate size (over 200 subjects) have been selected for review. One exception is the study by Costello et al. (1988b) of a pediatric primary care practice sample. Because of the different role of pediatricians in North America compared to most of the British Commonwealth, which still retains a general practitioner primary care system, this U.S. sample has many of the characteristics of a primary care, community-based, sample rather than a referred sample, as would be the case outside North America.

All studies have used parent or teacher reports or both, with or without child reports, and a dimensional system for measuring *severity* of pathology on multivariate-derived scales or categorical DSM-III or ICD 9 diagnosis to define "caseness." In all the studies, the questionnaires, interview schedules, and diagnostic criteria used were standardized instruments, making the methodology replicable and more reliable than most earlier studies, with the exception of those by Rutter et al. (1970, 1975a). The methods, instruments, and sample characteristics are shown in Table 11.1.

Prevalence

Despite the wide variation in ages, sample size, instruments, and diagnostic systems, there is considerable convergence across studies in prevalence, both for total morbidity and for individual disorders. When either DSM-III criteria or clinically validated results from dimensional systems are used, the rates for one or more disorders range from 17.6% to 22%, with Conduct (either socialized or unsocialized), Attention Deficit, and Anxiety disorders equally the most prevalent. In those studies in which Oppositional disorder was identified separately from Conduct disorders, the prevalence of the latter was generally less than in studies in which only conduct problems were identified. There is some evidence from reliability studies and from examining external correlates of Conduct and Oppositional disorders that Oppositional disorder may represent the less severe end of the spectrum of these conditions (Anderson et al., 1987; Rutter, 1989; Werry et al., 1983). Accordingly, these two categories can be combined, giving a prevalence range from 5.5% to 12.0%.

Attention Deficit disorder (with or without hyperactivity) has prevalence rates

Table 11.1. Recent Community-Based Prevalence Studies

Authors	No. of Children	Age	Measures	DSM-III Disorders*							
				ALL	ADD	CD	OPP	OAN	SAN	PHO	DEP
Anderson et al., 1987	792	11	CI, PQ, TQ	17.6	6.7	3.4	5.7	2.9	3.5	2.4	1.8
Bird et al., 1988	777	4–16	CI, PI	18.0	10.1	1.5	9.7	na	4.8	2.3	5.9
Costello et al., 1998b	789	7–11	CI, PI	22.0	2.2	2.6	6.6	4.6	4.1	9.2	2.0
Offord et al., 1987a	2679	4–16	CCL, PCL, TCL	18.1	6.2	5.5	na	9.9	emo	emo	emo
Valez et al., 1989	776	11–20	CI, PI	20.6	4.3	5.4	6.6	2.7	5.4	na	1.7
McGee et al., 1990	943	15	CI, PCL	22.0	2.1	7.3	1.7	5.9	2.0	4.7	2.3

Authors	No.	Age	Measures	ICD9*					
				ALL	NEU	CD/EM	CD	HYP	OTH
Verhulst et al., 1985	153	8–11	CI, PCL, TCL	26.0	na	na	na	na	na
Esser et al., 1990	216	8	CI, PI	16.2	6.0	0.9	0.9	4.2	4.2
Esser et al., 1990	191	13	CI, PI	18.0	5.8	2.6	5.8	1.6	2.1
Vikan 1985	1510	10	PQ, TQ, NQ	5.0	na	na	na	na	na

*Prevalence rates %

Abbreviations: Measures—CI = child interview; PI = parent interview; CQ = child questionnaire; PQ = parent questionnaire; TQ = teacher questionnaire; NQ = nurse questionnaire; CCL = child checklist; PCL = parent checklist; TCL = teacher checklist. Disorders—ADD = Attention deficit; CD = Conduct; OPP = Oppositional; OAN = Overanxious; SAN = Separation anxiety; PHO = Phobia; DEP = Depression/dysthymia; NEU = Neurotic; CD/EM = Conduct/Emotional; HYP = Hyperkinesis; OTH = Other.

ranging from 2.2% to 10.1% in those studies using DSM-III criteria and generally lower rates (1.6% to 4.2%) in studies using ICD 9 or a dimensional system.

Anxiety disorders, either as a generic anxious-withdrawn category or as the more refined DSM-III subtypes, show a prevalence rate almost equal to Conduct disorders. Uniformly less prevalent are other affective (mood) disorders (Depression, Dysthymia, Phobias), whereas Obsessive-Compulsive, Avoidant, and Psychotic disorders are rarely, if ever, identified in general population samples.

Prevalence rates for one or more disorders are higher than for earlier studies, but generally comparable with the Inner London Study of Rutter et al. (1975a). Precise prevalence rates are dependent on the number of informants, the instruments used, and cut-off points for severity of symptoms or syndromes. In addition, most diagnostic classifications include a weighting for handicap or disability to child or family resulting from the symptoms, and the studies described in this section have all been careful to include some such measure in their diagnoses. If one also includes severity or pervasiveness as criteria, the prevalence rates are significantly lower (Anderson et al., 1987). For cross-study comparisons it is important to know which severity, handicap, or pervasiveness criteria were used. The way in which information from different sources is combined to make diagnoses also affects prevalence rates, with relatively more importance given by some studies to some sources, such as parents rather than children, when sources conflict. This issue is one of the most important methodologic problems in epidemiologic studies of child disorder and is discussed in detail in the following section.

Informant Variance

The serious problem that arises when reports from parents, teachers, and children differ on whether a disorder is present, either as a syndrome or as individual symptoms, has been apparent since the early studies. Rutter, Tizard, and Whitmore (1970) found relatively low agreement between parents and teachers in the Isle of Wight Study, and later studies have confirmed these differences. When children are included as one source of information, these difficulties are compounded further. Children can be quite reliable informants about their own internal states and thus can give valuable information about emotional disorders, but they are less able to assess externalizing problems (Edelbrock et al., 1986). *Age* also affects a child's ability to report, and reliability studies between parents and children using similar structured interviews (Achenbach et al., 1987c; Edelbrock et al., 1985) report low reliability in the 6- to 11-year age group. The reliability improves markedly thereafter, however.

Solutions to the problems of informant variance have included using a psychiatric assessment as the "gold standard" by which to measure the reliability of other informants; using parent reports as the standard (on the reasonable assumption that they know their children better than anyone else); and combining information from all sources to get a "best estimate" diagnosis. In the studies reviewed here, varying ways of estimating the validity of "caseness" were used. For example, in the New Zealand study, Anderson et al. (1987) estimated the *probability* of caseness by the number of informants (parent, teacher, or child), ranging from high (independent full diagnosis from more than one source) to low (diagnostic threshold only reached by combining all the sources of information and accumulating symptoms). A significant number of cases were only identified by one source, with no corroborating information from either of the other two sources, and these cases were regarded as representing "situational" (as opposed to pervasive) disorder. Agreement between self-report of symptoms with either parent or teacher report was low (Williams et al., 1989). McGee et al. (1990) also used a combination of parent and self-reports on the same sample in midadolescence, producing confirmed (two sources) or unconfirmed diagnoses. Parents confirmed half of all self-reported Conduct and Oppositional disorders, but only one third of Anxiety or Depressive disorders.

In contrast, Offord and colleagues used a combination of sources to identify total prevalence rates, but examined risk factors and correlates for parent- and teacher-identified cases separately. They found some systematic differences that indicated the value of viewing parent-identified and teacher-identified disorder as separate subtypes of child and adolescent disorder (Boyle et al., 1987; Offord et al., 1987a, 1989). For prevalence estimates, both the Canadian (Offord et al., 1987a) and Puerto Rican (Bird et al., 1988) studies used cut-off points for interview symptom scores or for impairment of functioning to define caseness. The New York longitudinal study used a "best estimate," combining child and parent information for the initial stage with a later, more stringent dimensional score on scales derived from the original structured interview (Cohen et al., 1987; Velez et al., 1989).

The whole issue of informant variance has been reviewed in detail by Achenbach, McConaughy, and Howell (1987c). After examining data on inter-rater correlations in over 100 studies, they concluded that variability in reporting across situations was not necessarily error, but was to be expected. Different informants were needed to report on all the different situations in which the child functions. Correlations between informants seeing children in similar situations (i.e., parent-parent or teacher-teacher) show good agreement; accordingly, one informant from that situation is likely to provide good data. Achenbach, McConaughy, and Howell (1987c) criticize the practice of considering one informant's (e.g., a teacher's) ratings as "more reliable," given the likelihood that children behave differently in different situations and that the informant's own views about the importance or seriousness of the symptoms influence reporting. Accordingly, these differences should not be considered a source of unreliability.

In summary, informant variance is essentially situation variance. In choosing informants, the question needs to be asked: what information is needed for what purpose? In children who have little say over their destiny, adult views may miss much inner misery by concentrating largely on the child's nuisance behavior to adults. Teachers may miss important family and recreational problems, whereas parents miss learning and peer group disorders.

Missing Cases

One of the more difficult problems when assessing prevalence rates of disorder in general population samples is the effect of missing data. Whether samples are chosen randomly, by school, by area of residence, or by age (e.g., birth cohorts), there will always be children and adolescents for whom data are missing or incomplete. The direction and degree of bias introduced by this lack of information have not often been assessed. Studies both of population-based samples (Cox et al., 1977) and of school-based samples (Beck et al., 1984) have shown an increase in psychopathology among parents of children who do not participate and poorer social integration of their children (as measured from prior information given to the school by parents and teachers). In the New Zealand longitudinal study, McGee (unpublished data, 1985) found that non-participation at one age was more likely to be preceded by a marked increase in family adversity at the earlier ages. This adversity included poorer maternal mental health, low socioeconomic status (SES) single parenting following parental separation, poor family relationships, and large family size and was most marked for most recent refusers. Children who attended an interview but who did not complete the DISC-C at 11 years had significantly higher parent and teacher reports of symptoms, higher disadvantage scores, and lower self-esteem than those who completed the interview, but were not significantly different on IQ and educational tests (Williams et al., 1989).

At 15 years for those subjects with DISC-C data but no parent data, the prevalence of self-reported disorder was nearly 50%, twice that of the sample as a whole (McGee et al., 1990). Similar findings were reported by Offord et al. (1992), who found that nonresponders in a 4-year follow-up study had higher levels of family pathology and family risk factors in the original data compared to responders. Other studies have either found no differences between refusers and participants (Boyle et al., 1987; Esser et al., 1990; Verhulst et al., 1985) or differences indicating increased pathology among refusers or their families (Verhulst et al., 1990) depending on the method of data collection.

In summary, it is likely that most prevalence figures are conservative estimates for the populations from which the samples were drawn because missing cases are likely to be more disturbed.

Co-Morbidity

The extent to which disorders can occur together in general population samples has been apparent since the Isle of Wight studies that identified the need for a "mixed" disorder category (Rutter et al., 1970). This co-morbidity is found both within broad groups of disorders (e.g., externalizing or disruptive versus internalizing or emotional) and across the traditionally viewed discrete emotional and conduct categories. Recent studies have also described co-morbidity between DSM-III categories, which are much more refined than those used by Rutter and colleagues. Of these recent studies, the Puerto Rican survey (Bird et al., 1988) found Conduct/Oppositional, followed by affective (mood) disorders to be the most overlapping, whereas the New Zealand study (Anderson et al., 1987; McGee & Williams, 1988) found considerable overlap between Depression/Dysthymia and externalizing disorders and between ADHD and Conduct disorder at 11 years. At 15 there was still overlapping of disorders in approximately one in four children with a disorder, with Anxiety and Depression being the most overlapping, both with other Anxiety disorders and with ADHD and

Conduct/Oppositional disorders (McGee et al., 1990). Anderson et al. (1987, 1989) also described a small group of children (2% of the sample) who presented with multiple concurrent disorders, including Conduct or Oppositional disorder, ADHD, Depression/Dysthymia, and one or more Anxiety disorders.

The problems posed by the extent of co-morbid disorders are best seen when trying to untangle correlates and risk factors for individual disorders and when establishing diagnostic validity, as is described below. There is accumulating evidence that some patterns of co-morbidity may be more significant in terms of severity of disability, response to treatment, and long-term outcome than others. In particular, the combinations of ADHD with Conduct disorder and of Depression with Conduct disorder warrant further discussion.

Differentiating between ADHD and Conduct Disorder (CD) has long been a source of debate between DSM-III and ICD 9. The widely different prevalence rates for ADHD in both systems, which also correlate with sides of the Atlantic, have been shown to be due to differences in recognition and labeling of symptoms as hyperactive (United States) or conduct (United Kingdom), rather than a true difference (Prendergast et al., 1988; Taylor et al., 1986).

Much of the earlier confusion about the separateness of ADHD and CD arose from studies that failed to discriminate between the two. Better-designed studies (Lahey et al., 1980; Loney et al., 1978; McGee et al., 1985; Milich et al., 1982; Szatmari et al., 1989) have shown that ADHD and CD exist as separately identifiable disorders with separate correlates—Conduct disorders being related to adverse family and social background, whereas ADHD is related to other cognitive deficits (especially reading, spelling, and arithmetic) and to lower IQ levels (Werry et al., 1987). Both disorders, however, frequently co-occur, which clouds the picture, particularly in clinic attenders who often have adverse correlates of both disorders. In fact "pure" CD may be hard to find among clinical groups, which understandably are preselected for severity (Reeves et al., 1987). Children with both ADHD and CD form a distinctive group with major cognitive, social, and behavioral problems, as is discussed further in the section on correlates of disorder. (In ICD these children are recognized as such, i.e., hyperkinetic conduct disorder).

Another important group, both from a diagnostic and management standpoint, are those co-morbid for Conduct disorder and Depression or Dysthymia. There is difficulty untangling which disorder is the primary or more longstanding, which results in conflicting views about the primary or secondary nature of the depressive illness (Anderson et al., 1987; Fleming & Offord, 1990; Puig-Antich, 1982). Conduct disorder among adolescent girls may follow a history of preadolescent mood disorder (McGee et al., 1992), and among preadolescent boys, depression and aggression are known to coexist (Anderson et al., 1987; Bird et al., 1988; Cohen et al., 1985; Costello, 1989). In dimensional classification systems, depressed mood and aggression occur together in boys aged 6 to 11 (Edelbrock & Achenbach, 1980). Depression in preadolescence is also found frequently coexisting with anxiety disorders (Werry, 1991) and, to a lesser extent, with ADHD (Kovacs et al., 1984). Consequently, "pure" childhood depression (as a disorder) may be difficult to find except in specialized tertiary settings (Graham, 1979; Nurcombe et al., 1989; Pataki & Carlson, 1990; Puig-Antich, 1982; Seifer et al., 1989), as opposed to depressive symptoms, which are much more common (Carlson & Cantwell, 1980). This distinction between symptoms and disorder is not trivial; it has important treatment implications.

Among the anxiety disorders, the overlap is such that these disorders are combined as "one or more anxiety disorders" in many studies (Werry, 1991), and when this occurs it greatly increases the reliability of the category. This problem of co-morbidity is discussed for ICD 9 by Gould et al. (1988) and has been demonstrated in studies for DSM-III subgroups by Anderson et al. (1987), Bird et al. (1988), and McGee et al. (1990). Williams et al. (1989) have shown that not only do diagnosed disorders display significant degrees of overlap but so do symptoms that do not reach a diagnostic threshold. They coexist with other disorders more frequently than in children with no disorder. These findings, based on child self-reports, indicate that even so-called pure disorders may be associated with subdiagnostic but clinically important symptom loadings with other disorders. The degree of overlap found among diagnosed disorders in the study by Anderson et al. (1987) is fairly typical of reported co-morbidity in general population studies of pre-adolescents and is presented in Table 11.2.

Theoretical explanations for the high rates of co-morbidity have been well described by several authors (Biederman et al., 1991; Caron & Rutter, 1991; Rutter, 1989). These explanations include co-morbidity from artifact (e.g., as a result of overlapping diagnostic criteria), separate identification of early and late manifestations of the same disorder as two disorders, and splitting one disorder into several categories. True co-morbidity may arise from sharing common risk factors, overlapping risk, one disorder increasing the risk for another, or the co-morbid pattern representing a distinctive new syndrome.

In summary, co-morbidity, or lack of specificity, is a serious problem that erodes the value of other than broad categories. It probably derives from the nonspecific nature of many of the symptoms used for the diagnosis and from shared risk factors.

Risk Factors

Correlates also form a test of the validity of a disorder, in that a diagnosis should have a reasonably unique set of associated features and predictors that discrim-

Table 11.2. Overlap of Disorders

	Number of Cases			
	Attention Deficit	Conduct or Oppositional	Anxious or Phobic	Depression
Attention deficit	—			
Conduct or oppositional	25	—		
Anxious or phobic	14	19	—	
Depression or dysthymia	8	11	10	—
Total co-morbid	29	35	23	11
Total pure cases	24	37	36	3

Source: From Anderson et al. (1987).

inate it from other disorders, either by type of correlate or by the degree to which a feature or predictor is associated. Many studies reporting risk factors do so using correlational cross-sectional data (Jensen et al. 1990; Offord, 1990), which can be misleading because risk cannot always be established in such a design. Exceptions are the studies carried out by Anderson et al. (1987, 1989), McGee et al. (1990), Offord et al. (1992), and Velez et al. (1989), each of which used data collected prospectively at earlier ages (true risk factors), as well as at the time the disorder was identified. However, when correlates clearly antedate the disorder and can be shown to co-vary with the disorder, these variables also may be considered to be risk factors for that disorder.

A risk factor does not necessarily imply a direct causal relationship; it may simply identify an early marker for disorder. The more often an individual variable is identified as a risk factor, however, the higher the index of suspicion will be that the relationship between the marker variable and the disorder is indeed causal.

In child and adolescent psychopathology, disorders are seldom associated with only one risk factor, and the strength of association is rarely great enough to regard the risk factor as a necessary or sufficient precursor of disorder. Risk factors seem to exert their influence in a cumulative fashion, with the number of risk factors present being more important than the specific nature or type of each individual variable. Furthermore, the risk factors associated with the onset of disorder may not be the same as those associated with maintaining an already established emotional or behavioral problem.

Earlier studies identified many correlates (risk factors) for psychopathology in children, the most widely supported being male gender, low intelligence, educational disabilities (particularly reading), and a socially disadvantaged large family with a history of parental illness or criminality. Children with chronic physical illness, divorced or separated parents, violent or abusive families, or poor families and those from inner-city environments have also been shown to be more likely to develop psychological disorders either of an emotional or behavioral nature (Graham, 1979; Links, 1983; Rutter, 1989).

Recent community-based studies have examined correlates and risk factors for specific disorders. In the cross-sectional studies, externalizing disorder has been shown to be related to male gender, low SES, educational failure (repeating a grade), ethnicity (higher rates for black children), family dysfunction (including single parent), physical illness, and low family income or family on welfare (Achenbach et al., 1990a; Bird et al., 1989; Costello et al., 1988b; Offord et al., 1987b, 1989). Internalizing disorders, mainly anxiety disorders, were associated with parental stress or "nerves," chronic illness, family dysfunction, and female gender for older children (12 years upward), as well as family welfare status, especially for girls.

Longitudinal studies show similar risks, but generally with more attenuated associations than the cross-sectional studies. Common to all of the longitudinal studies were higher risk for any disorder with male gender in preadolescence and with female gender in adolescence, low IQ or repeating a grade, poor physical health, poor peer relationships, and dysfunctional and disadvantaged families—all of which preceded the identification of disorder (Anderson et al., 1987, 1989; Cohen & Brook, 1987; McGee et al., 1990; Offord et al., 1992;

Velez et al., 1989). However, distinguishing between individual disorders by risk factors is not so clear. For example, in the New Zealand study, Anderson et al. (1989) reported that the most clearly identified risk factors were found in the multiple disorders group, who were predominantly male; had reading, spelling, and low IQ problems; had poor global health, poor peer relations, and low self-esteem; and came from the most disadvantaged families. Other disorders had less distinctive correlates, although ADHD and Conduct disorder were separable by male gender (ADHD), cognitive and academic problems (ADHD), poor global health (ADHD), poor peer relations (CD), and family disadvantage (CD). Emotional disorders could be distinguished from ADHD or Conduct/Oppositional disorders because the former were less handicapping cognitively and socially. Correlates of disorder also differ according to who gives the information about the child or family. For example, Offord, Boyle, and Racine (1989) found that low family income was strongly associated with hyperactivity reported by teachers but not by parents. The implications of these results for the validity of diagnostic categories are discussed later.

Williams et al. (1990) examined the family and social risks in the New Zealand study in more detail and found that several factors distinguished any disorder from no disorder (male sex, maternal depression, marital status of parents, and child reading problems) as did the number of risk factors. There was less distinction, however, among types of disorder by specific risk factors. Children with one or more diagnoses had higher symptom scores on scales on which they did not reach diagnostic thresholds (Williams et al., 1989), indicating that the diagnostic groups were less distinct from each other symptomatically than they may seem. This lack of specificity and the extent of co-morbidity previously described for this sample make correlational studies difficult to interpret. The lack of clear distinctions among diagnostic groups according to specific correlates (Reeves et al., 1987; Werry et al., 1987) also raises questions about the diagnostic validity and distinctiveness of many DSM-III disorders. On the one hand, the disorder/no disorder distinction (caseness) and externalizing versus internalizing differences are supported consistently. On the other hand, there is only weak support for separating internalizing disorders into anxiety and depression (Fleming & Offord, 1990; Quay & La Greca, 1986) or for separating externalizing disorders into ADHD, Conduct, and Oppositional disorders (Quay, 1986). If, however, externalizing disorders are grouped as ADHD, Conduct disorder, and mixed ADD and CD, and Oppositional disorder is treated as CD, considerably better validity is attained (Anderson et al., 1989; Schachar & Wachsmuth, 1990; Werry et al., 1987; Williams et al., 1990).

Protective factors for children otherwise at risk for disorder have also been identified. "Getting along with others" and being a "good student" were the most powerful of these factors in the Canadian study (Offord et al., 1992; Rae-Grant et al., 1989). Other protective factors described include high IQ, having an "easy temperament" (e.g., active, alert, sociable, and actively eliciting warmth from caregivers), a cohesive family, a good relationship with another adult, and having skills in areas outside the family, such as at school, sports, or hobbies, which enhance self-esteem (Offord & Fleming, 1991; Werner, 1990; Werner & Smith, 1977). Some children display considerable resilience or seem invulnerable to high risk and adversity for reasons that are not well understood. Here too there is a relation with temperament, family support, or skills learnt outside the home, as described for Hawaiian children by Werner and Smith (1982). It is important to stress, however, that protection may not just be the absence or converse of risk; it may operate under different mechanisms that have yet to be elucidated.

In summary, male sex and a disadvantaged/disordered family or social background increase the risk of disorder in general, but especially for Conduct disorders, whereas female sex predisposes to emotional disorder. The overlap in disorders belies much of the precision in such risk factors. Protective factors are less often described, and more sophisticated statistical models are needed to unravel the relationships among risk, protection, and disorder.

Follow-Up and Stability of Disorder

Stability may also be viewed as a test of the validity of caseness or of diagnosis. The Isle of Wight study (Graham & Rutter, 1973) showed that between ages 10 to 11 years and 14 to 15 years there was a twofold increase in prevalence, with 40% of the previously identified cases still having a disorder. There are several other follow-up studies (Anderson et al., 1987, 1989; Cantwell & Baker, 1989; Esser et al., 1990; McGee et al., 1992; Offord et al., 1992; Velez et al., 1989; Verhulst et al., 1990) that, although differing in instruments and methods, have considerable similarities. The time interval averages 4 or 5 years, and the ages studied range from preadolescence to early adolescence in most, although that of the study by Anderson and colleagues went from 5 to 11 years. These studies have consistently shown a higher stability for externalizing disorders, particularly Conduct disorder, than for internalizing disorders. About 40% to 50% of children with Conduct disorder still have it or another externalizing disorder 4 to 5 years later, although a few do develop internalizing disorders. Conduct disorder is more persistent than ADHD in most studies. Some suggest that ADHD or hyperactivity declines with age, and some of the children with this diagnosis shift into other diagnostic groups (Anderson et al., unpublished data; Esser et al., 1990; McGee et al., 1990). In contrast, Cantwell and Baker (1989) reported ADHD to be among the most stable disorder in a study of younger children attending a speech clinic. However, these subjects are likely to have had both language and cognitive or neurologic disorders, which are associated with more severe ADHD. Internalizing disorders show less stability, with recovery rates over 4 to 5 years ranging from 60% to 75% and Anxiety disorders showing greater recovery rates than Depression.

Older children tend to have a worse prognosis than younger children. They have higher rates of continuing disorder at follow-up (Offord et al., 1992; Verhulst et al., 1990), and those with more than one disorder are twice as likely as those with a single disorder to have the condition persist (Anderson et al., unpublished data; McGee et al., 1992; Offord et al., 1992). Although children with any disorder were more likely than the nondisordered to have disorder at follow-up, the majority of cases in adolescence were new cases in all studies (from 60% to 80% of adolescent cases). Recovery was reported for more than half of the original cases, including some of the severe multiple disorders (Anderson et al., unpublished data). For some children abnormal behavior patterns can be identified in early childhood (5 or younger); notably, aggressive or hyperactive behavior in those who later develop externalizing or multiple disorders (Anderson et al., 1987). There are also gender differences in the continuity of disorder. McGee et al. (1992) found that externalizing disorders in boys were the most stable, followed by internalizing disorders in girls. Paradoxically, internalizing disorder in boys at 11 was a strong predictor for externalizing disorder at 15. This contrasts with the low stability for externalizing disorder in girls. With the high rates of co-morbidity at both symptom and disorder levels already described, it is difficult to be certain whether the onset of "new" cases is preceded by higher levels of symptoms than are noncases. Apparent shifts of diagnosis with age may also be preceded by higher levels of co-morbid symptoms for the second disorder, which is not detected until symptoms reach a diagnostic threshold.

In summary, most studies show rather low stability over time, with the exception of Conduct disorder, multiple disorders, and severe disorders.

Service Utilization

The proportion of children having handicapping conditions who receive help from medical, psychiatric, or educational services is quite low. Rutter, Tizard, and Whitmore (1970) found that approximately 10% of disturbed children were receiving help, whereas more recent studies show a range from 29% for all services (Anderson et al., 1987) to 16% for mental health (Costello et al., 1988a) or special education (Offord et al., 1987a). Referral rates for the whole array of services vary from 4% (Bird et al., 1989) to 12% (Anderson et al., 1987), but the figure is higher—as high as half of those with a disorder, or about 1 in 4 of the whole sample (McGee et al., 1990)—among adolescents, who can more easily get help from school counselors or family physicians without requiring parental assistance. Even so, McGee et al. (1990) found that the parent-instigated referral rate had risen to 40% of 15-year-olds with a disorder, whereas only 12% were self-referrals. Offord et al. (1987a) noted that referral to mental health or social services was more likely for children with disorder than those without (16% versus 4%), but no such differences were found in referrals for primary *medical* care. Neither urban-rural differences, age, nor sex affected service use. However, proportionately more children with disorder use services in urban areas. The fact that a substantial proportion of children without disorder are referred [(9% of the nondisorder group at 11 and 15) as calculated from Anderson et al. (1987) and McGee et al. (1990)] may reflect minor disorder, availability of services, a poor level of discrimination among referring agents, or the limited validity of diagnosis. Children with ADHD, aggression, or multiple disorder are those most likely to have been referred by age 11 (Anderson et al., 1987). In pediatric practice populations, approximately 25% of cases are identified, and 16% are referred (Costello et al., 1988b). This finding indicates that pediatricians are no more likely to identify and refer children with emotional and behavioral disorders than are parents, teachers, or family physicians. (The special case of pediatric clinic attenders is discussed further).

The New Zealand study reveals that boys with externalizing disorders and who have learning problems are identified from about age 5. Higher rates of referral at age 15 may reflect the fact that, as the adolescent becomes a more reliable source of information about his or her symptoms, referral patterns become more selective (Anderson et al., 1987; McGee et al., 1990).

In summary although children with disorder are more likely to be referred, too few are receiving service, although the proportion increases with age. Professionals may be concerned with the low referral rates, but it has to be remembered that except for a few disorders (Conduct and multiple), spontaneous remission is high and treatment for persistent disorders is not particularly effective.

Cross-Cultural Studies

Recent cross-cultural projects, using identical methods, have begun to address whether common syndromes are valid across societies. All have used the Child Behavior Checklist's (CBCL; Achenbach & Edelbrock, 1983, 1986, 1987) Parent or Teacher forms, and some have used the Youth Self-Report. The questionnaires have been translated, tested, and then used on large groups of randomly selected children. So far, comparisons have been reported between American children and Thai, Australian, Dutch, and Puerto Rican children. Although each non-American group has been compared to the American sample, they have not been compared with each other. Other prevalence studies in New Zealand, Canada, Puerto Rico, and America, although using somewhat different methods, also permit some comparisons of "caseness" for samples of varying ages.

The impression gained from these studies is one of considerable congruence for caseness, as well as for items on the CBCL. The comparisons of American children with Dutch, Australian, Thai, and Puerto Rican children (Achenbach et al., 1987a, 1987b, 1990a, 1990b; Weisz et al., 1987, 1989) consistently show boys having more symptoms and lower competence scores than girls on Parent and Teacher reports; younger children with more symptoms than older children (Dutch, Australian, American samples); and more problems for children from lower SES families.

Cross-national comparisons showed the American children had lower symptom scores than Thai, Australian, and Puerto Rican children and higher competence scores than all four comparison samples. Thai children had more problems with overcontrol (anxiety, withdrawal) and were reported to be especially prone to anxious, sulking, overdependent, and somatic problems. These national differences, which were more marked for boys, may reflect that Thai culture is less tolerant of aggressive, disobedient, or disrespectful behavior, resulting in the children internalizing anger and being afraid of teachers (Weisz et al., 1987, 1989). Australian children swore and talked about sex more, whereas Puerto Rican children had higher Parent and Teacher scores, but lower self-report of problems. The American children had higher numbers of problems than the Puerto Ricans in the Conduct disorder range (cruelty, drug abuse, stealing, and poorly socialized).

In most studies teachers reported more problems than parents and greater gender differences. This finding raises the issue of whether separate male and female norms are needed for teacher reports and whether boys are more socially troubled or disadvantaged in school. Other comparisons discussed by Achenbach et al. (1990a, 1990b) showed youth reports to be higher than parent reports for symptoms in American, Dutch, Puerto Rican, and German samples; Chilean and Canadian children had higher problem scores than American, Dutch, or Thai children; and South Pacific countries (including Hong Kong, Australia, and New Zealand) report high symptom scores on the same instruments.

Whether these differences represent some threshold effect or a truly different pattern of psychopathology across cultures can best be resolved by biculturally skilled observers. In interpreting such studies, one must guard against observer bias and the possibility that parent or teacher reporting may not be constant across cultures. Further, as noted in adult cross-cultural studies (Kleinman, 1987; Littlewood, 1990), the problems of ethnocentricity inherent in translating and using Western questionnaires on non-Western groups may make comparisons of limited value. Although the Achenbach studies do not claim to identify disorders that are equally meaningful in all cultures, they do assume that the items contained in the questionnaires have equal valence in all cultures.

These cautions may also apply to cultural subgroups within a traditionally Western culture, such as the aboriginal or indigenous nations that were colonized and culturally dominated by Caucasians until recently. Whether the children of different cultures truly behave differently, as opposed to parent and teacher thresholds of tolerance being different, calls for "culture-free" observations or universal markers of behavior, as is the case with many physical diseases. Such markers would ideally be biologic or biochemical, but careful observation by clinicians skilled in the nuances of different cultures would seem to be the next best way to make valid comparisons. The major issue facing such research is how to avoid ethnocentricity and imposing meaningless categories of disorder on other cultures while not lapsing into the despair of total cultural relativism, i.e., where no cultural group is seen as having enough in common with any other to learn from them and share solutions to similar problems.

In summary, cross-cultural studies, so far using one main method, have revealed generally similar patterns of disorder, with some minor variations. However, it is still not clear to what extent these are true cultural differences or artifacts of the method.

Disorders Not Found in Community Studies

Some serious disorders have not been subject to many epidemiologic studies because of their low incidence. Among these are infantile autism, childhood schizophrenia, obsessive-compulsive disorder, and anorexia nervosa. What little is known about the epidemiology of these conditions is discussed briefly in this section.

Infantile autism is a serious handicapping disorder with congenital or very early onset and a triad of severe disturbance in language development, poor social relationships, and bizarre behavioral rituals (Kanner, 1943). DSM-III adds the criteria of onset before 30 months of age, peculiar speech patterns (where speech is present), and absence of schizophrenic symptoms, such as hallucinations, delusions, incoherence, or loosening of association and thought. There are difficult boundary problems in distinguishing autistic children from (1) those with lesser degrees of the syndrome, (2) those who have improved sufficiently to no longer qualify fully, or (3) those who have severe brain damage as well (Prior & Werry, 1986).

The prevalence of "pure" autism in the general population is relatively constant at 4 to 5 cases per 10,000 children under 14 years, with half being severe cases. There are many more children who show some autistic features in association with brain damage. A recent study of all autistic children in a Swedish city (Steffenburg, 1991) found 35 children with autism, 17 with autistic-like disorders, and 164 with mental retardation who had some autistic features. The autistic children were mainly boys (6:1), and an extensive assessment found 90% to have major indications of brain damage or dysfunction—a frequency similar to that in severely mentally retarded children. Hereditary disorders and other known syndromes accounted for 46% of the abnormal findings. This study reinforces the increasing acceptance of the view that autism and autistic-like disorders are a result of brain dysfunction that affects processing of language and interpersonal information (Gillberg, 1988).

Childhood schizophrenia is also rare, with similar symptoms to the same disorder presenting in later life (Werry, in press). Prior and Werry (1986) assess the prevalence for this disorder as virtually nil before 5 years and around 1 per 1000 until midadolescence, after which the prevalence climbs 5- to 10-fold into early adult life. There are few studies of the disorder in childhood, and most cases are described as part of a series of adolescents or young adults. Onset for males seems to be earlier, particularly in the prepubertal age group, and the course is variable, but is similar to schizophrenia in adolescents and young adults. Unlike autism, childhood schizophrenia is not associated with mental retardation, and the association with brain damage is unclear. The role of parents and families in the etiology of autism or childhood schizophrenia is not now regarded as significant (see Prior & Werry, 1986, for a discussion of this role).

Obsessive-compulsive disorder is marked by disabling, repetitive, unwanted (intrusive) thoughts or rituals [compulsions] to relieve the anxiety of obsessions. It is reported in children in 0.2% in clinic populations and 1% of inpatients (Rapoport, 1986). There is, however, little literature on this disorder and few epidemiologic studies. The largest and only longitudinal study is the above NIMH sample of 30 cases, ranging from 3 to 14 years for age of onset. In this sample boys outnumbered girls by 2:1, had an earlier onset of disorder (by a mean of 2.5 years), and a history in most cases of sudden onset of problems over a few months, with no previous history of obsessive traits or abnormal development (Rapoport, 1986). Other studies cited by Rapoport also describe rapid onset of the disorder in children who, except for a tendency to anxiety and perfectionism, were previously unremarkable. Most commonly associated conditions were Tourette's syndrome, anorexia nervosa, motor tics and, less commonly, Conduct disorder, other anxiety states, and depression.

Anorexia nervosa is a distressing and potentially life-threatening condition that usually only appears at or after puberty and overwhelmingly in girls. The pathologic fear of obesity and obsessional dieting, to the point of emaciation despite objective evidence that the girl is not obese, are the major symptoms. Anorexia is diagnosed when 25% of the ideal body weight has been lost, thus distinguishing the disorder from weight loss to healthy levels in obese children.

Its prevalence has been estimated at 1% of 16-year-old girls, with anorexic-type behavior or unwise dieting being five to six times higher. The prevalence may have peaked about 1985 (Lucas et al., 1991). Associated disturbances in body image, so that even emaciated patients see themselves as obese, distinguish anorexia from other eating problems, as does the stated wish to continue to lose weight or the failure to regain it despite obvious thinness. Many anorexic girls have a history of obesity at some time in their past, and girls whose interests and hobbies include gymnastics, ballet, or modeling are especially at risk, because of their need for thinness or a prepubertal body shape in these activities. Associated problems are amenorrhea, increased body hair, induced vomiting with associated damage to the esophagus and teeth, and, in severe cases, emaciation and death. An unknown proportion of cases are associated with and may follow the onset of a major depressive illness, but the usual picture is overactivity, compliance in all behaviors except eating, maintaining academic progress until very thin, and an all-absorbing desire to be thin. Werry (1986) has described the epidemiology and its link to cultural and social values that perpetuate the pursuit of thinness in most Western cultures.

Special Populations

Pre-School Children

Interest in the distribution and correlates of disorders among preschool-aged children is relatively new in child psychiatry, and there have been few studies of individual symptoms (Richman, 1985). In one study of a general population sample, Richman et al. (1975) used standardized instruments in a two-stage design to distinguish between transient problems and more persistent disorder. The questionnaire designed for this study, the Behavior Screening Questionnaire (BSQ), has been used in several subsequent preschool population studies and has proven useful.

Commonly identified problems among 3-year-olds are overactivity, restlessness, attention-seeking and difficult-to-control behavior, bedwetting, daytime wetting, food fads, difficulty settling down at bedtime, and night waking. Less common are soiling, fearfulness, poor concentration, aggression, tantrums, being unhappy, and excessive worrying. Boys are more often overactive and have more sphincter control problems, whereas girls are more tearful.

In studies carried out in London, Hong Kong, the rural United States, and urban areas in the United States, prevalence rates for all disorders are 22% to 24% of 3-year-olds, with 5% to 7% having moderate to severe and 15% to 18% mild disorder (Campbell & Ewing, 1990; Earls, 1980b; Luk et al., 1991a; Richman et al., 1975). Fathers reported one third the number of problems reported by mothers and less association with family problems (Earls, 1980a). The most common findings were no gender differences (or boys having more problems; Luk et al., 1991a); no ethnic differences; language problems; and an association with maternal depression, poor family relationships, and marital disharmony (Earls, 1980a; Richman et al., 1975).

When preschool children are followed up to ages 8 or 9, externalizing disorders are more persistent than internalizing disorders for boys, as is hyperactivity. Their persistence is also associated with language delay, family problems, negative and controlling maternal behavior, ongoing family stress, and male gender. As many as two thirds of children with problems at 3 years still had them at ages 8 or 9, indicating considerable persistence (Campbell & Ewing, 1990; McGee et al., 1984a,b, and c; Richman et al., 1982). Improvement by age 6 predicted continuing good adjustment at 9 years (Campbell & Ewing, 1990).

Cross-cultural differences were noted in the Hong Kong Chinese children (Luk et al., 1991a and unpublished data), with less overactivity, better concentration, less frequent poor moods, less eating and sleeping problems, but more temper tantrums, more fearfulness, and more often sleeping with their parents reported compared to Western children. These differences again highlight possible cultural and temperament differences in early life between Asian and Western children.

In summary, these studies of preschoolers paint a consistent picture of early onset of persistent externalizing disorders in some children, especially boys, which are characterized by overactivity, impulsiveness, discipline problems, and early difficulty with peer aggression for some. The associated family characteristics of poor family and marital relationships, maternal depression, negative and controlling behavior toward the child, and ongoing stresses are associated with persistence of the behavior problems.

Pediatric Clinics

The prevalence and characteristics of mental health problems among children seen by pediatricians are of interest for two main reasons. First, the diagnostic and referral patterns of pediatricians play a major role in the identification, treatment, and referral of disturbed children. Second, there is a clear association between chronic illness and mental health problems, especially if the illness affects the central nervous system, e.g., epilepsy, head injury; see Breslau (1990).

In most general population studies, the prevalence rates of chronic or disabling illness are too low to assess the association with psychiatric disorder (Anderson et al., 1987, 1989; McGee et al., 1990). Yet, in studies with sufficient numbers of children with chronic illnesses, the association with higher rates of mental health problems is confirmed. Rutter, Tizard, and Whitmore (1970) found the highest rate of conduct and emotional problems among children with disorders affecting brain functioning and only a moderate increase in risk associated with non-neurologic disorders. In the Ontario Child Health Study, Cadman et al. (1987) found moderately increased risk for psychological problems associated with a chronic disorder of any type, rising to a higher risk of problems (three- to fourfold) if the disorder was disabling, as well as chronic. These investigators did not distinguish between brain and other disorders, so their findings are not directly comparable with those of Rutter, Tizard, and Whitmore (1970). There is little evidence that specific physical conditions are associated with specific psychiatric problems, although Conduct disorder is less common among children with disabling chronic illness (Cadman et al., 1987).

The epidemiology of psychiatric disorders among pediatric clinic attenders has been studied extensively by Costello and colleagues in Pittsburgh (Costello, 1989; Costello et al., 1988b and c). Their prevalence, correlates, and associated risk factors were described in an earlier section. Comparisons in diagnostic sensitivity and specificity between the primary care pediatrician's diagnoses and the research-generated diagnoses, and the implications for referral and management, remain to be discussed (Costello et al., 1988a; Dulcan et al., 1990). In these studies, the pediatrician and research team diagnosed mental health problems among children attending a primary care clinic at the same time, but independently of each other. The prevalence rate for one or more disorders of 22% by the research team was not reflected in either the pediatricians' diagnoses (5.7%) or in their referral rates for mental health evaluation in the previous year (3.6%; Costello et al., 1988b). Children identified as having emotional or behavioral problems by the pediatricians had approximately twice the rate of physical illness episodes as the nondisturbed group and were higher users of health services. This relationship did not hold, however, for the research-team-identified group, who had the same number of physical health visits as the nondisturbed children (Costello et al., 1988a). Pediatricians had a high *specificity* for identifying psychiatric disorder, but a low *sensitivity*. They failed to diagnose a mental health problem in 75% of cases and referred only one in six with disorder for a mental health assessment.

These findings raise the possibility that the reported association between mental health problems and high rates of service use for physical health problems may be partly due to identification and referral bias, at least with children. Primary care physicians, whether pediatricians in North America or family practitioners elsewhere, have a "gatekeeping" role in referring children to mental health services. Thus, it is important to recognize characteristics that may enhance or obstruct diagnosis and appropriate management. Dulcan et al. (1990) found that parental distress, family psychiatric history, and parents expressing their concerns to the primary care physician all enhanced the identification of behavioral and emotional problems in the Pittsburgh study, whereas physician attitudes toward psychological disorders and their willingness to entertain a psychological diagnosis influenced diagnosis and referral. In a study of pediatricians' descriptions of their own diagnostic, treatment, and referral practices for mental health problems, Goldberg et al. (1984) found very similar rates of identification of disorder (5%), with some variation by age, sex, and SES of between 4% and 8%. By contrast, children with chronic physical illnesses were diagnosed as having mental health problems more than twice as often (13%). These discrepancies between physician-identified disorder and community prevalence rates represents hidden morbidity among primary care patients (Costello et al., 1988c). Asking parents routinely about their concerns for their child's mental health may be a simple and effective way of raising diagnostic sensitivity.

Persistence of Disorder

Follow-up studies into adult life have shown that some childhood and adolescent disorders may persist, either in the same form or as a different disorder. Comprehensive reviews of follow-up, follow-back, and high-risk population studies by Rutter (1984; 1985a) have examined early precursors of adult disorder, continuities in personality, and the role of environmental changes in mediating adult disorders.

Adult Schizophrenia

Pre-existing abnormalities in childhood are found in approximately 50% of those who develop schizophrenia as adults, and these abnormalities are more marked if their onset is early (Foerster et al., 1991). Children who later developed schizophrenia were more likely to have poor neurodevelopmental skills (particularly motor skills), poor cognitive skills with attention deficits, and abnormal interpersonal relationships, especially "schizoid" and odd behavior that caused other children to reject them (Foerster et al., 1991; Rutter, 1985a; Werry, 1992). Preschizophrenic children were also more likely to be aggressive, but less likely to be involved in gross delinquent activity with peers and no more likely than other children to be anxious or withdrawn. It seems from these studies that preschizophrenic children were identified as unusual or eccentric in some way by others. These characteristics tended to be more pronounced in adolescence.

Adult and Child Depression and Anxiety Disorders

In contrast, in follow-back studies, adults with depression showed few characteristic behavior patterns as children, although depressed children and adolescents may go on to develop depressive illnesses as adults. These continuities, however, are less strong for depression and other emotional disorders than for conduct disorders or attention deficit disorder (McGee & Williams, 1988; Robins, 1983; Rutter, 1985a). Although most emotional disorder of childhood does not persist, when such children do develop a disorder in adult life, it is likely to be similar in type if not in content to the childhood disorder. Rutter (1985a) concludes that there is insufficient evidence to say if there are any systematic similarities or differences between childhood and adult emotional disorders.

Conduct Disorder and Antisocial Personality

The most persistent childhood disorder is conduct disorder (Loeber, 1991). In an early follow-up study of children seen at a Child Guidance clinic, Robins (1966) found that about half of the children with conduct disorders had persistent problems as adults, mainly in the form of antisocial personality disorders, with characteristic criminality, impaired social relationships, alcohol and drug abuse, and poor employment records (Robins, 1966, 1983; West, 1982). Risk factors that make adult antisocial personality disorder a more likely outcome for conduct-disordered children have been identified as being male, early onset of disorder, pervasive disorder, a high frequency and variety of antisocial behaviors, poor peer relationships, associated attention deficits, and continuing family dysfunction, particularly harsh, nonaffectionate parenting and parental criminality (Farrington, 1986; Robins, 1983).

Attention Deficit Disorder

The long-term outcome for children with ADHD has been studied by Weiss and colleagues, who followed a group of hyperactive boys into adult life (Weiss et al., 1978). These studies showed a diminution of hyperactivity after adolescence, but the continuation of inattention, impulsiveness, and academic problems despite treatment. Although the inattention and impulse control problems remain, most young adults find work within their attention span and maintain good employment records (Hechtman & Weiss, 1983; Hechtman et al., 1984; Weiss et al., 1978, 1979). Remaining problems include low self-esteem, more frequent traffic accidents, more moves and changes of job, but fewer antisocial or criminal problems unless the ADHD was associated with conduct disorder. Treatment in childhood seemed to improve the young adult's social skills compared to untreated young adults with a history of ADHD. Klein and Mannuzza's review (1991) concludes similarly, but reports somewhat higher rates of serious conduct disorder and drug abuse. This finding may be due to higher rates of both in the United States as a whole.

Autism

This rare and serious disorder of childhood persists into adult life, although there is usually some improvement in language skills, social interaction, and loss of rituals during adolescence for those who acquired language by 5 years of age. As adults they remain impaired in their ability to process information concerned with affect or social interactions and appear odd, eccentric, or isolated (Rutter, 1985b).

Mechanisms of Continuity

Mechanisms postulated to account for both continuities and discontinuities between childhood and adult disorders have been examined by Rutter (1984, 1985a). The role of development in the discontinuity of maladaptive behavior is recognized, as old patterns of behavior may become incompatible with newer cognitive skills or physical maturity. Further, environmental disadvantages may improve with time, reducing stress on the child or adolescent. Continuities of disorder do not follow a rigid or unvarying pattern because the child or adolescent continues to develop and interact with the environment. Changes in behavior patterns may act to elicit environmental responses from parents or teachers that can either enhance or reduce the maladaptive behaviors and limit or open up later opportunities for the child, particularly in education and employment or social interactions.

Rutter (1985a) has demonstrated how diverse disadvantages, such as losing a parent at a young age, being brought up in institutional care, or developing aggressive defiant behavior, can all set up cycles of interaction that may make the child more vulnerable to adult disorders, regardless of early mental health. Such vulnerability may require later psychological or social stress to precipitate an adult disorder. Patterson (1976) has also described how aggressive children may provoke maladaptive responses to their behavior from parents, precipitating escalating cycles of hostility between parent and child, referred to as "coercive spirals." Such behavior and response patterns become self-perpetuating, so that even when the original stimuli for the aggressive behavior have disappeared, the interactions continue unabated, perpetuating the worsening aggression. Similarly, anxious and overprotective responses to children's fears can, in themselves, escalate and prolong patterns of anxious and phobic behavior in children. These patterns may continue into adult life if a fearful view of the world as a dangerous and hostile place persists.

In such situations it is difficult to untangle the genetic, constitutional, and environmental components in the persistence of maladaptive behavior. Further indirect mechanisms in setting up vulnerability may be via the effect on self-concept, self-esteem, or the developing view of oneself as an active agent for change.

Recent interest in the long-term sequelae of childhood sexual abuse has arisen from the findings of poorer adult mental health (particularly anxiety and depressive disorders) among women sexually abused as children, compared to nonabused women, in general population studies. It is likely that the mechanisms for poorer adult outcome among abused children include the sense of powerlessness they experience and the damage to their self-esteem and their capacity to trust. Such damage may well lead to a poor choice of partners, poor educational achievement, and early unplanned pregnancies, each of which limits later opportunities for these women. The abuse experience acts not only as a direct trauma but also as a vulnerability factor, setting up later stresses and failures for the victim (Browne & Finkelhor, 1986; Finkelhor, 1984; Mullen, 1989; Mullen et al., 1988).

Labeling, either directly as in young persons adjudicated "delinquent" or "retarded" or indirectly, as occurs when a child is consistently seen as incompetent, bad, or inadequate in meeting normal challenges, may also set up adverse situations in later life through poor self-image, poor choices, and an external locus of control. It may result in exposure to the adverse social, occupational and interpersonal situations associated with higher risk of adult mental illness. Conversely, an improvement in self-esteem, establishing supportive social networks, and a good choice of partner can all protect a vulnerable adult from developing disorder. It is clear that the mechanisms for both continuity and discontinuity of disorder are complex and interactive and involve genetic, temperament, constitutional, family, social, and intrapsychic factors.

Conclusions

First, there is now a significant body of good research in the epidemiology of children's behavior and emotional disorders and problems.

Second, the field is still bedeviled by serious methodologic problems common to all psychiatry, stemming from a lack of coherent theory, imperfectly validated diagnostic entities, and disagreements among parents, children, teachers, and professionals as to who is sick or needs care.

Third, even so, certain trends are discernible. Cases are relatively common, especially among those with health problems, but are often missed by primary care physicians, although most cases are mild in degree.

Fourth, most problems come and go without treatment, but there is a core of persistent, disabling disorders—notably conduct disorder, multiple disorders, autism, and child schizophrenia—that merit special attention.

Fifth, like other child health problems, psychiatric disorders are most common among those disadvantaged by urban living, lower social class, family adversity, and male gender. Unfortunately, these children are least likely to receive help.

Sixth, the epidemiology of emotional and behavior problems in children is a complex area, not one for amateurs. As such, it requires skills in epidemiology, taxonomy, psychometrics, and psychiatry. Obtaining such skills requires specialized training in specialized centers with appropriate incentives for those who choose this tortuous path.

Seventh, there is a sufficient link between some child and serious adult disorders to warrant investment of considerable research funds to analyze this link and how to influence it. The economic and social benefit of such systematic knowledge could be inestimable.

References

Achenbach TM. DSM-III in light of empirical research on the classification of child psychopathology. *J Am Acad Child Psychiatry* 1980; 19:395–412.

Achenbach TM. The role of taxonomy in developmental psychopathology. In: Lamb ME, Brown AL, eds. *Advances in Developmental Psychology*. Vol 1. New Jersey: Lawrence Erlbaum; 1981: 159–198.

Achenbach TM, Edelbrock CS. The classification of child psychopathology: a review and analysis of empirical efforts. *Psychol Bull* 1978; 85:1275–1301.

Achenbach TM, Edelbrock CS. *Manual for the Child Behavior Checklist and Revised Child Behavior Profile*. Burlington, VT: University of Vermont; 1983.

Achenbach TM, Edelbrock CS. *Manual for the Teacher Report Form and Teacher Version of the Child Behavior Profile*. Burlington, VT: University of Vermont; 1986.

Achenbach TM, Edelbrock CS. *Manual for the Youth Self-Report and Profile*. Burlington, VT: University of Vermont; 1987.

Achenbach TM, Conners CK, Quay HC. *The ACQ Behavior Checklist*. Burlington, VT: University of Vermont; 1983.

Achenbach TM, Verhulst FC, Baron GD, Akkerhuis GW. Epidemiological comparisons of American and Dutch children: I. Behavioral/emotional problems and competencies reported by parents for ages 4 to 16. *J Am Acad Child Adolesc Psychiatry* 1987a; 26:317–325.

Achenbach TM, Verhulst FC, Edelbrock C, Baron GD, Akkerhuis GW. Epidemiological comparisons of American and Dutch children: II. Behavioral/emotional problems and competencies reported by teachers for ages 6 to 11. *J Am Acad Child Adolesc Psychiatry* 1987b; 26:326–332.

Achenbach TM, McConaughy SH, Howell CT. Child/adolescent behavioral and emotional problems: implications of cross-informant correlations for situational specificity. *Psychol Bull* 1987c; 101:213–232.

Achenbach TM, Conners CK, Quay HC, Verhulst FC, Howell CT. Replication of empirically derived syndromes as a basis for taxonomy of child/adolescent psychopathology. *J Abnorm Child Psychol* 1989; 17:299–323.

Achenbach TM, Bird HR, Canino G, Phares V, Gould MS, Rubio-Stipec M. Epidemiological comparisons of Puerto Rican and U.S. Mainland children: Parent, teacher and self-reports. *J Am Acad Child Adolesc Psychiatry* 1990a; 29:84–93.

Achenbach TM, Hensley VR, Phares V, Grayson D. Problems and competencies reported by parents of Australian and American children. *J Child Psychol Psychiatry* 1990b; 31:265–286.

American Psychiatric Association. *Diagnostic and Statistical Manual of Mental Disorders (DSM-III)*. 3rd ed. Washington, DC: American Psychiatric Association; 1980.

American Psychiatric Association. *Diagnostic and Statistical Manual of Mental Disorders (DSM-III)*. 3rd ed. Washington, DC: American Psychiatric Association; 1987.

Anderson JC, Williams S, McGee R, Silva P. DSM-III disorders in preadolescent children: prevalence in a large sample from the general population. *Arch Gen Psychiatry* 1987; 44:69–76.

Anderson JC, Williams SM, McGee RO, Silva P. Cognitive and social correlates of DSM III disorders in pre-adolescent children. *J Am Acad Child Adolesc Psychiatry* 1989; 28:842–846.

Beck S, Collins L, Overhoser J, Terry K. A comparison to children who receive and who do not receive permission to participate in research. *J Abnorm Child Psychol* 1984; 12:573–580.

Biederman J, Newcorn J, Sprich S. Comorbidity of attention deficit hyperactivity disorder with conduct, depressive, anxiety, and other disorders. *Am J Psychiatry* 1991; 148:564–557.

Bird H, Canino G, Rubio-Stipec M, Gould MS, Ribera J, Sesman M, Woodbury M, Heurtas-Goldman S, Pagan A, Sanchez-Lacay A, Moscoso M. Estimates of the prevalence of childhood maladjustment in a community survey in Puerto Rico: the use of combined measures. *Arch Gen Psychiatry* 1988; 45:1120–1126.

Bird HR, Gould MS, Yager T, Staghezza B, Canino G. Risk factors for maladjustment in Puerto Rican children. *J Am Acad Child Adolesc Psychiatry* 1989; 28:847–850.

Blashfield RK, Draguns JG. Toward a taxonomy of psychopathology: the purpose of psychiatric classification. *Br J Psychiatry* 1976; 129:574–583.

Boyle MH, Jones SC. Selecting measures of emotional and behavioral disorders of childhood for use in general populations. *J Child Psychol Psychiatry* 1985; 26:137–159.

Boyle MH, Offord DR, Hofmann HG, Catlin GP, Byles JA, Cadman DT, Crawford JW, Links PS, Rae-Grant NI, Szatmari P. Ontario child health study: I. methodology. *Arch Gen Psychiatry* 1987; 44:826–831.

Breslau NZ. Chronic physical illness. In: Tonge B, Burrows G, Werry JS, eds. *Handbook of Studies on Child Psychiatry*. Amsterdam: Elsevier; 1990: 371–384.

Browne A, Finkelhor D. Impact of child sexual abuse: a review of the research. *Psychol Bull* 1986; 99:66–77.

Cadman D, Boyle M, Szatmari P, Offord DR. Chronic Illness, disability and mental and social well-being: findings of the Ontario child health study. *Pediatrics* 1987; 79:805–813.

Campbell SB, Ewing LJ. Follow-up of hard-to-manage preschoolers: adjustment at age 9 and predictors of continuing symptoms. *J Child Psychol Psychiatry* 1990; 31:871–889.

Cantwell DP. The diagnostic process and diagnostic classification in child psychiatry—DSM III. *J Am Acad Child Psychiatry* 1980; 19:345–355.

Cantwell DP, Baker L. Stability and natural history of DSM-III childhood diagnoses. *J Am Acad Child Adolesc Psychiatry* 1989; 28:691–700.

Carlson G, Cantwell DP. A survey of depressive symptoms, syndrome and disorder in a child psychiatric population. *J Child Psychol Psychiatry* 1980; 21:19–25.

Caron C, Rutter M. Comorbidity in child psychopathology: concepts, issues and research strategies. *J Child Psychol Psychiatry* 1991; 32:1063–1080.

Cohen P, Brook J. Family factors related to the persistence of psychopathology in childhood and adolescence. *Psychiatry* 1987; 50:332–345.

Cohen P, Velez CN, Garcia, M. The epidemiology of childhood depression. Presented at the Annual Meeting of the American Academy of Child Psychiatry; October 1985; San Antonio, TX.

Cohen P, Velez CN, Kohn M, et al. Child psychiatric diagnosis by computer algorithm: theoretical issues and empirical tests. *J Am Acad Child Adolesc Psychiatry* 1987; 26:631–638.

Connell HM, Irvine L, Rodney J. The prevalence of psychiatric disorder in rural school children. *Aust NZ J Psychiatry* 1982; 16:43–46.

Costello EJ. Developments in child psychiatric epidemiology. *J Am Acad Child Adolesc Psychiatry* 1989; 28:836–841.

Costello EJ, Burns BJ, Costello AJ, Edelbrock C, Dulcan M, Brent D. Service utilization and psychiatric diagnosis in pediatric primary care: the role of the gatekeeper. *Pediatrics* 1988a; 82:435–441.

Costello EJ, Costello AJ, Edelbrock CS, Burns BJ, Dulcan MJ, Brent D, Janiszewski S. DSM-III disorders in pediatric primary care: prevalence and risk factors. *Arch Gen Psychiatry* 1988b; 45:1107–1116.

Costello EJ, Edelbrock CS, Costello AJ, Dulcan MK, Burns BJ, Brent D. Psychopathology in pediatric primary care: the new hidden morbidity. *Pediatrics* 1988c; 82:415–424.

Cox A, Rutter M, Yule B, Quinton D. Bias arising from missing information: some epidemiological findings. *Br J Prev Soc Med* 1977; 31:131–136.

Dulcan MK, Costello EJ, Costello AJ, Edelbrock C, Brent D, Janiszewski S. The pediatrician as gatekeeper to mental health care for children: do parents' concerns open the gate? *J Am Acad Child Adolesc Psychiatry* 1990; 29:453–458.

Earls F. The prevalence of behavior problems in 3-year-old children. Comparison of the reports of fathers and mothers. *J Am Acad Child Psychiatry* 1980a; 19:439–452.

Earls F. Prevalence of behavior problems in 3-year-old children: a cross-national replication. *Arch Gen Psychiatry* 1980b; 37:1153–1157.

Edelbrock C, Achenbach TM. A typology of child behavior profile patterns: distribution and correlates for disturbed children aged 6–16. *J Abnorm Child Psychol* 1980; 8:441–470.

Edelbrock C, Costello A. Structured psychiatric interviews for children. In: Rutter M, Tuma A, Lann I, eds. *Assessment and Diagnosis in Child Psychopathology*. London: Guilford Press; 1988: 87–112.

Edelbrock C, Costello AJ, Dulcan MK, Kalas R, Conover MC. Age differences in the reliability of the psychiatric interview of the child. *Child Dev* 1985; 56:265–275.

Edelbrock C, Costello AJ, Dulcan MK, Conover MC, Kalas R. Parent-child agreement on child psychiatric symptoms assessed via structured interviews. *J Child Psychol Psychiatry* 1986; 27:181–190.

Esser G, Schmidt MH, Woerner W. Epidemiology and course of psychiatric disorders in school-age children: results of a longitudinal study. *J Child Psychol Psychiatry* 1990; 1:243–263.

Farrington DP. The socio-cultural context of childhood disorders. In: Quay HC, Werry JS, eds. *Psychopathological Disorders of Childhood.* 3rd ed. New York: John Wiley and Son; 1986: 391–422.

Finkelhor D. Long term effects of childhood sexual abuse. In: Finkelhor D, ed. *Child Sexual Abuse.* New York: The Free Press, 1984: 188–199.

Fleming JE, Offord DR. Epidemiology of childhood depressive disorders: a critical review. *J Am Acad Child Adolesc Psychiatry* 1990; 29:571–580.

Foerster A, Lewis S, Owen M, Murray R. Premorbid adjustment and personality in psychoses: effects of sex and diagnosis. *Br J Psychiatry* 1991; 158:171–176.

Gillberg C. The neurobiology of infantile autism. *J Child Psychol Psychiatry* 1988; 29:257–266.

Goldberg ID, Roghmann KJ, McInerny TK, Burke JD. Mental health problems among children seen in pediatric practice: prevalence and management. *Pediatrics* 1984; 73:278–293.

Gould M, Shaffer D, Rutter M, Sturge C. UK/WHO study of ICD 9. In: Rutter M, Tuma A, Lann I, eds. *Assessment and Diagnosis in Child Psychopathology.* London: Guilford Press; 1988: 37–65.

Graham P. *Epidemiological Approaches in Child Psychiatry.* London: Academic Press; 1977.

Graham P. Epidemiological studies. In: Quay HC, Werry JS, eds. *Psychopathological Disorders of Childhood.* 2nd ed. New York: John Wiley and Sons; 1979: 185–209.

Graham P, Rutter M. Psychiatric disorder in young adolescents: a follow-up study. *Proc Roy Soc Med* 1973; 66:1226–1229.

Hechtman L, Weiss G. Long term outcome of hyperactive children. *Am J Orthopsychiatry* 1983; 53:532–541.

Hechtman L, Weiss G, Perlamn T, Amsel R. Hyperactive as young adults: initial predictors of adult outcome. *J Am Acad Child Psychiatry* 1984; 23:25–260.

Herjanic B, Reich W. Development of a structured psychiatric interview for children: agreement between child and parent on individual symptoms. *J Abnorm Child Psychol* 1982; 10:307–324.

Herjanic B, Herjanic M, Brown F, Wheatt T. Are children reliable reporters? *J Abnormal Child Psychol* 1975; 3:41–48.

Hewitt LE, Jenkins RL. *Fundamental Patterns of Maladjustment. The Dynamics of Their Origin.* Springfield, IL: State of Illinois; 1946.

Jenkins RL. Psychiatric syndromes in children and their relation to family background. *Am J Orthopsychiatry* 1966; 36:450–457.

Jensen PS, Bloedau L, Degroot J, Ussery T, Davis H. Children at risk: I. Risk factors and child symptomatology. *J Am Acad Child Adolesc Psychiatry* 1990; 29:51–59.

Kanner L. Autistic disturbances of affective contact. *Nerv Child* 1943; 2:217–250.

Kastrup M. Psychic disorders among preschool children in a geographically delimited area of Aarhus county, Denmark. *Acta Psychiatr Scand* 1976; 54:29–42.

Kendell RE. *The Role of Diagnosis in Psychiatry.* Oxford: Blackwell; 1975.

Klein R, Mannuza S. Long-term outcome of hyperactive children: a review. *J Am Acad Child Adolesc Psychiatry* 1991; 30:283–287.

Kleinman A. Anthropology and psychiatry. The role of culture in cross-cultural research on illness. *Br J Psychiatry* 1987; 151:447–454.

Kovacs M, Feinberg TL, Crouse-Novak MA, Paulauskas SL, Finkelstein R. Depressive disorders in childhood I. *Arch Gen Psychiatry* 1984; 41:229–237.

La Greca AM, Quay HC. Behavior disorders of children. In: Endler NS, Hunt J McV, eds. *Personality and the Behavior Disorders.* 2nd ed. New York: Wiley; 1984.

Lahey BB, Green KD, Forehand R. On the independence of ratings of hyperactivity, conduct problems and attention deficits in children: a multiple regression analysis. *J Consult Clin Psychol* 1980; 48:566–574.

Lahey BB, Loeber R, Stouthamer-Loeber M, Christ MG, Green S, Russo MF, Frick PJ, Dulcan M. Comparison of DSM-III and DSM-III-R diagnoses for prepubertal children: changes in prevalence and validity. *J Am Acad Child Adolesc Psychiatry* 1990; 29:620–626.

Links PS. Community surveys of the prevalence of childhood psychiatric disorders: a review. *Child Dev* 1983; 54:531–548.

Littlewood R. From categories to contexts: A decade of the "new cross-cultural psychiatry." *Br J Psychiatry* 1990; 156:308–327.

Loeber R. Antisocial behaviour: More enduring than changeable. *J Am Acad Child Adolesc Psychiatry* 1991; 30:393–397.

Loney J, Langhorne JE, Paternite CE. An empirical basis for subgrouping the hyperkinetic/minimal brain dysfunction syndrome. *J Abnorm Psychol* 1978; 87:431–441.

Lucas AR, Beard CM, O'Fallon WM, Kurland LT. 50 year trends in the incidence of anorexia nervosa in Rochester, Minn: a population-based study. *Am J Psychiatry* 1991; 148:917–922.

Luk SL, Leung PWL, Bacon-Shone J, Chung SY, Lee PWH, Chen S, Ng R, Lieh-Mak F, Ko L, Wong VCN, Yeung CY. Behaviour disorder in preschool children in Hong Kong—a two-stage epidemiological study. *Br J Psychiatry* 1991; 158:213–221.

Maxwell AE. Multivariate statistical methods and classification problems. *Br J Psychiatry* 1971; 119:121–127.

Maxwell AE. Difficulties in a dimensional description of symptomatology. *Br J Psychiatry* 1972; 21:19–26.

McGee R, Williams S. A longitudinal study of depression in nine year old children. *J Am Acad Child Adolesc Psychiatry* 1988; 27:342–348.

McGee R, Silva P, Williams S. Behaviour problems in a population of seven year old children: prevalence, stability and types of disorder. *J Child Psychol Psychiatry* 1984a; 25:251–259.

McGee R, Williams S, Silva P. Background characteristics of aggressive, hyperactive and aggressive-hyperactive boys. *J Am Acad Child Psychiatry* 1984b; 23:180–284.

McGee R, Williams S, Silva P. Behavioural and developmental characteristics of aggressive, hyperactive and aggressive-hyperactive boys. *J Am Child Psychiatry* 1984c; 23:270–279.

McGee R, Wiliams S, Silva P. The factor structure and correlates of ratings of inattention, hyperactivity and antisocial behaviour. *J Consult Clin Psychol* 1985; 53:480–490.

McGee R, Feehan M, Williams S, et al. The prevalence of DSM-III disorders in a large sample of adolescents. *J Am Acad Child Adolesc Psychiatry* 1990; 29:611–619.

McGee RO, Feehan M, Williams SM, Anderson JC: Mental health from age 11 to age 15. *J Am Acad Child Adolesc Psychiatry* 1992; 31:50–59.

Milich R, Loney J, Landau S. Independent dimensions of hyperactivity and aggression. A validation with playroom observation data. *J Abnorm Psychol* 1982; 91:183–198.

Miller FJW, Court SDM, Knox EG, Brandon S. *The School Years in Newcastle on Tyne.* London: Oxford University Press; 1974.

Mullen PE. The long-term influence of sexual assault on the mental health of victims. *J Forensic Psychiatry* 1989; 1:13–34.

Mullen PE, Romans-Clarkson SE, Walton VA, Herbison GP. Impact of sexual and physical abuse on women's mental health. *Lancet* 1988; 1:841–845.

Nurcombe B, Seifer R, Sciolo A, Tramontana MG, Grapentine WL, Beauchesne HC.

Is major depressive disorder in adolescence a distinct diagnostic entity? *J Am Acad Child Adolesc Psychiatry* 1989; 28:333–342.

Offord DR. Social factors in the aetiology of childhood psychiatric disorders. In: Tonge B, Burrows G, Werry JS, eds. *Handbook of Studies on Child Psychiatry*. Amsterdam: Elsevier; 1990: 55–68.

Offord DR, Fleming JE. Epidemiology. In: Lewis M, ed. *Child and Adolescent Psychiatry*. Baltimore: Williams & Wilkins; 1991: 1156–1168.

Offord DR, Boyle MH, Szatmari P, Rae-Grant NI, Links PS, Cadman DT, Byles JA, Crawford JW, Munroe Blum H, Byrne C, Thomas H, Woodward C. Ontario child health study: II. Six-month prevalence of disorder and rates of service utilization. *Arch Gen Psychiatry* 1987a; 44:832–836.

Offord DR, Boyle MH, Jones BR. Psychiatric disorder and poor school performance among welfare children in Ontario. *Can J Psychiatry* 1987b; 32:518–525.

Offord DR, Boyle MH, Racine Y. Ontario child health study: correlates of disorder. *J Am Acad Child Adolesc Psychiatry* 1989; 28:856–860.

Offord DR, Boyle MH, Racine YA, Fleming JE, Cadman DT, Monroe-Blum H, Byrne C, Links PS, Lipman EL, MacMillan HL, Rae-Grant NI, Sanford MN, Szatmari P, Thomas H, Woodward CA. Outcome, prognosis and risk in a longitudinal follow-up study. *J Am Acad Child Adolesc Psychiatry* 1992; 31:916–923.

Orvaschel H, Walsh G. *The Assessment of Adaptive Functioning in Children: A Review of Existing Measures Suitable for Epidemiological and Clinical Services Research*. Washington, DC: US Government Printing Office; 1984.

Orvaschel H, Sholomskas D, Weissman M. *The Assessment of Psychopathology and Behavioral Problems in Children: A Review of Scales Suitable for Epidemiological and Clinical Research*. Washington, DC: US Government Printing Office; 1983.

Pataki CS, Carlson GA. Affective disorders in children and adolescents. In: Tonge B, Burrows G, Werry J, eds. *Handbook of Studies on Child Psychiatry*. Amsterdam: Elsevier; 1990: 137–160.

Patterson GR. The aggressive child: victim and architect of a coercive system. In: Mash E, Hamerlynck L, Hardy L, eds. *Behaviour Modification in Families*. New York: Brunner/Mazel; 1976: 267–316.

Prendergast M, Taylor E, Rapoport JL, Bartko J, Donnelly M, Zametkin A, Ahearn MB, Dunn G, Wieselberg HM. The diagnosis of childhood hyperactivity. A U.S.-U.K. cross-national study of DSM-III and ICD-9. *J Child Psychol Psychiatry* 1988; 29:289–300.

Pringle MLK, Butler NR, Davie R. *11,000 Seven Year-Olds*. London: Longman; 1966.

Prior M, Werry JS. Autism, schizophrenia, and allied disorders. In: Quay HC, Werry JS, eds. *Psychopathology Disorders of Childhood*. 3rd ed. New York: Wiley and Sons; 1986: 156–210.

Puig-Antich J. Major depression and conduct disorder in prepuberty. *J Am Acad Child Psychiatry* 1982; 21:118–128.

Quay HC. Classification. In: Quay HC, Werry JS, eds. *Psychopathological Disorders of Childhood*. 2nd ed. New York: Wiley and Sons; 1979: 1–42.

Quay HC. Classification. In: Quay HC, Werry JS, eds. *Psychopathological Disorders of Childhood*. 3rd ed. New York: Wiley and Sons; 1986: 1–34.

Quay HC, La Greca AM. Disorders of anxiety withdrawal and dysphoria. In: Quay HC, Werry JS, eds. *Psychopathological Disorders of Childhood*. 3rd ed. New York: Wiley and Sons; 1986: 232–293.

Rae-Grant N, Thomas BH, Offord DR, Boyle MH. Risk, protective factors, and the prevalence of behavioral and emotional disorders in children and adolescents. *J Am Acad Child Adolesc Psychiatry* 1989; 28:262–268.

Rapoport JL. Annotation: childhood obsessive compulsive disorder. *J Child Psychol Psychiatry* 1986; 27:289–295.

Reeves J, Werry J, Elkind G, Zametkin A. Attention deficit, conduct, oppositional and anxiety disorders in children: II. Clinical characteristics. *J Am Acad Child Psychiatry* 1987; 6:144–155.

Reich W, Herjanic B, Welner Z, Gandhy P. Development of a structured psychiatric interview for children: agreement on diagnosis comparing child and parent interviews. *J Abnorm Child Psychol* 1982; 10:325–336.

Richman N. Disorders in pre-school children. In: Rutter M, Hersov L, eds. *Child and Adolescent Psychiatry*. London: Blackwell; 1985: 336–350.

Richman N, Stevenson JE, Graham PJ. Prevalence of behaviour problems in 3-year-old children: an epidemiological study in a London borough. *J Child Psychol Psychiatry* 1975; 16:277–287.

Richman N, Stevenson JE, Graham PJ. *Preschool to School: A Behavioural Study*. London: Academic Press; 1982.

Robins L. *Deviant Children Grown Up*. Baltimore: Williams & Wilkins; 1966.

Robins L. Continuities and discontinuities in the psychiatric disorders of children. In: Mechanic D, ed. *Handbook of Health, Health Care and the Health Professions*. New York: The Free Press; 1983: 195–219.

Rosen BM, Bahn AK, Kramer M. Demographic and diagnostic characteristics of psychiatric clinic outpatients in the USA, 1961. *Am J Orthopsychiatry* 1964; 34:455–468.

Ross DM, Ross SA. *Hyperactivity, Current Issues, Research and Theory*. 2nd ed. New York: John Wiley and Sons; 1982.

Rutter M. Classification and categorisation in child psychiatry. *J Child Psychol Psychiatry* 1965; 6:71–83.

Rutter M. Syndromes attributed to "Minimal Brain Dysfunction" in childhood. *Am J Psychiatry* 1982; 139:21–33.

Rutter M. Psychopathology and development: 1. Childhood antecedents of adult psychiatric disorder. *Aust NZ J Psychiatry* 1984; 18:225–234.

Rutter M. Psychopathology and development: links between childhood and adult life. In: Rutter M, Hersov L, eds. *Child and Adolescent Psychiatry*. London: Blackwell; 1985a: 20–739.

Rutter M. Infantile autism and other pervasive developmental disorders. In: Rutter M, Hersov L, eds. *Child and Adolescent Psychiatry*. London: Blackwell; 1985b: 545–566.

Rutter M. Isle of Wight revisited: twenty-five years of child psychiatric epidemiology. *J Am Acad Child Adolesc Psychiatry* 1989; 28:633–653.

Rutter M, Tizard J, Whitmore K. *Education, Health and Behaviour*. London: Longmore Inc; 1970.

Rutter M, Cox A, Tupling C, Berger M, Yule W. Attainment and adjustment in two geographical areas 1. *Br J Psychiatry* 1975a; 126:493–509.

Rutter M, Shaffer D, Shepherd M. *A Multiaxial Classification of Child Psychiatric Disorders*. Geneva: WHO; 1975b.

Rutter M, Tuma A, Lamm I, eds. *Assessment and Diagnosis in Child Psychopathology*. London: Guilford Press; 1988.

Schachar R, Wachsmuth R. Oppositional disorder in children: a validation study comparing conduct disorder and normal children. *J Child Psychol Psychiatry* 1990; 31:1089–1102.

Schwartz-Gould M, Wunsch-Hitzig R, Dohrenwendt B. Estimating the prevalence of childhood psychopathology. A critical review. *J Am Acad Child Psychiatry* 1981; 20:462–476.

Seifer R, Nurcombe B, Sciolo A, Grapentine WL. Is major depressive disorder in childhood a distinct diagnostic entity? *J Am Acad Child Adolesc Psychiatry* 1989; 28:935–941.

Skinner HA. Toward the integration of classification theory and methods. *J Abnorm Child Psychol* 1981; 90:68–87.

Steffenburg S. Neuropsychiatric assessment of children with autism: a population-based study. *Dev Med Child Neurol* 1991; 33:495–511.

Structured diagnostic interviews for children and adolescents. *J Am Acad Child Adolesc Psychiatry* 1987; 26:611–675.

Szatmari P, Boyle M, Offord D. Attention deficit disorder with hyperactivity and conduct disorder: degree of diagnostic overlap and differences among correlates. *J Am Acad Child Adolesc Psychiatry* 1989; 30:865–872.

Taylor E, Schachar R, Thorley G, Wieselberg M. Conduct disorder and hyperactivity: I. Separation of hyperactivity and antisocial conduct in British child psychiatric patients. *Br J Psychiatry* 1986; 149:760–777.

Velez CM, Johnson J, Cohen P. A longitudinal analysis of selected risk factors for childhood psychopathology. *J Am Acad Child Adolesc Psychiatry* 1989; 28:861–864.

Verhulst FC, Berden GFM, Sanders-Woudstra JAR. Mental health in Dutch Children: II. The prevalence of psychiatric disorder and relationship between measures. *Acta Psychiatr Scand* 1985; 72(suppl):1–45.

Verhulst FC, Koot HM, Berden GFMG. Four year follow-up of an epidemiological sample. *J Am Acad Child Adolesc Psychiatry* 1990; 29:440–448.

Vikan A. Psychiatric epidemiology in a sample of 1510 ten-year-old children: I. Prevalence. *J Child Psychol Psychiatry* 1985; 26:55–75.

Weiss G, Hechtman L, Perlman T. Hyperactives as young adults: school, employer and self-rating scales obtained during ten-year follow-up evaluation. *Am J Orthopsychiatry* 1978; 8:438–445.

Weiss G, Hechtman L, Perlman T, Hopkins J, Wener A. Hyperactivity in young adults. *Arch Gen Psychiatry* 1979; 36:675–681.

Weisz JR, Suwanlert S, Chaiyasit W, Weiss B, Achenbach TM, Walter BR. Epidemiology of behavioral and emotional problems among Thai and American children: parent reports from ages 6 to 11. *J Am Acad Child Adolesc Psychiatry* 1987; 26:890–897.

Weisz JR, Suwanlert S, Chaiyasit W, Weiss B, Achenbach TM, Trevathan D. Epidemiology of behavioral and emotional problems among Thai and American children: teacher reports from ages 6 to 11. *J Child Psychol Psychiatry* 1989; 30:471–484.

Werner EE. Protective factors and individual resilience. In: Meisels SJ, Shonkoff JP, eds. *Handbook of Early Childhood Intervention*. New York: Cambridge University Press; 1990; 97–116.

Werner EE, Smith RS. *Kauai's Children Come of Age*. Honolulu: University Press of Hawaii; 1977.

Werner EE, Smith RS. An epidemiologic perspective on some antecedents and consequences of childhood mental health problems and learning disabilities. *J Am Acad Child Psychiatry* 1979; 18:292–306.

Werner EE, Smith RS. *Vulnerable but Invincible*. New York: McGraw-Hill; 1982.

Werry JS. ICD 9 and DSM-III: classification for the clinician. *J Child Psychol Psychiatry* 1985; 26:1–6.

Werry JS. Physical illnesses, symptoms and allied disorders. In: Quay HC, Werry JS, eds. *Psychopathological Disorders of Childhood*. 3rd ed. New York: Wiley and Sons; 1986: 232–293.

Werry JS. Classification and epidemiology. In: Tonge B, Burrows G, Werry JS, eds. *Handbook of Studies on Child Psychiatry*. Amsterdam: Elsevier; 1990: 71–82.

Werry JS. Overanxious disorder: a taxonomic review. *J Am Acad Child Adolesc Psychiatry* 1991; 30:533–544.

Werry JS. Child and adolescent schizophrenia: a review in the light of DSM-III-R. *J Autism Dev Disord* 1992; 22:601–604.

Werry JS, Methven RJ, Fitzpatrick J, Dixon H. The inter-rater reliability of DSM-III in children. *J Abnorm Child Psychol* 1983; 11:341–354.

Werry JS, Reeves J, Elkind G. Attention deficit, conduct, oppositional and anxiety disorders in children: 1. A review of research on differentiating characteristics. *J Am Acad Child Adolesc Psychiatry* 1987; 26:133–143.

West DJ. *Delinquency—Its Roots, Careers, and Prospects*. Heinemann: London; 1982.

Williams S, McGee R, Anderson J, Silva PA. The structure and correlates of self-reported symptoms in 11-year-old children. *J Abnorm Child Psychol* 1989; 17:55–71.

Williams SM, Anderson JC, McGee RO, Silva P. Risk factors for behavioral and emotional disorder in pre-adolescent children. *J Am Acad Child Adolesc Psychiatry* 1990; 29:413–419.

Wing JK. Theory testing in psychiatric epidemiology. In: Wing J, Bebbington J, Robins LN, eds. *What is a Case*? London: Grant McIntyre; 1981: 1–8.

Yule W. The epidemiology of child psychopathology. In: Lahey BB, Kazdin AE, eds. *Advances in Clinical Child Psychology*. Vol 4. New York: Plenum Press; 1981: 1–51.

12

Suicide

David Shaffer and Roger Hicks

Although formal definitions of suicide are available, for epidemiologic purposes the most useful definition is an administrative one, i.e., whether or not death has been determined by a medical examiner, coroner or equivalent official to be a self-inflicted and intended death. The definition of attempted suicide, however, varies from study to study. In the work of the authors cited in this chapter, the definition requires that a behavior should have been self-initiated with the intent of causing death, but that, with or without outside intervention, death did not result. In some research on this topic, the terms "gestures" or "parasuicide" are found. These terms are used variably to define either very mild attempts, usually ingestions, or attempts in which the apparent intention was not to cause death, but rather to communicate in some fashion with an important other. In practice, it is difficult to gauge retrospectively the precise motivation of an individual patient. Most adolescents seen in the emergency room will say that they had intended to die, but will then minimize lethal intent when seen weeks or months later.

Epidemiologic methods are well suited to the study of suicide. Suicidal deaths are for the most part readily identifiable, and as a rule countries employ stringent methods to determine and record their occurrence. Investigating the uneven distribution of suicide in different populations provides information about the risk factors and suggests avenues through which it may be prevented.

Three methods have been used to study the epidemiology of suicide. The first method is examination of mortality statistics to identify differences in the suicide rate by age, sex, and nationality to identify both broad secular trends and acute epidemics: case-control studies, sometimes known as the psychological autopsy method, are used to identify the attributable risk of such features as mental illness or family characteristics. Because of the nature of suicide, case-control studies are inevitably retrospective. Third, prospective, controlled, follow-up studies of high-risk groups are conducted to identify the predictive characteristics of those who will go on to commit suicide. Although prospective studies avoid such limitations of retrospective studies as unreliable recall or inadequate knowledge of details that might only have been apparent to clinicians, their potential is limited because suicide is rare even in such high-risk groups as former psychiatric patients or suicide attempters.

Biologic Considerations

Several biologic correlates of suicide have been identified in adult suicides and suicide attempters (see Stanley & Mann, 1987, for a review). The most frequently replicated finding, first reported by Asberg et al. (1976), is the presence of significantly lower concentrations of the serotonin metabolite 5-HIAA in the cerebrospinal fluid of suicide attempters and completers than in age- and sex-matched nonsuicidal controls. These findings have been elaborated and include autoradiographic studies that show a low density of presynaptic serotonin receptors and high concentrations of postsynaptic receptors. There is some evidence that low serotoninergic states are associated with impulsive, labile, and aggressive behavior. These behavior traits may be found in individuals with a variety of different psychiatric disorders, as well as in those with no psychiatric abnormality. Low levels of serotonin metabolites are found in suicides who were schizophrenic, depressed, aggressive, etc., i.e., the neurochemical correlates of suicide seem to be quite independent of diagnosis.

Despite the large number of studies that have reported these abnormalities, several questions remain unanswered. The base rate for the reported abnormalities in representative or even replicable samples of suicide victims, attempters, or controls is not known. However, more surprisingly, the specific behavioral correlates of low serotonin states in suicides have yet to be documented by psychological autopsy techniques.

Patterns of Occurrence

One cannot assume that all suicides are reported accurately. Several investigators have noted potential underreporting (Farberow et al., 1977; Monk, 1987; O'Carroll, 1989). Wilkins (1970) studied deaths among 1311 individuals (all ages) who had contacted a suicide prevention program in Chicago 19 months or more previously. Seventeen had died, but only four of these had been certified as suicides. On reinvestigation, Wilkins concluded that an additional four to eight of the deaths were likely to have been suicides. The findings from this ingenious study are widely quoted as providing evidence for gross underreporting, but other researchers fail to support the phenomenon of underreporting.

It is likely that the possibility of suicide was at least raised during the investigation of many false-negative cases. In such instances the medical examiner or coroner may designate "undetermined whether death is accidental or purposefully inflicted" (*International Classification of Diseases*, 1968 and later versions). Thus, Barraclough (1973) suggests that the true rate is probably closer to the sum of undetermined and suicidal deaths. Shaffer and Fisher (1981) were interested in whether using that total would affect the estimate of the apparently very low rate of suicide in children under 15 years. Although the ratio of undetermined to suicidal deaths was greatest in the younger groups, adding undetermined to actual suicides made very little impact on the overall rate of suicide in the young. Suicide remained rare, and the ethnic and sex proportions were essentially unchanged.

If not designated "undetermined," most false-negative cases are likely to be classified as accidents. Shaffer (1974) reviewed coroners' inquest depositions on a cohort of British children (below age 15) who had died from the most common causes of suicide. Most accidental deaths from asphyxiation and ingestion occurred in the infant and toddler age groups, and therefore it is reasonable to assume that these deaths were not suicidal. Kleck (1988) also examined accidental deaths from firearms, asphyxiation, falling from a height, and ingestion using U.S. national data and estimated that the net undercount was probably no more than 26.5%. This figure was then reduced by accidental deaths that were misclassified as suicides (Littman et al., 1963), leaving, in Kleck's estimation, a net undercount of less than 10%.

Relatively few studies have demonstrated systematic distortion that may arise as a result of variations in ascertainment procedures and idiosyncratic practices among officials responsible for recording cause of death. Ascertainment methods vary both within certain countries, including the United States (Nelson et al., 1978), and between nations, and differences in procedure influence cross-national comparisons (see below). However, it seems likely that these effects are quite limited. Variations within a country have been studied by Sainsbury and Barraclough (1968), who showed that in Great Britain the incidence of suicide within a particular coroner's district was unaffected by a change in the coroner or the staff, such as the police and pathologist, who provide information to the coroner (Barraclough, 1976).

Distortions in suicide rates between countries have been examined by comparing the rank ordering of rates among immigrants in the United States (Sainsbury & Barraclough, 1968) and in Australia (Lester, 1972) with the rates in the immigrants' countries of origin. In both studies the rank ordering was largely similar. One is left to conclude from studies of this kind that idiosyncratic or biased reporting is not an important source of error and that suicide mortality rates are a moderately robust source of information.

Risk Factors

Age

The incidence of suicide varies markedly by age and sex between different countries and within a country between different cultural groups. This is well illustrated in Figure 12.1, which shows variations in incidence by age, gender, and ethnic group within the United States in 1988.

Suicide is uncommon in childhood and early adolescence. Its incidence increases markedly in the late teens and continues to rise until the early twenties. This pattern is remarkably consistent across different countries, as can be seen by the ratio of child to later adolescent suicides in the 25 countries with the highest adolescent suicide rates (Table 12.1).

These incidence data suggest that there are factors that either protect younger children from suicide or enhance risk in older adolescents. Because of the similarity of rates in different countries with quite discrepant cultures, it seems likely

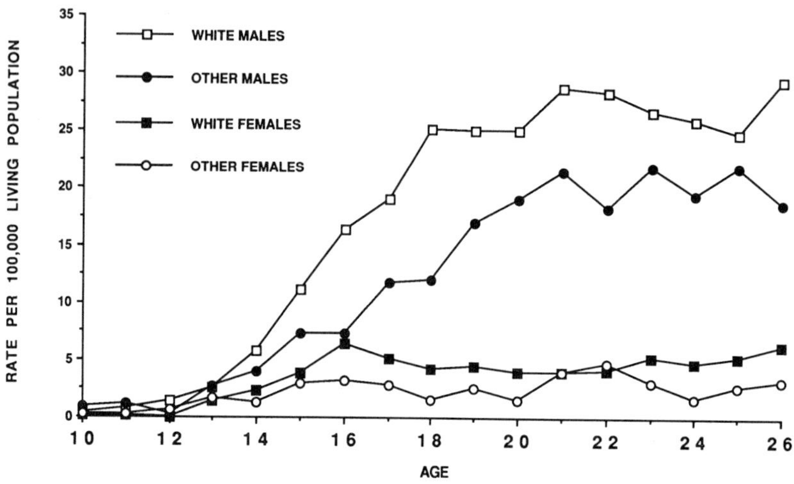

Fig. 12.1. Suicide rate per 100,000 Living Population, ages 10 to 26, 1988. (Data from the National Center for Health Statistics.)

Table 12.1. Countries with the Highest Youth Suicide Rates

Country	Year	Rate per 100,000		Ratio of
		5–14 yrs	15–24 yrs	5–14:15–24
1. Finland	1989	0.46	28.89	0.02
2. Iceland	1990	0.00	26.19	—.—
3. China	1989	0.61	21.30	0.03
4. New Zealand	1987	1.51	19.28	0.08
5. Australia	1988	0.28	16.37	0.02
6. Norway	1989	0.56	16.33	0.03
7. Canada	1989	0.68	15.80	0.04
8. Switzerland	1990	0.52	15.68	0.03
9. Austria	1990	0.33	15.52	0.02
10. Hungary	1990	1.68	14.27	0.12
11. USSR	1990	1.17	13.87	0.08
12. Luxembourg	1989	4.65	13.72	0.34
13. Singapore	1989	0.50	13.61	0.04
14. United States	1988	0.70	13.17	0.05
15. Sweden	1988	0.40	12.17	0.03
16. Trinidad/Tobago	1988	1.52	11.89	0.13
17. Belgium	1986	0.32	10.60	0.03
18. East Germany	1989	0.46	10.32	0.04
19. France	1989	0.43	10.25	0.04
20. Poland	1990	0.60	9.63	0.06
21. Czechoslovakia	1990	0.44	8.47	0.05
22. Yugoslavia	1989	0.75	8.23	0.09
23. South Korea	1987	0.51	8.11	0.06
24. Ireland	1989	0.00	7.97	0.00
25. United Kingdom	1990	0.28	7.23	0.04

Source: Data from World Health Organization. *World Health Statistical Annual*; 1986–1991.

that the age differential is independent of such psychosocial factors as expectations of moral conformity or academic or social success, which almost certainly vary in different countries. It is more likely to be a function of risk factors that appear only in late adolescence, such as the occurrence of depressive illness or the complications of drug and alcohol abuse, or of some universal feature of development.

One aspect of cognitive development that could explain the increase in both suicide and depression is that both are often associated—at least in adults—with hopelessness and despair. In turn, despair and hopelessness involve contemplating the future and finding neither pleasure nor solutions to alternative hypothetical outcomes. Projecting oneself into the future and weighing alternative hypotheses are often regarded as classic features of adolescent thinking, Piaget's "formal operations." An inability to experience hopelessness might therefore be protective. Although this would be a tidy developmental explanation, hopelessness has been reported in depressed children (Kovacs & Beck, 1977).

Another aspect of cognition—the ability to plan the successful execution of a suicide—might also be subject to developmental maturation. Although such methods as hanging may require privacy and planning, most children have some private areas available to them. The methods that are most favored by the young when they threaten suicide, such as jumping from a high place or running into traffic, are effective, readily accessible, and require little if any planning. However, they are rarely used.

Finally, there is a curiously illogical body of literature that suggests that the younger child's concept of the reversibility of death (Freud & Burlingham, 1944; Koocher, 1973; Nagy, 1965) is an important developmental factor. A child who believes that death is reversible will be less inhibited about engaging in suicidal behavior (see Schilder & Wechsler (1934) and McIntire et al. (1972) for reviews). If this were so, suicide should be *more* common in the young, which it is not.

There are, however, certain important conditions—specifically affective illness and alcohol abuse—that operate as risk factors both for adults (Barraclough et al., 1974; Robins et al., 1959) and adolescents (Brent et al., 1989; Gould et al., 1990; Shaffer et al., unpublished data) and that become significantly prevalent only in later adolescence. It seems most likely that these predisposing conditions account for the striking age gradient that is found for suicide.

Gender

In North America, Western Europe, Australia, and New Zealand, suicide is more common in males than in females at all ages except the very young. However, in several countries in Latin America and Asia, sex rates are equal, and, in some, the majority of suicides are committed by women (Barraclough, 1987; Table 12.2).

It is likely that both psychopathologic factors and sex-related method preferences contribute to the pattern of sex differences. Aggressive behavior and substance and alcohol abuse are very significant risk factors for suicide (see below), and both are more common in males than females. However, they can

Table 12.2. Youth Suicide Rates by Sex and Country*

Country	Year	5–14 yr Males	5–14 yr Females	M:F	15–24 yr Males	15–24 yr Females	M:F
1. Iceland	1990	0.0	0.0	—.—	46.7	4.8	9.73
2. Finland	1989	0.9	0.0	—.—	50.4	6.5	7.75
3. Australia	1988	0.5	0.1	5.00	27.8	4.5	6.18
4. United Kingdom	1990	0.1	0.0	—.—	12.2	2.1	5.81
5. Poland	1990	1.0	0.2	5.00	16.2	2.8	5.78
6. Luxembourg	1989	4.6	4.8	0.96	23.0	4.0	5.75
7. Canada	1989	1.0	0.3	3.33	26.4	4.7	5.62
8. Ireland	1989	0.0	0.0	0.00	13.3	2.4	5.54
9. United States	1988	1.0	0.4	2.50	21.9	4.2	5.21
10. Austria	1990	0.2	0.5	0.40	25.0	5.5	4.54
11. New Zealand	1987	2.6	0.4	6.50	31.2	6.9	4.52
12. Norway	1989	0.4	0.8	0.50	25.9	6.2	4.18
13. Switzerland	1990	0.0	1.1	0.00	24.8	6.3	3.94
14. USSR	1990	1.9	0.4	4.75	21.3	6.2	3.43
15. France	1989	0.6	0.2	3.00	15.8	4.6	3.43
16. East Germany	1989	0.9	0.0	—.—	15.5	4.9	3.16
17. Sweden	1988	0.6	0.2	3.00	18.2	5.9	3.08
18. Czechoslovakia	1990	0.6	0.2	3.00	12.2	4.3	2.83
19. Belgium	1986	0.5	0.2	2.50	15.5	5.5	2.82
20. Hungary	1990	2.5	0.8	3.12	20.1	8.2	2.45
21. Yugoslavia	1989	1.0	0.5	2.00	11.5	4.8	2.39
22. Trinidad/Tobago	1988	0.0	3.1	0.00	16.5	7.4	2.23
23. South Korea	1987	0.6	0.4	1.50	10.9	5.2	2.10
24. Singapore	1989	1.0	0.0	—.—	12.8	14.5	0.88
25. China	1989	0.5	0.8	0.62	14.0	29.1	0.48

*All rates/100,000. 25 countries with highest overall youth suicide rate are listed in descending order of 15–24 M:F ratio.

Source: Data from World Health Organization. *World Health Statistic Annual*; 1986–1991.

be balanced or added to by gender-related method preferences. In such disparate countries as the United States (National Center for Health Statistics, 1988) and India (Adityanjee, 1986), female suicides are most often committed by overdose or jumping from a height, whereas male suicides most often result from hanging or shooting. A similar choice of method may have quite different implications for lethalness in different societies. In countries with well-developed treatment facilities and strict regulation of potentially lethal ingestants, such as barbiturates, ingestions are rarely "successful." Many potential suicides who ingest a poison change their minds and inform someone shortly afterward so that effective treatment resources can then be brought to bear. However, in countries where such treatment resources are not readily available or when the chosen ingestant is untreatable, that method will have a higher lethal potential, which will in turn affect the male:female suicide ratio. In some South Asian and South Pacific countries, the rate of female suicide by poisoning is especially high, and the most commonly used ingestants are herbicides, such as paraquat (Haynes, 1987), for which no effective treatments are available.

Ethnicity and Social Class

Multiethnic countries, such as the United States, in which recording and reporting procedures are largely similar across different groups, offer an opportunity to examine cultural influences on suicide. In the United States, suicide is generally more common in whites than in non-whites in both the young (see Fig. 12.1) and in other age groups. Rates vary greatly among different Native American groups (May, 1987), with some having average rates whereas in other tribes suicide may be more than 20 times as common as the national average.

The relative risk for white and African-American teen suicide in the United States (1980) is 2.8. It ranges from 48 in the South Central states to 0.8 in the Mountain states. However, the areas where discrepancy is least (Mountain and West North Central), are also those where the black population is also very small and by extension where rates are most unreliable. The relationship of white-black differences to SES seems to be quite complicated. In whites and Hispanics, who have a similar suicide rate to whites, there is no relationship between socioeconomic status and adolescent suicide (Gould et al., unpublished data). It is therefore unlikely that the low African-American suicide rate can be attributed to a confounding between the low socioeconomic status that characterizes the African-American population as a whole and ethnicity. However, in a study in the New York City area—where African-American adolescent suicide rates are significantly lower than white rates—African-American adolescent suicides have a higher-than-expected socioeconomic status (Gould et al., unpublished data). This finding is compatible with the hypothesis that there is some element of traditional African-American culture that serves to protect teenagers (and their elders) from suicide, but that it is lost with deculturation and that socioeconomic status is a marker. These differences could in turn be a function of different attitudes toward suicide (e.g., that suicide cannot be justified as an expression of free will nor that it is a reasonable escape from life's burdens, or that it is a feature of insanity or cowardice) or the existence of more effective social support systems for African-Americans than whites in areas of traditional settlement (Bush, 1976; Gibbs & Martin, 1964; May, 1987).

Cultural differences are not obviously related to cultural sanctions or prohibitions against suicide. In Japanese Samurai families, suicide was condoned or even required in some circumstances, and one might have expected this value to affect attitudes toward suicide more generally within that country. However, the rate of teen suicide in Japan is well below that in the United States, and in most of Europe where suicide has never been condoned and where, until fairly recent times, many countries treated it as an illegal act. Although the Catholic church strongly prohibits suicide, suicide rates vary considerably in countries with predominantly Catholic populations (Table 12.1).

The mechanisms whereby suicide rates vary in different cultures have not been well explored. One possibility is that a culture's taboos against suicide protect almost all of those individuals who, because of character disorder or psychopathology, would otherwise be prone to suicide at times of personal stress. Quite subtle variations in the strength or nature of these taboos might then be more or less effective in maintaining low suicide rates. An alternative explanation—unrelated to attitudes or beliefs—is that contagion (see below) operates within a cultural group and modifies the attitudes toward suicide. Individuals who have had close contact with a suicide of the same cultural group would be more likely to commit suicide themselves. If the suicide rate is high in a given society or location, more people will know someone who has committed or attempted suicide, their inhibitions about suicide will be reduced, and the higher rate should maintain itself. This is in keeping with the quite stable regional differences that exist within and between countries.

Adolescence

Because adolescence is a relatively healthy period of life, suicide counts as one of the more important causes of adolescent death in both well-developed and underdeveloped countries. In the United States, it is the second leading cause of death in male whites aged 15 to 19 and the third leading cause among male African-Americans (Table 12.3).

Secular Changes

The suicide rate among male teens in the United States has increased markedly since the mid-1960s. Similar trends have been observed in some, but not all, of the other countries (Tables 12.4A and 12.4B). In the United States, the increase in male suicide has been regular and consistent over the past two decades, which, coupled with the fact that so many other countries report a similar trend, suggests that the increase is a real one and not the inadvertent result of some change in ascertainment procedures.

In reviewing U.S. and Canadian data in the late 1970s, some authorities interpreted the increase as a "cohort effect" (Murphy & Wetzel, 1980; Solomon & Heller, 1980), i.e., that the suicide rate could be expected to operate throughout the cohort's life. Yet, more recent data (National Center for Health Statistics, 1988) suggest that the increased incidence is present only through the second and third decades of life. Generations that had a high suicide rate in their teens and twenties show a suicide rate that is broadly comparable to those in earlier generations as they enter their fourth decade. Although this could be due to

Table 12.3. Leading Causes of Death in U.S. Males, 15–19 Years, 1988

Cause of Death	Rate per 100,000	% of all Deaths
	Whites	
Accidents	71.8	59.8
Suicide	19.6	16.3
Homicide	8.1	6.7
	African-Americans	
Homicide	77.4	47.1
Accidents	45.9	27.9
Suicide	9.7	5.8

Source: Data from National Center For Health Statistics, 1988.

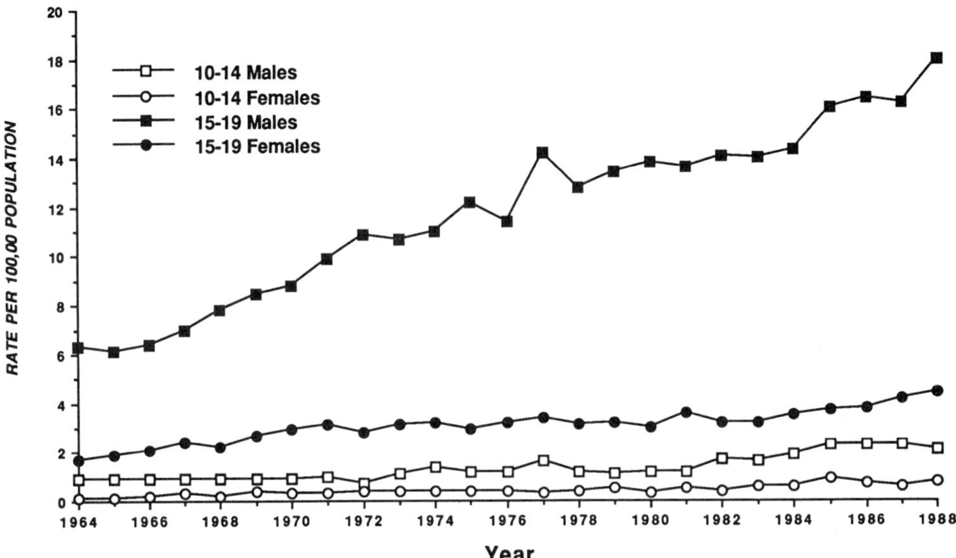

Fig. 12.2. Youth suicide in the United States, 1964 to 1988. (Data from the National Center for Health Statistics.)

the premature death of suicide-prone individuals at an early age, it is also compatible with the increase during adolescence being due to some etiologic factor, such as substance or alcohol abuse, the prevalence of which increased during this period, and that mainly affects the young.

Suicide Methods

The frequency with which a method is used to commit suicide seems to vary according to the victim's place of residence (Brent et al., 1991; Fisher et al., unpublished data; Moens et al., 1988). For example, in a demographically varied area surrounding New York City, hanging was common in all areas, but death by firearms was most prevalent in rural areas where firearms are commonly kept for hunting (Fisher et al., unpublished data). Self-asphyxiation, which usually involves feeding automobile exhaust back into a car parked in a garage, occurred most often in suburban areas, and jumping from a height occurred exclusively in urban areas.

If the choice of method is determined by availability, then one reasonable approach to prevention would be to limit access to a commonly used means for committing suicide. This strategy is discussed in greater detail below.

Risk Factors

Retrospective Case-Control Studies

The psychological autopsy method involves a detailed interview with a surviving informant and/or abstracting information from surviving records collected during

Table 12.4A. Twenty-Year Changes in the Youth Suicide Rate: Males

Country	Period	Mean rate Time 1*	Mean rate Time 2†	Percent Difference
1. Norway	1970–1989	7.4	25.4	243
2. Iceland	1971–1990	11.3	36.9	226
3. New Zealand	1970–1987	10.1	24.6	143
4. Belgium	1970–1986	8.1	15.8	95
5. Luxembourg	1971–1989	9.3	16.2	74
6. Australia	1970–1988	14.2	24.5	72
7. Finland	1970–1989	25.8	42.6	65
8. United States	1970–1988	14.4	21.6	50
9. France	1970–1989	10.0	14.8	48
10. Canada	1970–1989	18.0	26.3	46
11. Trinidad/Tobago	1971–1988	11.1	15.2	37
12. Bulgaria	1970–1990	9.3	12.4	33
13. Singapore	1970–1989	9.0	11.2	24
14. Denmark	1970–1990	12.4	14.9	20
15. Switzerland	1971–1990	23.1	26.4	14
16. Austria	1970–1990	23.5	26.4	12
17. Yugoslavia	1979–1987	10.6	11.7	10
18. Sweden	1970–1988	17.8	18.2	2
19. Ecuador	1971–1986	10.4	9.0	(13)
20. Poland	1970–1990	17.9	15.1	(16)
21. West Germany	1970–1989	19.9	16.0	(19)
22. Hungary	1970–1990	27.8	21.6	(22)
23. Uruguay	1971–1989	13.9	10.3	(26)
24. USSR‡	1970–1990	28.5	19.8	(30)
25. Czechoslovakia	1970–1990	28.9	13.3	(54)

*Mean annual rate for 3 years starting at beginning of period.

†Mean annual rate for 3 years preceeding end of period.

‡Time 1 data from 1970 and 1975.

Source: Data from World Health Organization, 1970–1991.

the suicide's life. Information has to be obtained through "psychological autopsy," i.e., retrospective history taken from surviving informants who knew the proband during life. This technique can be applied in an epidemiologic context by establishing a sample frame or a denominator, most commonly by conducting psychological autopsies on consecutively determined suicides in a predefined geographical area. The method can provide representative information that could not be obtained in any other way, but it has its limitations and the limits of its reliability are not known. The information gained is often *incomplete*, being limited to whatever the informant has observed. Informants are likely not to know about undetected illegal activities, and they may be insensitive to subjective mental states, such as depression or anxiety. Information not found in surviving records may have been truly absent or simply not noted. Despite these limitations, the psychological autopsy is often the only method available to study the detailed characteristics of suicide victims.

Uncontrolled psychological autopsy studies of child or adolescent suicides include those by Shaffer (1974), Sanborn et al. (1974) and Rich et al. (1988). Small sample-controlled studies used acquaintance controls (Shafii et al., 1985), psychiatric inpatients (Brent et al., 1988), both of which may be difficult to

Table 12.4B. Twenty-Year Changes in the Youth Suicide Rate: Females

Country	Period	Mean rate Time 1*	Mean rate Time 2†	Percent Difference
1. Luxembourg	1971–1989	2.8	4.9	75
2. Norway	1970–1989	3.4	5.5	62
3. New Zealand	1970–1987	4.6	6.7	46
4. Ecuador	1971–1986	5.8	8.0	38
5. Belgium	1970–1986	3.5	4.6	31
6. Bulgaria	1970–1990	4.3	5.6	30
7. Switzerland	1971–1990	5.9	7.2	22
8. Singapore	1970–1989	9.1	10.6	16
9. Canada	1970–1989	4.7	4.9	4
10. France	1970–1989	4.3	4.3	0
11. Australia	1970–1988	5.5	5.3	(4)
12. United States	1970–1988	4.5	4.3	(4)
13. Hungary	1970–1990	9.0	8.5	(5)
14. USSR‡	1970–1990	6.4	6.0	(6)
15. Finland	1970–1989	7.7	7.2	(6)
16. Austria	1970–1990	6.7	6.2	(7)
17. Sweden	1970–1988	7.5	6.5	(13)
18. Yugoslavia	1979–1987	6.0	5.1	(15)
19. Trinidad/Tobago	1971–1988	9.3	7.6	(18)
20. Denmark	1970–1990	6.1	4.6	(24)
21. Poland	1970–1990	3.8	2.7	(29)
22. Uruguay	1971–1989	5.1	3.4	(33)
23. West Germany	1970–1989	6.7	4.5	(33)
24. Iceland	1971–1990	3.5	1.6	(54)
25. Czechoslovakia	1970–1990	10.2	3.9	(62)

*Mean annual rate for 3 years starting at beginning of period.

†Mean annual rate for 3 years preceding end of period.

‡Time 1 data from 1970 and 1975.

Source: Data from World Health Organization, 1970–1991.

interpret. We are currently analyzing a large population-based psychological autopsy study of completed suicides under age 20 that occurred over a 2-year period in the New York metropolitan region (N = 173), with both a randomly selected age-, ethnic-, and sex-matched normal control group recruited by random telephone dialing in the same area and a similarly matched comparison group of suicide attempters. Of the 170 suicides recorded among children and adolescents aged 19 or under in the predefined area during the 2-year study period, 122 instances were examined in detail by structured interviews with surviving family members and teenage friends. Some relevant data from this sample are referred to below.

Terminal Events

According to several studies (Shaffer, 1974; Shafii et al., 1988), most suicides seem to be precipitated by a "disciplinary crisis," e.g., awaiting a punishment or other consequence of committing a crime or breaking school rules. The child or youth is most likely to commit suicide after the time of apprehension, but *before* the time when he or she would otherwise have found out about any punishment that might be received. Other common precipitants include a public humiliation, such as being ejected from a party when drunk, the threat of separation from a girl- or boyfriend, or reading or seeing a film about suicide (Shaffer, 1974). Suicide without an obvious precipitant is less common and is most often associated with a depressive illness. In a small number of cases, suicide occurs on the anniversary of a parental breakup or a friend's death. In one study (Shaffer, 1974), a significantly higher-than-expected number of young adolescents committed suicide within 2 weeks of their own birthdates.

Approximately half of all youth suicides are preceded by talk or threats of suicide. Previous attempts occur in about 50% of female and 25% of male teen suicides (Shaffer, unpublished data).

Associated Psychiatric Disorder

Suicide is rare in adults without psychopathology (Winokur & Tsuang, 1975), and high rates of psychiatric disorder have been found in retrospective psychological autopsy studies of consecutive suicides in adults (Barraclough et al., 1969; Dorpat & Ripley, 1960; Rich et al., 1988; Robins et al., 1959) and in the studies of children and teenagers referred to above.

In the New York study, psychiatric disorder was more prevalent in suicides than in controls. After making allowance for differences due to the number of informants, very few of the suicides were found to be free of significant psychiatric symptomatology, and approximately two thirds of each sex met DSM-III criteria for a psychiatric diagnosis. The remaining third, although not meeting diagnostic criteria, had numerous psychiatric symptoms, and most showed evidence of significant social or academic impairment before their death. Most cases showed chronic symptomatology, with only a small proportion having shown an onset of symptoms within 3 months of death. Approximately half of all suicides had had previous contact with a mental health professional.

Some sex differences were found in the type of psychiatric diagnosis. Approximately one third of each sex met criteria for an anxiety disorder. Conduct disorder and alcohol or drug abuse (often in combination with each other) were found in just under one half of the male teenagers. In contrast, none of the girls was found to have a significant substance abuse problem, and a somewhat smaller proportion than among the boys had a conduct disorder. The prevalence of alcohol abuse increased markedly with age, such that approximately two thirds of the older *male* teenagers (the group that accounts for the majority of cases) had a significant alcohol or substance abuse problem. Major depression was present in approximately one third of the girls, but in only half as many boys.

Most cases fell into one of three groups: (1) those who were irritable, impulsive, volatile, and sometimes physically aggressive; (2) those who were excessively anxious about forthcoming events, perfectionistic, and "rigid" and who experienced difficulties in adapting to new circumstances; (3) a group, made up mainly of girls, who were depressed and were, in several instances, being treated for this depression at the time of their death.

Findings that alcohol and drug abuse are important risk factors for boys and not for girls, taken together with the evidence that substance abuse has generally become more prevalent among male adolescents in the past 20 years, lends weight to the hypothesis that alcohol abuse is the determining factor in the recent increases in youth suicide. The value of this knowledge for prevention should be seen in perspective. The presence of substance abuse in the male adolescent population is approximately 5% or 5000 per 100,000. The incidence of substance- or alcohol-related suicide in older male adolescents is approximately 12 per 100,000. It follows that only 1 in 400 of male substance abusers in their late teens will commit suicide. This fraction is too small to be a useful predictor for preventive intervention.

Using findings from this study, along with age- and sex-specific base rate estimates (Fleiss, 1981), Gould, Shaffer, and Davies (1990) estimated that previous suicide attempts in males and/or depression in either sex are the most specific psychiatric risk factors for suicide. The extent of the excess risk can be illustrated by projecting the rate in various populations. The annual incidence of suicide in male adolescents is just under 15 per 100,000. However, the expected incidence of suicide among male suicide attempters would be 270 per 100,000 and among male depressives 100 per 100,000. The incidence in adolescent females is less than 4 per 100,000; among depressed female teens this would rise to 80 per 100,000, but because suicide attempts seem to be more common among girls and completions less common, the incidence among female attempters would be only 20 per 100,000.

Family History

Several studies (see Roy, 1983) have found that both suicide and suicide attempts are more common than expected in the families of adult suicides. Although not yet examined in the New York Study, twin registry (Roy et al., 1991) and adopted-away studies (Kety, 1986; Wender et al., 1986) suggest that genetic factors are important. In the twin registry study, concordance was six times as common (12%) in monozygous as in dizygous twins (2%). It is still not clear what is inherited, but it is most likely some predisposing psychiatric disorder or character trait.

Family Circumstances

In the New York study, two thirds of the control children who lived at home lived with two biologic parents, whereas only half of the suicides did so. Levels of friction in familial relationships (e.g., marital or parent-child conflict) were not significantly different between families of suicides and controls. However, even after adjusting for parent and adolescent psychopathology, patterns of family communication in the suicide sample were less good than in controls.

Prenatal and Perinatal History

In a controlled study of the obstetric records of consecutive youth suicides in Rhode Island, Salk et al. (1985) found a highly significant threefold excess of perinatal morbidity compared with controls. Not surprisingly, the excess of obstetric complications was associated with a reduced amount of prenatal care and higher levels of maternal smoking and alcohol consumption during pregnancy.

The association with suicide could therefore have been a function of some neurologic complication, exposure to teratogen during pregnancy, the heritability of psychopathology, or the later effects of inappropriate parenting by deviant mothers. The findings with respect to obstetric morbidity have been replicated in Sweden by Jacobson et al. (1987).

High-Risk Follow-Up Studies

As discussed above, retrospective studies may be limited by such distortions and deficiencies as simple forgetting, trying to assign meaning to a very traumatic event, or the absence of pertinent information. These limitations could, in principle, be remedied by collecting appropriate contemporaneous baseline information on an unselected sample and then examining that information in the light of a later suicidal outcome. However, given the low incidence of suicide, this is not a practical proposition. Although the strategy can be better used among high-risk individuals (e.g., patients with depression), because of the low incidence of suicide doing so would necessitate a large sample. Because the period of risk for subsequent suicide is not finite, long-term follow-up studies are likely to be more informative. Finally, the high-risk sample should be representative.

There have been several follow-up studies of adolescents who were initially hospitalized because of severe depression or a serious suicide attempt and on whom baseline information was obtained at the time of their original presentation (Garfinkel et al., 1982; Goldacre & Hawton, 1985; Motto, 1984; Otto, 1972; Spirito et al., 1989). Unfortunately, because of differences between attempters identified in clinics and in the community (see below), it is by no means clear that findings from these studies are representative of suicide attempters at large.

The subsequent suicide rate of hospitalized attempters seems to be considerably higher than that of the general population. Observed rates range from approximately 9% of a group of male teenagers admitted to a psychiatric inpatient unit who had been depressed or who had made a suicide attempt (Motto, 1984; Otto, 1972), to less than 1% of boys who presented at an emergency room after an overdose, but who were not admitted to a psychiatric hospital (Hawton & Goldacre, 1982). Similar proportions for females range from 1% for former psychiatric inpatients to 0.1% for those who received no inpatient psychiatric care. In general, male attempters seem to be from three to seven times as likely as female attempters to ultimately commit suicide. Among attempters who would ultimately commit suicide, Otto (1972) reported that 70% in the Swedish national sample of hospitalized attempters ultimately completed suicide with the same method that they had originally used. In the 5- to 15-year follow-up of a California sample described by Motto (1984), symptoms of severe depression (psychomotor retardation, difficulty in communicating, hopelessness, hypersomnia, feelings that they were going mad, etc.) were the best predictors of later suicide. In general, subsequent suicide has been associated with greater disturbances at the time of initial contact, is many times higher in psychiatrically hospitalized patients than in outpatients, and is more common in older teens. However, the prevalence of the predictors in noncompleters is also high, so that their specificity is limited.

Attempted Suicide

Prevalence

Research into the epidemiology of attempted suicide has lagged behind the study of completed suicide. Most descriptions of attempted suicides have been drawn from limited clinical samples. However, clinics vary in the type of cases they attract, and only a fraction of children or teenagers who self-report having made a suicide attempt receive treatment for it.

Relatively little is known about the characteristics of attempters whose attempt is not brought to clinical attention, and accordingly estimates of incidence vary considerably, reflecting different definitions and samples. The Centers for Disease Control (1991) surveyed over 11,000 high-school students ranging in age from 14 to 17 years regarding suicidal behavior in the past 12 months and found that 27% had thought about suicide, 16.3% had made a specific plan, 8.3% had made an attempt, and 2% had made attempts that required medical attention. Based on these results, the CDC estimated that almost 300,000 high-school students in the United States made a serious suicide attempt in 1990. Garrison et al. (1991) reported a very similar 1-year prevalence rate of attempts, i.e., between 1.5% and 2% in a school-based survey of 12- to 14-year-olds. Information about treated suicide is obtainable from Oregon, the first and only U.S. state to require registration of all suicide attempters under the age of 18 presenting for hospital treatment. This data indicate an annual hospital-treated attempt rate of 0.2% in 1988 (Andrus et al., 1991) or an incidence of 214 per 100,000, which is approximately 15 times the mortality incidence.

Studies in other countries have identified lifetime prevalence rates of between 2% and 4% for adolescents, but do not differentiate between attempts that require treatment and those that go unreported. In Canada, Pronovost et al. (1990) found a 3.5% lifetime attempt rate in a school-based survey of 2850 French-Canadian 12- to 18-year-olds from Quebec. Kienhorst et al. (1990) found that 2.2% of Dutch high-school and polytechnic students (aged 14 to 20 years) had made a suicide attempt at some point in their lifetime, and in Sweden Larsson et al. (1991) reported that 4% of a representative school-based sample of 605 13- to 18-year-olds had made an attempt during their lifetime. Two percent had made attempts in the past year.

Age

Although both attempts and ideation seem to be less common before puberty, findings about changes in incidence during adolescence are inconsistent. Dubow et al. (1989), in a study of 1384 junior high and high-school students in the Midwest, and Velez and Cohen (1988), in a longitudinal population probability sample in New York State, found no relationship between age during adolescence and attempt prevalence. In France, Choquet and Menke (1989) reported an increase in the frequency of suicidal ideation through adolescence in girls, but not boys.

Gender

In clinic samples in the United States (Piacentini et al., 1991), Hong Kong (Chung et al., 1987), and Great Britain (Sellar et al., 1990), female attempters present for treatment between three and seven times more often than males. Smaller sex differences have been found in community samples. In the Centers for Disease Control (CDC, 1991) survey, females outnumbered males by a factor of about 1.6 to 1 for all types of suicidal behavior. Small differences have also been found in unselected samples of U.S. college students (Meehan et al., 1992), native Americans (Blum et al., 1992), French-Canadian adolescents (Provonost et al., 1990), and French suburban adolescents (Choquet & Menke, 1989). However, in their survey of Swedish adolescents, Larsson et al. (1991) found that females were three times more likely than males (6% to 2%) to report a lifetime attempt. The sex differences in clinic and community samples may reflect a lesser degree of intentionality among females than males, but are more likely to reflect the means used to make the attempt. If a teenage boy tries to hang himself and fails, he is unlikely to need medical attention. However, if a girl takes an overdose and decides that she does not want to die or is inadvertently discovered, medical treatment will be sought to counteract any subsequent effects of the ingestant.

Ethnicity

In the CDC survey (1991), attempt rates were higher for Hispanics (12%) than either whites (7.9%) or African-Americans (6.5%), whereas in a survey of native Americans, Blum et al. (1992) reported a lifetime prevalence of 17%.

Social Class

In a community sample of almost 1400 U.S. seventh to twelfth graders, Dubow et al. (1989) reported low socioeconomic status among subjects at increased risk for both suicidal ideation and attempts.

Psychiatric Disorder

Community studies of teen suicide attempters suggest that, depending on the diagnostic criteria used, the prevalence of *depression* lies between 19% and 42% (Garrison, et al., 1991; Smith & Crawford, 1986; Velez & Cohen, 1988), which is well above the 1% to 4% prevalence reported for adolescents at large. Although affective disturbance is a potent risk factor for suicidal behavior, a substantial number of suicidal adolescents are not depressed. Several studies have found *aggression* and *antisocial behaviors* to be as or more common than depression in suicide attempters (Choquet & Menke, 1989; Garfinkle et al., 1982; Velez & Cohen, 1988). Although conduct disorder often co-occurs with childhood depressive illness (McGee et al., 1990), clinic studies indicate that many attempters have conduct problems without associated affective symptoms (Pfeffer et al., 1983). Despite the fact that substance abuse is common in clinic-identified attempters (see Shaffer & Piacentini, in press), the relationship has not been examined in representative community samples.

Other Characteristics

A large number of studies have found that the most common method used by suicide attempters who are referred for psychiatric treatment is a drug overdose. Studies of the precipitants that occur before an attempt, various gauges of seriousness and intention, natural history, and family functioning (including child abuse) have, almost without exception, been carried out on narrow clinical convenience samples derived from a single treatment center. The reader is referred to a comprehensive review elsewhere (Shaffer & Piacentini, in press) for a summary of information on these clinical samples.

Secular Change

Studies in the United Kingdom and Australia indicate a marked increase in referrals for treatment of attempted suicide between 1960 and the early 1980s (Hawton & Goldacre, 1982; Kreitman & Schreiber, 1979; Oliver et al., 1971). In the United Kingdom there is some evidence that the methods used among attempters who present to clinics have changed in recent years. Sellar, Hawton, and Goldacre (1990) in Oxford, England, found a significant decline between 1980 and 1985 in overdose with psychotropic-type substances among 16- to 20-year-old females, which they attributed to increased vigilance by physicians in prescribing psychotropic drugs.

Mechanisms

Imitation and Contagion

The bulk of epidemiologic research on suicide imitation is of an "ecologic" nature, i.e., there is a statistically robust link between the occurrence of a purported stimulus and a subsequent increase in the suicide or suicide-attempt rate among individuals exposed to the stimulus. However there is no evidence that the actual suicides that occur within the contingent period were exposed to the stimulus. Examples of such stimuli include newspaper or television reports of individual suicides. Morbidity has been reported to increase after newspaper reports of the suicide of prominent individuals (Bollen & Phillips, 1981, 1982; Phillips, 1974, 1979, 1980, 1984; Wasserman, 1984). It also increases after televised dramatizations that feature teen suicide (Gould & Shaffer, 1986; Gould et al., 1988; Holding, 1974, 1975) and after televised news stories of suicide (Schmidtke & Hafner, 1986). Children and adolescents are affected the most, increases in the number of suicides remain for 1 to 2 weeks after exposure, and the number of suicides is proportional to the number of times the stimulus has been shown (Phillips & Carstensen, 1986). Although several studies have failed to replicate findings on imitation (Berman, 1988; Gould et al., 1988), this lack of replication could be accounted for by variations in the age and size of the exposed viewership or the context in which the material was seen, e.g., whether or not the programs were accompanied by material that could direct a disturbed viewer to obtain help, etc.

Other evidence that supports a "contagion model" includes the occurrence of clusters or epidemic suicides, which may account for up to 4% of all teen suicides in the United States (Gould et al., 1989). Suicide clusters are defined as an unexpectedly high incidence of suicidal deaths that occur within a limited area over a short time period. Their occurrence seems unrelated to significant changes in the community. Little is known about individual suicides that occur in a cluster. In one study (Davidson et al., 1989), several of the victims had previously attempted suicide, and the supposition is that, during a cluster or epidemic, the threshold for suicide is reduced in individuals who are in any way vulnerable to the condition.

Models for Suicide

Psychodynamic

Psychodynamic models explain suicide as a consequence of either intrapsychic dynamics, such as the need to identify with or join a deceased love object; the internalization of anger; or of interpersonal goals, such as manipulation either to gain love or inflict punishment (Abraham, 1927; Zilboorg, 1936; Freud, 1950; Toolan, 1962). However, such phenomena as self-denigratory thought or morbid preoccupation with deceased loved ones can be reversed with antidepressant medication and may well be a consequence, rather than a cause, of a mood disturbance.

Sociologic

Sociologic models hold suicide to be an intended or understandable behavior in the light of an individual's life situation or position in society. Variations on the model variously implicate a lack of social integration or anomie; group dynamics, such as racial or sexual prejudice that foster or lessen identification with others; or political-economic pressures, such as cycles of unemployment or increases in cohort size, that increase pressure for educational and employment resources. In all such examples the individual is seen to be responding to social forces beyond his or her control.

This model cannot stand alone and does not suggest that *all* individuals in an anomalous position in society or experiencing a particular stress will seek suicide as a solution. Most of the evidence used to support sociologic models is ecologic, i.e., mortality statistics are found to be associated with such variables as total population, unemployment rates, phases in the economic cycle, ethnic mixtures in geographic units, immigration patterns, migration, crime and divorce rates, etc., without demonstrations that a significant proportion of suicides have been individually affected by the purported stress. A causal relationship cannot be inferred because when one factor—for example, unemployment rate—varies, others may vary with it, or the variation may occur against a backdrop of more general change. Studies of individual suicides have, in general, failed to find impaired access to educational or employment resources among suicide victims that could not be better explained as a consequence of deviant behavior or social drift.

Psychiatric Disease

The psychiatric disease model is supported by psychological studies positing that suicide occurs as a consequence of the distortions of perception and judgment that characterize a disturbance of mental state brought about by a psychiatric illness, such as depression or intoxication. Suicide is not seen as a disease, but rather as a symptom or sign of an underlying disturbance of mental state.

Heuristic

A model that takes account of many of the correlates described above and that is heuristic for prevention is shown in Figure 12.3 (see Shaffer et al., 1988).

It assumes that suicide does not occur capriciously and that it mainly affects predisposed individuals. Important predispositions include major mood disorder and certain personality types. Very few individuals who are not thus affected will be at risk for suicide. Predisposed individuals will usually make their suicide

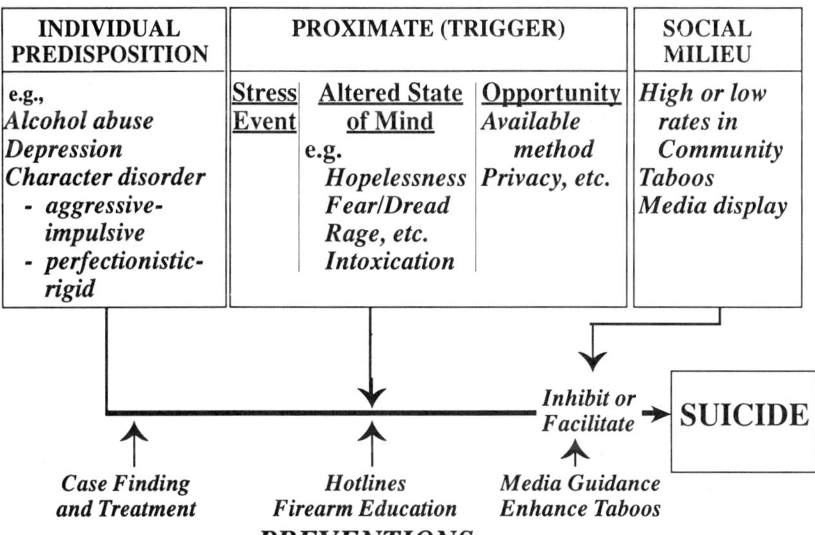

Fig. 12.3. Suicide: an heuristic model (Shaffer et al., 1988).

attempt or commit suicide after some stressful event—often a consequence rather than a cause of their disorder—has induced an extreme emotion, such as fear, unhappiness, hopelessness, or rage. This mental state may lead to suicide if judgment is impaired by drugs or alcohol or identification with a glamorously or heroically portrayed suicide model in a movie or on TV. Finally, the means to commit suicide in an acceptable and effective way will need to be at hand.

Prevention

Given this model, a logical strategy for prevention is to identify high-risk cases and provide them with optimal treatment and follow-up. Other prevention strategies that fit the model include intervening at the penultimate stage with crisis management or limiting access to potential methods for committing suicide.

Case-Finding

Case-finding can be either *indirect*, in which educational programs train pupils, teachers, and parents to spot the "warning signs" of suicide among their friends, pupils or children, or *direct*, in which risk status is ascertained directly from the teenagers themselves. There are two problems with the indirect approach: many at-risk teens do not show visible symptoms, and behaviors that denote risk, such as depression or alcohol abuse, are prevalent in nonsuicidal teens. In one study, there was no evidence that teenagers who had received systematic training in case-finding were any more likely to recommend treatment to their distressed friends than those who had not (Vieland et al., 1991).

A direct approach is more reasonable because older teenagers' self-identification of problems is highly correlated with a clinician's determination of need for treatment (Achenbach & Edelbrock, 1987; Bird et al., 1990; Kovacs 1981). Regardless of the method used, the value of case-finding will be restricted by the very high base rate of some high-risk conditions, such as alcohol abuse, anxiety disorders, and aggressive behavior; sparse treatment resources; and limited knowledge about optimal treatment.

Crisis Intervention

Crisis intervention was originally formulated on the assumption that suicide intent is usually associated with a stressful event that arises in the context of mental disturbance (Litman et al., 1965; Schneidman & Farberow, 1957). Crisis services are usually provided by telephone hotlines. Their efficacy has been tested by determining whether the establishment of a service in a given area results in a lower suicide morbidity. On balance, the evidence is that crisis services have no, or, at best, very limited effects on the suicide rate (Barraclough et al., 1977; Bridge et al., 1977; Jennings et al., 1978; Miller et al., 1984). Possible explanations for this lack of effect (see Shaffer et al. (1988) for a review) are the predominance of female callers (females are at relatively low risk for suicide);

the indifferent quality of much of the advice given (Apsler & Hodas, 1975; Bleach & Claiborn, 1974; Hirsch, 1981; Knowles, 1979; Slaiku et al., 1975); or the fact that a significant proportion of suicides occur when the victim is preoccupied or disorganized, under the influence of alcohol, or in an otherwise agitated state when he or she may not be able to summon the resources to make or benefit from an appropriate call. Furthermore, only a small proportion of teens know how to gain access to a hotline (Greer & Anderson, 1979; Litman et al., 1965).

Limiting Access to Methods

Because youth suicide is so often an impulsive act, it is reasonable to expect that limiting the availability of or access to any common method could reduce the teen suicide rate. The British experience (Hassall & Trethowan, 1972; Kreitman, 1976) is the most frequently cited example of how reducing access to the means of suicide can significantly reduce the suicide rate. Between 1957 and 1970, the carbon monoxide content of domestic gas was eliminated in Great Britain; the overall suicide rate declined by 26%, and suicide rates from carbon monoxide asphyxiation declined from 40% to 10% of all suicides. Almost all of the reduction could be attributed to the fall in deaths from domestic gas asphyxiation, with no compensatory increase in suicidal deaths by other methods, although the incidence of attempts by overdose increased (Johns, 1977). However, the impact of this reduction was limited because over the same period self-poisoning became progressively less lethal with the substitution of less dangerous drugs for the highly toxic barbiturates and improved methods of resuscitation. The British experience is not directly relevant to the United States where suicide by self-asphyxiation is rare and most suicides are committed with firearms. Yet, it is possible that the suicide rate would decline if access to firearms were better controlled or if appropriate education programs urged parents of vulnerable children not to maintain firearms in the home or, alternatively, to make sure that firearms are maintained under the most secure conditions.

Acknowledgments

This work was made possible by NIMH Research Training Grant MH 38198-11A2 and Research Training Grant MH 16434, NIMH Center Grant MH 4 3878 AI, the Centers for Disease Control Grant R49 CCR202598, NIMH Project Grants ROI MH 38198, ROI MH416898 and R18MH48059-02 and grants from the American Mental Health Foundation and the Leon Lowenstein Foundation.

References

Abraham K. *Notes on the Psychoanalytic Investigation and Treatment of Manic-Depressive Insanity and Allied Conditions*. London: Hogarth Press; 1927:137–156.

Achenbach TM, Edelbrock C. *Manual for the Youth Self-Report and Profile*. Burlington, VT: University of Vermont; 1987.

Adityanjee DR. Suicide attempts and suicides in India: cross-cultural aspects. *Int J Soc Psychiatry* 1986; 32:64–73.

Andrus JK, Flemming DW, Heumann MA, Wassell JT, Hopkins DD, Gordon J. Surveillance of attempted suicide among adolescents in Oregon, 1988. *Am J Pub Health* 1991; 81:1067–1069.

Apsler R, Hodas M. Evaluating hotlines with simulated calls. *Crisis Intervent* 1975; 6:14–21.

Asberg M, Traskman L, Thoren P. 5-HIAA in the cerebrospinal fluid: a biochemical suicide predictor. *Arch Gen Psychiatry* 1976; 33:1193–1197.

Barraclough BM. Sex ratio of juvenile suicide. *J Am Acad Child Adolesc Psychiatry* 1987; 26:434–435.

Barraclough BM. Differences between national suicide rates. *Br J Psychiatry* 1973; 122:95–96.

Barrouclough P. Influence of coroners' officers and pathologists on suicide verdicts. *Br J Psychiatry* 1976; 128:471–474.

Barraclough BM, Bunch J, Nelson B, et al. *The Diagnostic Classification and Psychiatric Treatment of 100 Suicides*. London; Proceedings of the Fifth International Conference for Suicide Prevention; 1969.

Barraclough BM, Bunch J, Nelson B, Sainsbury P. A hundred cases of suicide: clinical aspects. *Br J Psychiatry* 1974; 125:355–373.

Barraclough BM, Jennings C, Moss JR, Hawton K, Cole D, O'Grady J, Osborne M. Suicide prevention by the samaritans. *Lancet* 1977; 2:237–238.

Berman AL. Fictional depiction of suicide in television films and imitation effects. *Am J Psychiatry* 1988; 145:982–986.

Bird H, Yager T, Staghezza B, Gould M, et al. Impairment in the epidemiological measurement of childhood psychopathology in the community. *J Am Acad Child Adolesc Psychiatry* 1990; 29:796–803.

Bleach G, Claiborn WL. Initial evaluation of hot-line telephone crisis centers. *Comm Ment Health* 1974; 10:387–394.

Blum RW, Harmon B, Harris L, Bergeisen L, Resnick MD. American Indian-Alaska native youth health. *JAMA* 1992; 267:1637–1644.

Bollen KA, Phillips DP. Suicidal motor vehicle fatalities in Detroit: a replication. *Am J Sociol* 1981; 87:404–412.

Bollen KA, Phillips DP. Imitative suicides: a national study of the effects of television news stories. *Am Sociol Rev* 1982; 47:802–809.

Brent DA. Correlates of medical lethality of suicide attempts in children and adolescents. *J Am Acad Child Psychiatry* 1987; 26:87–91.

Brent DA, Perper JA, Goldstein C, Kolko D, Allan M, Allman C, Zelenak J. Risk factors for adolescent suicide: a comparison of adolescent suicide victims and suicide inpatients. *Arch Gen Psychiatry* 1988; 45:581–588.

Brent D, Kerr M, Goldstein C, Bozigar J, Wartella M, Allan M. An outbreak of suicide and suicidal behavior in a high school. *J Am Acad Child Adolesc Psychiatry* 1989; 28:918–924.

Brent D, Perper J, Allman C, Moritz G, Wartella M, Zelenak J. The presence and accessibility of firearms in the homes of adolescent suicides. *JAMA* 1991; 266:2989–2995.

Bridge TP, Potkin SG, Zung WW, Soldo BJ. Suicide prevention centers: ecological study of effectiveness. *J Nerv Ment Dis* 1977; 164:18–24.

Bush JA. Suicides and blacks: a conceptual framework. *Suicide Life-Threatening Behav* 1976; 6:216–222.

Centers For Disease Control. Attempted suicide among high school students-U.S., 1990. *MMWR* 1991; 40:633–635.

Choquet M, Mencke H. Suicidal thoughts during early adolescence: prevalence, associated troubles and help-seeking behavior. *Acta Psychiatr Scand* 1989; 81:170–177.

Chung SY, Luk SL, Lieh Mak F. Attempted suicide in children and adolescents in Hong Kong. *Soc Psychiatry* 1987; 22:102–106.

Davidson L, Rosenberg M, Mercy J, Franklin J, Simmons J. An epidemiologic study of risk factors in two teenage suicide clusters. *JAMA* 1989; 262:2687–2692.

Dorpat TL, Ripley HS. A study of suicide in the Seattle area. *Compr Psychiatry* 1960; 1:349–359.

Dubow EF, Kausch DF, Blum MC, et al. Correlates of suicidal ideation and attempts in a community sample of junior high and high school students. *J Clin Child Psychol* 1989; 18:158–166.

Farberow NR, MacKinnon DR, Nelson FL. Suicide: whose counting? *Pub Health Rep* 1977; 92:223–232.

Fisher P, Shaffer D. Facts about adolescent suicide: a review of national mortality statistics and recent research. In: Rotheram-Borus MJ, Bradley J, Oblolensky N, eds. *Planning to Live: Evaluating and Treating Suicidal Teens in Community Settings*. Tulsa: University of Oklahoma, National Resource Center for Youth Services; 1990.

Fleiss JL. *Statistical Methods for Rates and Proportions*. 2nd ed. New York: John Wiley; 1981.

Freud A, Burlingham D. *Infants Without Families*. New York: International Universities Press; 1944.

Freud S. *Mourning and Melancholia*. In: Jones E, ed. Collected Papers, Vol. IV. London: Hogarth Press; 1950: 152–170.

Garfinkel BD, Froese A, Hood J. Suicide attempts in children and adolescents. *Am J Psychiatry* 1982; 139:1257–1261.

Garrison CZ, Jackson KL, Addy CL, McKeown RE, Waller JL. Suicidal behavior in young adolescents. *Am J Epidemiol* 1991; 133:1005–1014.

Gibbs JP, Martin WT. *Status of Integration and Suicide*. Eugene, OR: University of Oregon Press; 1964.

Goldacre M, Hawton K. Repetition of self-poisoning and subsequent death in adolescents who take overdoses. *Br J Psychiatry* 1985; 146:395–398.

Gould MS, Shaffer D. The impact of suicide in television movies: evidence of imitation. *N Engl J Med* 1986; 315:690–694.

Gould MS, Shaffer D, Kleinman M. The impact of suicide in television movies: replication and commentary. *Suicide Life-Threatening Behav* 1988; 18:90–99.

Gould MS, Wallenstein S, Davidson L. Suicide clusters: a critical review. *Suicide Life Threatening Behav* 1989; 19:17–29.

Gould MS, Shaffer D, Davies M. Truncated pathways from childhood: attrition in follow-up studies due to death. In: Robins L, Rutter M. eds., *Straight and Devious Pathways from Childhood to Adulthood*. Cambridge: Cambridge University Press; 1990:3–10.

Greer S, Anderson M. Samaritan contact among 325 parasuicide patients. *Br J Psychiatry* 1979; 135:263–268.

Hassall C, Trethowan WH. Suicide in Birmingham. *Br Med J* 1972; 1:717–718.

Hawton K, Goldacre M. Hospital admissions for adverse effects of medicinal agents (mainly self-poisoning) among adolescents in the Oxford region. *Br J Psychiatry* 1982; 141:106–170.

Haynes RH. Suicide and social response in Fiji: a historical survey. *Br J Psychiatry* 1987; 151:21–26.

Hirsch S. A critique of volunteer-staffed suicide prevention centres. *Can J Psychiatry* 1981; 26:406–410.

Holding TA. The B.B.C. "Befriender" series and its effects. *Br J Psychiatry* 1974; 124:470–472.

Holding TA. Suicide and "the befrienders." *Br Med J* 1975; 3:751–753.

Jacobson B, Eklund G, Hamberger L, Linnarsson D, Sedvall G, Valverius M. Perinatal origin of adult self-destructive behavior. *Acta Psychiatr Scand* 1987; 76:364–371.

Jennings C, Barraclough BM, Moss JR. Have the samaritans lowered the suicide rate? A controlled study. *Psychol Med* 1978; 8:413–422.

Johns MW. Self-poisoning with barbituates in England and Wales during 1959–1974. *Br Med J* 1977; 2:1128–1130.

Kety S. Genetic factors in suicide. In: Roy A, ed. *Suicide*. Baltimore: Williams & Wilkins; 1986:41–45.

Kienhorst CWM, De Wilde EJ, Van Den Bout J, Diekstra RFW, Wolters WHG. Characteristics of suicide attempters in a population-based sample of Dutch adolescents. *Br J Psychiatry* 1990; 156:243–248.

Kleck G. Miscounting suicides. *Suicide Life Threatening Behav* 1988; 18(3):219–236.

Knowles D. On the tendency for volunteer helpers to give advice. *J Counsel Psychol* 1979; 26:352–354.

Koocher GP. Childhood, death, and cognitive development. *Dev Psychol* 1973; 9:369–375.

Kovacs M, Beck AT. An empirical-clinical approach toward a definition of childhood depression. In: Schulterbrandt JG, Raskin A, eds. *Depression in Childhood: Diagnosis, Treatment, and Conceptual Models*. New York: Raven Press; 1977.

Kovacs M. Rating scales to assess depression in school-aged children. *Acta Paedopsychiatr* 1981; 46:305–315.

Kreitman N. The coal gas story: United Kingdom suicide rates, 1960–71. *Br J Prev Soc Med* 1976; 30:86–93.

Kreitman N, Schrieber M. Parasuicide in young Edinburgh women, 1968–1975. *Psychol Med* 1979; 9:469–479.

Larsson B, Melin L, Breitholtz E, Andersson G. Short-term stability of depressive symptoms and suicide attempts in Swedish adolescents. *Acta Psychiatr Scand* 1991; 83:385–390.

Lester D. Migration and suicide. *Med J Australia* 1972; 18:941–942.

Litman R, Farberow N, Schneidman E, Heilig S, Kramer J. Suicide prevention telephone service. *JAMA* 1965; 192:107–111.

Litman RE, Curphey T, Schneidman E, Farberow N, Tabachnick N. Investigations of equivocal suicide. *JAMA* 1963; 184:924–929.

Littman et al., 1963.

May PA. Suicide and self-destruction among American Indian youths. *Am Indian Alaska Native Ment Health Res* 1987; 1:52–69.

McGee R, Feehan M, Williams S, Partridge F, Silva P, Kelly J. DSM-III disorders in a large sample of adolescents. *J Am Acad Child Adolesc Psychiatry* 1990; 29:611–619.

McIntire MS, Angle CR, Struempler LJ. The concept of death in midwestern children and youth. *Am J Dis Child* 1972; 123:527–532.

Meehan PJ, Lamb JA, Saltzman LE, O'Carroll PW. Attempted suicide among young adults. *Am J Psychiatry* 1992; 149:41–44.

Miller HL, Coombs DW, Leeper JD, et al. An analysis of the effects of suicide prevention facilities on suicide rates in the U.S. *Am J Pub Health* 1984; 74:340–343.

Moens GFG, Lycsch MJM, Van de Voorde H. The geographical pattern of methods of suicide in Belgium: implications for prevention. *Acta Psychiatr Scand* 1988; 77:320–327.

Monk M. Epidemiology of suicide. *Epidemiol Rev* 1987; 9:51–69.

Motto JA. Suicide in male adolescents. In: Segdak HS, Ford AB, Rushforth NB, eds. *Suicide in The Young*. Boston: John Wright PSG Inc; 1984:227–244.

Murphy GE, Wetzel RD. Suicide risk by birth cohort in the U.S., 1949–1974. *Arch Gen Psychiatry* 1980; 37:519–523.

Nagy ML. The child's view of death. In: Feifel H, ed. *The Meaning of Death*. New York: McGraw-Hill; 1965.

Nelson FL, Faberow NL, MacKinnon DR. The certification in eleven western states: an inquiry into the validity of reported suicide rates. *Suicide Life Threatening Behavior* 1978; 8(2):75–88.

O'Carroll P. A consideration of the validity and reliability of suicide mortality data. *Suicide Life Threatening Behav* 1989; 19(1):1–16.

Oliver RG, Kaminski Z, Tudor K, Hetzel BS. The epidemiology of attempted suicide as seen in the causalty department, Alfred Hospital, Melbourne. *Med J Aust* 1971; 1:833–839.

Otto U. Suicidal acts by children and adolescents: a follow-up study. *Acta Psychiatr Scand* 1972; 233(suppl):5–123.

Pfeffer CR, Plutchik R, Mizruchi MS. Suicidal and assaultive behavior in children: classification, measurement, and interrelations. *Am J Psychiatry* 1983; 140:154–157.

Phillips DP. The influence of suggestion on suicide: substantive and theoretical implication of the Werther effect. *Am Sociol Rev* 1974; 39:340–354.

Phillips DP. Suicide, motor vehicle fatalities, and the mass media: evidence toward a theory of suggestion. *Am J Sociol* 1979; 84:1150–1174.

Phillips DP. Airplane accidents, murder and the mass media: towards a theory of imitation and suggestion. *Social Forces* 1980; 58:1001–1004.

Phillips DP. Teenage and adult temporal fluctuations in suicide and auto fatalities. In: Sudak HS, Ford AB, Rushforth NB, eds. *Suicide in the Young*. Littleton: John Wright-PSG Inc; 1984:69–80.

Phillips DP, Carstensen LL. Clustering of teenage suicides after television news stories about suicide. *N Engl J Med* 1986; 315:685–689.

Piacentini J, Rotheram-Borus MJ, Trautman P, Graae F. Psychosocial correlates of treatment compliance in adolescent suicide attempters. Presented at the Association for Advancement of Behavior Therapy Meeting; 1991; New York.

Pronovost J, Cote L, Ross C. Epidemiological study of suicidal behavior among secondary school students. *Can Ment Health* 1990; 3:9–15.

Rich CL, Fowler RC, Fogarty LA, Young D. San Diego suicide study: III. Relationships between diagnosis and stressors. *Arch Gen Psychiatry* 1988; 45:589–592.

Robins E, Gassner S, Kayes J, et al. The communication of suicide intent: a study of 134 consecutive cases of successful (completed) suicide. *Am J Psychiatry* 1959; 115:724–733.

Roy A. Family history of suicide. *Arch Gen Psychiatry* 1983; 40:971–974.

Roy A, Segal NL, Centerwall BS, Robinette CD. Suicide in twins. *Arch Gen Psychiatry* 1991; 48:29–32.

Sainsbury P, Barraclough B. Differences between suicide rates. *Nature* 1968; 220(173):1252.

Salk L, Sturner W, Reilly B, et al. Relationship of maternal and perinatal conditions to eventual adolescent suicide. *Lancet* 1985; 1:624–627.

Sanborn DE, Sanborn CJ, Cimbolic P. Two years of suicide: a study of adolescent suicide in New Hampshire. *Child Psychiatr Human Dev* 1974; 3:234–242.

Schilder P, Wechsler D. The attitudes of children toward death. *J Gen Psychol* 1934; 45:406–451.

Schmidtke A, Hafner H. Die vermittlung von selbstmordmotivation und selbstmordhandlung durch fiktivemodelle. *Nervenarzt* 1986; 57:502–510.

Schneidman E, Farberow N. Statistical comparisons between attempted and committed suicides. In: Farberow N, Schneidman E, eds. *The Cry for Help.* New York: McGraw-Hill; 1965.

Sellar C, Hawton K, Goldacre MJ. Self-poisoning in adolescents: hospital admissions and deaths in the Oxford region 1980–1985. *Br J Psychiatry* 1990; 156:866–870.

Shaffer D. Suicide in childhood and early adolescence. *J Child Psychol Psychiatry* 1974; 15:275–291.

Shaffer D, Fisher P. The epidemiology of suicide in children and young adolescents. *J Am Acad Child Adolesc Psychiatry* 1981; 20:545–565.

Shaffer D, Piacentini J. Suicide and attempted suicide. In: Rutter M, Taylor E, eds. *Child Adolescent Psychiatry—Modern Approaches.* 3rd ed. (in press). Oxford: Blackwell Scientific Publications, Ltd.

Shaffer D, Garland A, Gould M, Fisher P, Trautman P. Preventing teenage suicide: a critical review. *J Am Acad Child Adolesc Psychiatry* 1988; 27:675–687.

Shaffer D, Vieland V, Garland A, Rojas M, Underwood M, Busner C. Adolescent suicide attempters: response to suicide prevention programs. *JAMA* 1990; 264:3151–3155.

Shaffer D, Garland A, Vieland V, Underwood M, Busner C. The impact of curriculum-based suicide prevention programs for teenagers. *J Am Acad Child Adolesc Psychiatry* 1991; 30:588–596.

Shafii M, Carrigan S, Whittinghill JR, et al. Psychological autopsy of completed suicide in children and adolescents. *Am J Psychiatry* 1985; 142: 1061–1064.

Shafii M, Steltz-Lenarsky J, Derrick AM, et al. Comorbidity of mental disorders in the post-mortem diagnosis of completed suicide in children and adolescents. *J Affective Disord* 1988: 227–233.

Slaiku KA, Tulkin SR, Speer DC. Process and outcome in the evaluation of telephone counseling referrals. *J Consult Clin Psychol* 1975; 43:700–707.

Smith K, Crawford S. Suicidal behaviors among "normal" high school students. *Suicide Life-Threatening Behav* 1986; 16:313–325.

Solomon MJ, Heller CO. Suicide and age in Alberta Canada, 1951–1977. *Arch Gen Psychiatry* 1980; 37:511–513.

Spirito A, Brown L, Overholser J, Fritz G. Attempted suicide in adolescence: a review and critique of the literature. *Clin Psychol Rev* 1989; 9:335–363.

Stanley M, Mann JJ. Biological factors associated with suicide. In Frances AJ, Holes RE, eds. *American Psychiatric Association Annual Review.* Washington, DC: American Psychiatric Press 1988; 7:334–352.

Tishler CL, McKenry PC, Morgan KC. Adolescent suicide attempts: some significant factors. *Suicide Life-Threatening Behav* 1981; 11:86–92.

Toolan JM. Suicide and suicide attempts in childhood and adolescence. *Am J Orthopsychiatry* 1962; 118:719–724.

Velez C, Cohen P. Suicidal behavior and ideation in a community sample of children: maternal and youth reports. *J Am Acad Child Adolesc Psychiatry* 1988; 27:349–356.

Vieland V, Whittle B, Garbard A, Hicks R, Shaffer D. The impact of curriculum-based suicide prevention programs for teenagers: an 18-month follow-up. *J Am Acad Child Adolescent Psychiatry* 1991; 30(5):811–815.

Wasserman IM. Imitation and suicide: a reexamination of the Werther effect. *Am Sociol Rev* 1984; 49:427–436.

Wender P, Kety S, Rosenthal D, Schulsinger F, Ortmann J, Lunde I. Psychiatric disorders in the biological and adoptive families of adopted individuals with affective disorders. *Arch Gen Psychiatry* 1986; 43:923–929.

Wilkins JA. Follow-up study of those who called suicide prevention center. *Am J Psychiatry* 1970; 127:155–161.

Winokur G, Tsuang M. The Iowa 500: suicide in mania, depression and schizophrenia. *Am J Psychiatry* 1975; 132:650–651.

World Health Organization. *World Health Statistic Annual*. Geneva: WHO; 1970–1991.

Zilboorg G. Consideration on suicide with particular reference to that of the young. *Am J Orthopsychiatry* 1936; 7:15–35.

PART IV

INJURIES AND VIOLENCE

13

Unintentional Injuries

FRED P. RIVARA

The problem of injuries to children is not a new one. In recent years, however, interest in trauma has dramatically increased for a number of reasons. Advances in medical care and public health have had a major impact on the mortality and morbidity from a wide variety of infectious and other acute diseases. Similar changes have not occurred in trauma, and consequently its relative importance has increased. An increasingly scientific approach to injury causation has led to progressively more effective prevention programs in specific areas. Finally, the interest of governmental agencies at the national and local level has been accompanied by an infusion of money for both research and prevention. As a result, the scientific and academic community has taken a greater interest in this problem, and in the last decade, a large number of important contributions have appeared (Baker et al., 1992; Robertson, 1992). Injuries, including intentional injuries, such as homicide, have come to be viewed as public health problems, rather than as problems of the motor vehicle industry, police, or criminologists (National Committee for Injury Prevention and Control, 1989). The application of the standard techniques of public health to the study of injury has been fruitful and is beginning to yield impressive results.

First, some definition of terms is necessary. This chapter focuses on and discusses injuries, i.e., physical, usually acute, trauma to an individual. The term "accident" is not used because of its connotation of random events, acts of God, and its sense of fatalism, as in the expressions, "Accidents happen," and "It was an accident." Such usage tends to undermine the current scientific approach in which the focus is on **injury control**—the attempt to reduce the morbidity and mortality from trauma through primary prevention, better acute care, and improved and more accessible long-term rehabilitation.

Patterns of Occurrence

The magnitude of the problem of childhood injuries can be measured in terms of mortality, morbidity, and cost.

Mortality

The most important measure of the magnitude of childhood trauma is fatal injuries, both because of their importance and because the data on these injuries are the most valid information available. Injury causes almost 40% of the deaths among children 1 to 4 years of age and almost 70% of deaths for those 5 to 19 years (Division of Injury Control, 1990). In 1986, unintentional injuries caused more than 17,000 deaths of children and adolescents in the United States (Table 13.1). Unintentional injuries cause more potential years of life lost than any other cause (Fig. 13.1).

Motor vehicle injuries lead the list of injury deaths at all ages during childhood and adolescence. Even in children under 1 year of age, motor vehicle crashes are an important cause of death (Baker et al., 1974). Motor vehicle occupant injuries account for the majority of injury deaths during childhood, as they do in adults (National Highway Traffic Safety Administration, 1992). However, among children in the 5- to 9-year age group, pedestrian injuries overshadow occupant injuries as a cause of death and in fact are the most common cause of death from trauma in this age group. During adolescence, occupant injuries are by far the leading cause of injury death, accounting for more than half of unintentional trauma deaths in this age group.

Drowning overall ranks second as a cause of trauma deaths, with peaks in the preschool and later teenage years. In some states of the United States, drowning is the leading cause of death from trauma for preschoolers (Wintemute, 1990). Although children 0 to 4 years make up only 26% of the U.S. population, they account for 36% of all drowning deaths. The causes of these drowning deaths vary with age and geographic area (Fig. 13.2). In young children, bathtub and swimming pool drowning predominate, whereas in older children and adolescents drownings occur predominantly in natural bodies of water while swimming or boating (Orlowski, 1987). Drowning during adolescence frequently involves alcohol use and abuse, as described further below. This secondary increase in drowning deaths among adolescents occurs only for boys (Wintemute, 1990) and occurs predominantly in rivers, lakes, canals, and beaches. Children with seizure disorders are at markedly increased risk of drowning compared to normal children, particularly bathtub drowning (Diekma et al., 1992).

Table 13.1. Violent Deaths in Children and Adolescents in the United States, 1986

	Age in Years				
	<5	5–9	10–14	15–19	Total
All injuries	4,607	2,133	2,776	12,895	22,411
Motor vehicle					
Occupant	658	397	643	5,714	7,412
Pedestrian	500	502	285	500	1,787
Drowning	754	326	323	659	2,062
Fire and burns	859	321	177	262	1,619
Homicide	660	134	245	1,838	2,877
Suicide	0	5	250	1,896	2,151

Source: Data from the Natural Center for Health Statistics, 1986.

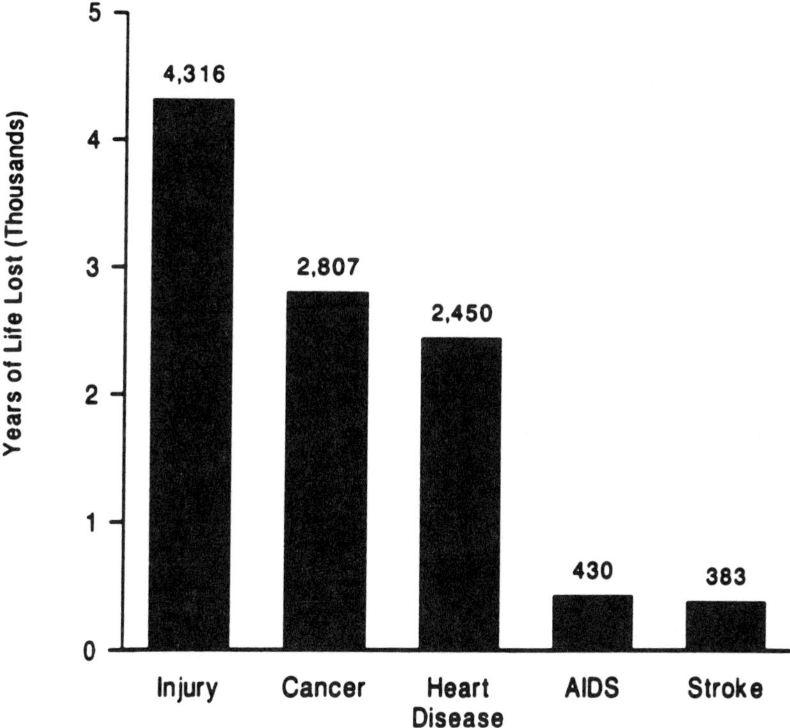

Fig. 13.1. Potential years of life lost before age 70 (Baker et al., 1992).

Fire and burn deaths account for nearly 10% of all trauma deaths and more than one in five in those under 5 years of age. The vast majority of these deaths (85%) are due to house fires and involve smoke inhalation and asphyxiation, rather than severe burns. Children and the elderly are at greatest risk of these deaths because of difficulty in escaping from burning buildings. Scalds and cloth-

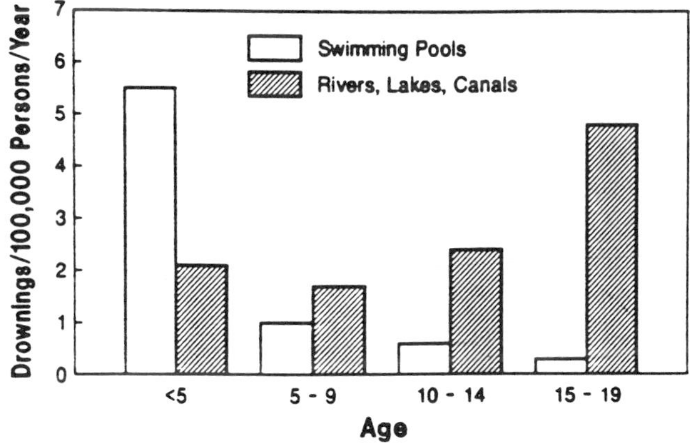

Fig. 13.2. Drowning rates by age at selected sites, Sacramento County, California: children ages 0 to 19, 1974 to 1984 (Wintemute et al., 1990).

ing ignition in the United States presently account for only 2.5% of burn deaths to children. The Flammable Fabrics Act of 1967, which made children's sleepwear flame retardant resulted in 90% reduction in burn unit admissions for sleepwear-related burns (McLoughlin et al., 1977).

Asphyxiation by choking accounts for approximately 40% of all unintentional deaths in children under 1 year of age. The majority of these deaths are caused by choking on food items, such as hot dogs, candies, grapes, and nuts (Baker & Fisher, 1980). Nonfood items that cause choking deaths include undersized infant pacifiers, small balls, and latex balloons.

Homicide is the leading cause of injury death for infants under 1 year and the fourth leading cause of death for ages 1 to 14. Homicide among children falls into two patterns: "infantile" and "adolescent" (Christoffel, 1990; See Chapter 14). Infantile homicide of children under the age of 5 represents child abuse, usually by a caregiver and mostly due to blunt trauma. In contrast, the adolescent pattern of homicide involves peers and acquaintances, and firearms are used in more than two thirds of cases (Jason, 1983). By far, a majority of these firearms are handguns. Children between these two ages experience homicides of both types.

Suicide is rare under age 10, and only 1% of suicides occur in children under 15 years of age (Baker et al., 1992; See Chapter 12). The suicide rate increases markedly after the age of 10 to become the second leading cause of death for 15- to 19-year-olds, accounting for more than 100,000 potential years of life lost (Hollinger, 1990). Native American teenagers have the highest risk, followed by white males; black females have the lowest rate of suicide in this age (Baker et al., 1992). Approximately 60% of teenage suicides involve firearms (Hollinger, 1990).

Morbidity

Mortality statistics, however, illustrate only part of the problem. Nonfatal injuries place a large burden on the health care system. Population-based studies indicate that approximately 25% of children and adolescents 0 to 19 years receive medical care for an injury each year (Rivara et al., 1989). Of these, 2.5% require hospitalization, and 55% have at least temporary disability from their injuries (Rivara et al., 1989).

The distribution of nonfatal injuries is very different from that of fatal injuries (Table 13.2). An estimated 600,000 children are hospitalized for trauma each year in the United States, and more than 15 million require emergency room care for trauma (Guyer & Ellers, 1990). Falls and sports are the leading cause of both emergency room visits and hospitalizations. Most of the serious falls are from heights greater than 10 feet; few serious injuries occur at heights of less than this distance (Chadwick et al., 1991). The leading cause of emergency room visits and hospitalizations involving sports is bicycle use, which annually accounts for more than 300,000 emergency room visits (Bicycle-related injuries, 1987). Motor vehicle occupant injuries are an important cause of emergency room visits and hospitalizations, but are not the leading cause as they are for deaths. Falls

Table 13.2. Estimates of the Incidence of Childhood Injuries in 1985

Cause of Injury	Hospital Inpatients	Emergency Department Visits
Motor vehicle		
Occupant	73,334	667,053
Pedestrian	23,974	111,411
Other	35,962	322,950
Burns	19,039	352,565
Drowning	1,410	NA
Sports	91,667	2,564,558
Falls	122,693	3,603,214
Suicide/self-inflicted	23,974	36,667
Homicide/violence	26,795	432,950
Other	174,872	7,611,877
Total	593,720	15,703,245

Source: Data from Guyer & Ellers (1990).

account for more than five times and sports injuries for almost four times the number of emergency room visits as motor vehicle occupant injuries.

The morbidity from some types of injuries should not be underestimated. Children with severe submersion incidents requiring cardiopulmonary resuscitation in the emergency department have a poor prognosis. Approximately 60% to 100% of survivors of these episodes are severely damaged (Wintemute, 1990). Burn victims frequently require skin grafting and multiple surgical procedures; many are left with disfiguring scars and emotional sequelae (Cooper & Thomas, 1988). Head injuries account for the majority of severe trauma to children and are the injury most likely to produce long-term sequelae (Brink et al., 1980). These sequelae include learning problems, emotional lability, memory loss, and resultant stress on parents and siblings (Jaffe et al., 1990).

Costs

The cost of trauma in the United States is enormous—an estimated $157 billion in 1985, of which children accounted for $13.8 billion (Rice et al., 1989). This figure includes direct costs, the expenditure for medical services; morbidity costs, the value of goods and services not produced because of injury-related illness and disability; and mortality costs, the lost wages and earnings from premature death. The highest direct medical care costs for childhood injuries are for falls, sports injuries, motor vehicle occupant injuries, and burns (Guyer & Ellers, 1990). Injuries that are most frequent, such as those due to falls and sports, contribute more to direct medical care costs, whereas fatal injuries such as motor vehicle occupant and pedestrian injuries, account for a greater portion of the indirect costs.

Geographic Variations

There are sizeable differences in the incidence of fatal injury between rural and urban areas and among different states and geographic regions of the United

States. Unintentional injury death rates are highest in rural areas for both motor vehicle and nonmotor vehicle related deaths (Baker et al., 1992). In contrast, the homicide rate is much higher in central cities than in other areas.

Geographic differences in injury rates are very large for some types of injuries. Injury death rates for children 0 to 14 years from 1980 to 1985 ranged from 11.2 per 100,000 in Massachusetts to 35.0 per 100,000 in Alaska (Waller et al., 1989). In general, the highest rates were in the Mountain States and in the South, and the lowest rates were in New England, the Midwest and the Mid-Atlantic states. House fire deaths had a distinct geographic pattern, with high rates in the East, especially the Southeast, and low rates in the West. These regional differences may be due to the use of noncentral heating equipment, such as kerosene heaters and wood-burning stoves, as well as differences in types of building materials used (Baker et al., 1992). Differences between states in drowning deaths reflect a variety of factors including exposure to boats and pools. The rates of drowning in Alaska are very high in large part due to the ubiquitious use of boats as a method of transportation. Drowning deaths among preschoolers are very high in California, Florida, and Arizona because of the number of pools in the immediate environment of young children.

These differences in death rates for childhood injury may suggest causal factors that would be amenable to intervention (Waller et al., 1989). The high death rate from fires in some states may reflect the need to promote smoke detectors. The high rate of drowning suggests the need for use of personal floatation devices in Alaska and four-sided pool fencing in California. The low motor vehicle death rates in Utah suggests that limiting alcohol use will further reduce motor vehicle fatalities.

Trends Over Time

The death rate for childhood injuries has declined throughout this century, with rather marked decreases in deaths from unintentional injuries over the last two decades. Compared to the years 1977 to 1979, childhood injury deaths in 1984 to 1986 were 25% to 30% lower (Baker et al., 1992). In contrast, adolescent suicide rates increased from 1950 to 1970 and have continued to do so for white males (Hollinger, 1990). Among black males aged 15 to 19, the firearm suicide rate doubled between 1982 and 1987, whereas the rate of suicide by other means declined (Fingerhut & Kleinman, 1989). Firearm suicide rates in 1985 for white males are more than threefold higher than in 1955. Many have attributed this increase in suicide rates to an increase in firearm suicides and a greater availability of guns (Boyd, 1983). Homicide is the only leading cause of childhood death to increase from 1950 to 1980, and handgun homicides have increased fivefold during the last three decades (Baker et al., 1992).

International Comparisons

Childhood injury mortality in the United States is higher than in most industrialized countries (Williams & Kotch, 1990) and is twice the rate of fatal injuries in Sweden (Bergman & Rivara, 1991). The rates of childhood injury deaths were similar in the United States and Canada at the beginning of the 1980s, but diverged markedly by the end of the decade (Fig. 13.3). Motor vehicle injuries account for a large portion of the gap between the United States and other countries. However, the fatality rate per vehicle miles driven is lower in the United States than in other countries; the higher rate of fatal motor vehicle crashes per population is due to the larger number of miles traveled in the United States (Lamm et al., 1985).

The teenage homicide rate in the United States is far higher than that of other countries. In 1985, the homicide rate among U.S. males aged 15 to 19 was approximately five times greater than rates for Canada and Australia and 18 to 20 times greater than those of European countries (Williams & Kotch, 1990). This increased rate is not limited to minority children; nonblack child homicide rates in the United States are twice the Canadian rate and three- to sixfold higher than rates for European countries.

Drowning deaths in the United States are also higher than in other countries, particularly for males aged 15 to 19 years. This is true for both white and nonwhite males (Williams & Kotch, 1990). Among the youngest children, fire-related deaths are especially high in North America relative to European countries. Deaths by fire are also common in Canada, possibly due to the use of wood stoves and fireplaces for heating.

Efforts to prevent childhood injuries have met with success, particularly in Sweden. Comprehensive programs of education, legislation, regulation, environmental modification, and safe product design have resulted in marked reductions in childhood injury mortality over the last 30 years and can serve as models for this and other countries (Bergman & Rivara, 1991).

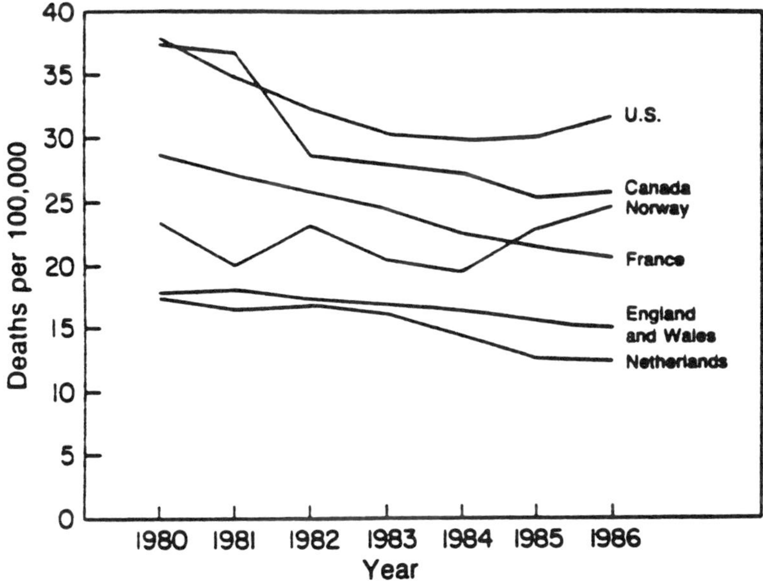

Fig. 13.3. Injury death rates 1980 to 1986, ages 1 to 19 years, for the United States and selected countries (Williams & Kotch, 1990).

Special Applications and Problems

Epidemiology is the keystone to injury control. It is used to define the problem, target high-risk groups, determine risk factors leading to injury, and evaluate the effectiveness of intervention programs. The injury field presents some special challenges for epidemiology, as well as some unique opportunities.

Surveillance

Surveillance provides the basic information on which injury research and prevention efforts are based. It can occur at many levels, each with its own advantages and disadvantages (Graitcer, 1987). Whenever injuries are identified, whether they be from a medical examiner's office, a hospital medical record department, or emergency room logs, they must be classified as to type and severity. The International Classification of Diseases (ICD) codes injuries in two different ways. Diagnosis codes, called "N" codes, are used to classify the nature of the injury, e.g., midshaft fracture of the femur, laceration of the spleen, or subdural hematoma. An external cause of injury, "E" code, is used to classify the etiology of the injury, e.g., fall from a height, pedestrian motor vehicle collision, or assault. The current Ninth Revision of the ICD for E codes is cumbersome at best, and inadequate at worst. The next version promises to be a major revision and should prove far more useful and user friendly than the current one.

Categorizing injuries by severity is necessary for priority setting and for comparison of the importance of different causes. The most commonly used scale is the Abbreviated Injury Scale (AIS; Committee on Injury Scaling, 1985) and its derivative, the Injury Severity Scale (ISS; Baker et al., 1974) for multiple trauma. The ISS has been shown to correlate well with the risk of mortality (MacKenzie, 1989). Recent studies have shown the AIS does correlate with risk of long-term disability (MacKenzie et al., 1988), but is less accurate for coding the severity of traumatic brain injury and for penetrating trauma, such as gunshot wounds. More importantly, it provides little discriminating power for the majority of less severe injuries to children or adolescents treated in the emergency room setting. New scales are needed that can accurately separate injuries with a significant impact on at least short-term disability and costs from those with little consequence other than the emergency room visit.

Surveillance of fatal injuries is relatively easy and complete. However, for every fatal injury that occurs, 28 children are admitted to hospital for trauma and 740 are treated in emergency rooms (Guyer & Ellers, 1990). Data on fatal injuries are also usually population based, thus allowing the calculation of rates. Yet, fatal injuries may be misclassified, particularly suicides, which may be classified as "accidental" injuries (Robertson, 1992). Misclassification may be a particular problem in some jurisdictions where the coroner is an elected official without medical training.

Hospital admissions, by virtue of the severity of the trauma, stem from an important subset of injuries and are usually feasible to identify; nevertheless, they represent only 2% to 3% of injuries presenting to an emergency room

(Rivara et al., 1989). Most hospitals serve a varying population, making calculation of rates difficult if not impossible. Referral patterns, particularly to trauma centers, can create biases in data collection and analysis (Payne & Waller, 1989). Trauma centers usually care only for severely injured patients; those with less severe injuries are likely to be treated elsewhere. Reliance solely on trauma center data can thus underestimate the effectiveness of injury prevention measures, such as bicycle helmets, motorcycle helmets, and seatbelts (Thompson et al., 1989).

More than half of the states in the United States have computerized hospital discharge summary databases. However, only six states currently mandate that all discharges for injury be E-coded, which identifies the etiology of injury. Without this crucial code, such data are much less useful for surveillance or research purposes. One study found the cost to hospitals for additional E-coding was minimal (Rivara et al., 1990). Universal coding of hospital discharges has been recommended by many groups and will be facilitated by the addition of fields for E-codes to currently used billing forms.

Injuries treated in the emergency room are very similar to those treated in physician's offices (Rivara et al., 1989) and probably represent the minimum severity of injury that deserves prevention; the collection of emergency room data can be labor intensive and thus expensive because of the large number of hospitals involved. Nevertheless, such ER data may be necessary for the study of less common types of injuries or injuries that do not routinely result in death or hospitalization, such as toy injuries, poisoning, and animal bites.

Specific surveillance systems have been developed by various agencies. The National Highway Traffic Safety Administration (NHTSA) operates a Fatal Accident Reporting System (FARS), which collects police report and medical data on all motor vehicle crashes in which a person dies within 30 days of an injury (NHTSA, 1992). NHTSA also operates a General Estimate System, which is a probability sample of all police-reported motor vehicle crashes in the United States, regardless of whether an injury occurred (NHTSA, 1990). The Federal Bureau of Investigation maintains data on a variety of crimes in the United States, including assaults and criminal homicides. The Consumer Product Safety Commission operates the National Electronic Injury Surveillance System based on a sample of hospital emergency rooms in the United States. This system collects information on consumer-product-related injuries treated in hospital emergency rooms and allows the calculation of national rates. However, it does not include information on motor vehicles or guns, since they do not come under the jurisdiction of the Commission. The Laboratory for Disease Control in Canada has recently instituted a surveillance of injuries to children treated in 13 hospital emergency rooms, the Childhood Injury Research and Prevention Program (CHIRPP). There are no equivalent general emergency room surveillance systems in the United States.

The Haddon Matrix

Epidemiologists commonly view variations in disease occurrence as a function of the classic triad of host, agent, and environment. William Haddon made an important contribution to the injury field when he demonstrated that the application of this epidemiologic paradigm would be much more useful if applied to the different phases in the pathway of injury occurrence (Haddon, 1972). Unlike other diseases, the occurrence of an event leading to an injury (pre-event phase) can and should be distinguished from the actual injury-producing event itself (event phase). Finally, the ultimate morbidity and mortality from trauma are affected by what happens after the injury occurs, the postevent phase. Haddon developed a matrix in which the interaction of all three dimensions can be displayed and considered (Figure 13.4). In addition, the physical environment is considered separately from the social environment in which children play, adults work, products are built, and laws are passed.

This paradigm is also based on the premise that injury occurs from the transfer of energy to people at rates and amounts that exceed the threshold to cause an injury. Thus, motor vehicles are the means by which this energy is transferred; it is the energy transfer, however, that causes the injury and not the crash itself. Barriers, such as airbags or padded dashboards, cannot prevent the crash from occurring, but can prevent the transfer of energy from exceeding human tolerances, thereby preventing the person from being injured (Haddon, 1980).

This matrix is useful for considering risk factors for the occurrence of injuries and their consequences, as well as for determining points for intervention in the causal sequence leading to disability from trauma. Epidemiologic studies of risk factors for injuries commonly concentrate on pre-event host factors, such as age or sex. However, injury prevention depends more on examining modifiable risk factors—pre-event factors in the agent or environment; event factors, such as crash protection afforded by cars; and postevent factors, such as the availability of emergency medical services, trauma center care, and long-term rehabilitation (Robertson, 1992).

		Epidemiologic Dimension			
		Human Factors	Agent or Vehicle	Physical Environment	Socio-Cultural Environment
Event Dimension	Pre-Event				
	Event				
	Post-Event				

Fig. 13.4. Matrix and conceptual framework for injury cause and prevention (Haddon, 1972).

Case-Control Studies

Despite the magnitude of the problem, injuries, particularly serious injuries of a specific type and mechanism, are relatively rare events. Prospective studies to determine the importance of risk factors for an injury would require large cohorts and/or long periods of follow-up (see Chapter 1). For example, the rate of hospitalization for head injuries related to bicycling among children is 13.5 per 100,000 (Kraus et al., 1987). To determine whether helmets are effective (i.e., whether they reduce the risk of head injury compared to unhelmeted riders), would require a large cohort of helmeted and unhelmeted children to be followed over a relatively long period of time, e.g., 1 year. This is expensive as well as difficult to do; in this example, helmet use is so uncommon as to require a huge population in order to obtain enough "exposed" cases. Retrospective cohort studies that rely on questionnaire or survey to ascertain exposure to risk factors may encounter recall bias. For example, 97% of people involved in a motor vehicle crash recalled the crash when interviewed within 3 months, but only 73% recalled the crash 9 to 12 months later (National Center for Health Statistics, 1972).

Nevertheless, some large cohort studies have been conducted and provide important information about childhood injuries. The two most useful studies involve data from the British Births Study (Bijur et al., 1988; Pless et al., 1989) and the Dunedin Child Development Study (Langley et al., 1980). In both cases, a large birth cohort was followed prospectively over time. These studies have provided useful information on risk factors for childhood injuries, especially social and behavioral factors (Bijur et al., 1988; Langley et al., 1980; Pless et al., 1989).

An alternative technique for the study of risk factors for injuries is the use of case-control designs (see Chapter 1). These designs are well known to epidemiologists, but have been underutilized in the injury field. Case-control designs are ideal for the study of relatively rare problems, such as head injuries from bicycle crashes, suicides from home ownership of guns, or motor vehicle crashes in individuals with certain medical risk factors. They allow one to measure the strength and direction of association between an injury and multiple risk factors. Often, they use existing records and data sources, making these studies much more economically feasible than prospective cohort studies. Finally, case-control studies do not require long-term follow-up.

The use of case-control studies in injury research, however, is not without its challenges. As with all such studies, a key issue is the proper selection of control subjects. The use of individuals with other injuries may be an appropriate control group when analyzing the protective effect of a specific intervention, such as bicycle helmets. However, such a control group may underestimate the true effect of helmets in that helmeted bicyclists may sustain no injuries at all in a crash and thus not be part of the control group (Thompson et al., 1989). A more appropriate control group would thus be one that sampled the entire population of cyclists who crashed, regardless of the presence or absence of injuries. This bias from the use of controls in medical settings will occur in any situation in which the hypothesized risk factor influences in some way the decision to seek medical care (Robertson, 1992).

Ecologic studies have also been used to assess risk factors for injuries. These studies correlate injury rates with characteristics of a community in one geographic area compared to another. They are best used to generate hypotheses, rather than to test them, and have important limitations (Morgenstern, 1982). Nevertheless, these studies have been useful, for example, in examining the potential effect of restrictive firearm regulations on the community rates of suicide (Sloan et al., 1990) and homicide (Sloan et al., 1988).

Exposure Measurement

A key element of any study design, whether it be a cohort or case-control study, is the proper measurement of risk. For child pedestrian injuries, such an exposure may be the number of motor vehicles encountered in some period of time—hour, day, week, year (Routledge et al., 1974). Children in urban areas may have a higher risk of pedestrian injury than those in rural areas solely because of an increased exposure to traffic; other risk factors may be similar once this difference is accounted (adjusted) for. The risk of childhood drowning is clearly related to exposure to water. However, it is also related to the type of exposure (swimming versus wading), the length of the exposure, and potentially the duration of exposure per episode, as well as the number of episodes per year. The apparent increased risk of some types of injuries, such as injuries to children in day care, may disappear when the number of hours of exposure are taken into account (Rivara et al., 1990).

Calculation of rates of injuries should ideally take these exposure measurements into consideration (Robertson, 1992). Motor vehicle fatalities are often reported both as per 100,000 population and as per 100 million vehicle miles traveled (NHTSA, 1992). Unfortunately, calculation of rates based on hours of exposure is difficult for most activities because of the general lack of availability of such data.

Evaluation of Interventions and Use of Proxies

One of the important uses of epidemiology in injury research is in the evaluation of interventions. The traditional evaluation of health promotion and disease prevention programs has been based on examining subsequent reductions in diseases and deaths. However, because injuries are rare diseases, reduction in the number of deaths for specific injury types, particularly locally, may not be statistically feasible. An examination of changes in hospital admissions, although more numerous, is hindered by the fact that most hospitals do not have a well-defined, specific population base, and changes in the actual occurrence of injuries may not be reflected in a hospital's admission census. Emergency-room-treated injuries are much more frequent (20- to 30-fold more common than hospitalizations) and represent a clearly defined event. A significant disadvantage to the use of emergency room data, however, is the expense of data collection. Most emergency rooms do not routinely code injury data for mechanism of injury. Ongoing surveillance systems may need to be established to collect the quality and type of data necessary for these evaluation studies.

At the other end of the outcome spectrum are surveys measuring changes in knowledge and attitudes. Although often used to measure the effectiveness of injury prevention programs, the available evidence argues against these being valid measures in injury research (Robertson, 1992). For example, the Centers for Disease Control regularly conducts telephone surveys to determine the prevalence of certain risk factors, including seatbelt use and drinking while driving (Anda et al., 1990). Comparison of these self-report data with actual observations of seatbelt use indicates that seatbelt use is overreported by an average of 21% (Mawson & Buindo, 1985; Robertson, 1992). Self-reported data on driving while intoxicated also do not correlate with the proportion of fatally injured drivers who are intoxicated. Self-reports of hazards in the home are not an accurate reflection of home safety as measured by actual inspections (Fergusson et al., 1982). More importantly, there seems to be little correlation between knowledge and behavior change. Educational programs can increase knowledge, but increased knowledge often does not translate into behavior change (McLoughlin et al., 1982).

One method that has proven very useful for the evaluation of injury prevention programs has been the use of proxies, i.e., changes in behavior that directly lead to prevention in injuries.

The evaluation of programs to increase seatbelt or child seat restraint use has depended heavily on observations of restraint use as a measure of effectiveness (Williams & Wells, 1981; Williams et al., 1987). Initial increases in seat restraint use were sufficiently small as to make meaningful analysis of reduction in injury and fatality rates difficult. However, once use rates increased sufficiently, evaluation of reductions in fatalities (Partyka, 1989), severity of injuries (Barancik et al., 1988), and costs and hospitalizations supported the effectiveness of seat restraints and programs to increase their use.

Observations of helmet use have been used to evaluate the effectiveness of community bicycle helmet programs. Bicycle helmet use among school-aged children increased from 2% to 16% in Seattle after the introduction of a comprehensive educational and discount buying program, whereas use remained at 2% to 3% in Portland, Oregon, a control community without a similar program (DiGuiseppi et al., 1989). More recently, helmet use has increased to 38% in Seattle and has been accompanied by a 50% reduction in admissions for bicycle-related head injuries. Helmet use increased from 4% to 47% in Howard County, Maryland after the introduction of a mandatory bicycle helmet use law (Cote et al., 1992). The sampling for these observations can be done in such a way as to allow analysis, for example, of differential effects of the campaign in poor as compared to nonpoor areas (DiGuiseppi et al., 1989).

Prevention of child pedestrian injuries has been approached in several ways. Many communities have used school-based pedestrian skills training programs to address this problem (Rothengatter, 1984). Observations of children before and after training have been used to evaluate the effectiveness of these programs. One recent study found only modest improvements in children's pedestrian skills, indicating the need for broader-based efforts to reduce pedestrian injuries (Rivara et al., 1991).

The effectiveness of legislation to reduce home water heater temperatures has been evaluated through a combination of observation of water heater temperature and an examination of changes in admission rates for tap water scald injuries. Five years after legislation requiring water heaters to be preset at 120°F, 84% of homes with postlaw water heaters had tap water temperatures in the safe range (Erdmann et al., 1991). This was accompanied by a 50% reduction in the admission rate for tap-water-related burns, as well as a reduction in the total body surface area burned, mortality, grafting, and length of hospital stay.

Risk Factors

The use of epidemiology has been critical in identifying risk factors for childhood injuries. These risk factors help pinpoint target populations for prevention programs and, using Haddon's matrix, delineate the key points for intervention.

Age

Injuries do not occur homogeneously throughout childhood. Infants are at greatest risk for burns, drowning, and falls. As these children increasingly acquire mobility and exploratory behavior, poisonings join the list. Young school-aged children are at greatest risk of pedestrian injuries, bicycle-related injuries (the most serious of which usually involve motor vehicles), motor vehicle occupant injuries, burns, and drowning. The teenage years see a markedly increased risk from motor vehicle occupant trauma, a continued risk from drowning and burns, and the new risk of intentional trauma, discussed in Chapter 12.

Injuries occurring at a particular age represent a window of vulnerability during which children or adolescents encounter a new task or hazard that they often do not have the developmental skills to handle successfully. For example, toddlers do not have the judgment to know that medications can be poisonous or that some house plants are not to be eaten; they cannot handle the hazard presented by a swimming pool or an open second-story window. For young children, parents may inadvertently "set up" this mismatch between the skills of the child and the demands of the task. A walker converts an infant into a mobile toddler and greatly increases contact with hazards. Many parents expect young school-aged children to walk home from school, the play field, or the local candy store, yet careful developmental studies indicate that children under the age of 9 or 10 do not have the developmental skills to handle traffic safely (Rivara, 1990).

The lack of skills and experience to handle many tasks during the teenage years contributes to teenagers' increased risk of injuries, particularly motor vehicle injuries. This age group has both the highest daytime and the highest nighttime crash rate (Robertson, 1981). Nighttime curfews for young drivers have been effective in decreasing motor vehicle crashes and fatalities for inexperienced drivers (Preusser et al., 1984). High-school driver education training does not seem to reduce individual drivers' risk of crashing, but increases the number of drivers licensed at an earlier age, thereby increasing the population at risk (Shaoul, 1975). A case-control study of driver licensure and crash records of teenagers in schools that eliminated driver training programs, compared to schools that retained such programs, found large reductions in the number of adolescents licensed before age 18 years and a reduction in the number of crashes in this age group (Robertson, 1980).

Younger teens seem to have a higher motor vehicle crash rate than older teens. Increasing the minimum age for licensure from 16 to 17 years could result in a 65% to 85% reduction in fatalities involving 16-year-old drivers without a concomitant increase in fatalities among 17- to 29-year-old drivers (Williams et al., 1983).

Returning to the Haddon matrix, age influences both the risk of injury during the event phase and the risk of long-term disability in the event phase. For example, young school-aged children have an inadequately developed pelvis; in a motor vehicle crash, the seat belt does not anchor onto the pelvis, but rides up onto the abdomen, resulting in the risk of serious abdominal injury (Anderson et al., 1991). Furthermore, age interacts with the vehicle characteristics in this instance in that most children ride in the rear seat, which until very recently have only been equipped with lap belts and not lap-shoulder harnesses. These abdominal injuries are distinctly unusual with lap-shoulder harnesses, but are not uncommon with lap belts (Anderson et al., 1991). Children under the age of 2 have much worse outcomes from closed head injuries than do older children and adolescents, potentially because of the relatively unmyelinated brain found in infants and toddlers (Bruce et al., 1979).

Sex

Beginning at approximately 1 to 2 years of age and continuing until the seventh decade of life, males have higher rates of injuries than do females. This difference during childhood does not seem to be due to developmental differences between the sexes, differences in coordination, or differences in muscle strength (Rivara et al., 1982). Rather, variation in exposure may account for the male predominance in some types of injuries. Boys in all age groups have higher rates of bicycle-related injuries (Rivara et al., 1982). However, correcting for exposure reduces this excess rate in boys. Therefore, for bicycles, boys have higher rates of injuries because they use them more frequently or for more hours. Similar results have been found in other studies on bicycle crashes (Chlapecka et al., 1975).

In contrast, Routledge and colleagues (1974) examined the difference in exposure to risk of pedestrian injury in children. They found that, at the peak ages for pedestrian injuries (5 to 8 years), boys and girls had equal exposure to risk, as measured by the number of roads crossed in the course of a day and the traffic densities on the road. Thus, the higher rate of pedestrian injuries among boys could not be explained by differences in exposure. This increased incidence may be due to differences in behavior. For example, their risk-taking behavior, combined with their greater frequency of alcohol use, may lead to the disproportionately high rate of motor vehicle crashes among teenage males.

Part of this difference between boys and girls, particularly in younger children, may lie in parental expectations and child-rearing practices. Parents of young boys tolerate, if not encourage, rough-and-tumble behavior, a type of behavior that may not be acceptable for little girls. The differences in injury rates do not seem to be due to differences in motor skills, since boys at all ages are more coordinated than girls, are stronger, and have faster reaction times (Maccoby & Jacklin, 1974).

Race

There are striking racial variations in injury mortality, including mortality during childhood. Blacks have much higher rates of injuries than whites, whereas Asians have lower rates and Hispanics are intermediate between blacks and whites (Division of Injury Control, 1990). Native Americans have the highest death rate from unintentional injuries (Baker et al., 1992). These discrepancies are even more pronounced for some injury problems. For example, the homicide rate in black teenagers 15 to 19 years was 50 per 100,000 in 1986 compared with 8 per 100,000 for whites. The suicide rate among Native American youth is twice the rate among whites and threefold greater than the rate among Asians (Baker et al., 1992). The rate of fire and burn deaths in black preschoolers is more than threefold higher than for whites—12 per 100,000 compared to 3.9 per 100,000 respectively.

The reasons for these racial differences seem to be related primarily to poverty. Studies that have examined racial discrepancies for homicide, for example, have found that rates for blacks are nearly equivalent to whites when adjusted for socioeconomic status (Griffith & Bell, 1989; Loftin & Hill, 1974).

Socioeconomic Status

One of the most important risk factors for childhood injuries is poverty. Injuries do not occur in the population at random, and those at greatest risk in general are poor children. This fact has been demonstrated in several studies. An analysis of child deaths in Maine for the years 1976 to 1980 found that poor children (defined as those receiving AFDC or food stamps) had more than twice the rate of trauma deaths of nonpoor children (Nersesian et al., 1985). The rate of deaths from fires and burns was fivefold higher and, from drowning, fourfold higher. Rivara and Barber (1985) compared census tracts in Memphis in which children sustained child pedestrian injuries to tracts without pedestrian injuries. By all socioeconomic parameters, the tracts experiencing pedestrian injuries were poorer than those without pedestrian injuries, as measured in a variety of ways: lower median family income, a higher proportion of children in poverty, a higher proportion of families headed by women, lower housing values, and more crowding. Pless has shown a similar relationship for traffic injuries in Montreal, where children from low-income areas at all age groups and for both sexes had higher rates of injury than children from middle- and upper-income areas of the city (Pless et al., 1987). Residential fire deaths occur predominantly in poor areas of inner cities (Mierley & Baker, 1983).

These same socioeconomic relationships are also found within racial groups. Both blacks and whites have an inverse relationship between income level and death rates. The higher the income level, the lower the death rate (Baker, 1974). Native Americans have especially high rates in low-income areas (Baker et al., 1992).

Environment

How does the important risk factor of poverty increase the risk of injury to children? One mechanism is through its effect on the environment. Children who are poor are at increased risk of injury to a large degree because they are exposed to more hazards in their living environments than other children. They live in more fire-trap housing and are less likely to be protected by smoke detectors. The roads on which they live are more likely to have high-speed traffic and higher traffic volumes and are more likely to be major thoroughfares. Their neighborhoods are more likely to be violent, and they are more likely to be victims of assault than are children and adolescents living in middle-class suburbs.

Focus on the environment is also important because it directs attention away from relatively immutable factors, such as family dynamics, poverty, and race, and directs it more toward factors that can be changed through appropriate efforts.

Interventions

Efforts at injury control have begun to meet with substantial success in recent years. They have occurred at all levels of prevention: primary, secondary, and tertiary.

Motor vehicle injuries, as the most important cause of trauma death for children and adolescents in the United States, has been the subject of a wide variety of injury prevention efforts. Properly used car safety seats seem to reduce the risk of severe injury or death by as much as 70% (Kahane, 1986); seatbelts for older children and adolescents reduce the risk by almost 50% (Evans, 1986). All 50 states now have laws requiring children to be properly restrained when riding in motor vehicles. These laws have been effective in increasing restraint use (Williams et al., 1987) and have decreased morbidity and mortality due to motor vehicle crashes (Campbell et al., 1991; Partyka, 1989; Wagenaar & Margolis, 1990).

Bicycle helmets have been found to be a very effective means of preventing head injury, the most common serious injury resulting in hospitalization or death in bicycle crashes. Bicycle helmets prevent 88% of brain injuries in bicycle crashes; unhelmeted riders are eightfold more likely to have a brain injury than are helmeted bicyclists (Thompson et al., 1989). Both educational programs

(Bergman et al., 1990) and mandatory use laws (Cote et al., 1992) have been successful in increasing helmet use.

Deaths in housefires can be prevented most easily through the use of smoke detectors, perhaps the single most cost-effective device for injury prevention a family can own. Clothing ignition, once an important source of fatal and severe burn injury, has been reduced by flame-retardant materials as mandated for children's sleepwear (McLoughlin et al., 1977). Most scald burns have proven difficult to prevent, with the exception of tap water scalds, which are fully preventable by turning down water heater temperatures (Erdmann et al., 1991).

There has been a marked reduction in childhood poisoning deaths in this country over the last 30 years (Baker et al., 1992). Efforts to reduce poisoning deaths stand as one of the success stories in pediatric injury control. Prevention has occurred at the primary, secondary, and tertiary levels. Reduction in the number of aspirin and iron tablets in one bottle to sublethal doses, the use of child-resistant packaging (Walton, 1982), the development of poison center networks and poison information lines (McIntire & Angle, 1983), the use of syrup of ipecac in the home, and the development of effective protocols for management of poisoning (Done, 1978) have all contributed to this remarkable reduction in death among preschool children.

Falls are the leading cause of nonfatal injury and have an enormous variety of causes. The majority of serious and fatal falls in children involve falls from heights, usually greater than 10 feet (Chadwick et al., 1991). These falls most often occur out of windows and can be prevented through the use of simple window guards (Speigel & Lindaman, 1977).

Prevention of drowning deaths must be approached through a variety of means. Childproof pool fencing that completely surrounds the pool is extremely effective in preventing drowning of young children (Wintemute, 1990). Pool barriers that use the residence as one side of the enclosure are not effective since they do not decrease access to the pool from the house. Bathtub drowning involves young children or children with seizure disorders and can only be prevented through appropriate supervision of children. Drowning of older children and adolescents is much more problematic. There is, unfortunately, inadequate evidence for the effectiveness of swimming training in reducing drowning (Pearn, 1985). Drowning among adolescents most commonly involves alcohol (Davis et al., 1985) and may be preventable through further restriction of access to alcohol by adolescents.

Injury control also involves care of the trauma patient, including emergency medical services, emergency room and hospital care, and rehabilitation for any injury sequelae. Advanced paramedic care at the scene has become the standard of care for trauma patients including children (Lewis, 1983). However, many of the procedures employed by paramedics—including fluids in the field (Kaweski et al., 1990), airway control, and the use of helicopters (Schiller et al., 1988; Schwartz et al., 1989)—have not been subjected to adequate rigorous randomized clinical trials. Unfortunately, such procedures may have become so well established as standard care that prospective randomized trials are currently not feasible.

Trauma center care has made a significant difference in the survival of seriously injured patients. Comprehensive trauma systems seem to reduce the number of preventable deaths by more than 50% (West & Cales, 1983).

Improvements in emergency medical services and acute care have increasingly enabled children to survive severe injury. However, many of these injuries to children result in substantial sequelae. Wesson et al. (1989) found that approximately 50% of children admitted to a hospital for the care of serious trauma have not yet returned to normal activities by 6 months after the injury. Unfortunately, only a small percentage of children receive appropriate rehabilitation care. A recent analysis of 4870 cases of head injury found that 58% of children with four or more impairments in the areas of vision, hearing, speech, self-feeding, bathing, dressing, walking, cognition, and behavior were discharged from acute care without rehabilitation management (DiScala et al., 1991).

Conclusions

The magnitude of the injury problem need not lead to paralysis of action. Epidemiology has and can continue to make important contributions to the development of effective interventions that can reduce the prime health problem among children today. We need only to look to a country, such as Sweden, to see what is possible. In 1954, 450 Swedish children aged 15 and under died from trauma; in 1988 that number had been reduced to 88 (Bergman & Rivara, 1991). Death rates from motor vehicle injuries are one third to one half that of the United States; deaths from fires and burns are one half the United States rate. This injury prevention effort began with a systematic campaign in the 1950s and is based on a program of injury surveillance and research, legislation and regulation to make the environment safer, and a broad-based safety education campaign. Although there are obvious differences between Sweden and other countries, particularly the United States, nevertheless many lessons can be learned from it. Sweden has demonstrated that "where there's a will, there's a way."

References

Anda RF, Waller MN, Wooton KG, et al. Behavioral risk factor surveillance, 1988. *MMWR CDC Surveillance Summaries* 1990; 39(2):1–21.

Anderson P, Rivara FP, Maier RV, Drake C. The epidemiology of seat belt-associated injuries. *J Trauma* 1991; 31:60–67.

Baker SP, Fisher RS. Childhood asphyxiation by choking or suffocation. *JAMA* 1980; 244:1343–1346.

Baker SP, O'Neill B, Haddon W, et al. The injury severity score: a method for describing patients with multiple injuries and evaluating emergency care. *J Trauma* 1974; 14:187.

Baker SP, O'Neill B, Ginsburg MJ, Li G. *The Injury Fact Book*. New York: Oxford University Press: 1992.

Barancik JI, Kramer CF, Thode HC, Harris D. Efficacy of the New York state seat belt law: preliminary assessment of occurrence and severity. *Bull NY Acad Med* 1988; 64:742–749.

Bergman AB, Rivara FP. Sweden's experience in reducing childhood injuries. *Pediatrics* 1991; 88:69–74.

Bergman AB, Rivara FP, Rogers LW et al. The Seattle children's bicycle helmet campaign. *Am J Dis Child* 1990; 144:727–731.

Bicycle-related injuries: data from the National Electronic Injury Surveillance System. *MMWR* 1987; 36:269–271.

Bijur P, Golding J, Haslum M, Kurzon M. Behavioral predictors of injury in school-age children. *Am J Dis Child* 1988; 142:1307–1312.

Boyd JH. The increasing rate of suicide by firearms. *N Engl J Med* 1983; 308:872–874.

Brink JD, Imbus C, Woo-Sam J. Physical recovery after severe closed head trauma in children and adolescents. *J Pediatr* 1980; 97:721–727.

Bruce DA, Raphaely RC, Goldberg AI, et al. Pathophysiology, treatment and outcome following severe head injury in children. *Child Brain* 1979; 5:174–191.

Campbell BJ, Stewart JR, Reinfurt DW. Change in injuries associated with safety belt laws. *Accid Anal Prev* 1991; 23:87–93.

Chadwick DL, Chin S, Salerno C, et al. Deaths from falls in children: how far is fatal? *J Trauma* 1991; 31:1353–1355.

Chlapecka TW, Schupack SA, Planek TW, et al. *Bicycle Accidents and Usage Among Elementary School Children in the United States*. Chicago: National Safety Council; 1975.

Christoffel KK: Violent death and injury in US children and adolescents. *Am J Dis Child* 1980;144:697–706.

Committee on Injury Scaling. *Abbreviated Injury Scale*. Evanston, IL, 1985.

Cooper MK, Thomas CM. Psychosocial care of the severely burned child. In: Carvajal HF, Parks DH, eds. *Burns in Children. Pediatric Burn Management*. Chicago: Year Book Medical Publishers; 1988:345–362.

Cote TR, Sacks JJ, Lambert-Huber DA, et al. Bicycle helmet use among Maryland children: effect of legislation and education. *Pediatrics* 1992; 89:1216–1220.

Davis S et al. Drownings of children and youth in a desert state. *West J Med* 1985; 143:196–201.

Diekma DS, Quan L, Holt VL. Epilepsy as a risk factor for submersion injury in children. *Am J Dis Child* 1992; 146:478 (abstr).

DiGuiseppi CG, Rivara FP, Koepsell TK, Polissar L. Bicycle helmet use by children: evaluation of a community-wide campaign. *JAMA* 1989; 262:2256–2261.

DiScala D, Osberg JS, Gans BM, et al. Children with traumatic head injury: morbidity and post-acute treatment. *Arch Phys Med Rehabil* 1991; 72:662–666.

Division of Injury Control. Childhood injuries in the United States. *Am J Dis Child* 1990; 144:627–646.

Done AK. Aspirin overdosage: incidence, diagnosis and management. *Pediatrics* 1978; 59:890–897.

Erdmann TC, Feldman KW, Rivara FP, Heimbach DM, Wall HA. Tap water burn prevention: the effect of legislation. *Pediatrics* 1991; 88:572–577.

Evans L. The effectiveness of safety belts in preventing fatalities. *Accid Anal Prev* 1986; 18:229–241.

Fergusson DM, Horwood LJ, Beautris AL, et al. A controlled field trial of a poisoning prevention method. *Pediatrics* 1982; 69:515–520.

Fingerhut LA, Kleinman JC: Firearm mortality among children and youth. *Advance Data* 1989; 178:1–6.

Graitcer L. The development of state and local injury surveillance systems. *J Safety Res* 1987; 18:191–198.

Griffith EEH, Bell CC. Recent trends in suicide and homicide among blacks. *JAMA* 1989; 262:2265–2269.

Guyer B, Ellers B. Childhood injuries in the United States. Mortality, morbidity and cost. *Am J Dis Child* 1990; 144:649–652.

Haddon W. A logical framework for categorizing highway safety phenomena and activity. *J Trauma* 1972; 12:193–207.

Haddon W Jr. Options for the prevention of motor vehicle crash injury. *Israel J Med Sci* 1980; 16:45–68.

Hollinger PC. The causes, impact and preventability of childhood injuries in the United States: childhood suicide in the United States. *Am J Dis Child* 1990; 144:670–676.

Jaffe KM, Brink JD, Hays RM, Chorzay AJL. Specific problems associated with pediatric head injury. In: Rosentahl M, Griffith ER, Bond JR, Miller JO eds. *Rehabilitation of the Adult and Child with Traumatic Brain Injury*. Philadelphia: FA Davis; 1990:539–557.

Jason J: Child homicide spectrum. *Am J Dis Child* 1983; 137:573–581.

Kahane CJ. *An evaluation of Child Passenger Safety: The Effectiveness and Benefits of Safety Seats*. NHTSA Report No. DOT HS 806 890. Washington, DC: US Department of Transportation; 1986.

Kaweski SM, Sise MJ, Virgilio RW. The efect of prehospital fluids on survival in trauma patients. *J Trauma* 1990; 30:1215–1219.

Kraus JF, Fife D, Conroy C. Incidence, severity and outcome of brain injury involving bicycles. *Am J Pub Health* 1987; 77:76–78.

Langley J, Silva PA, Williams S. A study of the relationship of 90 background, developmental, behavioral and medical factors to childhood accidents. *Aust Paediatr* 1980; 16:244–247.

Lamm R, Choueiri EM, Kloeckner JH. Accidents in the US and Europe, 1970–1980. *Accid Anal Prev* 1985; 17:429–438.

Lewis FR. Prehospital care: the role of the EMT-paramedic. In: West JG, Gazzaniga AB, Cales RH, eds. *Trauma Care Systems*. New York: Praeger, 1983.

Loftin C, Hill RH. Regional subculture and homicide: an examination of the Gastil-Mackney thesis. *Am Sociol Rev* 1974; 39:714–724.

Maccoby E, Jacklin C. The Psychology of Sex Differences. Palo Alto, CA: Stanford University Press; 1974.

MacKenzie EJ. Injury severity scales: overview and directions for future research. *Am J Emerg Med* 1989; 2:537–549.

MacKenzie EJ, Siegel JH, Shapiro S, et al. Functional recovery and medical costs of trauma: an analysis by type and severity of injury. *J Trauma* 1988; 28:281–297.

Mawson AR, Buindo JJ. Contrasting beliefs and actions of drivers regarding seat belts: a study in New Orleans. *J Trauma* 1985; 25:433–437.

McIntire MS, Angle CR. Regional poison control centers improve patient care. *N Engl J Med* 1983; 308:219.

McLoughlin E, Clarke N, Stahl K, Crawford JD. One pediatric burn unit's experience with sleep-wear related injuries. *Pediatrics* 1977; 60:405–409.

McLoughlin E, Vince CJ, Lee AM et al. Project Burn Prevention: outcome and implications. *Am J Pub Health* 1982; 72:241–247.

Mierley MC, Baker SP. Fatal house fires in an urban population. *JAMA* 1983; 249:1466–1468.

Morgenstern H. Uses of ecological analysis in epidemiological research. *Am J Pub Health* 1982; 72:1336–1344.

National Center for Health Statistics. *Optimum Recall Period for Reporting Persons Injured in Motor Vehicle Accidents*. Rockville, MD: US Department of Health, Education and Welfare, 1972.

National Committee for Injury Prevention and Control. Injury prevention. Meeting the challenge. *Am J Prev Med* 1989; 5:1–303.

National Highway Traffic Safety Administration. *General Estimates System*, 1988. Washington, DC: Department of Transportation; 1990.

National Highway Traffic Safety Administration. *Fatal Accident Reporting System, 1990*. Washington, DC: Department of Transportation; 1992.

Nersesian WS, Petit MR, Shaper R, et al. Childhood death and poverty. A study of all childhood deaths in Maine, 1976 to 1980. *Pediatrics* 1985; 75:41–50.

Orlowski J. Adolescent drownings: swimming, boating, diving and scuba accidents. *Pediatr Ann* 1987; 17:126–132.

Partyka SC. Lives Saved by Child Restraints From 1982 Through 1987. Washington, DC: National Highway Traffic Safety Administration; 1989.

Payne SR, Waller JA. Trauma registry and trauma center biases in injury research. *J Trauma* 1989; 29:424–429.

Pearn J. Current controversies in child accident prevention: an analysis of some areas of dispute in the prevention of child trauma. *Aust NZ J Med* 1985; 15:782.

Pless IB, Verreault R, Arsenault L, et al. The epidemiology of road accidents in childhood. *Am J Pub Health* 1987; 77:358–360.

Pless IB, Peckham CS, Power C. Predicting traffic injuries in childhood: a cohort analysis. *J Pediatr* 1989; 115:932–938.

Preusser DF, Williams AF, Zador PL, Blomberg RD. The effect of curfew laws on motor vehicle crashes. *Law Policy* 1984; 6:115–128.

Rice DP, MacKenzie EJ, et al. *Cost of Injury in the United States: A Report to Congress*. San Francisco, CA: Institute for Health and Aging, University of California and the Injury Prevention Center, Johns Hopkins University; 1989.

Rivara FP. Child pedestrian injuries in the United States. Current status of the problem, potential interventions and future research needs. Am J Dis Child 1990; 144:692–696.

Rivara FP, Barber M. Sociodemographic determinants of childhood pedestrian injuries. *Pediatrics* 1985; 76:375–381.

Rivara FP, Bergman AB, LoGerfo J, Weiss NS. Epidemiology of childhood injuries. II. Sex differences in injury rates. *Am J Dis Child* 1982; 136:502–506.

Rivara FP, Calonge N, Thompson RS. Population based study of unintentional injury incidence and impact during childhood. *Am J Pub Health* 1989a; 79:990–994.

Rivara FP, DiGuiseppi C, Thompson RS, Calonge N. Risk of injury to children less than 5 years of age in day care versus home care settings. *Pediatrics* 1989b; 84:1011–1016.

Rivara FP, Morgan P, Bergman AB, Maier RV. Cost estimates for statewide reporting of injuries by E-coding hospital discharge abstract data base systems. *Pub Health Rep* 1990; 105:635–638.

Rivara FP, Booth CL, Bergman AB, Rogers LW, Weiss J. Prevention of pedestrian injuries to children: effectiveness of a school training program. *Pediatrics* 1991; 88:770–775.

Robertson LS. Crash involvement of teenaged drivers when driver education is eliminated from high school. *Am J Pub Health* 1980; 70:599–603.

Robertson LS. Patterns of teenaged driver involvement in fatal MV crashes: implications for policy choice. *J Health Politics, Policy Law* 1981; 6:303–314.

Robertson LS. *Injury Epidemiology*. New York: Oxford University Press; 1992.

Rothengatter T. A behavioral approach to improving traffic behavior of young children. *Ergonomics* 1984; 27:147–160.

Routledge DA, Repetto-Wright R, Howarth CI. The exposure of young children to accident risk as pedestrians. *Ergonomics* 1974; 17:456–480.

Shaoul J. *The Use of Accidents and Traffic Offenses as Criteria for Evaluating Courses in Driver Education*. Salford, England: University of Shalford; 1975.

Schiller WR, Knox R, Zinnecker H, et al. Efect of helicopter transport of trauma victims on survival in an urban trauma center. *J Trauma* 1988; 28:1127–1134.

Schwartz RJ, Jacobs LM, Yaezel D. Impact of pre-trauma center care on length of stay and hospital charges. *J Trauma* 1989; 29:1611–1615.

Sloan JH, Kellerman AL, Reay DT, et al. Handgun regulations, crime and assaults, and homicide: a tale of two cities. *N Engl J Med* 1988; 319:1256–1262.

Sloan JH, Rivara FP, Reay DT, Ferris J, Kellermann AL. Firearm regulations and rates of suicide: a comparison of two metropolitan areas. *N Engl J Med* 1990; 322:369–373.

Speigel CN, Lindaman FC. Children can't fly: a program to prevent children's morbidity and mortality from window falls. *Am J Pub Health* 1977; 67:1143–1147.

Thompson RS, Rivara FP, Thompson DC. A case control study of the effectiveness of bicycle safety helmets. *N Engl J Med* 1989; 320:1361–1367.

Thompson DC, Thompson RS, Rivara FP. The incidence of bicycle-related injuries in a defined population. *Am J Pub Health* 1990; 80:1388–1389.

Wagenaar AC, Margolis LH. Effects of a mandatory safety belt law on hospital admissions. *Accid Anal Prev* 1990; 22:253–261.

Waller AE, Baker SP, Szocka A. Childhood injury deaths: national analysis and geographic variations. *Am J Pub Health* 1989; 79:310–315.

Walton WW. An evaluation of the Poison Prevention Packaging Act. *Pediatrics* 1982; 69:363–370.

Wesson DE, Williams JI, Spence LJ, et al. Functional outcome in pediatric trauma. *J Trauma* 1989; 29:589–592.

West JG, Cales RH. Methods of evaluation of trauma care. In: West JG, Gazzaniga AB, Cales RH, eds. *Trauma Care Systems*. New York: Praeger; 1983.

Williams AF, Wells JK. The Tennessee child restraint law in its third year. *Am J Pub Health* 1981; 71:163–165.

Williams AF, et al. Seat belt use law enforcement and publicity in Elmira, New York: a reminder campaign. *Am J Pub Health* 1987; 77:1450–1451.

Williams AF, Karpf RS, Zador L. Variations in minimum licensing age and fatal motor vehicle crashes. *Am J Pub Health* 1983; 73:1401–1404.

Williams BC, Kotch JB. Excess injury mortality among children in the United States: comparison of recent international statistics. *Pediatrics* 1990; 66:1067–1073.

Wintemute GJ. Childhood drowning and near-drowning in the United States. *Am J Dis Child* 1990; 144:663–669.

14

Intentional Injuries: Homicide and Violence

KATHERINE KAUFER CHRISTOFFEL

Currently, injury is a major contributor to mortality and morbidity in childhood and adolescence. Where diarrhea, measles, and other such infectious diseases have been controlled, injury has emerged as the leading killer and maimer of the young. Contemporary students of pediatric epidemiology must therefore become familiar with patterns of injury.

Injuries are commonly divided according to parameters that group related causal factors, e.g., motor vehicle versus nonmotor vehicle, occupational versus nonoccupational. One such grouping combines injuries in which human agency is salient as "intentional injuries"—the results of suicidal (see Chapter 12) or violent behavior. This chapter covers violent injuries, including child abuse (assault and neglect by care-giving adults), other assault (e.g., by strangers and peers), and homicide (the fatal form of the other two categories). The information presented concerns the United States primarily, because its extremely high prevalence of violent death has resulted in a large body of epidemiologic information. Where published studies permit, international comparisons are made, but government data from countries other than the United States are not included.

Methodologic Considerations

The study and description of violence, as that of any epidemiologic phenomenon, entails problems related to case definition, ascertainment biases, confounding, and other such issues. It is worth reviewing how these problems arise in the context of the study of violence before presenting the available data, so that the limitations of these data can be understood.

When studies are compared, differences in case definitions must be considered carefully (Payne, 1989). Description of a human interaction as "violent" generally implies a social judgment that it is inappropriate. In different contexts, however, the same behavior (e.g., spanking) might be described as "limit-setting," "discipline," "corporal punishment," "assault," or "abuse." These differences may reflect different hypotheses about spanking, e.g., spanking as a measure of child abuse versus spanking as a measure of the application of desirable limit-setting. They also reflect differences in methods for surveying adults, adolescents, and children. These differences will inevitably result in varying estimates of the frequency of occurrence. It may become easier to compare violence research in the future than it has been in the past if researchers follow recommendations in a recent report on standard definitions for injury research (Christoffel et al. 1992). One of the recommendations is that the social judgments involved in definitions of maltreatment (assault and child abuse) should be made explicit. The report proposes that maltreatment be officially defined as "behavior towards another person, which (a) is outside the norms of conduct *and* (b) entails a substantial risk of causing physical or emotional harm. The behaviors included will consist of actions and omissions, ones that are intentional and ones that are unintentional. They will have severe, mild, or no immediate adverse consequences."

The same social judgments that result in varying definitions of violence can also cause inconsistencies in case ascertainment. Because of social stigma associated with violence, both victims and perpetrators are reluctant to report accurately that violence is the cause of observed injury. Medical and other observers are also reluctant to consider violence as a possible cause of injury. Because victims are generally loath to report such events, cases that are correctly identified may well be atypical of all cases—that is, having differing relationships to perpetrators, more severe injury, or more or less chronic violence. The unwillingness of perpetrators to bring victims for care may increase the severity of injury, not only as a result of bias in care-seeking (with only the more severely injured brought for care) but also as a result of the consequences when care is not sought quickly. The effects of delayed care may need to be distinguished therefore from the primary effects of assault when data are used for planning prevention programs.

Methods exist to reduce underreporting of violence by victims and perpetrators. For example, surveys can be done in an anonymous manner, thereby reducing respondents' fear of legal or other consequences of disclosure. However, measures that enhance reporting may adversely affect data in other ways, e.g., anonymous data gathering may make it difficult to identify repetitive cases. Furthermore, these measures may also raise ethical issues: a promise of anonymity may be harmful when protection or criminal justice intervention on behalf of a victim is warranted by the information collected.

The hesitancy of health providers to identify violence as the cause of an injury can be overcome as in locales that have legal requirements for reporting child abuse, such as the Netherlands (Pieterse & Van Urk, 1989). However, such improvements in case recognition can also cause problems in the interpretation of data: it may be difficult to distinguish apparently increasing incidence rates from the effects of better recognition and reporting.

There are times when the social context of violence can, paradoxically, result in overreporting, rather than underreporting. For example, when social services are underfunded (as they so often are), a diagnosis of violent injury (e.g., child abuse or neglect), may provide access to services that would not otherwise be obtainable. In this instance, a problem that might be more appropriately identified as "in need of help in parenting" may be labeled as "violence."

Data Sources

The most salient methodologic issue in the epidemiology of violent injury is the sources of data used. There are five basic types of data: vital statistics (which come from death certificate diagnoses), medical records (office, hospital, medical examiner, or coroner), the criminal justice system (police, courts, etc.), other designated governmental reporting agencies, and special surveys. In the United States, the governmental agencies involved include state child protective service agencies for injuries involving child abuse; the injury surveillance system of the Consumer Product Safety Commission (CPSC) for injuries involving certain types of weapons; and the Bureau of Alcohol, Tobacco, and Firearms (BATF) for injuries involving certain aspects of firearm use.

Except for special surveys, each data source exists for a specific purpose and in no instance has as its primary goal the surveillance of violent injury. It is therefore not surprising that each source has limitations when used for this purpose and that estimates of these events differ depending on which data source is used. Combining data from various sources may not be possible if reference populations differ or if data are incompatible in other ways, e.g., when they use inconsistent geographic or age groupings.

Some of the limitations of U.S. data sources are listed in Table 14.1, and these undoubtedly apply to other countries as well, although system details inevitably will differ. One limitation that cuts across medical sources is that the standard method for coding injuries, the E-codes in the International Classification of Diseases (ICD), is not well suited to the identification of violent injury, e.g., a baby who has been badly shaken may be coded as such *or* as head trauma, but not as both. As a result, critical information contained in the medical record may be lost at the time of coding. In addition, since routine coding is often not done, arduous manual record reviews may be the only way to obtain these data.

Causal Issues

Prevention of violent injury requires the identification of personal and environmental risk factors, both to guide the development of prevention strategies and to target the implementation of such strategies toward high-risk groups. Many of the factors discussed affect risk factor identification, most notably case ascertainment biases. Particularly knotty definitional and prevention problems may arise when risk for violence involves earlier victimization of the perpetrator, e.g., when an abusive parent was an abused child. In these circumstances, it becomes essential to be clear at which level of victimization primary prevention and intervention (or secondary prevention) measures are aimed. In general, it is probably best to establish public health efforts for primary prevention of injury to the youngest potential victims. However, this effort may, at times, need to involve secondary prevention by targeting other victims, e.g., the child's battered mother.

Definitional problems and issues of confounding arise for specific risk factors, such as poverty or intoxication. Some of those important definitional issues are

Table 14.1. Violent Injury Surveillance: U.S. Data Sources and Limitations

Data Source	Limitations
Vital Statistics	Based on death certificates: filled out inconsistently (bias against identification of violence), excludes nonfatal injuries and, often, delayed deaths
Medical records	
Office	Practitioners may not recognize violence or record recognized violence, not E-coded anywhere
Hospital outpatient departments	Same as office medical records
Hospital inpatient	Practitioners may not recognize or record violence; E-coding variably present, well done
Medical examiner	Investigative constraints can result in "undetermined" classification in cases in which violence is likely but not certain
Coroner	Autopsies and findings may not be done by forensic pathologists in jurisdictions in which coroners are elected
Criminal justice	
Police	Only includes cases reported to police, perpetrator categories geared for adults, e.g., may lack such categories as "mother's boyfriend"
Courts	Only includes cases that go to court, i.e., cases in which charges are pressed and evidence is clear
Surveys	Exclude victims too young to interview (under 12 years in the Institute of Justices's Annual Crime Survey)
Government agencies	
Protective Services	Only includes children (<18 years old) harmed by caregiving adults
CPSC	Only includes emergency room visits, includes knives and nonpowder firearms, but not powder weapons (since 1981)
BATF	Focus is on weapons, not injuries

addressed in the NICHD report mentioned above, e.g., methods for measuring social class and objective standards for alcohol intoxication, which has often only been assessed subjectively (Christoffel et al., 1992).

Alcohol as a risk factor serves to illustrate potential confounding. Alcohol use by the victim or perpetrator (or both) is almost certainly a risk factor for violence. Yet, evidence of this relationship can be elusive. The prevalence of high alcohol levels in the blood of homicide victims, who are the most readily tested, does not suffice to establish a causal connection (Amaro et al., 1990; Budd, 1989). At a minimum, the rate of alcohol use must be shown to be higher in homicide victims than in uninjured individuals in similar situations, but non-intoxicated individuals in similar situations may be difficult to find (or, if found, to test). Optimally, alternative possibilities (e.g., that behavioral predispositions result in both violence and alcohol use) should be excluded. Although these explanations may be implausible, disproving them may be difficult. Another example of confounding arises with the contemporary phenomenon of HIV infection: rates have been reported to be higher among young assault victims than among other emergency room attenders, suggesting that multiple risk-taking behaviors exist in these victims that may muddy risk factor analyses and also cloud understanding of the causal sequence (Soderstrom et al., 1989).

Reconstruction of causal sequences is an important step in the development of prevention strategies for all injuries, including violent ones. Without details about violent interactions, it may be extremely difficult to intervene to interrupt the processes that lead to the injuries of interest. Methodologic issues that arise in causal sequence reconstruction include all those already discussed: definitions, ascertainment, and confounding, each of which affects the details, as well as the generalizability of the results of the reconstructions (see Chapter 1). Additional issues include reconciling inconsistent reports from multiple observers (victim, perpetrator, bystander) and absent information that is unknown to available reporters or is withheld by them.

Although one may ask whether it is even worthwhile to examine estimates of the incidence or prevalence of violent injury in light of these concerns, they are not unique to this field. As in other realms, it is necessary to generate the best available estimates of the scope of a problem while recognizing the limitations and working to overcome them. In the following sections, it is important to bear in mind that all incidence figures are underestimates and that they vary depending on the source of the data.

Patterns of Occurrence

Homicide

The contemporary problem of homicide in the United States has been described recently (Christoffel, 1990). The problem is large and growing, as evidenced by a 44% rise in years of potential life lost from 1968 to 1985. This figure includes a 93% increase in deaths due to firearms. From 1985 to 1988, firearm homicides among those 15 to 19 years again rose by more than 100% (Fingerhut et al., 1991). Childhood homicides occur in two recognizable patterns: infantile and adolescent. The former category applies to children under age 5; infantile homicides usually involve parents or care-givers; are often precipitated by neglect or disciplinary actions; and often involve beatings, burns, or arson. Adolescent homicides involve those 12 and older and are usually perpetrated by peers or gangs; they may be precipitated by arguments or crime; and involve gunshots, stabbing, strangulation, or hit-and-run fatalities.

Several established and suspected risk factors for homicide and assault have been identified (Table 14.2). It should be noted, however, that the evidence suggests that socioeconomic factors, wholly or in large part, explain the frequently observed relationship with race.

Based on vital statistics data, U.S. homicide rates for all races in 1986 ranged from a low of 0.8 per 100,000 for victims 5 to 9 years to a high of 9.9 per 100,000 for those 15 to 19 years (Table 14.3). These rates form a U-shaped curve. The peak at the lower ages reflects child abuse—the leading cause of injury death affecting U.S. infants (Waller et al., 1989). The peak at the older ages is due to assault, primarily with firearms. As is evident in Figure 14.1, which is based

Table 14.2. Violence Risk Factors: U.S. Children and Adolescents

Homicide	Assault
Established	Sexual, all types
Male (after age 1 year)	Female
Black race	Urban residence
Urban residence	Delinquent behavior, peers
Poverty	Sexual, severe
Possible (Adolescent)	Older adolescent
History of juvenile detention	Black race
Low educational level	Poverty
Intoxication (drugs or alcohol)	Crime
	Unmarried
	Male
	Age 12 to 24 years
	Black race
	Poverty

Source: Reprinted with permission from Christoffel (1990) (© 1990, American Medical Association).

on police data, the proportion of homicides due to firearms rises with the age of the victim and reaches 67% among those 15 to 19 years.

Total homicide rates obscure marked racial and sex differences, with rates consistently higher for boys (two to three times the rates for girls) and for blacks (about five times the rates for whites). More than two thirds of the victims were boys, and almost half were black. The lowest rate was for white girls 5 to 9 years (0.4) and the highest for black boys 15 to 19 years (50.7). Homicide is now the leading cause of death for teenage black boys in the United States.

Child Abuse and Neglect

Among the risk factors for child physical abuse that are now reasonably well accepted are young maternal age, an unwanted pregnancy, a history of family disturbance, foster care, and poverty. Table 14.4 gives U.S. child abuse incidence estimates, based on the second National Incidence Survey (NIS-2) in 1986 (NCCAN, 1988). The rates range from 6.3 per 1000 for 0- to 2-year-olds to 27.5 per 1000 for those 15 to 17 years. The pattern of increasing incidence with increasing age is, however, contrary to the clinical impression of hospital-based teams, presumably because the greater severity of injuries to infants—as a result of their physical vulnerability and/or frequent delays in care-seeking by adults (care-givers or perpetrators)—brings them more often to such centers.

The NIS-2 survey, which relied on health professionals' recognition of violence, estimated that 1.6 million children are abused in the United States each year. The majority of cases included were due to physical abuse, and over one third of the children identified as neglected had evidence of physical neglect. Physical abuse was more common than emotional or sexual abuse at all ages, but after age 11, the rate of emotional abuse greatly exceeded that for sexual abuse (5.5 versus 2.9 per 1000). Compared with the first survey conducted 6 years earlier, NIS-2 showed a marked increase in sexual abuse (more than twofold) and other abuse of moderate severity, but no similar increase in neglect

Table 14.3. Homicides Among Children by Age, Sex, and Race, United States, 1986

	Deaths in 1986	
Age (year)	No.	Annual Rate/100,000
All races and sexes		
0–4	660	3.6
5–9	134	0.8
10–14	245	1.5
15–19	1838	9.9
Total	2877	4.1
White males		
0–4	199	2.6
5–9	38	0.5
10–14	84	1.2
15–19	659	8.5
Total	980	3.3
White females		
0–4	155	2.2
5–9	30	0.4
10–14	71	1.1
15–19	249	3.3
Total	505	1.8
Black males		
0–4	167	12.1
5–9	26	1.9
10–14	60	4.6
15–19	710	50.7
Total	963	17.5
Black females		
0–4	120	9.0
5–9	34	2.6
10–14	26	2.0
15–19	168	12.2
Total	348	6.5

Source: Data from the National Center for Health Statistics, 1986 (E-codes: E960-E969) (Division of Injury Control, 1990).

or severe abuse. The American Humane Association has reported that 2.5 million children were reported in 1990 because of abuse or neglect, which is approximately 4% of all U.S. children—up 274% from 1976. It is impossible to know whether these changes reflect real changes in incidence, alterations in patterns of recognition and reporting (e.g., in response to increased attention to sexual abuse in some state laws), or a combination of these factors.

Assault

Assaults that are not child abuse are estimated to be 100 times more frequent than homicides. They include, in descending order of frequency, attacks by siblings, peers, and strangers.

Telephone surveys indicate that 80% of siblings behave violently to each other each year. These acts include mostly mild altercations (e.g., pushing or

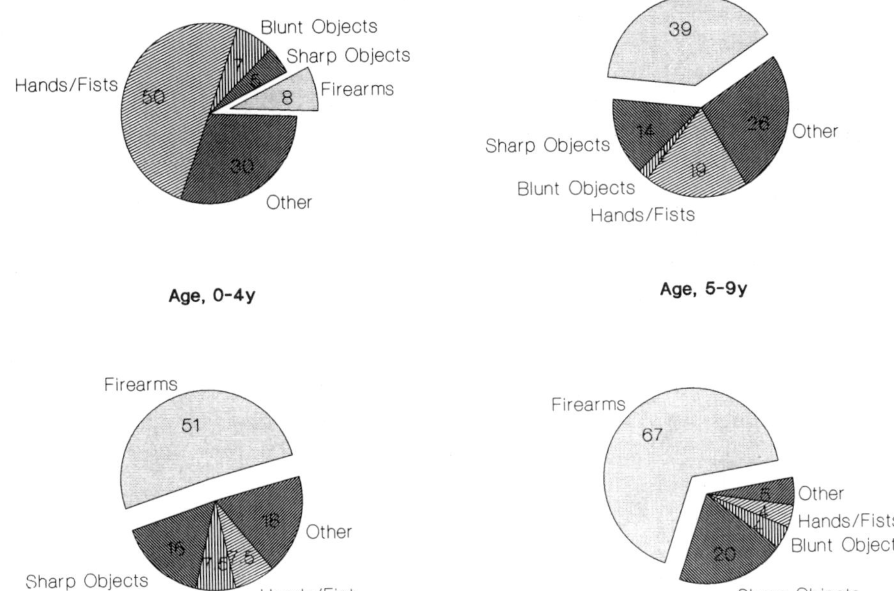

Fig. 14.1. Percent of weapons used to commit homicide on children aged 0 to 19 years in the United States, 1986 (*Uniform Crime Report*) (Division of Injury Control, 1990).

Table 14.4. Incidence Estimates: Assault and Child Abuse

Age (year)	All	Male	Female
	Violent Crime*		
12–15	54.1	72.2	35.3
16–19	67.2	87.8	46.3
	Child Abuse and Neglect†		
0–2	6.3	. . .	. . .
3–5	10.0	. . .	. . .
6–8	15.6	. .	. . .
9–11	15.1	. . .	. . .
12–14	22.6	. . .	. . .
15–17	27.5	. . .	. . .
0–17			
All abuse	10.7	8.4	13.1
Sexual abuse	2.5	1.1	3.9
All neglect	15.9	. . .	. . .

*The data are rates per 1000 population. Violent crime includes completed and attempted rape, robbery (with and without injury), and assault (aggravated and simple).

†The data are rates per 1000 population.

Source: Reprinted with permission from Christoffel (1990) (© 1990, American Medical Association).

shoving), but also some severe acts (e.g., threatening with a weapon in less than 5% of cases) and, not surprisingly perhaps, rates are highest for males (Gelles & Straus, 1988; Straus et al., 1980).

Table 14.4 shows estimated rates of violent crime, based on the U.S. Department of Justice's ongoing National Crime Survey of victims 12 and over. Such rates were high among teens, as compared with other age groups, although the likelihood that the crimes were reported to the police or that the resulting injuries were medically attended is low.

The Statewide Childhood Injury Prevention Project (SCIPP) monitored the incidence of injuries presenting for medical care in 14 Massachusetts communities outside Boston a decade ago (Guyer et al., 1989). SCIPP documented that 1 in 60 adolescents aged 15 to 19 presented for care after an assault, including 1 in every 42 boys in this age group. Most of these assaults did not involve weapons or involved knives if a weapon was used. The number of adolescents presenting for emergency room care for assault outnumbered deaths by over 500 to 1. The nature and extent of the role of gangs in adolescent violence varies in different eras and locales (Hagedorn, 1988).

Sexual Assault

Data on sexual assault (defined as "forced sexual behavior involving contact with the sexual parts of the body") in a sample of 12- to 18-year-olds based on the National Youth Survey's Sexual Abuse Project (Ageton, 1983) estimated that 700,000 to 1 million young women are assaulted annually. This is more than 50 times the rate based on police data. Eighty percent of assailants were known to the victims, with strangers committing the assault only among older teens. The assailants were usually dates or boyfriends, and often they were delinquents. Offenders identified alcohol and companions who approved of their assaultive behavior as factors fostering the assaults. The force used was most often verbal (50%) or "minimal physical" (27% to 40%), but too often, it was more severe, such as beatings, or including the presence of a weapon (15%).

Abductions

Stranger abductions are emphasized in U.S. media accounts, on milk cartons, in tollway pictures of "missing children," and in school curricula. All draw attention to "stranger danger." Yet, few data support the notion that such abductions are common. A recent report, commissioned by the U.S. Department of Justice, reviewed several surveys and police data to estimate the scope and nature of the problem of missing children. It defined five categories of cases and made estimates of the frequency of all instances, particularly those judged to be "severe" (Finkelhor et al., 1990). The five categories are: family abductions, nonfamily abductions, runaways, thrownaways, and missing.

Family abductions are defined as those in which children are taken (or are not returned) in violation of agreed-on custody or visitation agreements. Most perpetrators were noncustodial fathers or father figures, and the victims were typically 2 to 11 years. Few such episodes last longer than 3 days, with less than 10% lasting a month or more. Half of the time the care-givers knew where the children were, but had trouble obtaining them. There were an estimated 354,100 family abductions in 1988, 46% of which (163,200) were "severe," i.e., involved concealment, transportation out of state, or intent to alter custody permanently.

Nonfamily abductions include "coerced and unauthorized taking of a child into a building, a vehicle, or a distance of more than 20 feet; the detention of a child for . . . more than an hour, or the luring of a child for the purposes of committing another crime (e.g., sexual assault)." An estimated 3200 to 4600 such events were known to the police in 1988. The victims were typically teenagers and female; blacks and Hispanics were overrepresented, and sexual assault was involved in over 75% of cases. Most episodes lasted less than a day, and 12% to 21% lasted less than an hour. Of the several thousand nonfamily abductions, less than 10%—an estimated 200 to 300—were "stereotypical kidnappings" in which the abduction was by a stranger and the child was gone overnight, killed, transported 50 miles or more, or ransomed or in which there was evidence of intent to keep the child permanently. The FBI recorded between 43 and 147 abduction homicides per year between 1976 and 1987.

Runaways

Running away occurs when children leave home or stay away inappropriately overnight without permission. There were an estimated 446,700 runaways in 1988, and almost all were teenagers. They came disproportionately from households in which a parent was living with a stepparent, and the children ran to the home of a friend or relative. One half returned within 2 days, and for almost half, their whereabouts were known to their families. Of the over 400,000 runaways, an estimated 129,500 were "without a secure and familiar place to stay" during their time away. One tenth of the children went more than 100 miles from home; some traveled out of state. One percent were harmed physically, and 3% were sexually abused. Runaways from juvenile facilities, estimated to number 4000, tended to become involved in serious episodes, including prostitution, drug dealing, and arrest.

Thrownaway

Children were considered "thrownaway" if they had been told to leave the home, were refused permission to return, had run away without any subsequent care-giver effort to recover them, or had been abandoned or deserted. It was estimated that there were 127,000 of these episodes in 1988, of which 59,200 were without a secure and familiar place to stay for some period. Most were older teens. Children from households with both natural parents were underrepresented in this group. Thrownaways generally went to the homes of friends or relatives close to their own homes, and usually the parents or care-givers knew of the child's whereabouts.

Missing

Children who were lost, injured, or otherwise missing for periods ranging from a few minutes to overnight were estimated to number 438,200 in 1988. Of these, the police were called to intervene in 32% of cases, most of which involved children under age 4 or 16 to 17 years old. Six percent were injured, and 14% were abused or assaulted.

International Comparisons

Homicide

International homicide rates reported to WHO have been highly consistent over time in industrialized countries (Lester, 1989). These data reveal a tremendous difference between rates in the United States and those in other countries (Fingerhut & Kleinman, 1990; Tsuda et al., 1989). This difference reflects, above all, adolescent homicide rates (Fig. 14.2), which, in turn, reflect firearm rates (Table 14.5). In 1985, there were ten times as many homicides involving U.S. children 15 to 19 years than there were in six developed countries with a combined population 1.4 times that of the United States—Federal Republic of Germany, France, England and Wales, Sweden, Canada, and Japan (Division of Injury Control, 1990). It is clear that these patterns reflect society-wide differences in weapon use. For example, a recent survey of U.S. students indicated that almost one fourth of eighth to tenth grade boys carried knives to school,

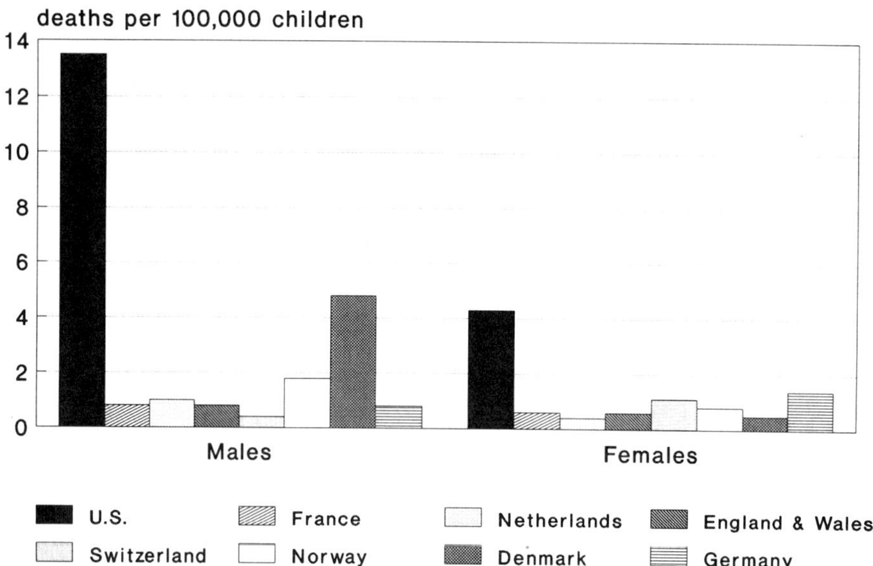

Fig. 14.2. International homicide rates for teenagers aged 15 to 19 years, 1985 (National Center for Health Statistics) (Division of Injury Control, 1990).

Table 14.5. International Homicide Incidence, 15- to 24-Year-olds

	Homicides* No. (rate/100,000)	Number of Firearm Homicides	Percent Firearm
United States	4223 (21.9)	3187	75
Australia	62 (2.9)	17	27
France	59 (1.4)	32	54
West Germany	49 (1.0)	3	6
England & Wales	48 (1.2)	3	6
Japan	47 (0.5)	8	17
Canada	34 (2.5)	11	32
Scotland	22 (5.0)	0	0
Sweden	14 (2.3)	3	21
Israel	13 (3.7)	5	38
Switzerland	7 (1.4)	1	14

*1985, 1986, or 1987.

Source: Data from Fingerhut & Kleinman (1990).

and 7% did so daily (Office of Disease Prevention and Health Promotion, 1989). Another survey of high-school students showed that nearly 20% of all students (31.5% of boys and 8.1% of girls) had carried weapons in the last month; 20.8% of these weapons were firearms (Division of Injury Control, 1991). It also revealed that 3% carried guns to school during the previous year and that 1% did so daily. Almost two thirds of boys and one fifth of girls actually reported using a firearm during the last year. In contrast, even the police in Great Britain do not carry firearms (Harper, 1991). The importance of firearms is related to their high lethality, as discussed below.

U.S. rates are also atypically high for fatal child abuse, as compared with the other developed countries studied. Based on 1970s vital statistics data, homicide rates involving children under age 5, presumed to be due overwhelmingly to child abuse, were found to be independent of adult homicide rates in developing countries, but correlated weakly with adult rates in developed countries (Christoffel & Liu, 1983; Christoffel et al., 1981). It may be that societies in developed countries confront toddlers and preschoolers with more adult situations or expectations than they face in developing countries.

Assault

Studies of interpersonal violence in Argentina, Australia, Denmark, and Great Britain make it clear that the social patterns contributing to this problem are the same as in the United States (Aalund et al., 1989; Breiting et al., 1989; Hedeboe et al., 1985; Hocking, 1989; Scott, 1990; Shepherd et al., 1988). Major risk factors for assault invariably include male gender, intoxication, and low socioeconomic status. In contrast and not surprisingly, in countries where war or internal tyranny are common, these factors play an overriding role in the epidemiology of this form of injury (Aalund et al., 1990; Herman, 1988).

Child Abuse and Neglect

Child abuse is recognized around the world, but in most countries the relevant medical literature only emphasizes the importance of recognition, e.g., clinical descriptions and case series (Baeza-Herrera et al., 1986; Fraser & Kilbride, 1980; Nazer et al., 1988), much as the literature in the United States did 20 or more years ago. Other countries have recently established reporting systems that will form the basis of surveillance in years to come. The most extensive research has come from the United States and Great Britain, where recognition is widespread and registries exist. Risk factors, clinical patterns, and methodologic issues do not seem to vary substantially from those in the United States (Sharma & Sunderland, 1988). International perspectives on child abuse were reviewed in 1979 and 1983 (Gelles & Cornell, 1983; Taylor & Newberger, 1979).

Risk Factors

Culture of Violence

Violence is not new: filicide was recorded in biblical times, and Shakespeare's plays make it clear that bloody battles fascinated people in his time as they do today. Yet, the context of contemporary violence is different from that of violence in other eras. Because any reduction in violence requires intervention in the specific context in which it occurs, the recognition that violence is not novel is less important than recognizing the factors that foster it today, which may or may not be novel.

Violent injury is the result of a combination of factors that increase the *frequency* of violent incidents and those that affect their *severity*. Table 14.6 lists "4 Ms and 2 Ps" that succinctly summarize the factors that experts most often identify as contributing to the frequency of violence. It is believed that some influences, such as the media (Centerwall, 1992), affect both the population at large and specifically those who are psychosocially at high risk, thereby exerting a small effect on many and a large effect on a few.

These factors can be thought of as those affecting the incidence of violence and hence those that must be addressed for primary prevention. Haddon's injury

Table 14.6. Factors Contributing to the Incidence of Violence

Factor	How It Works to Provoke Violence
Machismo	Fosters bravado and physical battle
Media	Model and glorify violence; may disinhibit, cause insensitivity to the consequences of violence
Metal (knives, guns)	Availability helps arguments escalate
Mind alteration	Drugs and alcohol affect judgment, may disinhibit
Parents	May model violent interaction; through abuse, may promote maladaptive behavior
Poverty	Promotes anger, deprivation, and hopelessness, which may disinhibit

prevention matrix (Haddon & Baker, 1981) divides the phases of injury occurrence (and prevention opportunities) into pre-event, event, and postevent; factors that promote violence operate at the pre-event stage.

Factors affecting the severity of violent incidents are listed in Table 14.7. Although there are several factors, they are less numerous than those that affect incidence. In Haddon's matrix, these factors operate at the event and postevent stages. Most prominent among them in the United States is weaponry, an event stage factor, and specifically, the availability of firearms of ever-increasing firepower. Their importance in the United States and the possibility that this pattern might be exported to other nations warrant a closer look at the rudiments of ballistics and the biomechanics and sociology of firearm use.

Firearms

Firearms are designed to convey kinetic energy (ke) efficiently to a missile (generally a bullet), which transfers it to the victim according to the formula, $ke = \frac{1}{2} mv^2$, where m is the mass of the missile and v is its velocity. Although the mass of the missile is small, the velocity with which it exits the firearm muzzle is large (hundreds to thousands of feet per second), and so the energy conveyed is extremely large. If a bullet exits the body, the velocity that affects the amount of energy conveyed is the difference between the entrance and the exit velocity.

Firearms are often divided into handguns and long guns (rifles and shotguns). In the United States, most such injuries are caused by handguns, although more long guns are owned. This presumably reflects the portability of handguns and the fact that many are kept or carried for protection, i.e., ready to fire.

In earlier centuries, firearms were extremely cumbersome to use: there were no manufactured bullets and no multiple-fire weapons. Therefore, gunpowder had to be measured and loaded between each firing of the weapon. Subsequently, multiple-fire weapons and prefabricated bullets came on the scene. Until fairly recently, however, it was still necessary to reload frequently and to depress the trigger for each firing. Fully automatic weapons continue to fire as long as the trigger is held. These guns have been banned in the United States for some time, but semiautomatic weapons, which accommodate large self-feeding bullet supplies and which fire each time the trigger is pulled (at momentary intervals),

Table 14.7. Factors Affecting the Severity of Violent Injury

Factor	How It Works to Increase Severity
Victim age/development	Infants and elderly more physically vulnerable
Delay in care-seeking	Unattended victims may suffer secondary damage, e.g., from hypoxia
Victim alcohol use	Affects body's response to injury and surgery
Perpetrator steroid use	Affects muscle strength brought to bear in beatings
Weaponry	Gunshot wounds more often fatal than knife wounds; semiautomatic weapons can kill many quickly; muzzle velocity and bullet characteristics affect extent of tissue damage

are increasingly available, both as rifles and handguns. Much political controversy in the early 1990s has involved "semiautomatic assault rifles," which are favored by urban gangs and which have been used in an increasing number of killings over the past few years. Regrettably, many U.S. manufactured weapons of this type are exported to other countries.

The damage caused when a bullet enters tissue depends on several factors: the strength of the tissue (e.g., a higher muzzle velocity is needed to penetrate bone than soft tissue), the tissue penetrated (more deadly damage is done if the brain, heart, or a major artery is hit than if a leg muscle or mesentery is struck), and the ballistic properties of the missile (Barach et al., 1986a and b; Hollerman et al., 1990). All bullets cause damage by direct contact (creating a permanent cavity) and by the crushing created by the tissues' absorption of the traversing bullet's energy, which causes a temporary cavity. Each type of bullet has its own unique path through tissue (e.g., with more or less tumbling), which affects the extent of the ultimate injury. By international convention, bullets that can be used in war must be full metal jacketed, because this type of construction maximizes the chances that the bullet will exit from the victim, thus reducing the destructive energy conveyed. Therefore, victims are likely to be either dead or salvageable. Bullets available for civilian use are often not of this construction and are marketed to emphasize destructive features, e.g., large quantities of gunpowder and protruding tips that maximize the tissue damage victims suffer.

An important consideration in prevention is that bullets are consumable goods. Accordingly, regulatory or other interventions that impede bullet acquisition or affect bullet design may reduce injury patterns more quickly than similar steps involving firearms themselves (unless home manufacture would suffice, as some have suggested). At present in the United States, there are no regulations, analogous to those covering so many other consumer products, governing the design of either firearms or bullets.

Social conditions that have resulted in widespread crime have also led many citizens to seek to protect themselves with firearms. An estimated 200 million firearms, including 60 million handguns, are kept in half of U.S. homes. Epidemiologic studies indicate that firearms kept in the home are far more likely to result in suicidal, unintentional, or homicidal death of a family member than to kill an intruder (Kellerman & Reay, 1986). This information has not yet been fully appreciated by the U.S. population. Many citizens believe that the second amendment to the U.S. Constitution protects individual firearm ownership, as claimed by firearm advocacy groups. However, federal courts have consistently ruled that it does not, but rather that it protects the states' rights to muster militias.

Because violent firearm injury is the result of intentional actions (albeit often later regretted by individuals who were, at the time, distraught or intoxicated), education regarding the safe handling of weapons is not likely to markedly reduce this type of injury. Because firearms are designed to kill efficiently, there are probably major limitations on the extent to which modifications in their design (e.g., loading indicators or automatic trigger safety devices) could reduce injury, particularly when there are large arsenals of existing weapons that lack any improved design features. Therefore, efforts to reduce firearm injury now focus on reducing the availability of those weapons to those who are most likely to use them violently. Since most homicides involve handguns and are the result of impulsive actions during arguments with peers, and most perpetrators are neither known criminals nor adjudicated mentally ill, many prevention planners and policy analysts believe that the reduction of these injuries requires reduced handgun ownership by all segments of the population.

Prevention

Efforts to prevent firearms injuries are primarily intended to reduce the lethality of violent acts. Such measures can reduce the morbidity and mortality from violent injuries, but will not reduce their incidence. To do so will require measures to reduce the risk for such encounters, including those listed in Table 14.8. There are now scores of programs in schools and communities designed to reduce the incidence of youth violence by teaching nonviolent conflict resolution, stress reduction, and related skills to teachers and young people. None has yet been adequately evaluated; the results of evaluations now in progress will be highly instructive (Cohen & Wilson-Brewer, 1991; Wilson-Brewer et al., 1991).

Table 14.8 lists potential primary and secondary violence prevention approaches. They include strategies aimed at the community and others aimed at individuals. They are intended to reduce risk not only in the population at large but also in those at high risk. Police approaches are not included because of the intimate nature of most violent interactions and also because there is insufficient evidence that the criminal justice system has been an effective deterrent to initial or subsequent attacks. The primary prevention strategy for child abuse that has been most studied and that seems to be effective is based on weekly home visits to mothers before and for some time after (in one study, a total of 2 years) delivery (Olds et al., 1986). The high costs of such a program must be weighed against the extreme social, as well as direct fiscal, costs of abuse. Early training

Table 14.8. Violence Against Children and Adolescents: Possible Prevention Approaches

Primary Prevention	Secondary Prevention
Assault	
Gun control	Restrictive licensure for guns
Reduce toy gun play	After-care for assault victims
Peer-/school-based education on drugs, conflict resolution, and guns	Peer-/school-based education
	Metal detectors
Gun safety education	Liability suits against gun manufacturers
Child Abuse and Neglect	
Parent aids	Parent aids
Ecologic support	Ecologic support
Parenting education	Parenting education
Parental stress relief	Parental stress relief
Child self-protection	Foster care
Child education regarding child development	Psychotherapy
Legal proscriptions of certain behaviors	Legal testimony methods

Source: Reprinted with permission from Christoffel (1990) (© 1990, American Medical Association).

of children in nonviolent ways to deal with troublesome infants has not been tried as a means of preventing child abuse, but seems promising.

Because the patterns of other types of childhood homicide make it clear that victims are injured when they find themselves in situations they are developmentally ill-equipped to handle, it also may be fruitful to train youngsters in ways to recognize high-risk situations and how to get out of them before trouble arises. Such training should target boys, who are at the highest risk for most

Table 14.9. Violent Injury to U.S. Children and Adolescents: Research Needs

Cross-Cutting Issues
Subgroup analyses by narrow age groupings and other variables
Intervention typology e.g., primary vs. secondary, behavior enhancing or restraining
Information on nonvictims
Details on circumstances, e.g., who was doing what with whom and under what circumstances?
Analysis of relationship, if any, of violence to family disruption
Information on prevalence of deranged and stranger perpetrators
Analysis of reasons for regional differences in violence rates
Analysis of how poverty increases risk (possibilities include crime, hopelessness, crowding, substance abuse, lack of policing, family dissolution)
Relationship between child abuse and adolescent peer violence
Discrimination between increased incidence and increased recognition when surveillance indicates rising rates
Interpersonally sensitive data-gathering methods
Assault
Analysis of effects of firearm ordinances at federal, state, and local levels, involving toy guns, nonpowder firearms, handguns, long guns, and assault weapons
Information on development of behaviors involved in firearm use
Evaluation of gun safety educational efforts
Survey of gun owners who favor gun control as to what approaches they prefer
Origin of firearms used in assaults
Prevalence and types of firearms in homes, correlates of possession, and access by children and adolescents
Exploration of possible needs for improvements in acute management of young firearm injury victims
Analysis of cohort effects in homicide rates
Evaluation of educational interventions to promote nonviolent conflict resolution
Risk assessment beyond demography, e.g., alcohol use by perpetrators, victims
Information on victim-perpetrator relationships in sexual assault and adolescent assault/homicide
Child Abuse
Clear goals: lower incidence vs. lowest severity vs. more mild sequelae vs. all of these
Standard definitions
Replication of home visitor interventions, with subgroups of adequate size
Evaluation of sexual abuse prevention training programs, particularly as to effects on behavior
Case-control study of fatal and nonfatal protective service cases: can optimal case management approaches be identified?
Prospective detailed evaluation of various intervention and prevention approaches for child abuse
Adequate funding of interventions and research
Analysis of risk factors and how they increase risk
Relationship of sexual exploitation of women and sexual abuse of girls
Information on sequelae of abuse carefully distinguishing those from consequences of correlates of abuse
Information on early experiences of abused adolescents
More detailed information on sexual development

Source: Reprinted with permission from Christoffel (1990) (© 1990, American Medical Association).

types of violent injury. It must be recognized, however, that this strategy challenges social patterns that foster the protection of girls but encourages risk-taking by boys.

In the realm of secondary prevention, it is sobering to realize that assault victims routinely leave medical attention without receiving social service help of the kind that is now routinely provided to suicide attempters. Indeed, lack of experience has resulted in few models of the kind of after-care that may be most effective. This is an area in which increased clinical experience will be needed to guide prevention planning (Spivak et al., 1988).

Conclusions

Table 14.9 indicates how much we still do not know about violence, despite the fact that it is a leading cause of morbidity and mortality among children. Perhaps the taboos related to violence, which affect victim reporting and clinician recognition, also have inhibited the development of scientific inquiry needed for control of this major killer. One can only hope that violence will not become the leading killer in many places—as it is in some groups in the United States—before scientists and public policy-makers provide for a greatly expanded violence research effort, one that will be neither easy nor quickly rewarding.

References

Aalund O, Danielsen L, Katz E, Mazza PH. Injuries due to deliberate violence in areas of Argentina. I. The extent of violence. Copenhagen Study Group. *Forensic Sci Int* 1989; 42:151–163.

Aalund O, Danielsen L, Sanhueza RO. Injuries due to deliberate violence in Chile. *Forensic Sci Int* 1990; 46:189–202.

Ageton SS. *Sexual Assaults Among Adolescents*. Lexington, MA: Lexington Books; 1983.

Amaro H, Fried LE, Cabral H, Zuckerman B. Violence during pregnancy and substance abuse. *Am J Pub Health* 1990; 80:575–579.

Baeza-Herrera C, Hoque S, James SM, Franco-Vázquez R. Sindrome del niño maltratado. Espectro de un problema. *Bol Med Hosp Infant Mex* 1986; 43:71–77.

Barach E, Tomlanovich M, Nowak R. Ballistics: a pathophysiologic examination of the wounding mechanisms of firearms: Part I. *J Trauma* 1986a; 26:225–235.

Barach E, Tomlanovich M, Nowak R. Ballistics: a pathophysiologic examination of the wounding mechanisms of firearms: Part II. *J Trauma* 1986b; 26:374–383.

Breiting VB, Aalund O, Albrektsen SB, Danielsen L, Helweg-Larsen K, Jacobsen J, Kjaerulff J, Staugaard H, Thomsen JL. Injuries due to deliberate violence in areas of Denmark. I. The extent of violence. *Forensic Sci Int* 1989; (4):183–199.

Budd RD. Cocaine abuse and violent death. *Am J Alcohol Abuse* 1989; 15:375–382.

Centerwall BS. Television and violence: the scale of the problem and where to go from here. *JAMA* 1992; 267:3059–3063.

Christoffel KK. Violent death and injury in US children and adolescents. *Am J Dis Child* 1990; 144:697–706.

Christoffel KK, Liu K. Homicide death rates in childhood in 23 developed countries: U.S. rates atypically high. *Child Abuse Negl* 1983; 7:339–345.

Christoffel KK, Liu K, Stamler J. Epidemiology of fatal child abuse: international mortality data. *J Chronic Dis* 1981; 34:57–64.

Christoffel KK, Scheidt PC, Agran PF, Kraus JF, McLoughlin E, Paulson JA. Standard definitions for childhood injury research: excerpts of a conference report. *Pediatrics* 1992; 89:1027–1034.

Cohen S, Wilson-Brewer R. *Violence Prevention for Young Adolescents: The State of the Art of Program Evaluation*. Washington, DC: Carnegie Council on Adolescent Development, Carnegie Corporation of New York; 1991.

Division of Injury Control, Center for Environmental Health and Injury Control, Centers for Disease Control. Childhood injuries in the United States. *Am J Dis Child* 1990; 144:627–646.

Division of Injury Control, Center for Environmental Health and Injury Control, Centers for Disease Control. Weapon-carrying among high school students, United States, 1990. *MMWR* 1991; 40:681–683.

Fingerhut LA, Kleinman JC. International and interstate comparisons of homicide among young males. *JAMA* 1990; 263:3292–3295.

Fingerhut LA, Kleinman JC, Godfrey E, Rosenberg H. Firearm mortality among children, youth, and young adults 1–34 years of age, trends and current status: United States 1979–88. *Monthly Vital Stat Rep NCHS* 1991; 39:1–15.

Finkelhor D, Hotaling G, Sedlak A. *Missing, Abducted, Runaway and Thrownaway Children in America. First Report: Numbers and Characteristics, National Incidence Studies*. Washington, DC: U.S. Department of Justice, Office of Juvenile Justice and Delinquency Prevention; 1990.

Fraser G, Kilbride PL. Child abuse and neglect—rare, but perhaps increasing, phenomena among the Samia to Kenya. *Child Abuse Negl* 1980; 4:227–232.

Gelles RJ, Cornell CP. International perspectives on child abuse. *Child Abuse Negl* 1983; 7:375–386.

Gelles RJ, Straus MA. *Intimate Violence*. New York: Simon & Schuster Inc; 1988.

Guyer B, Lescohier I, Gallagher SS, Hausman A, Azzara CV. Intentional injuries among children and adolescents in Massachusetts. *N Engl J Med* 1989; 321:1584–1589.

Haddon W, Baker SP. Injury control. In: Clark DW, MacMahon B, eds. *Preventive and Community Medicare*. Boston: Little, Brown and Co; 1981.

Hagedorn JM. *People and Folks: Gangs, Crime, and the Underclass*. Chicago: Lakeview Press; 1988.

Harper T. Armed with respect: most of Britain's bobbies still don't pack guns and don't want to. *Chicago Tribune* 10/18/1991; Sec. 5, p 1.

Hedeboe J, Charles AV, Nielsen J, Grymer F, Møller BN, Møller-Madson B, Jensen SE. Interpersonal violence: patterns in a Danish community. *Am J Pub Health* 1985; 75:651–653.

Herman AA. Political violence, health, and health services in South Africa. *Am J Pub Health* 1988; 78:767–768.

Hocking MA. Assaults in south east London. *J Roy Soc Med* 1989; 82:281–284.

Hollerman JJ, Fackler JL, Coldwell DM, Ben-Menachem Y. Gunshot wounds: 1. Bullets, ballistics, and mechanisms of injury. *Am J Roetgenol* 1990; 155:685–690.

Kellerman AL, Reay DT. Protection or peril? An analysis of firearm-related deaths in the home. *N Engl J Med* 1986; 314: 1557–1560.

Lester D. National suicide and homicide rates: correlates vs. predictors. *Soc Sci Med* 1989; 29:1249–1252.

National Center on Child Abuse and Neglect. *Study Findings: Study of National Incidence and Prevalance of Child Abuse and Neglect, 1988*. Washington, DC: U.S. Department of Health and Human Services; 1988.

Nazer H, Daradkeh T, Mohamed S, Shamayleh A-Q, Marei O. A diagnostic dilemma in Jordan: two child abuse case studies. *Child Abuse Negl* 1988; 12:593–599.

Office of Disease Prevention and Health Promotion, Office of the Assistant Secretary for Health, National Institute on Drug Abuse, ADAMHA. Division of Adolescent and School Health, Center for Chronic Disease Prevention and Health Promotion, Centers for Disease Control. Results from the National Adolescent Student Health Survey. *MMWR* 1989; 38:147–150.

Olds DL, Henderson CR, Chamberlin R, Tatelbaum R. Preventing child abuse and neglect: a randomized trial of nurse home visitation. *Pediatrics* 1986; 78:65–78.

Payne MA. Use and abuse of corporal punishment: a Caribbean view. *Child Abuse Negl* 1989; 13:389–401.

Pieterse JJ, Van Urk H. Maltreatment of children in The Netherlands: an update after ten years. *Child Abuse Negl* 1989; 13:263–269.

Scott KW. Homicide patterns in the West Midlands. *Med Sci Law* 1990; 30:234–238.

Sharma A, Sunderland R. Increasing medical burden of child abuse. *Arch Dis Child* 1988; 63:172–175.

Shepherd J, Scully C, Shapland M, Irish M, Leslie IJ. Assault: characteristics of victims attending an inner-city hospital. *Injury* 1988; 19:185–190.

Soderstrom CA, Furth PA, Glasser D, Dunning RW, Groseclose SL, Cowley RA. HIV infection rates in a trauma center treating predominantly rural blunt trauma victims. *J Trauma* 1989; 29:1526–1530.

Spivak H, Prothrow-Stith D, Hausman AJ. Dying is no accident: adolescents, violence, and intentional injury. *Pediatr Clin North Am* 1988; 35: 1339–1347.

Straus MA, Gelles RJ, Steinmetz SK. *Behind Closed Doors*. New York: Anchor Press, 1980.

Taylor L, Newberger EH. Child abuse in the international year of the child. *N Engl J Med* 1979; 301:1205–1212.

Tsuda R, Ito Y, Inoue T, Hara M. Statistical survey of medico-legal activities for the murderous and accidental death (40 cases) by use of fire arms. *Acta Med* 1989; 59:23–28.

Waller AE, Baker SP, Szocka A. Childhood injury deaths: national analysis and geographic variations. *Am J Publ Health* 1989; 79:310–315.

Wilson-Brewer R, Cohen S, O'Donnell L, Goodman IF. *Violence Prevention for Young Adolescents: A Survey of the State of the Art*. Washington, DC: Carnegie Council on Adolescent Development, Carnegie Corporation of New York; 1991.

PART V

CHRONIC DISORDERS

15

Asthma

TERRY NOLAN

Asthma is the most common chronic disorder in children. Despite its frequency, however, there is a long history of research and debate, not only about its causes but also, at an even more basic level, about what asthma is. One epidemiologist wrote that despite the enormous amount of information that has been amassed, "it is still impossible to construct a coherent synthesis of the epidemiology of asthma" (Gregg, 1986). The basic reason for such a pessimistic outlook is the difficulty in defining asthma with precision. In a sense, it is one of the most elusive classifications in the history of modern medicine. Its definition has changed over time, influenced by beliefs about its etiology and underlying pathophysiology.

Biologic Considerations

These beliefs have, at various times, been superseded by increasingly better understanding of the underlying disease processes, such that the definition itself has changed. For example, Barbee (1987) pointed out that for the better part of this century, virtually all definitions began with the phrase, "an allergic disease." This focus led many researchers and clinicians to be preoccupied with identifying allergic factors in order to classify an individual as having asthma.

A further example of a commonly held belief and its impact on both clinical care and community perceptions of asthma is that of the natural history of the disorder. It was not until long-term cohort studies had been carried out that the lifelong nature of asthma was appreciated. Here and elsewhere, the importance of epidemiologic research as the basis of sound clinical practice has been demonstrated repeatedly.

Epidemiologic studies have, to date, provided strong evidence for the role of environmental factors in the *modification* of asthma, and yet, there has been relatively little focus on environmental factors that might *cause* asthma. By contrast, enormous energy has been directed at elucidating its pathogenesis and molecular basis, especially with respect to atopy. Epidemiology has more recently been brought to bear to define three fundamental questions that are of both practical and theoretical importance: (1) What is asthma?, (2) What causes it?, and (3) What are the effects of its treatment in the aggregate and in the long term?

Definition

The American Thoracic Society and the American College of Chest Physicians define asthma as *a disease characterized by an increased responsiveness of the airways to various stimuli manifested by slowing of forced expiration which changes in severity either spontaneously or as a result of therapy* (American College of Chest Physicians & American Thoracic Society, 1975). The World Health Organization (1975) offers a similar definition that, however, does not include the requirement for a level of therapeutic response: *a chronic condition characterized by recurrent bronchospasm resulting from a tendency to develop reversible narrowing of the airway lumina in response to stimuli of a level or intensity not inducing such narrowing in most individuals*. Because these definitions are essentially clinical, operationalizing them for community-based epidemiologic studies is difficult.

Further complexity was introduced when the terms *intrinsic* and *extrinsic* asthma became popular. The former was used to describe asthma associated with respiratory infections and the latter for that associated with atopy. This distinction has never been shown to have an unambiguous basis in either immunologic or clinical studies, however, and may therefore compound the problem. Similarly, the term *exercise-induced asthma* is no more specific than describing exercise as one precipitant of asthma episodes, and it has not been demonstrated to be a separate entity.

In what was later to become an enormously influential study, Williams and McNicol (1969) studied over 3000 7-year-old Melbourne schoolchildren, of whom 401 were selected for longitudinal study. Of these, 113 had asthma (wheeze not associated with symptoms of respiratory infection on at least one occasion), 107 had wheezy bronchitis (≥5 episodes of wheeze with bronchitis), 75 had mildly wheezy bronchitis (<5 wheeze episodes with infection), and 106 served as controls. In comparing the proportions of the three wheeze groups to controls with respect to a past history of recurrent bronchitis, persistent or recurrent nasal discharge, and hay fever, each had a significantly higher rate than the controls (Table 15.1). A similar pattern was observed in relation to examination findings of nasal eosinophilia, skin test reactivity to rye grass or house dust, and a serum histamine-binding test.

However, the actual rates of these characteristics were two to three times higher in the *asthma* group compared to the *wheezy bronchitis* groups, with the exception of history of bronchitis, nasal discharge, and histamine binding. Nevertheless, on the basis of this uniformity of significant differences between the three groups and controls, Williams and McNicol (1969) concluded that "children with wheezy bronchitis and asthma were from the same population with the same underlying basic disorder."

Several other studies subsequently also showed that the inclusion of those children whose symptoms were consistent with a definition of asthma that emphasized airways flow reversibilty or wheeze substantially increased the preva-

Table 15.1. Results of Study of 3000 7-Year-Old Children in Melbourne

	Asthma %	Wheezy Bronchitis (%)	Mild Wheezy Bronchitis (%)	Controls (%)
Number	113	107	75	106
Recurrent bronchitis	87.3	97.2	90.5	38.1
Nasal discharge	73.6	66.0	49.3	21.3
Hayfever	45.5	19.8	12.0	1.0
Nasal eosinophilia	58.9	28.3	22.7	8.3
Rye grass	59.4	22.7	16.4	6.4
House dust	57.4	20.6	17.8	3.2
Histamine binding	80.5	72.1	60.0	36.3

Source: Data from Williams & McNichol (1969).

lence of asthma. Despite the clinical caveat that "all that wheezes is not asthma," such studies as these have profoundly influenced clinical practice, as well as the direction of etiologic research. However, it is possible that an adverse effect of this "unitary hypothesis" has been to gloss over potentially informative heterogeneity in the modifiers and risk factors associated with virus-induced wheeze compared to other triggers, such as specific allergens (Wilson, 1989).

Epidemiologic Methods in Asthma Research

Prevalence surveys have been used predominantly for three types of investigation: studies of changes in prevalence over time, studies of putative causal factors, and impact studies that focus on the morbidity associated with a child having asthma. Case-control studies have only recently been extensively used to investigate epidemics of asthma mortality. Cohort studies have been used to track the natural history of asthma and to study its longer-term impact. At least one cohort study has also served as a data base from which to mount a nested case-control study of asthma deaths (see Chapter 1).

Central to all research designs is the question of case definition and ascertainment, and although questionnaire methods have, for logistic as well as theoretical reasons, been the mainstay of epidemiologic study, clinical examination, pulmonary function testing, and, more recently, assessment of bronchial hyperresponsiveness (challenge testing) have also been employed.

Limitations of Prevalence Studies

There are several limitations of prevalence studies that are well illustrated in the case of asthma. First, the nosologic difficulties inherent in accurately defining asthma mean that population studies cannot be based on asking respondents whether they or their child have asthma. Rather, the studies must ask whether the child has a set of symptoms that are consistent with asthma with reasonable sensitivity and specificity. The possible misclassification of bronchitis and wheezy bronchitis has been sidestepped since the early 1970s with the acceptance of the symptom wheeze for the classification of asthma. For studies of medically diagnosed asthma, changes in coding practices and in physician diagnostic styles or conventions have plaqued examinations of changes in asthma over time.

The second epidemiologic difficulty to arise from these labeling constraints is which frequency parameter to employ. Published reports have used prevalence (without qualification), point prevalence, period prevalence, cumulative prevalence, cumulative risk, and lifetime prevalence, to name only a few (see Chapter 1). A further difficulty is that recall bias becomes an important problem in defining retrospectively changes in symptoms over time. In a large birth cohort study conducted in Britain since 1958, parents were asked cross-sectionally at subject ages 7, 11, and 16 years whether their child had ever experienced "asthma, wheezing, or wheezy bronchitis." The lifetime prevalence reported at each of these study points was 18.3%, 12.1%, and 11.6% (Anderson et al., 1986); (see Chapter 2).

Third, the age of the subjects studied in a prevalence survey is critical whenever the frequency of the condition varies with age. This variation is not linear in asthma because it may increase or decrease over time. Finally, the relationship between asthma (however defined) and its modifiers and determinants is least well established with the cross-sectional design of the prevalence survey because of the ever-present danger of misconstruing time sequences in this design.

Of the dozens of community surveys that have been performed in the past 30 years, there have been almost as many survey instruments used. Most such parent-completed tools have used items that have rarely been formally validated or even justified in terms of their content. Items used can be broadly grouped under three headings: questions about whether a child has been diagnosed as having asthma, questions about wheeze in various situations, and questions about other respiratory symptoms or conditions, such as nocturnal cough or bronchitis. The temporal reference period for these questions has varied from lifetime ("symptom ever") questions to those that refer to a specific, recent period, such as the preceding 12 months. Because asthma is a condition that requires the passage of time to permit the development of symptoms, this reference period has been critical to such survey research. Table 15.2 lists the questions used in a recent replication survey in Melbourne, Australia. This questionnaire is an adaptation of the International Union Against Tuberculosis (IUAT) questionnaire that was the result of an international working party's efforts to standardize an instrument for use in adult research. The adaptations reflect its use for a pediatric population. Similar instruments have been previously validated (Clifford et al., 1989; Mitchell & Miles, 1983).

Spirometry

The use and value of pulmonary function tests for epidemiologic studies are limited by two factors—cost and validity. Although modern, portable spirometers have greatly facilitated field measurements, the staff and time required to carry out standard tests, such as FEV, and FVC, pose cost constraints for large-scale screening surveys. More importantly, however, pulmonary function

Table 15.2. Screening Instrument Used in 1990 Melbourne Study

In the last 12 months:

1. Has your child had a wheezing or asthma attack?
2. How frequent were the wheezing or asthma attacks? (*None/less than 4 attacks/4 to 12 attacks/ more than 12 attacks*)
3. Has any wheezing or asthma attack woken your child at night?
4. Has any wheezing or asthma attack been severe enough to limit speech to only one or two words at a time between breaths?
5. Has your child sounded wheezy during or after exercise?
6. Has your child had a dry cough at night? (Apart from a cough associated with a cold or chest infection)
7. Has your child usually brought up any phlegm or mucus from the chest first thing in the morning?
8. Has your child woken with a feeling of tightness in the chest first thing in the morning?
9. Has your child had tightness in the chest or become short of breath when near animals, feathers, or dust?
10. Has your child been treated at any time with any of the following medications:

Ventolin	Bricanyl	Neulin	Somophyllin
Respolin	Berotec	Theodur	Elixophyllin
			Slo-bid

Source: From Robertson et al. (1991).

tests on their own do little to enhance the diagnosis or classification of asthma. They do provide, however, an important, static measure of airway function that can be related to symptoms and level of treatment.

Skinprick Tests

The assessment of atopy is best and most conveniently carried out by skin reactivity tests to indicator allergens, such as house dust mite, rye grass, pollen, and animal antigens. As discussed earlier, atopy is neither synonymous with nor a sine qua non for asthma classification. Cost and ethical constraints of using such tests also apply and limit their use in population surveys.

Bronchial Challenge Testing

The concept of bronchial hyperresponsiveness (BHR) was defined long ago in relation to its use in clinical settings, especially with exercise or histamine. The application of this technique to epidemiologic research is a recent phenomenon, and its importance and role are still uncertain. Methacholine is often preferred to histamine as the provocative agent because of its less unpleasant side effects, such as hoarse voice. The challenge is carried out with increasing doses of aerosolized agent administered via nebulizer. FEV_1 is subsequently measured, and a fall of 20% or more over the baseline value results in cessation of the test (at 7.8 mmol/L in the case of histamine challenge). This is the $PD_{20}FEV_1$ value. Arbitrary categorization of BHR severity has been made at histamine doses of $\leq$1 mmol/L (severe), 0.11–0.8 mmol/L (moderate), 0.81–3.2 mmol/L (mild),

3.21–7.8 mmol/L (slight), and normal responsiveness at no $PD_{20}FEV_1$ level (Peat et al., 1989). In Figure 15.1, the percent fall in FEV_1 can be seen in relation to clinically defined levels of responsiveness.

There is a strong, albeit imperfect, relationship between BHR and the respiratory symptoms of asthma and asthma treatment. This relationship is strongest for cases of severe or moderate BHR, in which in a recent cohort study of children between the ages of 8 and 14 years, 87% had current respiratory symptoms and 73% were using asthma medication (Peat et al., 1989). However, in this cohort of children studied three times over 6 years, 27% of those with current respiratory symptoms at 12 to 14 years had had no BHR at any of the three assessments. In several studies the relationship between BHR and atopy has been found to be strong. For example, in a recent Chinese study, odds ratios for having, respectively, mild, moderate, or severe BHR were 5.9, 21.0, and 30.4 for atopy as measured by allergen skinprick tests (Zhong et al., 1990).

The use in large-scale community studies of exercise-induced bronchoconstriction as a marker for bronchial hyperresponsiveness remains attractive but not yet fully evaluated. However, a South African study of a 6-minute exercise test had poor sensitivity (31%) for questionnaire-ascertained respiratory symptoms, but no parallel evaluation has been carried out with allergen provocation of BHR (Terblanche & Stewart, 1990).

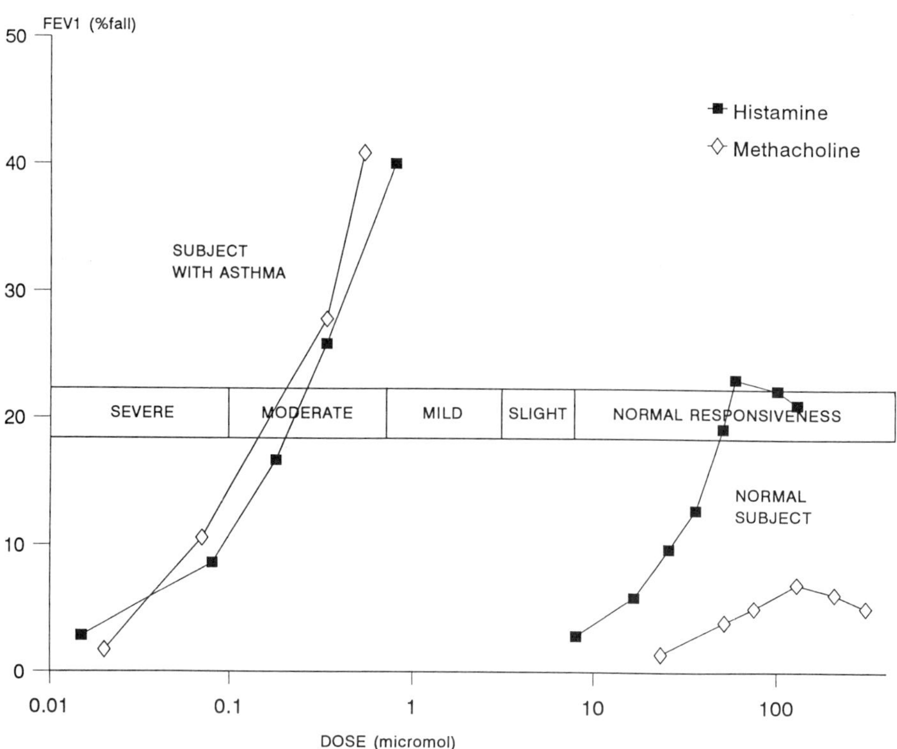

Fig. 15.1. Typical dose response curves to histamine and metacholine showing a 40% fall at a dose less than 1 mmol in an asthmatic patient and a smaller response at higher doses in a normal patient (redrawn from Woolcock & Peat, 1989).

Clinical Diagnosis and Medication Usage

There is ample evidence that parent report of a medical diagnosis of asthma prescription and use of asthma medications is an inadequate measure for epidemiologic study of asthma's prevalence or incidence. The factors that make such measures inadequate include different levels of access to medical care, differing criteria for diagnosis by clinicians, recall bias by parents, and poor communication between clinician and patient.

Severity

The assessment of severity of asthma has received much attention, and as with other chronic illnesses, it has proved difficult to achieve consensus or uniformity. An important epidemiologic complication in severity assessment in any setting is confounding by treatment, which arises from the fact that, at least in theory, the better the treatment, the fewer the symptoms. If that were all that mattered, then some measure of symptoms, combined with a score for the optimal level of treatment in subjects, would suffice. However, the determination of what level of treatment is optimal remains problematic, especially in community studies. Moreover, the possibility of overtreatment, as well as undertreatment, needs to be considered, especially in societies subjected to aggressive marketing of asthma medication. Another generic difficulty when using parent-reported criteria, such as restriction of activity, to assess severity is the possibility that parents may themselves determine the level of activity they permit a child to undertake, based on their instructions or beliefs about the risks of such activity in a child with asthma.

Notwithstanding these difficulties, the conceptualization of a domain of function in respect of daily living (or chronic asthma severity), together with coding a level of physiologic disturbance in an acute asthma episode, represent important first steps. The separation of innate disease activity (intrinsic severity) from the child's current functional status and disease symptoms, regardless of innate activity or treatment, assists in defining the purpose for which asthma severity assessment is to be used.

The simplest measure of severity classifies children into levels of asthma activity (namely, the frequency of episodes) and the presence of intercurrent wheeze—episodic, frequent episodic, persistent, persistent with frequent episodes (Williams & McNicol, 1969). Other severity indicators that reflect asthma's impact on daily living include school absence, sleep interference because of wheeze or cough, the presence of early morning wheeze, and exercise sensitivity. Finally, medical care indicators, such as admissions to a hospital, intensive care unit admissions, emergency room visits, and physician visits, have been used.

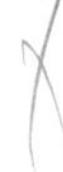

Some studies identify, cluster, and weight such potential indicators to produce a scale that could be used in both research and clinical practice. Most, however, fail to make any serious attempt to assess the scale's validity or reliability (see Chapter 1). One such attempt used cluster analysis to produce the scale illustrated in Table 15.3 (Donnelly et al., 1987). Ascending grades of severity were

Table 15.3. Asthma Severity Scale

	Symptom Frequency				
	Yearly	3-monthly	Monthly	Weekly	Daily
1. Wheeze	1	2	3	4	5
2. Cough	1	2	3	4	5
3. Shortness of breath	1	2	3	4	5
4. Tightness of chest	1	2	3	4	5
	Lifestyle Interference				
5. School missed (days) per	(1–5)	(6–10)	(11–15)	(61–20)	(21+)
year	1	2	3	4	5
6. Sleep missed (nights) per	(1–7)	(8–14)	(15–21)	(22–28)	(29+)
year	1	2	3	4	5
7. Hospital admissions	(1)	(2)	(3)	(4)	(5)
(number)	1	2	3	4	5
8. Physical activity tolerated	(very strenuous)	(strenuous)	(moderate)	(light)	(quiet play)
	1	2	3	4	5

Source: From Donnelly et al. (1987).

allocated to scores in the following way: Grade 1 (1–10), 2 (11–16), 3 (17–22), 4 (23–37), 5 (28–32), and 6 (33–40). Limited validation was performed based on current treatment.

Patterns of Occurrence

Incidence

Few prospective longitudinal studies have been carried out to document the age at which onset of wheezing occurs. In the very low prevalence area of Finland, incidence was calculated at 1.6 per 1000 per year between the ages of 3 and 18 years over a 6-year observation period (Pöysa et al., 1991). Analysis of the 1958 British birth cohort (National Child Development Study) of 8806 children followed to age 16 (Anderson et al., 1986) showed that 24.7% of subjects had asthma or wheezing at some point in their lives. Only about one in six of those whose wheezing started before age 8 continued to wheeze in adolescence. One quarter commenced wheezing between the ages of 8 and 16 years. Factors that predicted later onset were male sex; mother aged 15 to 19 at the child's birth; history of pneumonia, whooping cough, throat or ear infections, or tonsillectomy; atopy; and recurrent abdominal pain. A 10% random sample of a Tasmanian birth cohort of 8410 children was studied to age 20 years and provided data suggesting that the incidence of asthma falls into three phases: a high rate from birth to 3 years, a moderate phase until 5 years, and a declining phase thereafter (Giles et al., 1984).

Prevalence

Asthma prevalence surveys can be grouped broadly into two types: (1) those that focus on hospital admissions or visits for the treatment of asthma and (2) community samples, usually school-based, that have used parent questionnaires.

Community-based studies from Finland, Denmark, England, the Isle of Wight, Sweden, Scotland, the United States, and Australia in the 1950s and 1960s showed considerable variation in the prevalence estimates of asthma. This variation reflected many of the classification difficulties mentioned above and, in particular, the medical diagnoses of wheezy bronchitis and of asthma being treated by some as the same condition and by others as different. The Williams and McNicol study (1969), among other influences, led to an opening up of the epidemiologic definition of asthma. This effectively resulted in question designs that incorporated notions of wheeze or whistling in the chest, with or without breathlessness or atopic symptoms, in defining asthma for population surveys.

International and Secular Variations in Prevalence

It is now well demonstrated that the prevalence of asthma in children is substantially lower in developing countries (Cookson, 1987). For example, in Papua, New Guinea, Dowse et al. (1985) found a 0.2% prevalence in those under age 20, based on any past history of wheeze or intermittent breathlessness and/or wheeze accompanied by significant bronchial hyperresponsiveness. Such differences are not explained by methodologic differences in ascertainment. More recent studies, however, in Third World countries that are rapidly adopting Western lifestyles have shown prevalence rates much closer to the high rates observed in nearby developed nations. For example, in Fiji, a population-based study using identical methods to those employed in Western studies found a 12-month wheeze prevalence of 21% in 7- to 11-year-old children (Flynn, 1992).

However, there is also substantial variation among Western countries that remains to be explained. This is especially the case for Scandinavia. In Sweden in 1985, a study of 10,527 children aged 7 to 16 years revealed a 4% total prevalence of current wheeze or cough (Bråbäck et al., 1988), whereas in Norway in 1980 to 1981, Skarpaas and Gulsvik (1985) found that the prevalence of current wheeze was 8.3% (7 years), 8.1% (11 years), and 4.3% (15 years).

In addition to these unexplained differences, there is now overwhelming evidence of an increase in the prevalence of asthma in children over the past 30 years or longer and a less well-documented case for this increase occurring over the past century. Gregg (1986) cites a thesis on asthma written in 1882 in London in which the author noted that over a period of 20 years, only 21 of the 20,000 admissions made during that period were because of asthma. Anecdotal reports from pediatricians who practiced in the 1940s also suggest that asthma was a relatively rare disease at that time (Howard Williams, personal communication).

More recent evidence comes from both hospital admission studies and community-based studies using the same questionnaire items that had been used previously. In a careful replication of the Williams and McNicol study carried out 26 years earlier, Robertson et al., (1991) demonstrated an increase in the rate of parent-reported wheeze or asthma from 19.1% to 46.0% in 3325 7-year-olds. The 1-year period prevalence of wheeze was 21.1%, 21.7%, and 18.6% among 7-, 12-, and 15-year-olds, respectively. A comparison with other studies that have also used 12-month period prevalence of wheeze is shown in Table 15.4.

A similar repeat survey in the same population was carried out among 12-

Table 15.4. Twelve-Month Period Prevalence (%) of Wheeze in Recent British, New Zealand, and Australian Studies

Study and Year	7 Years	Age 12 Years	15 Years
Southampton, 1986	11.9	12.3	—
Dunedin, NZ, 1987	19.5	—	—
Tyneside, 1987	—	—	8.6
Cardiff, 1988	—	15.2	—
Melbourne, 1990	23.1	21.7	18.6

Source: From Robertson et al. (1991).

year-olds in Cardiff in 1973 and 1988 (Burr et al., 1989). The prevalence of "wheeze ever" had increased from 17% to 22%, and "current asthma" (reported to have had asthma and to have wheezed within the previous 12 months) had more than doubled from 4% to 9%. Moreover, the prevalence of a marked exercise response (⩾35% fall in peak expiratory flow rate) increased by 156% (from 0.9% to 2.3%) over the 15-year period, suggesting that the proportion with more severe asthma had also increased. Burney and colleagues (1990) analyzed data from a national British study of health and growth of around 6600 children aged 4 to 12 years and found a definite and highly significant increase in the 12-month prevalence of parent-reported wheeze or asthma between 1973 and 1986. The increase in asthma was significantly greater for girls (378%) than for boys (138%) and was accompanied by a smaller, but still significant decrease in the prevalence of reported bronchitis (47% for boys, 52% for girls). Parallel increases in parent-reported symptoms made it unlikely that these increases could have been fully explained by changes in diagnostic patterns.

A large number of hospital admission studies also document increases in asthma admission rates that are only partly explained by changes in discharge diagnosis coding practices, either as a result of changes in the International Classification of Diseases (ICD) codes or by changes in medical diagnosis itself, e.g., after the McNicol and Williams paper (1969) recommending the aggregation of asthma, wheezy bronchitis, and bronchitis with wheeze into a single rubric.

In the United States, Halfon and Newacheck (1986) showed that between 1970 and 1984 there was a 145% increase in hospital admissions for those under 15, and at the same time National Health Interview Survey reports demonstrated a 28% rise in parent-reported asthma for 6- to 16-year-olds. Although transition from ICD-8 to ICD-9 explained 30% to 40% of the increase between 1978 and 1979, clear increases remained apparent within homologous ICD segments of 1970 to 1978 and 1979 to 1983. Other studies confirm that diagnostic transfer does not fully explain the increase seen (Gergen & Weiss, 1990). In Washington, D.C. between 1961 and 1981, there was a 19-fold increase in asthma admissions, although there was only a 1.5-fold increase in the pediatric population (Mullally et al., 1984). In Montreal, Canada, the admission rate for 3-year-olds increased from 720 per 100,000 per year in 1980 to 1981 to 1190 in 1984 to 1985 (Infante-Rivard et al., 1987).

Several British studies show similar increases in hospital admission rates, especially in the 0- to 4-year age range (Anderson, 1989). In Christchurch (New

Zealand) between 1974 and 1989, there was a 4.5- to fivefold increase in admission rates (Horwood et al., 1991), although there has been a recent downward trend for school-aged children. The 1989 rates were approximately 800 per 100,000 per year for boys and 500 per 100,000 per year for girls 0 to 13 years. The rates for young children were strikingly high, e.g., 1,400 per 100,000 per year for boys 0 to 4 years. These changes were shown not to be attributable to diagnostic transfer or changes in admission policy.

One Australian study that has found a large part of the observed increase to have been attributable to ICD and coder practice changes was reported by Carman and Landau (1990). Between 1971 and 1987, there was an increase from 325 per 100,000 per year to 1000 in 1983, the rate thereafter remaining stable. The rate for children aged 0 to 4 years rose to 1652 per 100,000 per year in 1987. By contrast, another Australian study in New South Wales found that with consistent use of ICD 9 codes the admission rate for 1- to 5-year-olds increased from 839 per 100,000 per year to 1238 between 1979 and 1986 (Bauman et al., 1990).

Only one study has specifically addressed whether this increase has been associated with changes in the proportion of severe cases, it having been argued that larger numbers of milder cases were being admitted because of changes in admission thresholds and community expectations of care. At the Christchurch Hospital in New Zealand, the observed increase was not associated with an increase in admissions of milder cases. In fact, based on a retrospectively assessed clinical scoring system, a significant increase in the proportion with severe asthma was observed—from 19% in 1975 to 51% in 1985 (Dawson, 1987).

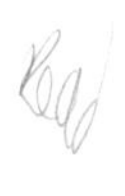

Natural History

Asthma is a disease the activity of which varies with time. This variation may occur from day to day or from year to year. It has therefore been necessary to carry out prospective cohort studies to define properly this temporal variation. There have now been several such studies, but the first to progress well into adult life was that begun by Williams and McNicol in Melbourne in 1964. From the initial prevalence survey of over 3000 7-year-old schoolchildren described above, 401 were selected for longitudinal study and followed initially until 10 years of age. This cohort was subsequently studied at 14, 21, and 28 years of age (Kelly et al., 1987; Martin et al., 1980; McNicol & Williams, 1973). Although the cohort was not followed from birth and had too few controls to document the incidence of asthma reliably, several important findings emerged. First, the persistence of wheeze to 10 years was highly correlated with early age of onset and with the frequency of episodes in the first year of symptoms. During adolescence, most subjects had improved such that 55% of those whose wheezing had ceased before adolescence remained wheeze-free in early adult life. Conversely, 45% of those who had ceased to wheeze by 14 years experienced minor recurrences until age 21, although in 44% the wheeze frequency increased once more by the age of 28 years. Seventy-three percent of those who were wheeze-free at 14 had little or no asthma at 28. During adolescence and early adult life, the preponderance of boys with troublesome asthma diminished.

These findings of improvement in adolescence with reactivation in early adulthood, especially in those with troublesome early-onset asthma, have been confirmed in Swedish (Jönsson, et al., 1987), Japanese (Mauro et al., 1990), Tasmanian (Giles et al., 1984), and English (Blair, 1977) studies.

Mortality

Death from asthma is a rare event. However, its prospect motivates an urgency and seriousness in medical care that are rivaled only by a few other pediatric conditions. The reason for this is probably the fear of sudden and relatively unexpected deterioration in respiratory function and concern about the "locked lung" or state of treatment refractoriness. It has been claimed that the sudden and fulminating attack of asthma is a relatively new phenomenon in this century (Roe, 1984), but data are not available to verify this claim. It is true that a large proportion of children who die from asthma do so in this way. Robertson et al. (1990), in an uncontrolled mortality survey over a 1-year period in the mid-1980s (based on information from family physicians and parents), showed that of the 19 deaths in those aged 0 to 19 years, 15 were judged to have only mild or moderate severity of previous asthma, and 15 also experienced a sudden collapse and died less than 20 minutes after the onset of the attack, with little apparent warning. This paradox highlights the dilemma whether the absence or delay in appropriate treatment versus the acute or long-term toxic effects of the treatment itself underlies asthma deaths.

In fact, the mortality from asthma has shown a modest but consistent increase in young people over the past 30 years. Against the backdrop of this increase, there have been two verified epidemics of asthma deaths.

The first epidemic began in the first half of the 1960s (Fig. 15.2) in at least six countries—Australia, England, Ireland, New Zealand, Scotland, and Wales). It was most marked in children, adolescents, and young adults, in whom the mortality rate increased two- to fourfold. The second epidemic occurred only in New Zealand, beginning in 1976, and peaked at a rate in 5 to 34 year olds of 4 per 100,000 per year in 1980. The cause of these epidemics remains hotly debated, with high-dose, metered dose inhaler beta-agonists with less beta-2 receptor selectivity being strongly implicated—isoprenaline forte in the 1960s and fenoterol in the 1970s. The 1960s epidemic only occurred in countries with the high-dose isoprenaline forte was used, with the exception of two countries where sales were low (Belgium and the Netherlands). Unfortunately, case-control studies were not done at the time of this first epidemic because it had declined before there was time to conduct them. Learning from this lesson, three case-control studies were performed in New Zealand during the second epidemic (Crane et al., 1989; Grainger et al., 1991; Pearce et al., 1990). These studies strongly implicate another potent formulation from the beta-agonist group; namely, fenoterol. A recent nested case-control analysis of a cohort study from Saskatchewan in Canada, where no epidemic had been observed, also identified fenoterol as a significant risk factor for asthma death (Spitzer et al., 1992). Additionally, however, other beta-agonists were also associated with increased mortality risk. Although a major issue in all these studies has been the possible

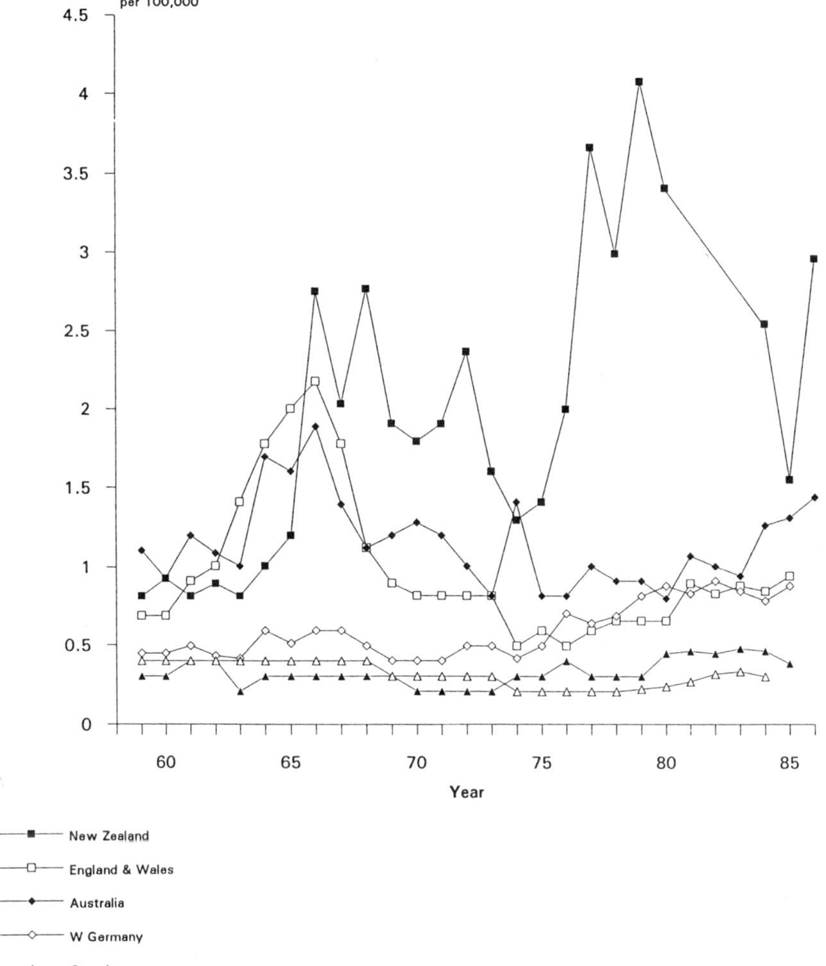

Fig. 15.2. Two verified epidemics of asthma deaths, the first in six countries in the 1960s, and the second in New Zealand in the 1970s (redrawn from Beasley et al., 1991).

confounding by asthma severity, adjustment for severity has not diminished the odds ratios. It seems that the most popular hypothesis about why these drugs might be associated with an increased risk of death—namely, the so-called drug-induced delay hypothesis—may not be able to account for the epidemics that have been observed. The alternative explanations, direct toxicity during an acute episode or chronic effects after long-term use, remain to be evaluated precisely (Pearce et al., 1991).

Explaining the background increase in asthma mortality has proved to be an even more difficult puzzle for several reasons (Burney, 1988a). First, the rate of increase has not been great. Second, the background increase in prevalence is a confounding factor. Third, it is hard to find an untreated comparison group for assessing the possible association with drug therapy. Finally, adjustment for severity as a possible confounder may not be possible if, as is suspected by some, beta-agonists may increase asthma severity with long-term use and therefore severity may be an intermediate factor in the relationship between a particular drug and death (see Chapter 1). Sears and colleagues (1990) recently demonstrated deterioration in asthma control with daily fenoterol use over a 6-month period compared to on-demand use in a double-blind crossover trial. This deterioration was associated with an increase in bronchial hyperresponsiveness. Although there are some earlier reports of medium-term adverse respiratory effects of lower-dose agents, such as salbutamol, controlled trials over longer periods in children remain to be carried out.

In the United States during the 1980s, asthma mortality increased by 6.2% per annum, with the increase being greater in children aged 5 to 14 years than in adolescents and young adults aged 15 to 34 years (Wiess & Wagener, 1990). There is evidence that, for children, changes in death coding practices do not explain increased mortality, and there is little evidence to support alternative hypotheses of increased atopic exposure in severely affected individuals or increased severity of chronic asthma (Friday & Fireman, 1988).

Apart from this focus on possible iatrogenic factors, a renewed search is now under way for possible environmental factors that may be associated with the risk of sudden and unexpected death. A recent case-control study from the Mayo Clinic has implicated aeroallergen from the common mold *Alternaria alternata* as a risk factor for respiratory arrest in young asthmatics (O'Hallaren et al., 1991). Ten of eleven cases (aged 11 to 25 years) of respiratory arrest before attendance and ascertainment (two of which were fatal and all of whom had sudden, unexpected, and overwhelming asthmatic episodes) had positive skin tests to this mold compared to 31% of 99 asthmatic controls. After adjustment for confounding by age, the odds ratio was 189.5 (95% CI, 6.5–5,535). This is one of the most common atmospheric mold spores throughout the United States, and the *Alternaria* season corresponds with the peak asthma mortality period of June through August. *Alternaria* has been shown to provoke immediate and late asthmatic responses and to increase bronchial hyperresponsiveness markedly.

Morbidity

Morbidity attributable to asthma is substantial. The increasing rates of hospitalization underline its community impact, as well as the family disruption, days of parent work lost, and costs involved. Length of hospital stay has fallen over the past 30 years, and although average stays of 2.5 days or less are often found in major centers, longer inpatient stays are reported in regional or district hospitals (Nolan et al., 1989). In the aggregate, asthma is responsible for more hospital bed days than any other condition. A broader description of the morbidity attributable to asthma has been provided from community-based studies, such as Anderson's report of 9-year-olds in a London borough (Anderson et al., 1983). They found that 27% of children reported to have wheezing or asthma had had their home activities restricted in the previous 6 months because of their illness. Fifteen percent had spent more than 5 days in bed in the previous year, and 24% reported limitation of games or physical education. Compared to controls, the 12-month period prevalence rate ratio for eczema was 1.5, allergic rhinitis 4.1, frequent headaches 1.7, and recurrent abdominal pain 1.7. Twenty-nine percent missed more than 10 days from school because of wheezing illness in the previous year. The impact on the family was demonstrated by 42% of the mothers reporting an effect on their activities: 29% had made special arrangements for the child's bedroom, and 20% had removed a pet from the home. On the other hand, they reported little effect on the child's social activities (club membership, swimming) compared to controls.

The impact of asthma on emotional adjustment has been the subject of many studies that have documented increased risks of maladjustment compared to controls (Graham et al., 1967; McNicol et al., 1973), including our own unpublished results from the 1990 Melbourne survey of 10,000 schoolchildren. Adjustment has been measured in these studies using parent and child interviews with unvalidated questions (McNicol et al., 1973) or formal, validated, parent- and/or teacher-report questionnaires (Graham et al., 1967; Nolan et al., unpublished data). Risk ratios for maladjustment have varied between 1.6 to 2.0, and there seems to be a positive linear relationship between asthma severity and risk of maladjustment. Some have argued that the unpredictability of the clinical course of chronic illnesses, such as asthma, may also be an important determinant of maladjustment (Jessop & Stein, 1985).

Risk Factors

Although the causes of asthma are not known, much is understood about risk factors and effect modifiers. The identification of a single dominant gene for atopy (Cookson et al., 1989) is a recent, encouraging development in the unraveling of the asthma mystery. It may allow a better understanding of the separate genetic and environmental determinants of wheezing illnesses. Unfortunately, the potential overlap between factors that might initiate asthma and those that exacerbate an already sensitized individual has made the search for an explanatory framework difficult.

Family Size

Strachan (1989) analyzed hay fever and eczema data (but not wheezing) on more than 17,000 subjects from the 1958 British birth cohort (National Child Development Study) at ages 7, 11, and 23 years. He found highly significant relationships between these conditions and small family size after adjusting for social class, breast feeding, and cigarette smoking. An only child was up to four times more likely to have hay fever than a child with four or more siblings. Such observations as these have led to the "increasing hygiene" hypothesis that conflicts with data linking infant viral infections with risk for later asthma (see Chapter 18). It is argued that diminishing family size and improvement in domestic hygiene have resulted in less opportunity for children to be exposed to "unhygienic" nasal secretion contacts between a young child and older children. Such exposure is thought to result in education of the immune system not to react to exogenous irritants, such as pollens. Strachan (1989) also speculated whether an as-yet unknown virus, perhaps a retrovirus, might infect an infant's mast cells and render them permanently less reactive (Gamlin, 1990).

Sex

Many studies have shown males to be at substantially higher risk for asthma than females in childhood, although, as stated above, this inequality is substantially reduced during adolescence and continues at a lower level into adult life (Kelly et al., 1987; Martin et al., 1980).

Social Class

There is conflicting evidence that childhood asthma is associated with poverty or other forms of social deprivation. Analysis of data from the British National Child Development Study failed to demonstrate significant associations with household crowding, social class, absence of one or more parents, or tenure of accommodation (Anderson et al., 1987). By contrast, the U.S. National Health and Nutrition Examination Survey (NHANES II) analysis revealed odds ratios of 1.98 (95% CI, 1.13–2.13) for asthma comparing the lowest income tertile to the highest and 1.25 (95% CI, 0.98–1.6) for current wheeze (Schwartz et al., 1990).

Race and Region

There is evidence from migration studies that the risk of asthma is acquired in the newly adopted country, suggesting strong environmental determination. Children born in India and Pakistan were found to have a much lower prevalence of asthma than British children or British-born Asian children (Smith et al., 1971). In South Africa, 0.15% of Xhosa children living in rural areas had exercise-induced wheeze compared to a rate of 3.2% among those who had moved to Cape Town townships (van Niekerk et al., 1979). In the Pacific Tokelau Islands, a prevalence of 11% was found in resident native children contrasted with a rate of 25% in children who had emigrated to New Zealand (Waite et al., 1980). A multivariate analysis of data from NHANES II attempted to control for social class and poverty in examining the increased relative risk for asthma in African-American children compared to white children. However, statistical control was unable to reduce the odds ratio below 1.7 (95% CI, 1.2–2.1; Schwartz et al., 1990). After taking other factors into account, living in the inner city was associated with asthma for both whites and African-Americans.

Viral Infection

There is a well-established association between respiratory syncytial virus (RSV) or parainfluenza type 3 infection (bronchiolitis) in the first year of life and the later development of asthma. Over 50% of such infants go on to wheeze in later childhood. However, although this relationship is also associated with increased bronchial hyperresponsiveness, no association with atopy has been demonstrated (Duiverman et al., 1987). An historical cohort study in Rochester, New York, suggested that the etiologic fraction of wheeze at 8 years of age due to bronchiolitis was 9.4% (McConnochie & Roghmann, 1984).

Genetics

Twin studies, pedigree analyses, and family concordance analyses from population prevalence surveys have been used with varying degrees of statistical sophistication to investigate the genetic contribution to asthma and atopy. For example, Edfors-Lubs (1971) analyzed data from a Swedish twin registry of 6996 twin pair responders. She found 19.0% concordance for asthma among monozygotic twins and 4.8% among dizygotic twins. From these and other results in her study, she concluded that the environmental contribution to asthma was very substantial (see Chapter 5).

Recently, Cookson and co-workers (Cookson & Hopkin, 1988; Cookson et al., 1989) showed that atopy seemed to be inherited as an autosomal dominant trait and then produced a molecular genetic linkage analysis identifying the gene locus on chromosome 11. Exactly which aspect of atopy is governed by this gene is not yet known. Further studies have suggested that the genetic determinants of atopy and asthma are different and possibly that atopy enhances the chance of a genetic predisposition to asthma being expressed (Sibbald, 1991).

Environmental: Tobacco Smoke

Substantial evidence implicates passive inhalation of environmental tobacco smoke as a cause of wheezing episodes (Burchfiel et al., 1986; Martinez et al., 1992; McConnochie & Roghman, 1989; Murray & Morrison, 1988; Strachan et al., 1990; Weitzman et al., 1990). Murray and Morrison (1988) found a highly significant dose-response relationship in 7- to 17-year-olds among the number of cigarettes the mother smoked in the house, pulmonary function, and BHR. Whether or not the increase in prevalence in wheezing illness is related to passive smoke effects is not known, but clearly reduction or elimination of this factor is an important public health objective.

Pollution and Atmospheric Factors

There is good laboratory evidence of the bronchoconstrictive capacity of sulfur dioxide in asthmatics with and without an atopic disposition. Several epidemiologic studies used ecologic data to relate ambient sulfar dioxide levels to respiratory symptoms, such as cough. Such studies have sometimes found effects at levels lower than demonstrated in the laboratory, which has been attributed to co-pollutants, such as acid aerosols, the levels of which parallel those of sulfur dioxide. On the other hand, some studies have shown confusing results with some pollutants. A recent study found a significantly higher prevalence of asthma in children living near a coal-fired power station (Henry et al., 1991a and b), but asthma symptoms were related neither to levels of sulfur dioxide nor nitrous oxide, another gas less reliably shown to induce bronchospasm. Airborne particulate matter levels have also been related to hospital admissions for asthma, such as, for example, after forest fires. Rennick and Jarman (1992) reported an association between asthma visits in the emergency room of the Royal Children's Hospital in Melbourne, Australia, and days reported by the environmental protection authority as exhibiting high levels of airborne particulates (smog alert days).

Seasonal variations in hospital admission rates of asthma have been described in many studies, with a moderate peak in the spring and a larger peak in the autumn. Weather change has also been a focus for investigation since it is often reported by parents as precipitating wheeze episodes in children with asthma. In another hospital admission study, Beer and colleagues (1991) showed that asthma attendances were related to afternoon gradients of air temperature and modified heat content factor (the energy required to heat the air water vapor to the ambient temperature), but not to the absolute values of air temperature and water content.

Two recent studies have suggested a mechanism to explain the relationship between weather and epidemics of asthma. Bellomo et al. (1992) studied the association between thunderstorms and asthma epidemics, demonstrating a five- to tenfold rise in asthma presentations to hospital immediately after thunderstorms. They also demonstrated a significant association with rye grass sensitivity in cases sampled from attendees at the time of the thunderstorms compared to clinic controls. More specifically, they demonstrated skin sensitivity to the starch granule extract that is derived from rye grass. Botanists from the same group subsequently identified the rye grass pollen allergen *Lol pIX* within intracellular starch granules inside the pollen grains (Suphioglu et al., 1992). It was shown that *Lol pIX* is a potent bronchoconstrictor. Rye grass pollens rapidly rupture during the osmotic shock of rainfall exposure, each grain releasing about 700 starch granules, each of which is less than 3 μm in diameter—small enough to penetrate to the lower airways. Atmospheric samples on a dry day without rain in the previous 24 hours averaged 910 (sd 149) starch granules/m^3, whereas samples on a dry day after rain on the previous day were more than 50 times higher, with 53,982 (sd 6,107) granules/m.

Breast Feeding and Cow's Milk

Breast feeding does not seem to protect from the later development of asthma. A survey in the Isle of Wight found similar rates of asthma in 4-year-olds who were exclusively breast fed in infancy compared to those who were bottle fed (Soothill et al., 1976). Schwartz et al.'s (1990) analysis of NHANES II data suggested that breast feeding was a protective factor, but they were unable to control for either pre- or postnatal maternal smoking. Analysis of the British National Child Development Study 1958 birth cohort found that breast feeding was not a predictor of wheeze at 7 to 16 years of age (Anderson et al., 1987). Similarly, data from another large British birth cohort study (Child Health and Education Study) failed to demonstrate any effect on asthma or current wheeze of breast feeding after adjustment for maternal smoking and parental asthma (Taylor et al., 1983).

Individual case reports of cow's milk-induced asthma are reported and well known to clinicians, but results from a recent randomized controlled trial make interpretation of the other epidemiologic data difficult at this time. Miskelly et al. (1988) randomized 487 newborn infants at high risk of allergic disease to receive either soy-based milk formula or conventional cow's milk-derived formula. Although follow-up was limited in this report to 1 year, both groups had similar rates of wheeze. However, breast feeding for any length of time was associated with a reduced incidence of wheezing.

Salt

In 1986, Burney proposed that dietary sodium chloride might be the "Westernizing factor" responsible for international variation in asthma prevalence and mortality (Burney, 1987). He demonstrated a strong ecologic relationship between child asthma mortality for England and Wales between 1969 and 1973 and table salt purchases ($r = 0.82$, $P < .05$). He also showed a strong relationship between urinary sodium excretion and bronchial hyperresponsiveness in 43 adult subjects with reactions to 8 mmol/L of histamine or less, after controlling for height, urinary creatinine, and smoking. Subsequently, Medici and Vetter (1991) conducted a crossover challenge trial in 14 asthmatic subjects and demonstrated that salt intake worsened symptoms ($P = 0.06$), increased the use of inhaled steroids ($P < .05$), and worsened FEV_1 ($P < .01$). Burney et al. (1989) showed experimentally that a low-sodium diet reduced bronchial hyperresponsiveness in male, but not female asthmatic adults, although Javaid et al. (1988) demonstrated a similar effect in both sexes. This promising lead requires further investigation with both epidemiologic and clinical studies in children.

Selenium

The element selenium is required for the function of the enzyme, glutathione peroxidase, that modulates arachidonic acid metabolism, which is important to the inflammatory process. The high prevalence of asthma in New Zealand, together with the knowledge that it is a country with low dietary selenium intake, motivated a recent case-control study in subjects with asthma (Flatt et al., 1990). Odds ratios of 1.9 (95% CI, 0.6–5.6) and 5.8 (95% CI, 1.6–21.2) were found for asthma in subjects with the lowest whole blood selenium levels and glutathione peroxidase activity, respectively.

Prevention

Primary prevention of asthma is an ambitious goal that has proved elusive in the absence of a comprehensive understanding of its basic pathogenesis. Attempts to intervene in early infancy to reduce the incidence of viral infection seem attractive, but must be balanced against concern generated by the "hygiene" hypothesis that such efforts might increase the incidence later. The reduction of environmental tobacco smoke exposure is one new opportunity, but its impact remains to be studied empirically. The iatrogenic hypotheses of possible detrimental class effects of agents active against beta-receptors will be tested as such agents are withdrawn or further controlled studies are carried out. Much research remains to be done on dietary, atmospheric, and other environmental factors, especially on the interaction between such factors and pollens and other allergens. A more incisive and analytic approach is needed for future epidemiologic research in order to unravel further the complex story that remains to be told.

References

American College of Chest Physicians & American Thoracic Society. Pulmonary terms and symbols. *Chest* 1975; 67:583–593.

Anderson HR. Increase in hospital admissions for childhood asthma: trends in referral, severity, and readmissions from 1970 to 1985 in a health region of the United Kingdom. *Thorax* 1989; 44:614–619.

Anderson HR, Bailey PA, Cooper JS, et al. Morbidity and school absence caused by and wheezing illness. *Arch Dis Child* 1983; 58:777–784.

Anderson HR, Bland JM, Patel S, et al. The natural history of asthma in childhood. *J Epidemiol Comm Health* 1986; 40:121–129.

Anderson HR, Bland JM, Peckham CS. Risk factors for asthma up to 16 years of age. *Chest* 1987; 87(suppl):27S–130S.

Barbee RA. The epidemiology of asthma. 1987; *Monogr Allergy* 21:21–41.

Bauman A, Lyle D, Taylor L, et al. The use of medical records in epidemiology: a case study using asthma hospitalisations in New South Wales. 1979–86. *Am Med Rec J* 1990; 20:101–105.

Beasley R, Pearce N, Crane J, et al. Asthma mortality and inhaled beta agonist therapy. *Aust NZ Med J* 1991; 21:753–763.

Beer SI, Kannai YI, Waron MJ. Acute exacerbation of bronchial asthma in children associated with afternoon weather changes. *Am Rev Respir Dis* 1991; 144:31–35.

Bellomo R, Gigliotti P, Treloar A, et al. Two consecutive thunderstorm associated epidemics of asthma in the city of Melbourne. *Med J Aust* 1992; 156:834–837.

Blair H. Natural history of childhood asthma. 20 year follow-up. *Arch Dis Child* 1977; 52:613–619.

Bråbäck I, Kälvesten L, Sundström G. Prevalence of bronchial asthma among schoolchildren in a Swedish district. *Acta Paediatr Scand* 1988; 77:821–825.

Burchfiel CM, Higgins MW, Keller JB, et al. Passive smoking in childhood. *Am Rev Respir Dis* 1986; 133:966–973.

Burney PGJ. The causes of asthma—does salt potentiate bronchial activity? Discussion paper. *J Roy Soc Med* 1987; 80:364–367.

Burney PGJ. Asthma deaths in England and Wales 1931–85: evidence for a tr in asthma mortality. *J Epidemiol Comm Health* 1988a; 42:316–320.

Burney PGJ. Why study the epidemiology of asthma? *Thorax* 1988b; 43:425

Burney PGJ, Neild JE, Twort CHC, et al. Effect of changing dietary sod airway response to histamine. *Thorax* 1989; 44:36–41.

Burney PGJ, Chinn S, Rona RJ. Has the prevalence of asthma increased in children? Evidence from the National Study of Health and Growth 1973–86. *Br Med J* 1990; 300:1306–1310.

Burr ML, Butland BK, King S, et al. Changes in asthma prevalence: two surveys 15 years apart. *Arch Dis Child* 1989; 64:1452–1456.

Carman PG, Landau LI. Increased paediatric admissions with asthma in Western Australia—a problem of diagnosis? *Med J Aust* 1990; 152:23–26.

Clifford RD, Radford M, Howell JB, et al. Prevalence of respiratory symptoms among 7 and 11 year old schoolchildren and association with asthma. *Arch Dis Child* 1989; 64:1118–1125.

Cookson JB. Prevalence rates of asthma in developing countries and their comparison with those in Europe and North America. *Chest* 1987; 91(suppl):97s–103s.

Cookson WO, Sharp PA, Faux JA, Hopkin JM. Linkage between immunoglobin E responses underlying asthma and rhinitis and chromosome 11q. *Lancet* 1989; i:1292–1294.

Cookson WO, Hopkins JM. Dominant inheritance of atopic immunoglobin-E responsiveness. *Lancet* 1988; i:86–87.

Crane J, Flatt A, Jackson R, et al. Prescribed fenoterol and death from asthma in New Zealand, 1981–83: case control study. *Lancet* 1989; 1:917–922.

Dawson KP. The severity of asthma in children admitted to hospital: a 20 year review. *NZ Med J* 1987; 100:520–521.

Donnelly WJ, Donnelly JE, Thong YH. Guidelines for maintenance treatment of childhood asthma: development of a score card system by multivariate cluster analysis. *Soc Sci Med* 1987; 25:1033–1038.

Dowse GK, Smith D, Turner KJ, et al. Prevalence and features of asthma in a sample survey of urban Goroka, Papua New Guinea. *Clin Allergy* 1985; 15:429–438.

Duiverman EJ, Neijens HJ, van Strick R, et al. Lung function and bronchial responsiveness in children who had infantile bronchiolitis. *Pediatr Pulmonol* 1987; 3:38–44.

Edfors-Lubs M-L. Allergy in 7,000 twin pairs. *Acta Allergologica* 1971; 26:249–285.

Flatt A, Pearce N, Thomson CD, et al. Reduced selenium in asthmatic subjects in New Zealand. *Thorax* 1990; 45:95–99.

Flynn M. Respiratory symptoms in Fijian and Indian children in sura city. Presented at the Annual Scientific meeting of the Thoracic Society of Australia and New Zealand; April 1992; Canberra.

Friday GA, Fireman P. Morbidity and mortality of asthma. *Pediatr Clin North Am* 1988; 35:1149–1162.

Gamlin L. The big sneeze. *New Scientist* June 2, 1990:19–23.

Gergen PJ, Weiss KB. Changing patterns of asthma hospitalization among children: 1979 to 1987. *JAMA* 1990; 265:1688–1692.

Giles GG, Lickiss N, Gibson HB, et al. Respiratory symptoms in Tasmanian adolescents: a follow up of the 1961 birth cohort. *Aust NZ J Med* 1984; 14:631–637.

Graham PJ, Rutter ML, Yule W, Pless IB. Childhood asthma: a psychosomatic disorder? Some epidemiological considerations. *Br J Prev Soc Med* 1967; 21:78–85.

Grainger J, Woodman K, Pearce N, et al. Prescribed fenoterol and death from asthma in New Zealand, 1981–7: a further case-control study. *Thorax* 1991; 46:105–111.

Gregg I. Epidemiological research in asthma: the need for a broad perspective. *Clin Allergy* 1986; 16:17–23.

Halfon N, Newacheck PW. Trends in the hospitalization for acute childhood asthma, 1970–84. *Am J Pub Health* 1986; 76:1308–1311.

Henry RL, Abramson R, Adler JA, et al. Asthma in the vicinity of power stations. I. A prevalence study. *Pediatr Pulmonol* 1991a; 11:127–133.

Henry RL, Bridgman HA, Wlodarczy KJ, et al. Asthma in the vicinity of power stations. II. October air quality and symptoms. *Pediatr Pulmonol* 1991b; 11:134–140.

Horwood LJ, Dawson KP, Mogridge N. Admission patterns for childhood acute asthma: Christchurch 1974–89. *NZ Med J* 1991; 104:277–279.

Infante-Rivard C, Sukia SE, Roberge D, et al. The changing frequency of childhood asthma. *J Asthma* 1987; 24:283–288.

Javaid A, Cushley MJ, Bone MF. Effect of dietary salt on bronchial reactivity to histamine in asthma. *Br Med J* 1988; 297:454.

Jessop DJ, Stein REK. Uncertainty and its relation to the psychological and social correlates of chronic illness in children. *Soc Sci Med* 1985; 20:993–999.

Jönsson JA, Boe J, Berlin E. The long-term prognosis of childhood asthma in a predominantly rural Swedish country. *Acta Paediatr Scand* 1987; 76:950–954.

Kelly WJW, Hudson I, Phelan PD, Olinsky A. Childhood asthma in adult life: a further study at 28 years of age. *Br Med J* 1987; 294:1059–1062.

Martin AJ, McLennan LA, Landau LI, Phelan PD. The natural history of childhood asthma to adult life. *Br Med J* 1980; 1397:1–10.

Martinez FD, Cline M, Burrows B. Increased incidence of asthma in children of smoking mothers. *Pediatrics* 1992; 89:21–26.

Maruo H, Hashimoto K, Shimanuki K. Long-term follow up studies of bronchial asthma in children. *Arerugi* 1990; 39:621–630.

McConnochie KM, Roghman KJ. Bronchiolitis as a possible cause of wheezing in childhood: new evidence. *Pediatrics* 1984; 74:1–10.

McConnochie KM, Roghmann KJ. Wheezing at 8 and 13 years: changing importance of bronchiolitis and passive smoking. *Pediatr Pulmonol* 1989; 6:138–146.

McNicol KN, Williams HE, Allan J, McAndrew I. Spectrum of asthma in children. III. Psychological and social components. *Br Med J* 1973; 4:16–20.

Medici TC, Vetter W. Bronchial asthma und kochsalz. *Schweiz Med Wschr* 1991; 121:501–508.

Miskelly FG, Burr ML, Vaughn-Williams E, Fehily AM. Infant feeding and allergy. *Arch Dis Child* 1988; 63:388–393.

Mitchell C, Miles J. Lower respiratory tract symptoms in Queensland schoolchildren. The questionnaire: its reliability and validity. *Aust NZ J Med* 1983; 13:264–269.

Mullally DI, Howard WA, Hubbard TJ, et al. Increased hospitalizations for asthma among children in the Washington, DC area during 1961–1981. *Ann Allergy* 1984; 53:15–19.

Murray AB, Morrison BJ. Passive smoking and the seasonal difference of severity of asthma in children. *Chest* 1988; 94:701–708.

Nolan TM, Phelan PD, McNamara J. Changes in hospital length of stay in Victoria. *Aust Paediatr J* 1989; 10:334.

O'Hollaren MT, Yunginger JW, Offord KD, et al. Exposure to an aeroallergen as a possible precipitating factor in respiratory arrest in young patients with asthma. *N Engl J Med* 1991; 324:359–363.

Pearce N, Grainger J, Atkinson M, et al. Case-control study of prescribed fenoterol and death from asthma in New Zealand, 1977–81. *Thorax* 1990; 45:170–175.

Pearce N, Crane J, Burgess C, et al. Beta agonists and asthma mortality: deja vu. *Clin Exp Allergy* 1991; 21:401–410.

Peat JK, Salome CM, Sedgwick CS, et al. A prospective study of bronchial hyperresponsiveness and respiratory symptoms in a population of Australian schoolchildren. *Clin Exp Allergy* 1989; 19:299–306.

Pöysa L, Korppi M, Pietikuäinen M, et al. Asthma, allergic rhinitis and atopic eczema in Finnish children and adolescents. *Allergy* 1991; 46:161–165.

Rennick GJ, Jarman FC. Are children with asthma affected by smog? *Med J Aust* 1992; 156:837–841.

Robertson CF, Rubinfeld AR, Bowes G. Deaths from asthma in Victoria: a 12 month survey. *Med J Aust* 1990; 152:511–517.

Robertson CF, Heycock E, Bishop J, et al. Prevalence of asthma in Melbourne schoolchildren: changes over 26 years. *Br Med J* 1991; 302:1116–1118.

Roe W. "Science" in the practice of medicine: its limitations and dangers. As exemplified by a study of the natural history of acute bronchial asthma in children. *Biol Med* 1984; 27:386–400.

Schwartz J, Gold D, Dockery DW, et al. Predictors of asthma and persistent wheeze in a national sample of children in the United States. *Am Rev Respir Dis* 1990; 142:555–562.

Sears MR, Taylor DR, Print CG, et al. Regular inhaled beta-agonist treatment in bronchial asthma. *Lancet* 1990; 336:1391–1396.

Sibbald B. Genetics of asthma and atopy: an overview. *Clin Exper Allergy* 1991; 21 (suppl 1): 178–181.

Skarpaas IJK, Gulsvik A. Prevalence of bronchial asthma and respiratory symptoms in schoolchildren in Oslo. *Allergy* 1985; 40:295–299.

Smith JM, Harding LK, Cumming G. The changing prevalence of asthma in schoolchildren. *Clin Allergy* 1971; 1:57–61.

Soothill JF, Stokes CR, Turner MW, et al. Predisposing factors and the development of reaginic allergy in infancy. *Clin Allergy* 1976; 3:305–309.

Spitzer WO, Suissa S, Ernst P, et al. The use of b-agonists and the risk of death and near death from asthma. *N Engl J Med* 1992; 326:301–306.

Storr J, Barrell E, Lenny W. Rising asthma admissions and self-referral. *Arch Dis Child* 1988; 63:774–779.

Strachan DP. Hay fever, hygiene, and household size. *Br Med J* 1989; 299:1259–1260.

Strachan DP, Jarvis MJ, Feyerabend C. The relationship of salivary cotinine to respiratory symptoms, spirometry, and exercise-induced bronchospasm in seven-year-old children. *Am Rev Respir Dis* 1990; 142:147–151.

Suphioglu C, Singh MD, Taylor P, et al. Mechanism of grass-pollen-induced asthma. *Lancet* 1992; 339:562–572.

Taylor B, Wadsworth J, Golding J, Butler N. Breast feeding, eczema, asthma and hayfever. *J Epidemiol Comm Health* 1983; 37:95–99.

Terblanche E, Stewart RI. The prevalence of exercise-induced bronchoconstruction in Cape Town schoolchildren. *S Afr Med J* 1990; 78:744–747.

van Niekerk CH, Weinberg EG, Shore SC, Heese H de V, van Schalkwyk DJ. Prevalence of asthma: a comparative study of urban and rural Xhosa children. *Clin Allergy* 1979; 9:319–324.

Waite DA, Eyles EF, Tonkin SF, O'Donnell TV. Asthma prevalence in Taukelauan children in two environments. *Clin Allergy* 1980; 10:71–75.

Weitzman M, Gortmaker S, Sobol A. Racial, social, and environmental risks for childhood asthma. *Am J Dis Child* 1990; 144:1189–1194.

Wiess KB, Wagener DK. Changing patterns of asthma mortality. *JAMA* 1990; 264:1683–1687.

Williams H, McNicol KN. Prevalence, natural history, and relationship of wheezy bronchitis and asthma in children. An epidemiological study. *Br Med J* 1969; 4:321–325.

Wilson NM. Wheezy bronchitis revisited. *Arch Dis Child* 1989; 64:1194–1199.

Woolcock AJ, Peat JK. Epidemiology of bronchial hyperresponsiveness. *Clin Rev Allergy* 1989; 7:245–256.

World Health Organization. Epidemiology of chronic non-specific respiratory diseases. *Bull WHO* 1975; 52:251–259.

Zhong NS, Chen RC, O-Yang M, et al. Bronchial hyperresponsiveness in young students of southern China: relation to respiratory symptoms, diagnosed asthma, and risk factors. *Thorax* 1990; 45:860–865.

16

Malignancies

Charles A. Stiller

Although the incidence of cancer in childhood is very low compared with that among adults, it accounts for a substantial proportion of deaths among children in industrialized countries. In England and Wales during 1989, the age-standardized mortality rate for neoplasms among children aged 1 to 14 was 40 per million. Neoplasms were certified as the underlying cause of 16% of all deaths in this age range, making them the second most important cause of death after accidents. All but 3% were malignant.

Biologic Considerations

A neoplasm is any abnormal proliferation of cells the growth of which exceeds that of normal tissue and continues irrespective of external stimuli. Malignant neoplasms, or cancers, have the potential to metastasize (i.e., to spread and to grow in tissue remote from the site of origin), whereas benign neoplasms are confined to the site at which they arise. Both malignant and benign neoplasms occur in children, but this chapter is concerned almost entirely with the malignant types for three main reasons:

1. Malignant neoplasms are a much more important cause of death.
2. Population-based incidence data are widely available for cancer in childhood, but hardly ever for benign tumors.
3. The etiology of childhood cancer has been studied very much more intensively than that of benign neoplasms.

Data on cancer incidence and mortality in adults are generally grouped according to the International Classification of Diseases (ICD), in which cancers other than leukemias, lymphomas, and melanomas are categorized solely by site of origin. Childhood cancers exhibit a great diversity of histologic type as well as primary site, but the most common cancers among Western adults—carcinomas of lung, female breast, stomach, and large bowel—are hardly ever seen in children. Consequently, it is more appropriate for childhood tumors to be classified according to their histology. A classification scheme has been developed (Birch & Marsden, 1987) in which groups are defined according to the codes for morphology and topography given in the first edition of the *International Classification of Diseases for Oncology* (ICD-O; WHO, 1976). The scheme contains 12 major diagnostic groups: leukemias, lymphomas, brain and spinal tumors, sympathetic nervous system tumors, retinoblastoma, kidney tumors, liver tumors, bone tumors, soft-tissue sarcomas, gonadal and germ-cell tumors, epithelial tumors, other and unspecified malignant neoplasms. This scheme has become the standard classification for the presentation of childhood cancer incidence data. Sine the ICD-O was published in 1976, further types of neoplasm have been recognized, including some that occur predominantly in children. Most of these additional tumor types have been allocated codes in the recently published second edition of ICD-O (Percy et al., 1990), which also includes a major revision of the coding for lymphomas. Work is in progress on a new version of the classification scheme, in which the groups will be defined according to codes in the second edition of ICD-O. For this chapter, however, the scheme based on first edition codes is used, but with a few modifications to admit new histologic entities and to take account of current clinical opinion. The principal modifications are as follows:

Megakaryocytic leukemia has been transferred from Other and unspecified leukemia to Acute nonlymphocytic leukemia.

Langerhans cell histiocytosis, formerly known as histiocytosis X, was a subgroup of Lymphomas in the original classification scheme, but has been omitted, because this group of diseases is not now regarded as neoplastic.

Primitive neuroectodermal tumor of the central nervous system is classified with Medulloblastoma.

Neuroectodermal tumor of bone is classified with Ewing's sarcoma.

Neuroectodermal tumor or Askin's tumor of other sites is classified with Other sympathetic nervous system tumors.

Bone-metastasizing renal tumor of childhood (clear-cell sarcoma of the kidney) and rhabdoid tumor are classified with Wilms' tumor.

An extra category has been created for Skin carcinoma.

Pancreatoblastoma is classified with Other and unspecified malignant neoplasms.

Patterns of Occurrence

In Western populations only 1 in 200 of all cancers occurs in children aged under 15. The incidence rate for all types of childhood cancer combined is typically in the range of 110 to 130 per million children per year—equivalent to a risk of 1 in 600 that a child will be affected during the first 15 years of life. Thus in the United Kingdom (child population of 11 million), 1200 new cases of childhood cancer can be expected each year. In the United States about 7000 cases will be diagnosed each year.

The largest population-based series of childhood cancers in the world is the National Registry of Childhood Tumors (NRCT), which covers England, Scotland, and Wales and is maintained at the Childhood Cancer Research Group in Oxford. Since 1962, copies of all notifications to the national cancer registration system for children aged under 15 have been sent to the Registry, as have death certificates for all children certified as having died of neoplasms. Starting in varying years, notifications have also been received from specialist childhood cancer registries that are maintained locally in several health service regions, from clinical trials organizers, and from the register of patients treated by pediatric oncologists who are members of the United Kingdom Children's Cancer Study Group. The diagnoses for children in the Registry are verified against medical records and amended where necessary. Table 16.1 shows the registration rates, based on notifications from all sources, for Great Britain during 1975 to 1984, when the average child population was 11.6 million. Registration is not complete, but from study of the patterns of ascertainment from multiple sources it seems that well over 95% of childhood cancers are included.

One third of all childhood cancers are leukemias. Of these, 80% are acute lymphoblastic leukemia (ALL), which thus accounts for 26% of all childhood cancers and is the most common single type. Between one quarter and one fifth are brain and spinal tumors, among which more than a third are astrocytomas. The four main malignant embryonal tumors of childhood—neuroblastoma, retinoblastoma, Wilms' tumor or nephroblastoma, and hepatoblastoma—together account for 14% of all registrations. Eleven percent of cases are lymphomas, 6% are soft-tissue sarcomas, 5% are bone tumors, and 3% are malignant germ-cell tumors.

Age

Within the childhood age range, cancer is more common at younger ages, with half the cumulative risk occurring within the first 6 years of life. The age distribution varies considerably among diagnostic groups (Fig. 16.1). The peak incidence of ALL occurs at age 2 to 3. Among the embryonal tumors, neuroblastoma, retinoblastoma, and hepatoblastoma all have their highest incidence in the first year of life, whereas Wilms' tumor is most common during the second year. The incidence of acute nonlymphocytic leukemia (ANLL) and rhabdomyosarcoma is also highest in early childhood. By contrast, Hodgkin's disease and malignant bone tumors are extremely rare among young children, but show a marked increase in incidence with age that continues into adolescence and early adulthood. Non-Hodgkin's lymphoma (NHL) is also rare before age 2, but the incidence is relatively constant thereafter. Yet another pattern of incidence relative to age occurs with fibrosarcoma: there is a peak in infancy, largely accounted for by so-called infantile or congenital fibrosarcoma, which is followed by a very low incidence between ages 1 to 9 and a higher rate at ages 10 to 14. Gonadal germ-cell tumors also have their lowest incidence during the middle years of childhood, but the age distribution differs markedly between the sexes. Among boys, the commonest type is orchioblastoma or testicular yolk-sac tumor, which occurs mostly in very early childhood; malignant testicular teratomas are relatively common after age 15, but are only occasionally seen before then. Among girls, ovarian tumors, again of the yolk-sac type, occur rarely in early childhood. Yet, the increase in incidence in the years after puberty takes place at an earlier age than among boys, and a variety of histologic subtypes are seen,

Table 16.1. Registration Rates for Childhood Cancer in England, Scotland and Wales, 1975 to 1984

Diagnostic Group	Total Registrations	Annual Rates Per Million for Age Group				Total (Age Standardized)	Sex Ratio† (M/F)
		0	1–4	5–9	10–14		
Total	12758	146.4	159.7	92.7	88.9	116.5	1.2
I. *Leukemias*	4228	29.2	68.5	31.7	21.7	40.0	1.2
Acute lymphoblastic	3363	14.3	59.3	26.4	14.6	32.2	1.3
Acute nonlymphocytic	684	10.5	6.9	4.5	5.8	6.1	1.1
Chronic myeloid	99	1.3	1.4	0.5	0.8	0.9	1.7
Other & unspecified	82	3.1	0.9	0.4	0.5	0.8	0.7
II. *Lymphomas*	1394	3.6	7.2	12.0	16.5	11.2	2.3
Hodgkin's disease	595	—	1.3	4.4	9.1	4.5	2.3
Non-Hodgkin's‡	755	2.1	5.7	7.4	7.0	6.3	2.5
Other reticuloendothelial	44	1.5	0.2	0.2	0.5	0.4	1.1
III. *Brain & Spinal*	2983	24.1	30.1	26.9	22.4	26.4	1.2
Ependymona	353	5.3	5.3	2.2	2.0	3.4	1.2
Astrocytoma	1107	6.1	10.4	10.0	9.2	9.6	0.9
Medulloblastoma	604	5.2	6.8	6.2	3.4	5.5	1.8
Other & unspecified	919	7.4	7.6	8.5	7.7	7.9	1.2
IV. *Sympathetic nervous*	742	30.4	14.1	2.8	1.0	7.9	1.2
Neuroblastoma	721	30.0	13.9	2.7	0.8	7.7	1.1
Other	21	0.4	0.2	0.1	0.3	0.2	
V. *Retinoblastoma*	327	19.9	6.5	0.4	0.0	3.7	1.0
VI. *Kidney*	727	12.9	17.0	3.6	0.8	7.7	1.0
Wilms' tumor	714	12.8	17.0	3.5	0.6	7.6	1.0
Renal carcinoma	13	0.1	0.0	0.0	0.2	0.1	

VII. *Liver*	108	4.5	1.6	0.4	0.4	1.1	0.8
Hepatoblastoma	76	4.3	1.4	0.1	0.1	0.8	0.8
Hepatic carcinoma	32	0.1	0.2	0.3	0.3	0.3	0.8
VIII. *Bone*	677	0.1	0.9	4.6	11.0	5.0	1.0
Osteosarcoma	352	—	0.3	1.5	6.7	2.5	0.8
Ewing's sarcoma	287	0.1	0.5	2.8	3.8	2.2	1.1
Other & unspecified	38	—	0.1	0.3	0.5	0.3	1.3
IX. *Soft-tissue sarcomas*	782	11.6	8.3	6.3	5.5	7.1	1.3
Rhabdomyosarcoma	523	7.1	6.7	4.6	2.6	4.9	1.4
Fibrosarcoma§	110	2.4	0.4	0.8	1.2	0.9	0.9
Other & unspecified	149	2.1	1.2	0.8	1.7	1.3	1.4
X. *Gonadal & Germ-cell*	367	8.2	3.9	1.4	3.6	3.3	0.8
Nongonadal germ-cell	154	4.0	1.7	0.7	1.3	1.4	0.8
Gonadal germ-cell	195	4.0	2.1	0.7	1.9	1.7	1.0
Other & unspecified	18	0.1	0.0	0.0	0.3	0.1	
XI. *Epithelial*	389	1.3	1.3	2.6	5.7	3.0	0.7
Adrenocortical carcinoma	28	0.6	0.4	0.2	0.1	0.3	0.2
Thyroid carcinoma	55	—	0.0	0.3	1.0	0.4	0.4
Nasopharyngeal carcinoma	48	—	0.1	0.2	0.9	0.3	2.3
Skin carcinoma	61	—	0.0	0.4	1.0	0.4	0.7
Other carcinoma	88	0.1	0.2	0.6	1.4	0.7	0.9
Malignant melanoma	109	0.6	0.6	0.9	1.3	0.9	0.7
XII. *Other*	34	0.6	0.2	0.2	0.4	0.3	1.2

*Total rates are standardized to world population.

†Sex ratio of age-standardized incidence rates calculated for diagnostic groups with over 25 cases.

‡Including Burkitt's and unspecified lymphoma.

§Including malignant fibrous histiocytoma and neurofibrosarcoma.

Source: Data from the National Registry of Childhood Tumors.

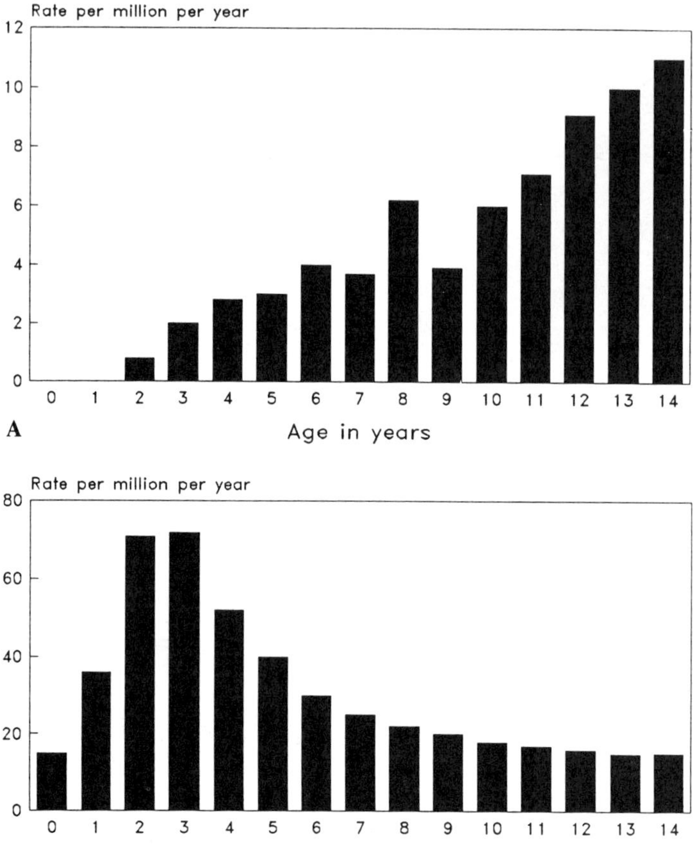

Fig. 16.1. Age distribution of various types of cancer in England, Scotland, and Wales, 1971 to 1984. Data from the National Registry of Childhood Tumors. **A**. Hodgkin's disease. **B**. Acute lymphoblastic leukemia. Figure continues.

including dysgerminoma, teratoma, and mixed tumors, as well as those of pure yolk-sac type. Generally, brain and spinal tumors are slightly more common at ages 1 to 9 than during infancy or in the 10 to 14 age group, but the age distribution varies among subtypes. Ependymoma, for example, is markedly less common after age 5, whereas the incidence of astrocytoma is lowest in infancy but fairly constant thereafter.

Sex

Cancer is about one third more common among boys than among girls, but again there is considerable variation in the sex ratio among diagnostic groups. The largest male excess is found in the lymphomas (M/F = 2.5:1 for both Hodgkin's disease and NHL), and there is also a distinct male predominance in leukemia, brain and spinal tumors, neuroblastoma, and soft-tissue sarcomas. Retinoblastoma, Wilms' tumor, liver, and bone tumors occur with roughly equal

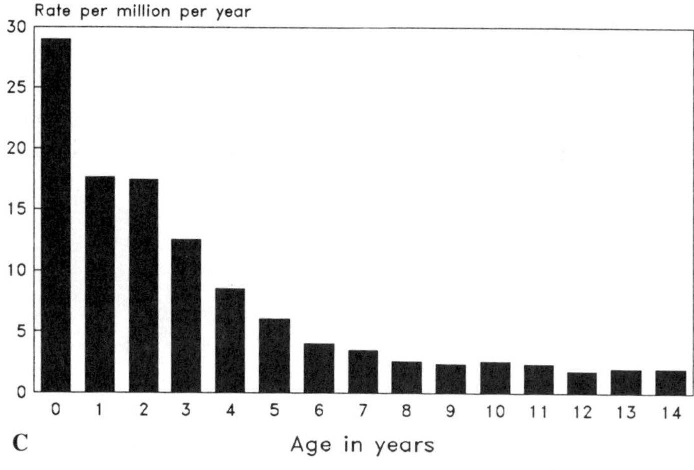

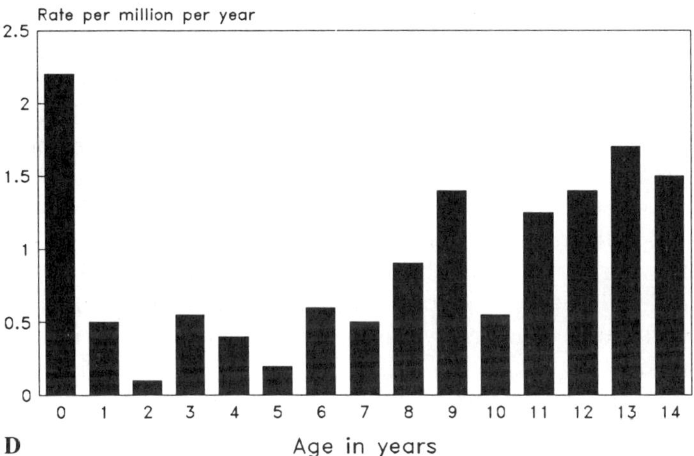

Fig. 16.1. Continued. **C**. Neuroblastoma and ganglioneuroblastoma. **D**. Fibrosarcoma, neurofibrosarcoma, etc.

frequency among boys and girls. There is an excess of girls with germ-cell tumors of both gonadal and other sites, carcinomas of the adrenal cortex and thyroid, and malignant melanoma. With the striking exception of gonadal germ-cell tumors discussed above, there is little variation in the sex ratio with age.

Temporal Trends

Between 1968 and 1978 in Britain there was a significant increase in the incidence of ALL that was most marked among boys aged under 5 (Stiller & Draper, 1982), but rates have since stabilized at the level reached in the mid-1970s (Stiller et al., 1991a). Increases have also been observed at varying times in Sweden, Denmark, and the Netherlands (Coebergh et al., 1989; Gustafsson & Kreuger, 1982; Hansen et al., 1983), but in the latter two countries, rates have subsequently fallen.

There is little evidence for time trends in any of the other major childhood cancers. In Denmark a significant increase in the recorded incidence of neuroblastoma between 1943 and 1980 was attributed to improved diagnosis (Carlsen, 1986).

The patterns of incidence described here are similar to those found among most populations of predominantly white Caucasian children throughout Europe, North America, and Oceania. Geographic, ethnic, and socioeconomic variations in incidence are described in the following sections.

Geographic and Ethnic Variations

Over the past two decades there have been several systematic studies of geographic and ethnic variations in the occurrence of childhood cancer. Nearly all of these studies were unsatisfactory because they included too few cases, the diagnoses were classified by ICD categories rather than by histology, or they were based on mortality rather than incidence data. Recently, however, the International Agency of Research on Cancer (IARC) coordinated the first comprehensive, worldwide study in which incidence data were collected wherever possible from population-based registries. Each series included at least 200 cases, and the diagnoses were classified according to the standard scheme of Birch and Marsden (1987), i.e. with groups defined according to histology. Registries in 50 countries contributed to the study. In some regions, principally in Africa and Asia, where population-based data were not available, large case series were contributed by hospitals or pathology departments. The method of the study is described in detail in a monograph (Parkin et al., 1988a), which also contains detailed results from each registry, including numbers of cases, incidence rates where these could be calculated, a brief description of the registry, and commentary on any notable features of the data. The following review of geographic and ethnic variations in incidence is based largely on the IARC monograph, although use is also made of other recent studies.

In most regions leukemia is the most common childhood cancer, accounting for about one third of all cases. In the predominantly white Caucasian populations of Europe, North America, and Oceania, the age-standardized incidence is in the range of 35 to 50 per million per year. Around three quarters of all cases are ALL, and most of the remainder are ANLL.

Few population-based data were available from Africa, but all three registries from which rates could be calculated had an incidence of leukemia of under 20 per million, with no sign of a peak for ALL in young children. Black populations in the United States had an incidence of all leukemias combined of 20 to 30 per million; the rate for ALL was only half that in whites, and the peak in incidence at age 2 to 3 years, although present, was less marked.

In Japan, the total incidence of leukemia was similar to that in white Caucasian populations, and there was a peak in early childhood. A much larger proportion of cases, 25% to 30%, were registered as ANLL. A recent study has concluded, however, that many cases of childhood ALL had been systematically misclassified as ANLL (Bessho, 1990). If this is correct, then the pattern of incidence of childhood ALL in Japan may be similar to that in other industrialized nations.

Elsewhere in East Asia, ANLL was relatively common, and the peak in early childhood was less marked. In South and West Asia leukemia had a lower incidence, and the rate for all types combined of 33 per million among Israeli Jews was the only one to approach those commonly seen in Europe and North America. The pattern of incidence of childhood leukemia in general, and particularly the peak for ALL in early childhood, among children of Asian (Indian subcontinent) ethnic origin in Britain seems to be similar to that among white children (Stiller et al., 1991b).

The worldwide pattern of a less marked age peak in the incidence of ALL in populations with a lower total incidence of this disease is consistent with the hypothesis of a constant underlying incidence across different regions and ethnic groups, but with selective underdiagnosis, particularly of the "common ALL" immunophenotype, in populations of lower socioeconomic status (Greaves & Chan, 1986).

Hodgkin's disease was the only diagnostic group in the IARC study to show systematic variation among populations of predominantly European origin: countries of lower latitude and thus with warmer climates tended to have higher incidence rates. The highest incidence of childhood Hodgkin's disease was observed in North Africa and West Asia, extending beyond the Mediterranean at least as far as western India. Throughout East Asia the incidence was low. Two distinct patterns were observed in relation to age. In industrialized Western countries the incidence increased steeply with age and was low in childhood compared with that in young adults. In the developing countries of the Caribbean, South America, Africa, and Asia, and in Japan, the excess among older children was less marked, and in some series there was even a peak at age 5 to 9. On the basis of this study, the age distribution of Hodgkin's disease seems to be related to levels of socioeconomic development, but the total incidence seems to be determined more by ethnic and environmental factors. Asian children in Britain, however, seem not only to have a high incidence compared with white Caucasians but also to have an especially marked excess in early childhood, implying that their age distribution for Hodgkin's disease is similar to that found in Asia (Stiller et al., 1991b).

By far the highest incidence of Burkitt's lymphoma occurred in tropical Africa and in Papua New Guinea, and in some areas of these regions it is the commonest childhood cancer. Elsewhere, Burkitt's lymphoma was rare, although the incidence was higher in Mediterranean and Middle Eastern countries than in other areas (Stiller & Parkin, 1990). There was no consistent pattern in the incidence of other non-Hodgkin's lymphomas, except for a tendency toward higher rates around the Mediterranean and in some Latin American countries, and a low incidence in Japan.

In Western industrialized countries and in Japan, brain and spinal tumors are the second most common type of childhood cancer after leukemia. In developing countries they are probably outnumbered by lymphomas, but comparisons of incidence rates are difficult because of variations in completeness of ascertainment and in the frequency of biopsy and autopsy.

Neuroblastoma has been thought to be relatively rare among black children in both Africa and the United States. This view was based partly on the low ratio of neuroblastoma to Wilms' tumor in these populations, together with the belief that Wilms' tumor had a constant incidence worldwide. In the IARC study, neuroblastoma seemed to have a low incidence in Africa, but this was probably due in part to underdiagnosis. The true rate may differ little from that among blacks in the United States, where the incidence was three quarters that recorded among whites. Neuroblastoma also seemed to have a low incidence in Central and South America and throughout much of Asia; in the latter continent, only Japan and Israel had rates approaching those in Western countries.

The incidence of retinoblastoma was high among black populations in Africa and the United States, and also in Brazil. Relative frequencies suggested that retinoblastoma also had a high incidence in much of Asia. No direct information was available on whether cases were heritable or nonheritable. The evidence from the few series with reasonably complete data on laterality of retinoblastoma suggested that in high-incidence areas the excess is accounted for by unilateral (mainly nonheritable) cases, and hence that in those countries there may be an increased level of environmental factors causing retinoblastoma.

As mentioned above, Wilms' tumor was formerly regarded as an "index tumor of childhood" because it was thought to have a relatively constant incidence throughout the world (Innis, 1972). It is now clear, however, that the incidence of Wilms' tumor varies greatly, with age-standardized rates ranging from over 10 per million in American and Nigerian black populations to 7 to 9 per million among white Caucasians, 4 per million in Bombay, and around 3 per million in several countries of East Asia. Age distributions were similar among white Caucasians and blacks, with the highest incidence in the second year of life. In East Asia about a third of all cases are in infants under 1 year, and Wilms' tumor also tends to occur at an earlier age among Asian children in the United States (Breslow et al., 1988). In Britain, there is an excess of Wilms' tumor among Afro-Caribbean children and a deficit among those of Indian subcontinent ethnic origin (Stiller et al., 1991b). These variations along ethnic rather than geographic lines suggest that genetic predisposition is important in the etiology of Wilms' tumor.

The incidence of hepatoblastoma showed little international variation. Hepatocellular carcinoma was very rare among children in Western industrialized countries, but was more frequent than hepatoblastoma in several countries in Eastern Asia and Latin America and throughout sub-Saharan Africa. The highest frequency of hepatocellular carcinoma was recorded in Papua, New Guinea, where it accounted for 8.5% of all childhood cancers. This elevated frequency of hepatocellular carcinoma in children in countries where it is common among adults is well known, and many of the affected children are chronic HBsAg carriers.

The incidence of osteosarcoma showed little international variation, although it is rather more common among blacks than whites in the United States and the incidence may also be higher in sub-Saharan Africa. Ewing's sarcoma, by contrast, is extremely rare among blacks both in the United States and in Africa, and the incidence is also very low in East Asia. Throughout southern and western Asia, from Bangladesh to Israel, and among the predominantly Arab populations of North Africa, there was no evidence that the incidence differs from that in white Caucasian populations.

Rhabdomyosarcoma had a higher incidence among whites than blacks in the

United States, and it seemed to be low in southern and eastern Asia. There were no clear geographic patterns in the incidence of fibrosarcoma, although, in contrast to rhabdomyosarcoma, this tumor was more common among blacks than whites in the United States. In most parts of the world, Kaposi's sarcoma is virtually never registered in children, but in eastern and southern Africa (Uganda, Tanzania, Malawi, and Zimbabwe) it accounted for 25% to 50% of soft-tissue sarcomas or 2% to 10% of all childhood cancer. In contrast to the "endemic" nodular, cutaneous form that is common among adult men in these countries, in children the disease often involves the lymph nodes, and in the IARC study a third of cases were among girls.

The numbers of cases of germ-cell tumors were generally small, rendering estimates of incidence rates and relative frequencies unstable. Gonadal germ-cell tumors, however, did seem to have a somewhat higher incidence in East Asia.

Malignant epithelial tumors are generally rare in childhood. There are nevertheless some striking international variations. Among registries reporting more than five cases of adrenocortical carcinoma, the annual incidence in Sao Paulo, Brazil, was 1.0 per million for boys and 2.0 for girls—about three times the rates in other countries. In Chinese populations and in Southeast Asia, which are known areas of high risk for nasopharyngeal carcinoma in adults, this tumor had a low relative frequency and incidence in children. In North Africa, which is an area of intermediate risk to adults, the frequency of childhood nasopharyngeal carcinoma was quite high, and in Tunisia and Sudan it accounted for 20% of all cancers at age 10 to 14. In Tunisia there was also a very high relative frequency of skin carcinoma, accounting for 9% of all registrations; the great majority (90%) were diagnosed in children with xeroderma pigmentosum. In Bangladesh, 3.2% of all registrations were for oral carcinoma, and there were also substantial numbers of unspecified malignant tumors in this site. Oral carcinoma has a high incidence among adults in Bangladesh, where chewing of tobacco and betel is frequent (Rahim, 1986), but it is not known whether this practice also accounts for the high incidence of oral carcinoma in children.

Relatively high rates for malignant melanoma, around 4 per million, were recorded in New South Wales and among the non-Maori population of New Zealand. The incidence of melanoma in adults is known also to be high in Australia and New Zealand, and so the registration rates among children in those countries may be an accurate reflection of the true incidence. In Queensland, Australia, however, where there is a specialist children's cancer registry, the age-standardized rate for malignant melanoma was only 0.35 per million (McWhirter & Petroeschevsky, 1990), and in some European countries, including Denmark, a large proportion of children registered as having malignant melanoma in fact only had benign nevi (Partoft et al., 1989).

Socioeconomic Variations

In a study of over 6000 cases of childhood ALL diagnosed in Britain from 1966 to 1983, there was a significantly higher incidence in higher socioeconomic areas as defined by percentages of households that were owner-occupied and possessed a car and the percentage of economically active men who were employed (Draper et al., 1991; Rodrigues et al., 1991). The excess was present when socioeconomic score was measured at the level both of county district (average child population 25,000) and of census tract (average child population 200). These results agreed with several other, smaller studies that had found a greater risk associated with higher socioeconomic status. A higher incidence of Hodgkin's disease among older children and young adults has been associated with higher socioeconomic status in many studies (Alexander et al., 1991). Data from Denmark (Carlsen, 1986) and the United States (Davis et al., 1987) have suggested that neuroblastoma may have a higher incidence among groups of lower socioeconomic status.

Risk Factors

Hardly anything is known about the etiology of childhood cancer. Familial aggregations of cancers and observed associations with various other inherited diseases and congenital abnormalities indicate a genetic component in some childhood cancers. The early age peak in incidence and the cell types of origin also suggest that for many diagnostic groups any causative factors operate before birth or even before conception and studies of possible environmental risk factors have therefore dealt largely with exposures occurring in utero.

Genetic Factors

The best-known and most comprehensively studied childhood cancer with a clear genetic component to its etiology is retinoblastoma (see Chapter 5). The genetics of this tumor have been reviewed by Cowell (1991). Retinoblastoma can be explained as the result of two successive mutations as described in the "two-hit" mutational model of Knudson (1971). In heritable cases the first mutation is prezygotic, which is inherited in about one third of cases and appears as a new germinal mutation in the remaining two thirds; in nonheritable cases the first mutation is postzygotic. This theory accounts for the frequent bilateral involvement and early age of onset in heritable cases. The retinoblastoma suppressor gene, RB1, has been assigned to chromosome region 13q14. The heritable form can be identified by the presence of bilateral tumors or a positive family history. Using these criteria it is estimated that about 40% of cases in Western populations are heritable. The characteristic deletion of 13q may, however, also be present constitutionally in 5% of patients with apparently nonheritable retinoblastoma (Bunin et al., 1989a), and with the addition of these cases the proportion of retinoblastoma that is genetic in origin is about 45%. The pattern of inheritance is essentially mendelian autosomal dominant with 90% penetrance. This pattern has been confirmed in follow-up studies of survivors; for example, that of Hawkins et al. (1989) in which 23 of 52 (44%) offspring of survivors of heritable retinoblastoma themselves developed the tumor. Survivors also have an extremely high risk of developing second primary tumors, especially osteosarcoma, for which the incidence is hundreds of times that in the general population (Draper et al., 1986). Many other types of second primary tumors also occur, with the elevated risk persisting well into adulthood (Sanders et al., 1989). Although some second primary tumors arise at the site of previous radiotherapy, in many cases they cannot be attributed to treatment previously given for retinoblastoma.

In comparison to retinoblastoma, familial aggregations of other embryonal tumors are rare, and correspondingly fewer cases can be regarded as genetic on the basis of family history. In the U.S. National Wilms' Tumor Study, a family history was found in only 37 of 3442 cases (1.1%; Breslow et al., 1988). Even with the relatively recent improvement in survival rates, the proportion of Wilms' tumors with a family history of the same cancer will fall well short of that for retinoblastoma (Li et al., 1988a). A few familial aggregations of neuroblastoma have been reported, but the heritable component is probably low (Kushner et al., 1986). The association between hepatoblastoma and familial adenomatous polyposis coli (Kingston et al., 1983) is well documented.

In the Li-Fraumeni syndrome, members of the same family are at increased risk for a wide variety of cancers, including soft-tissue sarcoma, adrenocortical carcinoma, premenopausal breast cancer, brain tumors, osteosarcoma, and carcinomas of the larynx and lung (Li et al., 1988b). Nearly 1% of childhood cancers may be part of this syndrome. In a follow-up study of 24 Li-Fraumeni families, the risk of cancer at age 0 to 19 among family members unaffected at the time of ascertainment was 21 times that in the general population, and the elevated risk seemed to persist, although at a lower level, until at least age 45 to 59 (Garber et al., 1991). Germ line mutations in the p53 tumor suppressor gene on chromosome 17p13 were identified in members of all five of a series of Li-Fraumeni families, suggesting that the syndrome was attributable to inherited alterations of this gene (Malkin et al., 1990). In a later study of affected members of eight Li-Fraumeni families, mutations in the defined region of p53 were only detected in two, indicating that the p53 mutation might be the primary lesion in only some families with this syndrome (Santibanez-Koref et al., 1991).

Much of the following discussion of the relationship between childhood cancer and other genetic disease is based on a recent study of data from the NRCT with literature review (Narod et al., 1991).

Among children with von Recklinghausen's neurofibromatosis (NF-1), the risk of brain and spinal tumors is over 40 times that in the general population, and the risk of optic nerve glioma is increased 1000-fold. The majority of childhood cases of neurofibrosarcoma are associated with NF-1, and there is also an increased risk of rhabdomyosarcoma; the relative risk for all types of soft-tissue sarcoma combined is over 50. There is a fourfold increased risk of leukemia among children with NF-1. The relative risk is particularly high, about 70, for chronic myeloid leukemia; the cases occurring in children with NF-1 are of the so-called juvenile form, which is negative for the Philadelphia chromosome. NF-1 is inherited as an autosomal dominant, but many cases result from new mutations.

Various other familial cancer syndromes account for much smaller numbers of childhood cancers. These include multiple endocrine neoplasia type 2 (medullary thyroid carcinoma), dysplastic nevus syndrome (malignant melanoma), basal cell nevus syndrome or Gorlin's syndrome (medulloblastoma and basal cell carcinoma), and Turcot's syndrome (brain tumors and carcinoma of the colon).

A substantial proportion of pairs of childhood cancers within a sibship are associated with the familial cancer syndromes described above and with other known genetic conditions. In the absence of any defined genetic syndrome, however, the risk of childhood cancer in a sibling of an affected child is approximately doubled (Draper et al., 1977). The causes of this increased risk are presumably largely genetic, although shared environmental exposures could also play a part. There is an especially high concordance rate among twins for leukemia in early childhood. Sometimes both of the identical twins who develop leukemia at an early age have the same cytogenetic abnormalities, strongly indicating that the origin of their disease is antenatal, although not necessarily prezygotic since twins have shared circulation in utero (Chaganti et al., 1979).

Among non-neoplastic genetic conditions, the one most frequently associated with childhood cancer is Down syndrome (see Chapter 4). Affected children have a 20-fold increased risk of leukemia, with the relative risk being higher for ANLL than for ALL and highest of all for the rare megakaryoblastic subtype of ANLL. Boys with Down syndrome are apparently also at increased risk of malignant testicular germ-cell tumors (Mann et al., 1989). There is no evidence of an increased risk of other cancers in children with Down syndrome.

Children with tuberous sclerosis have a relative risk of 75 for brain tumors and 50 for rhabdomyosarcoma, resulting in an 18-fold risk for all cancers combined. Xeroderma pigmentosum, an inherited syndrome of faulty DNA repair, carries a greatly increased risk of skin carcinoma, which is most striking in Tunisia (Miller, 1977).

Several rare, genetically determined immune deficiency syndromes also have an increased risk of childhood cancer. Most of these cancers are lymphomas occurring in children with ataxia telangiectasia, more than one tenth of whom develop cancer before age 15 (Morrell et al., 1986). Leukemia, lymphomas, and other cancers have also been seen in children with Wiskott-Aldrich's syndrome, Chediak-Higashi syndrome, hypogammaglobulinemia, IgA deficiency, and severe combined immunodeficiency.

Several congenital abnormalities are associated with Wilms' tumor (Breslow & Beckwith, 1982). Slightly more than 1% of cases occur in children with aniridia. In Britain one third of children with Wilms' tumor and aniridia had bilateral tumors, compared with 5% among children without aniridia. The Wilms' tumor-aniridia syndrome is associated with a chromosomal deletion at 11p13. Some children with this syndrome also have genitourinary abnormalities, hemihypertrophy, or mental retardation. Wilms' tumor without aniridia is also associated with hemihypertrophy, sometimes as part of the Beckwith-Wiedemann syndrome. The association of nephropathy, Wilms' tumor, and genital abnormalities, known as Drash syndrome, is likely to be of genetic origin, but there are no readily detected deletions within the 11p13 region (Jadresic et al., 1991). In one large population-based series, there was an 11-fold excess of cardiac septal defects in children with Wilms' tumor (Stiller et al., 1987); Bonaiti-Pellié et al. (1992) also found an excess of congenital heart defects with Wilms' tumor, but it was no more marked for septal defects than for other cardiac abnormalities.

Hemihypertrophy and Beckwith-Wiedemann syndrome are also associated with hepatoblastoma and adrenocortical carcinoma (Sotelo-Avila et al., 1980). Neural tube defects are more common among children with germ-cell tumors (Birch et al., 1982).

Other Birth Characteristics

Several birth characteristics that do not have exclusively genetic or environmental causes have been associated with childhood cancer in various case-control studies. In one study, (van Steensel-Moll et al., 1985) several indicators of maternal fertility problems were associated with ALL, whereas in a series of over 6000 childhood cancers in Japan there were nine cases among children conceived after induced ovulation, of whom four had neuroblastoma and none had leukemia, although there were two children with lymphoma (Kobayashi et al., 1991). Neuroectodermal tumors had previously been reported in five children born after in-vitro fertilization or artificial insemination in Australia (White et al., 1990). The suggested association of neuroblastoma and other neuroectodermal tumors with ovulation induction, assisted conception, and infertility or with drugs used under these circumstances requires further investigation, possibly by means of a follow-up study of as large a cohort as possible of children born after induced ovulation or assisted conception.

In a case-control study (see Chapter 1) of 103 young persons with rhabdomyosarcoma, there was a trend of increasing risk of this tumor with increasing number of mother's prior stillbirths (Ghali et al., 1992).

Parental Age

Possible effects of parental ages have been investigated in several studies, but few consistent results have emerged. In three European and North American series, children with heritable retinoblastoma but no family history of the disease had older parents than expected (Bunin et al., 1989b; Der Kinderen et al., 1990; Pellié et al., 1973), although no parental age effect was found in a larger series from Japan (Matsunaga et al, 1990).

Birthweight

The literature on birthweight and childhood cancer was reviewed by Daling et al. (1984). In their own series of 681 cases, as in the majority of other published studies, there was an increased risk of cancer in heavier babies. There was, however, only limited consistency among studies as to the types of cancer to which this applied, and in one of the largest studies (Salonen & Saxen, 1975) no association was found. The finding of a significantly raised relative risk for birthweight exceeding 3.8 Kg in children with ALL diagnosed before age 4 years (Kaye et al., 1991) agreed with a number of earlier reports linking high birthweight with an increased risk of leukemia. Otherwise, there has been a continued absence of consistent findings on possible associations of birthweight and childhood cancer.

Length of Gestation

A similar lack of consistency attends the findings on length of gestation. In one study of deaths from neuroblastoma there was a significant protective effect for gestation under 37 weeks and a significant excess risk for low birthweight after 37 weeks or longer gestation (Cole Johnson & Spitz, 1985), but no effect was found in another study of incident cases (Neglia et al., 1988). An excess risk of osteosarcoma before age 25 has been associated with preterm delivery and length at birth below the first quartile (Operskalski et al., 1987). In a study that included all types of childhood cancer (Hartley et al., 1988), children with germ-cell tumors had a slightly longer gestation then their controls, and there was an increased risk of Ewing's sarcoma for children of low birthweight. However, no association with length of gestation or birthweight was found for any other diagnostic group. If any of these associations are genuine, it seems likely that birthweight and length of gestation are markers for other, unknown risk factors, rather than themselves directly affecting a child's risk of developing cancer.

Other Genetic or Environmental Factors

There is some inconsistency among the several studies of dermatoglyphics and childhood leukemia, but it is possible that young children with certain abnormalities of palmar creases may be at greater risk of ALL in early childhood (Edelstein et al., 1991). Palmar creases are determined in utero, but aberrant patterns can have genetic or environmental causes.

Among over 30,000 twins in the Connecticut Twin Registry, the incidence of childhood cancer was significantly lower than among single-born children (Inskip et al., 1991). The deficit was similar to that in previous studies and applied both to leukemia and to other cancers. Boys, especially those aged under 4 years, had a particularly pronounced deficit. Suggested explanations were the relatively low birthweight of twins and the possible selective early mortality of twin fetuses or neonates who might have developed cancer had they survived.

Radiation

The carcinogenic risk of antenatal obstetric irradiation was first established over 30 years ago (Stewart et al., 1958), and it remains the only environmental factor certain to be the cause of more than a handful of cases of childhood cancer. The British data on cancer after prenatal x-ray exposure were comprehensively reviewed by Mole (1990). For births during 1958 to 1961, the odds ratio for childhood cancer deaths after irradiation in the third trimester was 460 per million live births per cGy fetal whole body dose (95% CI 80-950; see Chapter 1). At that time, exposure to diagnostic x-rays in utero may have caused 5% of all childhood cancers. The proportion will have declined since then with improved radiographic techniques and a reduction in the frequency of x-ray examination. Most obstetric imaging in pregnancy is now done by ultrasound, which two studies have concluded is not associated with any increased risk of cancer (Cartwright et al, 1984; Kinnier Wilson & Waterhouse, 1984).

Radiotherapy for cancer (Kingston et al, 1987; Meadows et al., 1985) and in the past also for benign childhood conditions, such as "enlarged thymus" (Hempelmann et al., 1975) and tinea capitis (Ron et al., 1988), can give rise to subsequent malignant neoplasms. The numbers of children irradiated have been small, however, and the majority of the radiation-induced cancers occurred in adulthood. Thus, radiotherapy can only have caused a very small proportion of childhood cancers.

In addition to the carcinogenic effects of irradiation of the child for medical purposes, whether before or after birth, it has also been suggested that radiation in the environment generally could be a cause of childhood cancer, particularly leukemia. Among children who survived the atomic bombs at Hiroshima and Nagasaki, an increased risk of leukemia appeared by 1 to 3 years after exposure, reached a peak at 6 to 7 years after, and declined steadily thereafter (Shimizu et al., 1990). A significant excess of leukemia was also observed among children in the areas of Utah that received the highest doses of fallout from the Nevada nuclear weapons tests (Stevens et al., 1990).

Excesses of childhood leukemia have been confirmed in areas near both of the nuclear reprocessing plants in Britain: Sellafield (Black, 1984) and Dounreay (COMARE, 1988). Although the population near Sellafield is highly mobile, the excess in Seascale, the village nearest to the plant, was confined to children born to mothers who were living there at the time of the birth (Gardner et al., 1987). An increased incidence of childhood leukemia and other childhood cancers has also been found in an area surrounding two military sites in Berkshire at which radioactive material is handled (COMARE, 1989). Mortality from 1969 to 1978 has been studied in relation to proximity to a range of 15 nuclear installations (mostly power stations) throughout England and Wales (Cook-Mozaffari et al., 1989a). A significant excess mortality among persons aged 0 to 24 from leukemia and Hodgkin's disease was found in districts near an installation. Intriguingly, a similar excess was later found in districts near sites where the building of several installations had been proposed but not proceeded with by the end of the study period (Cook-Mozaffari et al., 1989b). These British studies, together with others in the United States, Canada, France, and Germany, have been reviewed by Hill and Laplanche (1991). There was no evidence of excess mortality near nuclear installations studied in any of the latter four countries.

On the basis of current radiobiologic theory, the measured levels of environmental radiation around nuclear plants could not directly account for a detectable increase in the incidence of childhood malignant disease. Indeed, the contribution of discharges from the plants to total environmental exposure is small in comparison to natural background radiation. Consequently, other explanations have been sought for the well-substantiated excess numbers of cases that have been found in the vicinity of certain installations. Two possible causes have been studied in detail—occupational factors among the parents of affected children and the unusual degree of mixing of populations with differing experiences of infection that has occurred around several of the plants. The data currently available on these factors are discussed below.

Concern has also been expressed about the possible carcinogenic effects of the radioactive discharges into the atmosphere arising from the accident at the Chernobyl nuclear power station in the Ukraine in 1986, which resulted in increased background radiation over much of Europe. The occurrence of an unusually large number of infants with leukemia in Scotland has already been linked with Chernobyl (Gibson et al., 1988). As with the discharges from other nuclear plants discussed above, the predicted increase in childhood cancer incidence attributable to Chernobyl would be too small to detect by comparison with normal variability, even in parts of Central and Eastern Europe where background radiation levels doubled. Some uncertainty, however, still attaches to the risk predictions, and IARC is coordinating a study of childhood leukemia incidence in Europe after the Chernobyl accident (Parkin, 1990).

Radon

There is some indication that the incidence of childhood leukemia in Britain may be related to radon exposure, although there is considerable uncertainly over the nature of any such relationship and the excess annual incidence may only be of the order of 0.2 cases/Bq/m^3 (Alexander et al., 1990; Muirhead et al., 1991). Mortality from cancer, and especially leukemia, among children in North Carolina was higher in areas where there were higher concentrations of radon in drinking water, but this result could be due to confounding with other factors (Collman et al., 1991).

Electromagnetic Fields

There has also been considerable public concern about the possible health effects of the low-frequency alternating electromagnetic fields (EMF) emitted by electric power transmission lines and domestic wiring. The most recent, comprehensive reviews of studies in this area are by Dennis et al. (1991) and by Poole and Trichopoulos (1991). Some, though not all, showed an increased risk of childhood cancer associated with higher levels of ambient EMF in or near the home. When increased risks have been detected, possible confounding factors (see Chapter 1) have included maternal smoking and degree of access to medical care, both of which are linked to socioeconomic status, as well as to road traffic density. Considered together, the studies are inconclusive, but any risk attributable to EMF is unlikely to be large.

Drugs

A great range of drugs taken by mothers during pregnancy have been identified as possible causes of childhood cancer, but the risks have been substantiated for very few. Exposure in utero to diethylstilbestrol (DES), a hormone that was given to pregnant women with threatened abortion, is known to have caused clear-cell adenocarcinoma of the vagina or cervix predominantly in young women, although a very few cases have also been diagnosed in girls under age 15 (Vessey, 1989).

There have been several case reports of neuroblastoma in children of mothers who took the antiepileptic drug phenytoin during pregnancy, although this association has not been confirmed in any large series, perhaps because of the low frequency of use of phenytoin. The most recent report (Koren et al., 1989) includes a review of the previous literature. In a cohort study of over 2500 children born in Denmark whose mothers had previously been hospitalized for epilepsy and who were thus presumably exposed to anticonvulsants in utero, there was no excess of cancer overall nor of any specific tumor type (Olsen et al., 1990). In a case-control study of over 8000 children, a significantly increased relative risk with maternal epilepsy was not associated with exposure to anticonvulsant drugs (Gilman et al., 1989).

Many other drugs taken during pregnancy or labor, including barbiturates, diuretics, antihistamines, analgesics, antipyretics, and antibiotics, have been associated with an increased risk of particular childhood cancers or all cancers combined in various case-control studies (Gilman et al., 1989; Gold et al., 1979; Kramer et al., 1987; McKinney et al., 1987; Preston-Martin et al., 1982; Zack et al., 1991). None of these findings, however, has been repeated. Recently, a significantly elevated relative risk of ANLL has been reported among children of mothers who took marijuana during pregnancy (Robison et al., 1989). The association predominantly involved the myelomonocytic and monocytic subtypes of ANLL, but this finding has yet to be replicated and, if real, may be due to pesticide contamination, rather than the drug itself.

Drugs taken by children have also been reported as risk factors for cancer. Three (7.5%) of a series of 40 children given the alkylating agent chlorambucil for juvenile rheumatoid arthritis developed ANLL (Buriot et al., 1979). Alkylating agents used to treat cancer are themselves carcinogenic, but as with radiotherapy, the proportion of childhood cancer caused by these drugs must be very low. Three percent of a series of 100 children who received immunosuppressive drugs after a heart transplant developed non-Hodgkin's lymphoma at intervals of 2 to 18 months posttransplant (Michalski et al., 1990). Use of the antibiotic chloramphenicol by children in Shanghai has been associated with an increased risk of acute leukemia, both ALL and ANLL (Shu et al., 1988). This drug is less widely used in Western countries, and the finding has yet to be repeated.

Other Chemical and Occupational Factors

Analyses of the possible link between parental smoking and childhood cancer are discussed in the report on the most recent such study (John et al., 1991). The results of that study were suggestive of a possible risk arising from parents' prenatal smoking, but the number of cases in each diagnostic group was small and the slightly raised odds ratios were generally not statistically significant (see

Chapter 1). In the largest study with results published during the past decade, no consistent association was found (Buckley et al., 1986). Similarly, in a cohort of nearly 500,000 births including 327 childhood cancers, there was no evidence of increased cancer risk with maternal smoking (Pershagen et al., 1992). The evidence for a carcinogenic effect of parental smoking is inconclusive and must remain so in the absence of studies that include very large numbers of cases.

Household Products

Many other domestic environmental exposures have been linked with childhood cancers, but relatively few have been reported in more than one study. These include pesticides (Buckley et al., 1989; Infante et al., 1978; Lowengart et al., 1987), incense (Lowengart et al., 1987; Preston-Martin et al., 1982), and hair dyes (Bunin et al., 1987; Kramer et al., 1987). In general, there has been little consistency in the findings of such studies. It is notable, however, that several substances that have been associated with an increased risk of brain tumors after maternal exposure in pregnancy, including incense, contain nitrosamines; the association of brain tumors with in utero exposure to N-nitroso compounds is also supported by experimental evidence (see Preston-Martin, 1989). Children whose mothers used incense during pregnancy may also have an increased risk of leukemia (Lowengart et al., 1987), but this association, if real, could be due to other constituents of incense, such as aldehydes or polycyclic aromatic hydrocarbons.

Parental Occupations

There have been numerous studies of parental occupation and cancer. The most recent review is by O'Leary et al. (1991), who considered 32 published studies. They found some consistency in reports of excess risk associated with hydrocarbon-related occupations and other chemical industries, although there was little firm evidence of an association with any specific exposure or occupation. Their review specifically excluded consideration of the possible effects of occupational radiation exposure.

A moderately raised risk of certain cancers in the children of fathers in some occupations where they might have been exposed to ionizing radiation was reported by Hicks et al. (1984), but no details were obtained on the dose of radiation, if any, received by individual fathers. In a case-control study of young people born in the West Cumbria district of England (which includes the Sellafield nuclear reprocessing plant) who were diagnosed with leukemia or lymphoma while living there, there was a significantly high relative risk for children of fathers employed at Sellafield at the time of their conception (Gardner et al., 1990). There were six cases with fathers who worked at the plant and for whom dose information was obtained. The fathers of five of these six cases each had higher radiation doses before their child's conception than all of the matched control fathers; this suggested that exposure of men to ionizing radiation may be leukemogenic in their offspring. No excess cancer risk had previously been found in the children of men who had been exposed to radiation from the atomic bombs or who had received radiotherapy, but this might be explained by differences in the timing of exposure relative to the date of conception.

Another case-control study of children with leukemia or NHL in the area around the Dounreay reprocessing plant in Scotland found no association with parental preconception irradiation (Urquhart et al., 1991). In Shanghai a significant trend was found in the risk of leukemia with the number of paternal preconception diagnostic x-ray exposures (Shu et al., 1988). This result should be interpreted with caution, however, because the information on paternal x-ray exposure was apparently derived largely from interviews with the children's mothers and was not validated from medical records. It has recently been shown that alpha-particle irradiation of a cell may induce a transmitted chromosomal instability, resulting in genetic abnormalities later in the same cell line (Kadhim et al., 1992). Any possible risk of childhood leukemia related to paternal gonadal irradiation, however, is unlikely to be substantiated without larger epidemiologic studies incorporating detailed records of exposure.

Infection

Exposure to infection undoubtedly plays a part in the etiology of some childhood cancers. The classic example, and the one that to date accounts for by far the largest number of affected children, is that of Burkitt's lymphoma in tropical regions where this tumor has a very high incidence. The great majority of Burkitt's lymphoma patients in high-incidence regions have raised antibody titers for Epstein-Barr virus (EBV), whereas few patients in low-incidence areas have raised EBV titers. It is believed that malaria, which is endemic in the high-incidence regions, causes a continuous intense antigenic stimulus that alters the response to EBV infection, thus giving rise to Burkitt's lymphoma. Epidemiologic evidence for this theory is provided by a study in Tanzania, where a malaria suppression program, involving the distribution of chloroquine tablets to all children under 10, apparently contributed to a fall in the incidence of Burkitt's lymphoma during the study period to one quarter of its pretrial level (Geser et al., 1989). In regions where hepatitis B infection is common, there is a well-known related high incidence of hepatocellular carcinoma among adults. Children also have a relatively high incidence of hepatocellular carcinoma in these regions, and many, if not all, of the children with this tumor are chronic HBsAg carriers (Perilongo et al., 1990). In Western countries where hepatocellular carcinoma is rare in childhood, the proportion of affected children who are HBsAg positive is smaller, although still larger than in the general population (Leuschner et al., 1988; Perilongo et al. 1990).

Infection with human immunodeficiency virus (HIV) confers an enormously increased risk of Kaposi's sarcoma and certain types of lymphoma in adults. Before age 20, NHL is 360 times more common in AIDS patients than in the general population (Berel et al., 1991). Among a hospital series of 100 HIV-infected children, 3 developed primary CNS lymphoma within 18 months of follow-up (Epstein et al., 1988). Of the first seven cancers diagnosed in children enrolled in the Italian Register for HIV Infection in Children, five were B-cell malignancies: two CNS lymphomas, two abdominal lymphomas, and one leukemia (Arico et al., 1991). Although lymphomas are the commonest cancers among children with HIV infection, Kaposi's sarcoma also occurs (Arico et al., 1991; Buck et al., 1983). After the diagnosis of leiomyosarcoma in two HIV-infected children, it has been postulated that HIV infection may sometimes play a role in the etiology of this extremely rare tumor (Chadwick et al., 1990). Hepatoblastoma has also been recorded in an HIV-infected child (Arico et al., 1991). Doubtless cases of other childhood neoplasms will be reported in association with HIV, but it remains to be seen whether HIV infection increases risk for all types of childhood cancer.

Greaves (1988) has hypothesized that the "common" immunophenotype of ALL may be the result of two spontaneous mutations. The first mutation would be associated with antenatal proliferation and self-mutagenic activity of B-cell precursors. If immune stimulation of mature lymphoid tissue generates a positive feedback proliferation signal to the B-cell precursors, whose turnover in the bone marrow is highest in early infancy, then the greater immunologic challenge resulting from delayed exposure to infection may produce a less regulated proliferative stress. This would then bring about the second mutation in a cell of a clone that had already expanded after the first mutation, and this second mutation would precipitate clinically overt leukemia. Under this hypothesis, children with ALL might be expected to have relatively few infections in early infancy and correspondingly more shortly before the onset of leukemia, and the risk of ALL could also vary with the number of immunizations and the duration of breast feeding.

In one case-control study, children with ALL had fewer serious infections during the first year of life (van Steensel-Moll et al., 1986), but in another study children with leukemia or lymphoma had an excess of virus infections under the age of 6 months (McKinney et al., 1987). A protective effect of immunizations has been found in two studies (Hartley et al., 1988; Kneale et al., 1986), and this effect obtained for other cancers, as well as for leukemia. In another case-control study, children who were breast fed for over 6 months were found to have had a significantly reduced risk of all cancers combined and of lymphomas in particular, and there was a nonsignificant halving of the relative risk for ALL with prolonged breast feeding (Davis et al., 1988). Three other studies including larger numbers of children with leukemia and NHL, however, have produced no evidence for a protective effect of breast feeding (Magnani et al., 1988; McKinney et al., 1987; van Duijn et al., 1988). The recent finding of increased risk of ALL among children who were born at least 5 years after their preceding sibling, possibly reducing the opportunity for exposure to infections at an early age via the sibling, is also consistent with Greaves's hypothesis (Kaye et al., 1991). However, in the same study there was no evidence of increased risk among first-born children, who would, of course, have had no exposure to infections from siblings during infancy.

Support for Greaves's hypothesis is provided by the finding from a large population-based survey of leukemia that ALL among children aged 1 to 7 had an incidence in isolated towns and villages more than twice as great as in built-up areas (Alexander et al., 1990)—if children in isolated communities do indeed experience reduced antigenic challenge during infancy.

Another hypothesis, proposed by Kinlen (1988), is that leukemia in children is a rare response to a postulated widespread virus infection, possibly one that does not even produce any overt symptoms in most persons who are infected. It would then be predicted that leukemia would be more common in areas where there is a high level of population mixing, resulting in a low level of herd immunity. The communities near Sellafield and Dounreay are isolated and have experienced large population movements in connection with the nuclear plants and would thus be expected to have a higher-than-average incidence of childhood leukemia. In the first study of Kinlen's hypothesis, the New Town of Glenrothes was identified as the only other place in Scotland to have experienced isolation and population growth comparable to the area around Dounreay. During the period of fastest increase in the population in Glenrothes, there was a significant excess mortality from leukemia at ages 0 to 24, which was entirely accounted for by a greater excess below age 5 (Kinlen, 1988). A significant excess below age 5 has also been found in a group of four New Towns in England and Wales that, like Glenrothes, experienced rapid population growth but did not acquire their new populations predominantly from a single, nearby urban area, making them comparable with respect to population mixing (Kinlen et al., 1990). In both of these studies no excess of leukemia deaths was found in the period from the mid-1960s to the mid-1980s, when the population of the New Towns were growing much more slowly. Yet, these latter results should be treated with caution as they rely on mortality data for a period of marked improvements in survival for childhood leukemia.

In the first study of the hypothesis to use registration data (Kinlen et al., 1991), another index of population mixing was used; namely, the level of increase in employment-related commuting across a town's boundaries. Among the 28 towns in England for which comparable data were available on commuting levels from the 1971 and 1981 censuses, a significant excess incidence of childhood leukemia from 1972 to 1985 was found in the five that had experienced the greatest increase in commuting. These five towns included Reading, but the excess of leukemia was unaffected by its exclusion from the analysis. This is of particular interest because Reading is in the area near the Aldermaston and Burghfield nuclear plants, in which an excess of childhood leukemia had previously been found. From 1950 to 1953, when the number of men in England and Wales doing national military service was very large and had recently increased, there was a significant excess of childhood mortality from leukemia in the districts with the highest proportion of servicemen in their population (Kinlen & Hudson, 1991). As childhood leukemia at that time was almost invariably rapidly fatal, mortality and incidence were virtually equivalent. The excess was greatest in children under 1 year, suggesting transmission of infection among adults and thence to the fetus, rather than among the children themselves.

Trends in Survival

As recently as a quarter of a century ago, the prognosis for most childhood cancers was poor. Of the major diagnostic groups, only Hodgkin's disease, retinoblastoma, astrocytoma, craniopharyngioma (a nonmalignant tumor), and fibrosarcoma had a 5-year survival rate in excess of 50%. Fewer than 10% of children with leukemia survived for 5 years. Table 16.2 shows the population-based 5-year survival rates for children in the main diagnostic groups in Britain who were diagnosed in successive 3-year periods from 1962 to 1985, as calculated from National Registry data. Following standard cancer registry practice, the few cases notified by death certificate alone were not included in these analyses. By 1962 to 1970, survival rates were already very high for retinoblastoma. From 1962 to 1970, substantial improvements also took place in survival rates for Hodgkin's disease and Wilms' tumor, and the beginning of the increase in survival rates for childhood ALL was apparent. For other diagnostic groups, however, there was little improvement in prognosis. Yet, between 1971 and 1985 the outlook improved considerably for almost all types of childhood cancer (Stiller & Bunch, 1990). The most striking increases in survival rates took place in ALL and NHL, with more than two thirds of the children in each of these groups surviving at least 5 years. There were large improvements in the survival rates for rhabdomyosarcoma and for gonadal germ-cell tumors. ANLL and neuroblastoma also showed considerable improvements, although more than half the children with these diagnoses still died within 5 years. More modest increases in survival rates took place for children with Hodgkin's disease, Wilms' tumor, ependymoma, and medulloblastoma. In the 1980s there was a sizeable increase in the survival rate for osteosarcoma. Ewing's sarcoma was the only major diagnostic group for which there was no significant improvement from 1971 to 1985 and for which 5-year survival remained below 50%.

Since 1970 there have been considerable advances in the treatment of many childhood cancers, with the development of modern techniques of combination chemotherapy playing an especially important role. Undoubtedly, these advances were the principal cause of the increase in survival rates. Simultaneously, there were also major changes in the referral patterns for children with cancer, with treatment becoming more centralized and an increasing proportion of children being treated by specialists in pediatric oncology and entered in national and international clinical trials and studies. There have been several analyses of the effects of patterns of referral and entry to clinical trials on the survival rates for various childhood cancers, mainly in Britain and the United States. The data have been reviewed in detail elsewhere (Stiller, 1992). For many types of childhood cancer, it is clear that greater clinical experience and standardization of treatment, whether because of treatment at specialist centers or entry in clinical trials, were associated with an improved survival rate.

Interventions

Hitherto, the major impact on childhood cancer mortality has been the improved survival rates that have resulted from the development of effective treatment. This topic has been covered earlier in the chapter, and this section is concerned with other forms of intervention.

It is difficult to see at present how there could be a great reduction in childhood cancer incidence resulting from the avoidance of environmental risk factors because the causes of most cases are still unknown. The reduction in antenatal obstetric x-ray examinations that took place in the late 1950s was

Table 16.2. Five-Year Survival Rates for Principal Types of Childhood Cancer in Britain Diagnosed Between 1962 and 1985

Diagnostic Group	1962–64	1965–67	1968–70	1971–73	1974–76	1977–79	1980–82	1983–85
Acute lymphoblastic leukemia	2	8	14	37	47	53	65	70
Acute nonlymphocytic leukemia	2	2	3	4	7	18	20	28
Hodgkin's disease	37	50	69	76	83	88	90	90
Non-Hodgkin's lymphoma	19	17	20	22	28	39	56	69
Brain and spinal tumors	35	38	36	42	43	45	51	56
Neuroblastoma	19	18	18	15	19	25	37	43
Retinoblastoma	84	88	84	87	88	89	86	89
Wilms' tumor	26	31	44	58	64	76	76	79
Osteosarcoma	19	12	22	17	24	28	34	52
Ewing's sarcoma	19	29	21	39	38	34	34	44
Rhabdomyosarcoma	23	32	19	26	40	46	48	60
Malignant gonadal germ-cell	58	48	58	51	57	72	84	88

Source: Data for 1971 to 1985 from Stiller & Bunch (1990), with follow-up extended to the end of 1990.

prompted by concerns about their teratogenic rather than carcinogenic potential (Mole, 1990), and any consequent reduction in the incidence rate can only have been very small. Similarly, discontinuing the use of DES in pregnancy will have had a negligible effect on the total incidence of childhood cancer.

The incidence rate would also be expected to decline if there were to be a reduction in the proportion of the childhood population at high risk of cancer because of some other inherited condition. Although the incidence of Down syndrome among births to women aged 35 and over (the group with by far the highest incidence of this chromosomal abnormality) has decreased with the widespread use of antenatal screening, this decrease has been largely offset by a rise in the proportion of all births to older women. Also, the mortality rate from infections that were the major cause of death among children with Down syndrome has been reduced dramatically (see Chapter 3). There is no evidence of any change in the annual number of cases of childhood leukemia associated with Down syndrome, which in any event only accounts for 2% to 3% of all childhood leukemia.

Wider availability of genetic counseling might reduce slightly the numbers of children with heritable retinoblastoma, although only a third of cases occur in families with a previous history of the disease.

The objective of screening (see Chapter 1) for cancer is to reduce mortality and morbidity by detecting disease at an earlier stage than if it were to present clinically. Screening can be carried out either by examination of the small numbers of persons who are in identifiable high-risk groups or by mass screening.

For some years children with a family history of retinoblastoma have been offered regular ophthalmic examinations under anesthetia to diagnose tumors as early as possible, thus in many cases allowing sight to be preserved by less aggressive treatment of very early stage tumors. Advances in molecular genetics will soon permit the identification of members of retinoblastoma families who are gene carriers (Cowell, 1991); thus, frequent examinations of all relatives of retinoblastoma patients would no longer be necessary, and clinical resources could be concentrated on patients who are carriers.

Among children with aniridia, hemihypertrophy, Beckwith-Wiedemann syndrome, or Drash syndrome—all of whom are at increased risk of Wilms' tumor—the prognosis might be improved by early detection of the tumor resulting from routine abdominal examination and other investigations at intervals during early childhood (Mulvihill, 1989).

Neuroblastoma is the only childhood cancer for which population screening might be practicable. Cases can be detected at a presymptomatic stage by the presence of increased quantities of catecholamine metabolites in urine. Screening began in Japan in the 1970s and has been available nationally there since 1985. The history of neuroblastoma screening in Japan is reviewed by Sawada et al. (1991), and studies have also begun in North America and Britain. There are many problems in the interpretation of data on neuroblastoma screening (Goodman, 1991). These include the detection of cases that would never have presented clinically; lead-time bias, whereby screened patients have a longer survival from time of diagnosis only because they were diagnosed earlier; and length-time bias, which occurs if the screening test preferentially detects patients with slower-growing tumors that have a longer asymptomatic phase and a better prognosis (see Chapter 1). Although cases of neuroblastoma may be detected at an early stage by screening and these patients have an excellent prognosis, those with biologically unfavorable features, such as amplification of the n-myc oncogene, are apparently less likely to be detected. In a recent report of spontaneous regression of a case of neuroblastoma detected by screening at 6 months of age, the authors suggested that the clinical course of their patient was not exceptional (Matsumura et al., 1991). The impact of neuroblastoma screening on mortality from this disease is still unproven and can only be assessed by comparison of mortality rates in screened and unscreened populations (Murphy et al., 1991). If screening is everywhere offered as a service before such studies can be carried out, it will never be possible to assess its effectiveness and some children will die from the complications of treatment for neuroblastoma, which would otherwise have regressed with no need for medical intervention.

Acknowledgments

I am very grateful to Mrs. E. M. Roberts for secretarial assistance and to Mr. T. J. Vincent for producing the graphs. The Childhood Cancer Research Group is supported by the Department of Health and the Scottish Home and Health Department.

References

Alexander FE, Ricketts TJ, McKinney PA, Cartwright RA. Community lifestyle characteristics and risk of acute lymphoblastic leukaemia in children. *Lancet* 1990; 336:1461–1465.

Alexander FE, Ricketts TJ, McKinney PA, Cartwright RA. Community lifestyle characteristics and incidence of Hodgkin's disease in young people. *Int J Cancer* 1991; 48:10–14.

Arico M, Caselli D, D'Argenio P, et al. Malignancies in children with human immunodeficiency virus type 1. *Cancer* 1991; 68:2473–2477.

Beral V, Peterman T, Berkelman R, Jaffe H. AIDS-associated non-Hodgkin lymphoma. *Lancet* 1991; 337:805–809.

Bessho F. Acute non-lymphocytic leukemia is not a major type of childhood leukemia in Japan. *Eur J Cancer Clin Oncol* 1989; 25:729–732.

Birch JM, Marsden HB. A classification scheme for childhood cancer. *Int J Cancer* 1987; 40:620–624.

Birch JM, Marsden HB, Swindell R. Pre-natal factors in the origin of germ cell tumors of childhood. *Carcinogenesis* 1982; 3:75–80.

Black D. *Investigation of the Possible Increased Incidence of Cancer in West Cumbria.* London: HMSO; 1984.

Bonaiti-Pellié C, Chompret A, Tournade M-F, et al. Genetics and epidemiology of Wilms' tumor: the French Wilms' Tumor Study. *Med Pediatr Oncol* 1992; 20:284–291.

Breslow NE, Beckwith JB. Epidemiological features of Wilms' tumor: Results of the National Wilms' Tumor Study. *J Natl Cancer Inst* 1982; 68:429–436.

Breslow N, Beckwith JB, Ciol M, Sharples K. Age distribution of Wilms' tumor: report from the National Wilms' Tumor Study. *Cancer Res* 1988; 48:1653–1657.

Buck BE, Scott GB, Valdes-Dapena M, Parks WP. Kaposi sarcoma in two infants with acquired immune deficiency syndrome. *J Pediatr* 1983; 103:911–913.

Buckley JD, Hobbie WL, Ruccione K, Sather HN, Woods WG, Hammond GD. Maternal smoking during pregnancy and the risk of childhood cancer. *Lancet* 1986; 2:519–520.

Buckley JD, Robison LL, Swotinsky R, et al. Occupational exposures of children with acute nonlymphocytic leukemia: a report from the Children's Cancer Study Group. *Cancer Res* 1989; 49:4030–4037.

Bunin GR, Kramer S, Marrero O, Meadows AT. Gestational risk factors for Wilms' tumor: results of a case-control study. *Cancer Res* 1987; 47:2972–2977.

Bunin GR, Emanuel BS, Meadows AT, Buckley JD, Woods WG, Hammond GD. Frequency of 13q abnormalities among 203 patients with retinoblastoma. *J Natl Cancer Inst* 1989a; 81:370–374.

Bunin GR, Meadows AT, Emanuel BS, Buckley JD, Woods WG, Hammond GD. Pre- and postconception factors associated with sporadic heritable and nonheritable retinoblastoma. *Cancer Res* 1989b; 49:5730–5735.

Buriot D, Prieur A-M, Lebranchu Y, Messerschmitt J, Griscelli C. Leucémie aigue chez trois enfants atteints d'arthrite chronique juvenile traités par le Chlorambucil. *Arch Franc Pédiat* 1979; 36:592–598.

Carlsen NLT. Epidemiological investigations on neuroblastomas in Denmark 1943–1980. *Br J Cancer* 1986; 54:977–988.

Cartwright RA, McKinney PA, Hopton PA, et al. Ultrasound examinations in pregnancy and childhood cancer. *Lancet* 1984; 2:999–1000.

Chadwick EG, Connor EJ, Guerra Hanson IC, et al. Tumors of smooth-muscle origin in HIV-infected children. *JAMA* 1990; 263:3182–3184.

Chaganti RSK, Miller DR, Mayers PA, German J. Cytogenetic evidence of the intrauterine origin of acute leukemia in monozygotic twins. *N Engl J Med* 1979; 300:1032–1034.

Coebergh JWW, van der Does-van den Berg A, van Wering ER, et al. Childhood leukemia in The Netherlands, 1973–86: temporary variation of the incidence of acute lymphocytic leukaemia in young children. *Br J Cancer* 1989; 59:100–105.

Cole Johnson C, Spitz MR. Neuroblastoma: case-control analysis of birth characteristics. *J Natl Cancer Inst* 1985; 74:789–792.

Collman GW, Loomis DP, Sandler DP. Childhood cancer mortality and radon concentration in drinking water in North Carolina. *Br J Cancer* 1991; 63:626–629.

Committee on Medical Aspects of Radiation in the Environment (COMARE). *Second Report: Investigation of the Possible Increased Incidence of Leukaemia in Young People near Dounreay Nuclear Establishment, Caithness, Scotland*. London: HMSO; 1988.

Committee on Medical Aspects of Radiation in the Environment (COMARE). *Third Report: Report on the Incidence of Childhood Cancer in the West Berkshire and North Hampshire area, in Which are Situated the Atomic Weapons Research Establishment, Aldermaston and the Royal Ordnance Factory, Burghfield*. London: HMSO; 1989.

Cook-Mozaffari PJ, Darby SC, Doll R, et al. Geographical variation in mortality from leukaemia and other cancers in England and Wales in relation to proximity to nuclear installations, 1969–78. *Br J Cancer* 1989a; 59:476–485.

Cook-Mozaffari P, Darby S, Doll R. Cancer near potential sites of nuclear installations. *Lancet* 1989b; 2:1145–1147.

Cowell JK. The genetics of retinoblastoma. *Br J Cancer* 1991; 63:333–336.

Daling JR, Starzyk P, Olshan AF, Weiss NS. Birth weight and the incidence of childhood cancer. *J Natl Cancer Inst* 1984; 72:1039–1041.

Davis MK, Savitz DA, Graubard BI. Infant feeding and childhood cancer. *Lancet* 1988; 2:365–368.

Davis S, Rogers MAM, Pendergrass TW. The incidence and epidemiologic characteristics of neuroblastoma in the United States. *Am J Epidemiol* 1987; 126:1063–1074.

Dennis JA, Muirhead CR, Ennis JR. Epidemiological studies of exposure to electromagnetic fields: II. Cancer. *J Radiol Prot* 1991; 11:13–25.

Der Kinderen DJ, Koten JW, Tan KEWP, Beemer FA, van Romunde LKJ, den Otter W. Parental age in sporadic hereditary retinoblastoma. *Am J Ophthalmol* 1990; 110:605–609.

Draper GJ, Heaf MM, Kinnier Wilson LM. Occurrence of childhood cancers among sibs and estimation of familial risks. *J Med Genet* 1977; 14:81–90.

Draper GJ, Sanders BM, Kingston JE. Second primary neoplasms in patients with retinoblastoma. *Br J Cancer* 1986; 53:661–671.

Draper GJ, Vincent TJ, O'Connor CM, Stiller CA. Socio-economic factors and variations in incidence rates between County Districts. In: Draper GJ, ed. *The Geographical Epidemiology of Childhood Leukaemia and Non-Hodgkin Lymphoma in Great Britain, 1966–83. Studies on Medical and Population Subjects, No. 53.* London: HMSO; 1991:37–45.

Edelstein J, Amylon M, Berkman Walsh J. Dermatoglyphics and acute lymphocytic leukemia in children. *J Pediatr Oncol Nurs* 1991; 8:30–38.

Epstein LG, Di Carlo FJ, Joshi VV, et al. Primary lymphoma of the central nervous system in children with acquired immunodeficiency syndrome. *Pediatrics* 1988; 82:355–363.

Garber JE, Goldstein AM, Kantor AF, Dreyfus MG, Fraumeni JF, Li FP. Follow-up study of twenty-four families with Li-Fraumeni syndrome. *Cancer Res* 1991; 51:6094–6097.

Gardner MJ, Hall AJ, Downes S, Terrell JD. Follow-up study of children born to mothers resident in Seascale, West Cumbria (birth cohort). *Br Med J* 1987; 295:822–827.

Gardner MJ, Snee MP, Hall AJ, Powell CA, Downes S, Terrell JD. Results of case-control study of leukaemia and lymphoma among young people near Sellafield nuclear plant in West Cumbria. *Br Med J* 1990; 300:423–429.

Geser A, Brubaker G, Draper CC. Effect of a malaria suppression program on the incidence of African Burkitt's lymphoma. *Am J Epidemiol* 1989; 129:740–752.

Ghali MH, Yoo K-Y, Flannery JT, Dubrow R. Association between childhood rhabdomyosarcoma and maternal history of stillbirths. *Int J Cancer* 1991; 50:365–368.

Gibson BES, Eden OB, Barrett A, Stiller CA, Draper GJ. Leukaemia in young children in Scotland. *Lancet* 1988; 2:630.

Gilman EA, Kinnier Wilson LM, Kneale GW, Waterhouse JAH. Childhood cancers and their association with pregnancy drugs and illnesses. *Paediatr Perinat Epidemiol* 1989; 3:66–94.

Gold E, Gordis L, Tonascia J, Szklo M. Risk factors for brain tumors in children. *Am J Epidemiol* 1979; 109:309–319.

Goodman SN. Neuroblastoma screening data. An epidemiologic analysis. *Am J Dis Child* 1991; 145:1415–1422.

Greaves MF. Speculations on the cause of childhood acute lymphoblastic leukemia. *Leukemia* 1988; 2:120–125.

Greaves MF, Chan LC. Is spontaneous mutation the major 'cause' of childhood acute lymphoblastic leukaemia? The paucity of evidence for environmental and genetic factors in acute lymphoblastic leukaemia. *Br J Haematol* 1986; 64:1–13.

Gustafsson G, Kreuger A. Incidence of childhood leukemia in Sweden 1975–1980. *Acta Paediatr Scand* 1982; 71:887–892.

Hansen NE, Karle H, Jensen OM. Trends in the incidence of leukemia in Denmark, 1943–77: an epidemiologic study of 14,000 patients. *J Natl Cancer Inst* 1983; 71:697–701.

Hartley AL, Birch JM, McKinney PA, et al. The Inter-Regional Epidemiological Study of Childhood Cancer (IRESCC): past medical history in children with cancer. *J Epidemiol Comm Health* 1988; 42:235–242.

Hawkins MM, Draper GJ, Smith RA. Cancer among 1348 offspring of survivors of childhood cancer. *Int J Cancer* 1989; 43:975–978.

Hempelmann LH, Hall WJ, Phillips M, Cooper RA, Ames WR. Neoplasms in persons treated with X-rays in infancy: fourth survey in 20 years. *J Natl Cancer Inst* 1975; 55:519–530.

Hicks N, Zack M, Caldwell GG, Fernbach DJ, Falletta JM. Childhood cancer and occupational radiation exposure in parents. *Cancer* 1984; 53:1637–1643.

Hill C, Laplanche A. Cancer mortality around nuclear sites. *Eur J Cancer* 1991; 27:815–816.

Infante FF, Epstein SS, Newton WA. Blood dyscrasias and childhood tumors and exposure to chlordane and heptachlor. *Scand J Work Environ Health* 1978; 4:137–150.

Innis MD. Nephroblastoma: possible index cancer of childhood. *Med J Aust* 1972; 1:18–20.

Inskip PD, Harvey EB, Boice JD, et al. Incidence of childhood cancer in twins. *Cancer Causes Control* 1991; 2:315–324.

Jadresic L, Wadey RB, Buckle B, Barratt TM, Mitchell CD, Cowell JK. Molecular analysis of chromosome region 11p13 in patients with Drash syndrome. *Hum Genet* 1991; 86:497–501.

John EM, Savitz DA, Sandler DP. Prenatal exposure to parents' smoking and childhood cancer. *Am J Epidemiol* 1991; 133:123–132.

Kadhim MA, Macdonald DA, Goodhead DT, Lorimore SA, Marsden SJ, Wright EG. Transmission of chromosomal instability after plutonium α-particle irradiation. *Nature* 1992; 355:738–740.

Kaye SA, Robison LL, Smithson WA, Gunderson P, King FL, Neglia JP. Maternal reproductive history and birth characteristics in childhood acute lymphoblastic leukemia. *Cancer* 1991; 68:1351–1355.

Kingston JE, Herbert A, Draper GJ, Mann JR. Association between hepatoblastoma and polyposis coli. *Arch Dis Child* 1983; 58:959–962.

Kingston JE, Hawkins MM, Draper GJ, Marsden HB, Kinnier Wilson LM. Patterns of multiple primary tumors in patients treated for cancer during childhood. *Br J Cancer* 1987; 56:331–338.

Kinlen L. Evidence for an infective cause of childhood leukaemia: comparison of a Scottish New Town with nuclear reprocessing sites in Britain. *Lancet* 1988; 2:1323–1327.

Kinlen LJ, Hudson C. Childhood leukaemia and poliomyelitis in relation to military encampments in England and Wales in the period of national military service, 1950–63. *Br Med J* 1991; 303:1357–1362.

Kinlen LJ, Clarke K, Hudson C. Evidence from population mixing in British New Towns (1946–85) of an infective basis for childhood leukaemia. *Lancet* 1990; 336:577–582.

Kinlen LJ, Hudson CM, Stiller CA. Contacts between adults as evidence for an infective origin of childhood leukaemia: an explanation for the excess near nuclear establishments in West Berkshire? *Br J Cancer* 1991; 64:549–554.

Kinnier Wilson LM, Waterhouse JAH. Obstetric ultrasound and childhood malignancies. *Lancet* 1984; 2:997–999.

Kneale GW, Stewart AM, Kinnier Wilson LM. Immunizations against infectious diseases and childhood cancers. *Cancer Immunol Imunother* 1986; 21:129–132.

Knudson AG. Mutation and cancer: statistical study of retinoblastoma. *Proc Nat Acad Sci USA* 1971; 68:820–823.

Kobayashi N, Matsui I, Tanimura M, et al. Childhood neuroectodermal tumors and malignant lymphoma after maternal ovulation induction. *Lancet* 1991; 338:955.

Koren G, Demitrakoudis D, Weksberg R, et al. Neuroblastoma after prenatal exposure to phenytoin: cause and effect? *Teratology* 1989; 40:157–162.

Kramer S, Ward E, Meadows AT, Malone KE. Medical and drug risk factors associated with neuroblastoma: a case-control study. *J Natl Cancer Inst* 1987; 78:797–804.

Kushner BH, Gilbert F, Helson L. Familial neuroblastoma. Case reports, literature review and etiologic considerations. *Cancer* 1986; 57:1887–1893.

Leuschner I, Harms D, Schmidt D. The association of hepatocellular carcinoma in childhood with hepatitis B virus infection. *Cancer* 1988; 62:2363–2369.

Li FP, Williams WR, Gimbrere K, Flamant F, Green DM, Meadows AT. Heritable fraction of unilateral Wilms' tumor. *Pediatrics* 1988a; 81:147–149.

Li FP, Fraumeni JF, Mulvihill JJ, et al. A cancer family syndrome in twenty-four kindreds. *Cancer Res* 1988b; 48:5358–5362.

Lowengart RA, Peters JM, Cicioni C, et al. Childhood leukemia and parents' occupational and home exposures. *J Natl Cancer Inst* 1987; 79:39–46.

Magnani C, Pastore G, Terracini B. Infant feeding and childhood cancer. *Lancet* 1988; 2:1136.

Malkin D, Li FP, Strong LC, et al. Germ line p53 mutations in a familial syndrome of breast cancer, sarcomas and other neoplasms. *Science* 1990; 250:1233–1238.

Mann JR, Pearson D, Barrett A, Raafat F, Barnes JM, Wallendszus KR. Results of the United Kingdom Children's Cancer Study Group's Malignant Germ Cell Tumor Studies. *Cancer* 1989; 63:1657–1667.

Matsumura M, Tsunoda A, Nishi T, Nishihira H, Sasaki Y. Spontaneous regression of neuroblastoma detected by mass screening. *Lancet* 1991; 338:447–448.

Matsunaga E, Minoda K, Sasaki MS. Parental age and seasonal variation in the births of children with sporadic retinoblastoma: a mutation-epidemiologic study. *Hum Genet* 1990; 84:155–158.

McKinney PA, Cartwright RA, Saiu JMT, et al. The inter-regional epidemiological study of childhood cancer (IRESCC): a case control study of aetiological factors in leukaemia and lymphoma. *Arch Dis Child* 1987; 62:279–287.

McWhirter WR, Petroeschevsky AL. Childhood cancer incidence in Queensland, 1979–88. *Int J Cancer* 1990; 45:1002–1005.

Meadows AT, Baum E, Fossati-Bellani F, et al. Second malignant neoplasms in children: an update from the Late Effects Study Group. *J Clin Oncol* 1985; 3:532–538.

Michalski A, Radley-Smith R, Crawford D. Non-Hodgkin's lymphoma in a cardiac transplant patient—successful management without chemotherapy. *Med Pediatr Oncol* 1990; 18:503–509.

Miller RW. Ethnic differences in cancer occurrence: genetic and environmental influences with particular reference to neuroblastoma. In: Mulvihill JJ, Miller RW, Fraumeni JF, eds. *Genetics of Human Cancer*. New York: Raven Press; 1977:1–14.

Mole RH. Childhood cancer after prenatal exposure to diagnostic X-ray examinations in Britain. *Br J Cancer* 1990; 62:152–168.

Morrell D, Cromartie E, Swift M. Mortality and cancer incidence in 263 patients with ataxia-telangiectasia. *J Natl Cancer Inst* 1986; 77:89–92.

Muirhead CR, Butland BK, Green BMR, Draper GJ. Childhood leukaemia and natural radiation. *Lancet* 1991; 337:503–504.

Mulvihill JJ. Clinical genetics of pediatric cancer. In: Pizzo PA, Poplack DG, eds. *Principles and Practice of Pediatric Oncology*. Philadelphia: JB Lippincott; 1989:19–37.

Murphy SB, Cohn SL, Craft AW, et al. Do children benefit from mass screening for neuroblastoma? Consensus statement from the American Cancer Society workshop on neuroblastoma screening. *Lancet* 1991; 337:344–346.

Narod SA, Stiller C, Lenoir GM. An estimate of the heritable fraction of childhood cancer. *Br J Cancer* 1991; 63:993–999.

Neglia JP, Smithson WA, Gunderson P, King FL, Singher LJ, Robison LL. Prenatal and perinatal risk factors for neuroblastoma: a case-control study. *Cancer* 1988; 61:2202–2206.

O'Leary LM, Hicks AM, Peters JM, London S. Parental occupational exposures and risk of childhood cancer: a review. *Am J Industr Med* 1991; 20:17–35.

Olsen JH, Boice JD, Fraumeni JF. Cancer in children of epileptic mothers and the possible relation to maternal anticonvulsant therapy. *Br J Cancer* 1990; 62:996–999.

Operskalski EA, Preston-Martin S, Henderson BE, Visscher BR. A case-control study of osteosarcoma in young persons. *Am J Epidemiol* 1987; 126:118–126.

Parkin DM. The European Childhood Leukemia/Lymphoma Incidence Study. *Radiation Res* 1990; 124:370–371.

Parkin DM, Stiller CA, Bieber A, Draper GJ, Terracini B, Young JL, eds. *International Incidence of Childhood Cancers.* IARC Scientific Publications No. 87. Lyon: IARC; 1988a.

Parkin DM, Stiller CA, Draper GJ, Bieber CA. The international incidence of childhood cancer. *Int J Cancer* 1988b; 42:511–520.

Partoft S, Osterlind A, Hou-Jensen K, Drzewiecki KT. Malignant melanoma of the skin in children (0 to 14 years of age) in Denmark, 1943–1982. *Scand J Plast Reconstr Surg* 1989; 23:55–58.

Pellié C, Briard M-L, Feingold J, Frezal J. Parental age in retinoblastoma. *Humangenetik* 1973; 20:59–62.

Percy C, Van Holten V, Muir C, eds. *International Classification of Diseases for Oncology.* 2nd ed. Geneva: WHO; 1990.

Perilongo G, Pontisso P, Basso G. Can primary cancer of the liver in western countries be prevented? Pediatric point of view. *Med Pediatr Oncol* 1990; 18:57–60.

Pershagen G, Ericson A, Otterblad-Olavsson P. Maternal smoking in pregnancy: does it increase the risk of childhood cancer? *Int J Epidemiol* 1992; 21:1–5.

Poole C, Trichopoulos D. Extremely low frequency electric and magnetic fields and cancer. *Cancer Causes Control* 1991; 2:267–276.

Preston-Martin S. Epidemiological studies of prenatal carcinogenesis. In: Napalkov NP, Rice JM, Tomatis L, Yamasaki H, eds. *Perinatal and Multigeneration Carcinogenesis.* IARC Scientific Publications No. 96. Lyon: IARC; 1989:289–314.

Preston-Martin S, Yu MC, Benton B, Henderson BE. N-nitroso compounds and childhood brain tumors: a case-control study. *Cancer Res* 1982; 42:5240–5245.

Rahim MA. Bangladesh: cancer epidemiology research programme, 1978–1981. In: Parkin DM, ed. *Cancer Occurrence in Developing Countries.* IARC Scientific Publications No. 75. Lyon: IARC; 1986:195–198.

Robison LL, Buckley JD, Daigle AE, et al. Maternal drug use and risk of childhood nonlymphoblastic leukemia among offspring: an epidemiologic investigation implicating marijuana. A report from the Children's Cancer Study Group. *Cancer* 1989; 63:1904–1911.

Rodrigues L, Hills M, McGale P, Elliott P. Socio-economic factors in relation to childhood leukaemia and non-Hodgkin lymphomas: an analysis based on small area statistics for census tracts. In: Draper G, ed. *The Geographical Epidemiology of Childhood Leukaemia and Non-Hodgkin Lymphoma in Great Britain, 1966–83. Studies on Medical and Population Subjects No 53.* London: HMSO; 1991:47–56.

Ron E, Modan B, Boice JD, et al. Tumors of the brain and nervous system after radiotherapy in childhood. *N Engl J Med* 1988; 319:1033–1039.

Salonen T, Saxen T. Risk indicators in childhood malignancies. *Int J Cancer* 1975; 15:941–946.

Sanders BM, Jay M, Draper GJ, Roberts EM. Non-ocular cancer in relatives of retinoblastoma patients. Br J Cancer 1989; 60:358–365.

Santibanez-Koref MF, Birch JM, Hartley AM, et al. p53 germline mutations in Li-Fraumeni syndrome. *Lancet* 1991; 338:1490–1491.

Sawada T, Sugimoto T, Kawakatsu H, Matsumara T, Matsuda Y. Mass screening for neuroblastoma in Japan. *Pediatr Hematol Oncol* 1991; 8:93–109.

Shimizu Y, Schull WJ, Kato H. Cancer risk among atomic bomb survivors: the RERF Life Span Study. *JAMA* 1990; 264:601–604.

Shu XO, Gao YT, Brinton LA, et al. A population-based case-control study of childhood leukemia in Shanghai. *Cancer* 1988; 62:635–644.

Sotelo-Avila C, Gonzalez-Crussi F, Fowler JW. Complete and incomplete forms of Beckwith-Wiedemann syndrome: their oncogenic potential. *J Pediatr* 1980; 96:47–50.

Stevens W, Thomas DC, Lyon JL, et al. Leukemia in Utah and radioactive fallout from the Nevada test site. *JAMA* 1990; 264:585–591.

Stewart A, Webb J, Hewitt D. A survey of childhood malignancies. *Br Med J* 1958; 1:1495–1508.

Stiller C. Survival of patients in clinical trials and at specialist centres. In: Williams CJ, ed. *Introducing New Treatments for Cancer: Practical, Ethical and Legal Problems.* Chichester: Wiley; 1992:119–136.

Stiller CA, Bunch KJ. Trends in survival for childhood cancer in Britain diagnosed 1971–85. *Br J Cancer* 1990; 62:806–815.

Stiller CA, Draper GJ. Trends in childhood leukaemia in Britain 1968–1978. *Br J Cancer* 1982; 45:543–551.

Stiller CA, Parkin DM. International variations in the incidence of childhood lymphomas. *Paediatr Perinat Epidemiol* 1990; 4:302–323.

Stiller CA, Lennox EL, Kinnier Wilson LM. Incidence of cardiac septal defects in children with Wilms' tumour and other malignant diseases. *Carcinogenesis* 1987; 8:129–132.

Stiller CA, Draper GJ, Vincent TJ, O'Connor CM. Incidence rates nationally and in administratively defined areas. In: Draper G, ed. *The Geographical Epidemiology of Childhood Leukaemia and Non-Hodgkin Lymphoma in Great Britain, 1966–83. Studies on Medical and Population Subjects No. 53.* London: HMSO; 1991a:25–35.

Stiller CA, McKinney PA, Bunch KJ, Bailey CC, Lewis IJ. Childhood cancer and ethnic group in Britain: a United Kingdom Children's Cancer Study Group (UKCCSG) study. *Br J Cancer* 1991b; 64:543–548.

Urquhart JD, Black RJ, Muirhead MM, et al. Case-control study of leukaemia and non-Hodgkin's lymphoma in children in Caithness near the Dounreay nuclear installation. *Br Med J* 1991; 302:687–692.

van Duijn CM, van Steensel-Moll HA, van der Does-van den Berg A, et al. Infant feeding and childhood cancer. *Lancet* 1988; 2:796–797.

van Steensel-Moll HA, Valkenburg HA, Vandenbroucke JP, van Zanen GE. Are maternal fertility problems related to childhood leukaemia? *Int J Epidemiol* 1985; 14:555–560.

van Steensel-Moll HA, Valkenburg HA, van Zanen GE. Childhood leukemia and infectious diseases in the first year of life: a register-based case-control study. *Am J Epidemiol* 1986; 124:590–594.

Vessey MP. Epidemiological studies of the effects of diethyl stilboestrol. In: Napalkov

NP, Rice JM, Tomatis L, Yamasaki H, eds. *Perinatal and Multigeneration Carcinogenesis.* IARC Scientific Publications No. 96. Lyon: IARC; 1989:335–348.

White L, Giri N, Vowels MR, Lancaster PAL. Neuroectodermal tumours in children born after assisted conception. *Lancet* 1990; 336:1577.

World Health Organization. *International Classification of Diseases for Oncology.* Geneva: WHO; 1976.

Zack M, Adami H-O, Ericson A. Maternal and perinatal risk factors for childhood leukemia. *Cancer Res* 1991; 51:3696–3701.

17

Cerebral Palsy

FIONA J. STANLEY AND EVE BLAIR

This chapter focuses on one of the most common motor handicaps in childhood: the cerebral palsies. They are the most frequently occurring cause of motor handicap (Pharoah, 1985) and there is considerable interest in their trends and causes and whether their occurrence can be reduced by improved perinatal care. In recent years there has been a proliferation in the number of reports on cerebral palsy: "Reviewing the published work in cerebral palsy over the past 5 years, one is tempted to organize it into 'Epidemiology' and 'the Rest' and the epidemiologic papers outnumber 'the Rest'" (Robinson, 1991). Much of the former work has been stimulated, first, by the need to know the proportion of cerebral palsy that is due to birth asphyxia and is possibly preventable by obstetric care and, second, by increasing concerns about motor and other handicaps among the significant number of very low birthweight infants who are now surviving the neonatal period after having received intensive care. For this chapter pertinent publications since 1984 have been reviewed, because a major review monograph covered the earlier period (Stanley & Alberman, 1984).

Biologic Considerations

Cerebral palsy is defined as a group of nonprogressive disorders of movement or posture due to a defect or lesion of the developing brain (Bax, 1964). These disorders are characterized by aberrant control of movement or posture appearing in early life and are not the result of recognized progressive disease (Nelson & Ellenberg, 1978). Many syndromes, many of which are very rare, have as part of their clinical picture a chronic, nonprogressive motor handicap. As defined, interference with the developing brain includes the period from conception to well into childhood (by which time cerebral palsy has usually been diagnosed). Thus, causes can be genetic or related to prepartum (early pregnancy), perinatal, or postnatal problems. This broad grouping of children with similar handicaps due to such a variety of causes has been useful for management and service planning. In addition to their various etiologies, the cerebral palsies are also heterogeneous in terms of cerebral pathology, timing of interference or damage, type and location of motor handicap (i.e., spastic or athetoid, hemiplegia, or diplegia) and the presence of other associated disabilities (Table 17.1). A considerable epidemiologic challenge is created by grouping such heterogeneity together under one rubric, as is discussed throughout this chapter.

Several conferences on the epidemiology of cerebral palsy have debated diagnostic criteria ("what is a case?") and how best to describe motor handicap to enable international epidemiologic comparisons (Evans et al., 1986, 1989). Although most cerebral palsy surveys have excluded known congenital malformation complexes and genetic syndromes of which the motor dysfunction is only a part, others have included such defects as hydrocephalus, particularly that after intracranial hemorrhage (secondary), and other primary intracerebral malformations. Most studies identify those cases of obvious postneonatal origin that occur in children whose development was normal and in whom a well-documented postnatal brain-damaging insult, such as an accident or infection, preceded the motor disorder (Stanley & Blair, 1984). When, however, the interest in cerebral palsy is in identifying perinatal and antenatal causes or relating occurrence to medical care, the latter group of children are usually excluded. Yet, they are important to keep in mind because those cases are the most preventable of all the cerebral palsies.

Although these variable diagnostic criteria may seem unsatisfactory from the point of view of comparing prevalence data from different studies or over time, the majority of cases have no known cause or are thought to be of perinatal origin. Furthermore, many studies attempt to identify all those cases of motor handicap of cerebral origin that are diagnosed in early life, irrespective of the cause.

Patterns of Occurrence

The rate of cerebral palsy is usually calculated per 1000 live births or neonatal survivors (see Chapter 3). This suggests that this rate be viewed as an incidence

Table 17.1. Heterogeneity of the Cerebral Palsies

Motor (clinical) entities
Site
Type
Severity
Presence of other handicaps
Neuropathologic entities
Site of lesion
Type of lesion
Timing of "damage"/defect
Early pregnancy
Late pregnancy
Intrapartum
Postnatal
Putative cause
Inherited
Metabolic
Infection
Cerebrovascular
Asphyxia
Other

rate because it covers new cases diagnosed in a birth cohort (Paneth & Kiely, 1984). However, as the usual method of data collection for cerebral palsy is to ascertain the number of cases prevalent in a population of a certain age and to relate this number to the population of births, the rate is best viewed as a prevalence figure, i.e., the rate of cerebral palsy at a certain age per 1000 live births or neonatal survivors (see Chapter 1). For cohorts that are followed closely from birth and in which all new cases of cerebral palsy are identified, including those who die and those whose motor handicap is not permanent—as with certain high-risk groups, for example, low birthweight babies—the rates are more like true cumulative incidence rates. However, even these rates exclude fetuses and infants with possibly similar pathology who die in utero or in early postnatal life and who might have developed a motor disability had they survived. Thus, we suggest that "prevalence" is the best expression for rates in a birth cohort. If a comparison is being made of trends over time, how the data were collected, inclusions and exclusions, and how complete the ascertainment was thought to be should be stated. Better ascertainment may masquerade as increases in cerebral palsy rates.

The risk of cerebral palsy is best calculated per 1000 neonatal *survivors*, thereby excluding neonatal deaths from the denominator because they are not at risk for the outcome (see Chapter 1). The exclusion of deaths only makes a significant difference in low birthweight categories, where neonatal deaths are high. The denominator generally used in the studies reviewed here was live births and because neonatal death rates were seldom presented, it was not possible to calculate survival rates for all studies.

International Comparisons

Data on the frequency of cerebral palsy were published in a review by Paneth and Kiely (1984) of population studies in industrialized nations between 1950 and 1983. The rates of cerebral palsy per 1000 live births varied between 1 and 4. Most rates were between 2 and 3 per 1000. A preponderance of these reports were from Europe, particularly Scandinavia, with only one study from the United States. Approximately 10% of cases were estimated to be due to postneonatal events.

If the data collections had been ongoing from birth and had included early deaths among those already described as having cerebral palsy and those in whom motor impairment had resolved, a cumulative incidence rate would have been obtained that would have been considerably higher. This has since been confirmed by reports from northern Finland (Rantakallio & von Wendt, 1985, 1986) based on a regular follow-up of a complete cohort of births in two provinces to the age of 14 years. Of 12,058 live births (96% of the total), only 14 could not be traced at this age, and all were children who had weighed more than 2500 g at birth and had emigrated out of Finland. Such isolated countries have obvious advantages when conducting epidemiologic studies of this nature. In this cohort 69 children were diagnosed as having cerebral palsy (5.7 per 1000 live births), and 57 of these were alive at age 14 (4.8 per 1000 live births). Postnatal causes were identified in 13, but removing these cases still results in a rate (3.6) that is higher than other population estimates for the same time period. Whether this higher rate is due to more thorough ascertainment methods or to a higher occurrence in this population cannot be determined, although contemporary rates in southwest Finland of 1.6 in 1968 to 1972 and 2.5 in 1978 to 1982 (Riikonen et al., 1989) tend to support the former explanation.

An earlier (1955) Finnish cohort (Amnell, quoted in Rantakallio & von Wendt 1985) also showed a rate of 5.9 per 1000 live births in 94% of children traced to 14 years. Data from the United States on birth cohorts from several areas between 1959 and 1963, with follow-ups at 1 and 7 years, also showed a rate of 5.2 per 1000 live births (Nelson & Ellenberg, 1978). Thus, the rate of cerebral palsy occurring in birth cohorts from the 1950s to the late 1970s varies depending on the method of follow-up and is at least 2 and possibly as high as 6 per 1000 live births.

Prevalence data published since 1983 relating to birth cohorts since 1970 are shown in Table 17.2. These rates should be compared with Table II in Paneth and Kiely (1984) because the methods of data collection usually do not include following a birth cohort throughout childhood. The rates from the most recent cohorts vary between 1.0 and 5 and thus are not too different from those published for earlier periods. It is worth noting, however, that major changes have occurred in maternal risk factors and obstetric and neonatal care over this time.

Few American studies have been published giving the population prevalence of cerebral palsy related to a live birth cohort (Paneth & Kiely, 1984). A 1978 survey of 97% of households in Copiah County, Mississippi (Haerer et al., 1984), identified 50 individuals with cerebral palsy among 23,842 residents (2.1 per 1000 people). Of these, nine cases were under 5 years—a prevalence rate of 3.7 per 1000 for birth cohorts 1972 to 1977. Cerebral palsy deaths before the

Table 17.2. Prevalence of Cerebral Palsy from Total Population Studies Published Since 1983

Country	Birth Cohort (years)	Age of Ascertainment (years)	Rate/1000* Live births
Sweden (Hagberg et al., 1989a)	1979–82	4	2.2
United Kingdom			
Mersey (Pharoah et al., 1987)	1982–84	>4	2.1
S.E. Thomas (Evans et al., 1985)	1970–74	>4	2.2
National (Edmond et al., 1989)	1970	7	2.5
Northeast England (Jarvis et al., 1985)	1960–75	5+	1.6
Finland (Riikonen et al., 1989)	1979–82	5+	2.5
Ireland (Dowding & Barry, 1988)	1976–81	4	1.7
Japan			
Tottori (Takeshita et al., 1989)	1975–80	3	1.2
	1981–84	3	1.2
Tokyo (Suzuki H, personal communication)	1980s	>4	2.0
Denmark (Holst et al., 1989)	1978	4	5.0
Western Australia (Stanley & Watson, 1988)	1975–78	5	1.9
	1979–82	5	1.98
	1983–85	5	2.2

*Cases with postneonatal cause excluded.

survey were not included, and those cases with a postneonatal cause were not listed separately for this age group.

A registry of moderate and severe cerebral palsy was established in California (Grether et al., 1991) for children born from 1983 to 1985. The prevalence by 3 years of age was 1.24 per 1000 live births. This is comparable to 1.23 per 1000 live births for similarly classified children in the same years in Western Australia (Watson & Stanley, unpublished data).

Temporal Trends

The trends in total cerebral palsy rates from three population-based registries and other total population data available from 1959 to 1985 are shown in Figure 17.1, from which it appears that the proportion of children with cerebral palsy has either remained steady or has risen. Western Australia (WA) had the highest rates and Japan the lowest, but ascertainment may vary in these surveys.

The stillbirth, neonatal death, and cerebral palsy proportions per 1000 from 1956 to 1985 for WA, with percentages of women delivered by cesarean section superimposed, are shown in Figure 17.2. Whereas the proportions of stillbirths and neonatal deaths have fallen between 1956 and 1985, cerebral palsy rates have remained steady. Cesarean section, electronic fetal monitoring, and in-

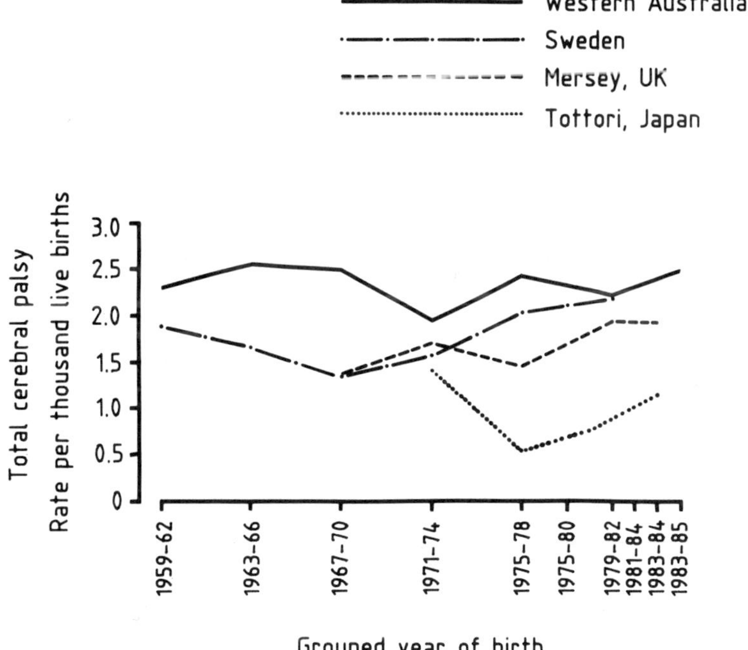

Fig. 17.1. Cerebral palsy rates per thousand live births from registries in Western Australia, Sweden, Mersey, United Kingdom, and Tottori, Japan, between 1959 and 1985 in grouped years (Hagberg et al., 1989a; Pharoah et al., 1990; Takeshita et al., 1989).

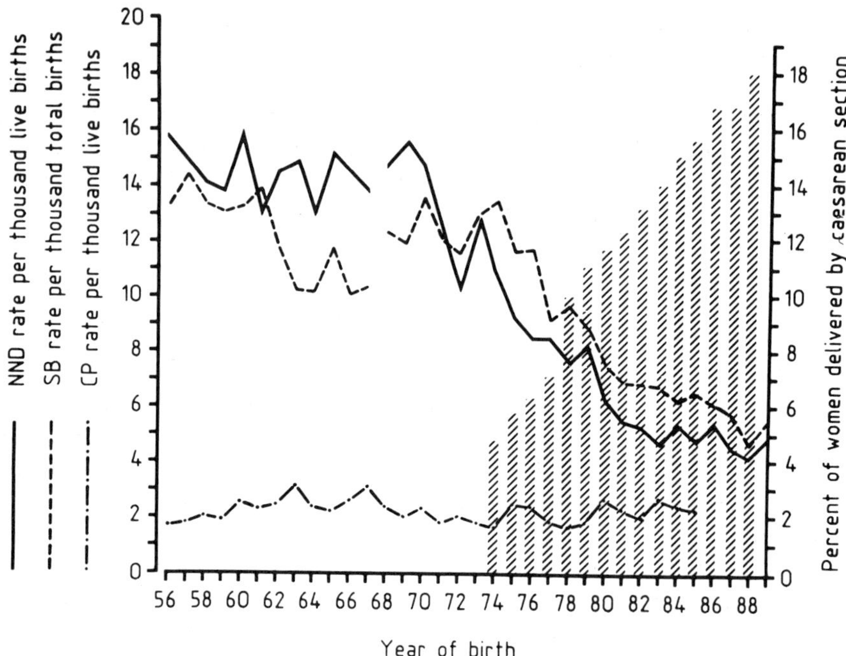

Fig. 17.2. Stillbirth, neonatal death, and cerebral palsy rates per thousand, 1956 to 1989, shown against the percentage of women having cesarean sections, 1980 to 1989, in Western Australia (Gee, 1990).

duction of labor for fetal distress—all aimed at reducing the adverse effects of birth asphyxia—were used more frequently during this time (Notzon, 1990; Read et al., 1990; Stanley & Watson, 1988).

Cerebral Palsy by Birthweight

Total cerebral palsy rates mask the recent significant increases in very low birthweight infants (see Chapter 3). This is because the proportion of all children with cerebral palsy of very low birthweight is still small, and these increases have made only a small contribution to the total rate. Furthermore, in some series there has been a coincident fall in the proportion of cerebral palsy among heavier babies.

The proportions of very low birthweight (<1500 g) cerebral palsy in three different populations are shown in Figure 17.3A as rates per 1000 live births and in Figure 17.3B as rates per 1000 neonatal survivors, with Sweden included (rates calculated by live births were not available for Sweden). The trends in WA are similar to those in Sweden and Liverpool. In the WA data, although there was no significant time trend for cerebral palsy rates, there were significant differences for the trend in the different birthweight groups, with highly significant increases in rates for survivors under 1500 g and no change in the rates over this weight. These patterns coincide with the increased survival of very low

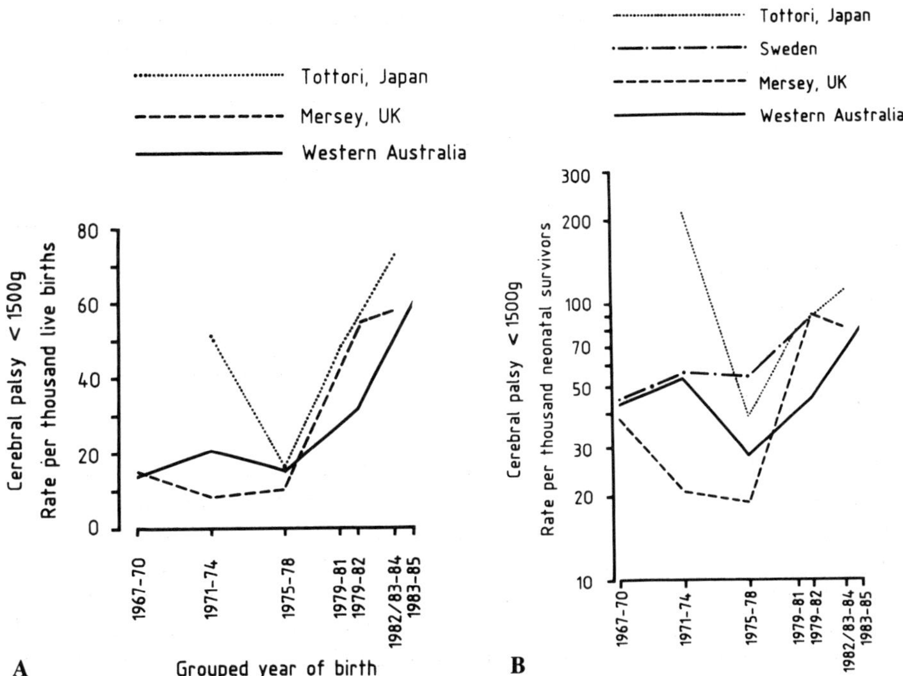

Fig. 17.3. A. Very low birthweight cerebral palsy (<1500 g) rates per thousand live births from registries in Western Australia, Mersey, United Kingdom, and Tottori, Japan, between 1967 and 1985 in grouped years (Pharoah et al., 1990; Takeshita et al., 1989). B. Very low birthweight cerebral palsy (<1500 g) rates per thousand neonatal survivors from registries in Western Australia, Sweden, Mersey, United Kingdom, and Tottori, Japan, between 1967 and 1985 in grouped years (Hagberg et al., 1989a; Pharoah et al., 1990; Takeshita et al., 1989).

birthweight infants over the same time period: in WA survival of babies under 1500 g rose from 20% in 1975 to 80% in 1985.

The risk of cerebral palsy rises as birthweight falls, and as more of these children survive, the numbers with cerebral palsy must also rise (Paneth et al. 1981). There have been gains as well as losses from the increased low birthweight survival from neonatal intensive care—gains in more low birthweight survivors who do not have cerebral palsy, as well as the observed increases in those with it (Hagberg et al., 1989b). Extrapolated figures for WA in Table 17.3 for under 1500 g infants show that in 1000 births there would be an additional 41 children with cerebral palsy and 359 survivors without cerebral palsy after the introduction of neonatal intensive care (Stanley & Blair, 1991).

Categories of Cerebral Palsy and Trends by Birthweight

The categorization of cerebral palsy syndromes into spastic hemiplegia, diplegia, quadriplegia, and other nonspastic syndromes is difficult and not often reliably reproducible (Blair & Stanley, 1985). There are quite marked differences in the rates of the different spastic syndromes, particularly quadriplegia or tetraplegia

Table 17.3. Extrapolated Number of Survivors with and without Cerebral Palsy Before and After Neonatal Intensive Care for Liveborn Infants with Birthweights of Less than 1500 g

	Before Neonatal Intensive Care, 1968–1971 (rate per 1000)	After Neonatal Intensive Care, 1982–1985 (rate per 1000)	Difference
No. who survived 28 days	325	725	+400
No. with cerebral palsy at 5 years of age	14	55	+41
No. of survivors without cerebral palsy	311	670	+359

Source: Data from Western Australia (Stanley & Blair, 1991).

in the Swedish, British, and Australian data. It seems that there have been increases in the rates of all spastic categories in very low birthweight infants. Early studies of these infants who subsequently were noted to have cerebral palsy reported that most had spastic diplegia that was often mild and not associated with significant other handicaps; in particular, they were often of normal intelligence (Hagberg et al., 1984; MacDonald, 1967). In the recent series quoted here, the rise in rates of cerebral palsies among infants of very low birthweight seems to be in all spastic syndromes and to be associated with multiple handicaps (sensory, intellectual, or epileptic) and with many being classified as severe (Hagberg et al., 1989a; Pharoah et al., 1990, Stanley & Blair, 1991). Recent neuropathologic studies of white matter necrosis among very low birthweight babies suggest a much broader distribution of necrosis beyond that in the periventricular region, with widespread involvement into the subcortex and elsewhere (Leviton & Paneth, 1990; Paneth et al., 1990).

Is this rise in cerebral palsy rates in low birthweight infants due only to the postnatal complications of prematurity, or is there a rising incidence due to the increased survival of antenatally brain-damaged infants? This question is of considerable import and not just of academic interest. If the increase is due to more infants surviving with antenatal brain damage or abnormal development who previously would have died, then there is little that neonatal intensive care can do to avoid this increase, and we must expect that these children will be born in increasing numbers. A reduced incidence may only result from knowledge about the antenatal causes of their CNS problems and by preventing them or from more accurate prognosis and selective nontreatment. If, however, the main reason for the rise is due to neonatal cerebral damage from complications of prematurity, then there is a possibility that different neonatal care practices could influence the occurrence of cerebral palsy in these infants.

Kitchen has expressed this dilemma eloquently:

> It is apparent that cerebral palsy is a widespread problem among very low birthweight and immature infants who graduate from modern intensive care units. We speculate that there may be a high rate of fetal aberration associated with the abnormal event of premature birth and that although modern perinatal care has a large impact on mortality there may be little influence on the occurrence of cerebral palsy. To accept this view absolves the perinatologists of

blame but is an anathema to those striving to improve outcome by ever more strenuous efforts to optimize care (Kitchen et al., 1987).

There is suggestive evidence of both antenatal and neonatal contributions to the rising rate of low birthweight cerebral palsy. Data from Liverpool (Cooke, 1991; Pharoah et al., 1990) suggest that antenatal factors are most important, whereas those from Sweden (Hagberg et al., 1989b) suggest that increases in neonatal complications of preterm birth, such as cerebral hemorrhage, are responsible. Figure 17.4 shows the numbers of stillbirths, neonatal deaths, neonatal survivors, and children with cerebral palsy in birth cohorts from 1975 to 1986 in WA (Stanley, 1992). The increase in low birthweight neonatal survival has come mainly from a decrease in neonatal mortality, but other contributing factors include a reduced number of stillbirths and an increase in the proportion of all live births of low birthweight—5.3% in 1975 to 5.9% in 1985. Both of these may have resulted from the earlier detection and delivery of at-risk fetuses.

Thus, the rise in cerebral palsy in low birthweight infants could be due to a combination of antenatal and perinatal problems in these children coincident with increased survival. Until we have better markers for antenatal brain damage, epidemiologic studies cannot contribute much more useful information to this important problem. Nevertheless, complete follow-up of all low birthweight

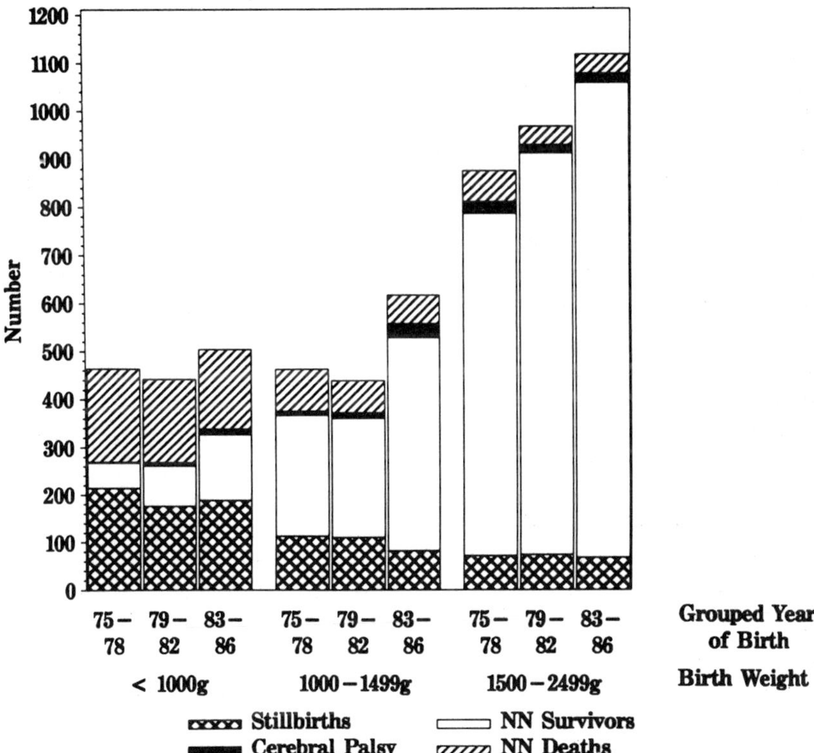

Fig. 17.4. Numbers of stillbirths, neonatal deaths, and cerebral palsy in low birthweight infants in Western Australia, 1975 to 1986, in grouped years (Stanley, 1992).

live births, with good documentation of possible brain-damaging events, remains very important (Wariyar & Richmond, 1989).

Escobar, Littenberg, and Pettiti (1991) reviewed 1136 studies in an attempt to summarize the international literature on low birthweight survival and neurologic handicap. Only 85 met their criteria for adequate methods with cerebral palsy as an outcome, and few of these were from the United States where neonatal intensive care is used more aggressively than elsewhere. They concluded that the best estimate of the rate of cerebral palsy in infants under 1500 g was 77 per 1000 (1960 to 1988), that there have been no changes over time, but that there were serious methodologic flaws in most studies. A later follow-up study from Liverpool of 761 under 1500 g survivors to 2 years from 1142 liveborn infants in 1980 to 1986 reported 81 children with cerebral palsy (70.9 per 1000 live births, 106.4 per 1000 neonatal survivors). Thus about 7% of these very low birthweight surviving infants can be expected to have a significant handicap, although it may be higher in the United States because more very low birthweight infants survive there than in those countries where most studies have been done.

Risk Factors

In searching for risk factors, it is important to stress again that the cerebral palsies comprise many disability syndromes, and in describing a single risk factor profile we may dilute relationships that exist for individual syndromes. The difficulty for epidemiologists working with data from one population, such as the WA or Swedish registers, is that the numbers of any one definable syndrome—for example, spastic diplegia in preterm infants—are too small to investigate properly. Consequently, data are pooled between centers to overcome this problem and to look for etiologic and clinical patterns in larger numbers of cases. When doing such combined analyses, it is important to be aware that criteria and descriptions of each syndrome may differ between observers, as mentioned earlier, and methods may need to be developed to overcome this problem.

Little (1862) and Freud (1968) both described the "syndromes" of diplegia in preterm infants and "rigidity" or spastic quadriplegia with dyskinesia in term asphyxiated infants (Ingram, 1984). Since then, many have tried to relate the clinical picture to antenatal and perinatal risk factor profiles. Hagberg summarized the patterns for the main motor syndromes observed in the 681 Swedish cases born from 1959 to 1976 in their population register (Hagberg & Hagberg, 1984). They wrote, "Our analyses have revealed a large degree of complexity and overlaps of causation both between and within the various (motor) syndromes. However, some general features can be distinguished." These are summarized in Table 17.4.

Since 1976 there have been dramatic changes in the survival of very low birthweight infants and significant increases in the use of obstetric interventions to reduce birth asphyxia. Have these been reflected in changing profiles of cerebral palsy subtypes? In the most recent Swedish data (Hagberg et al., 1989a), increases were observed in both term and preterm cerebral palsy rates, but particularly in the latter. They found that these preterm cerebral palsy children

Table 17.4. Summary of Features of Cerebral Palsy Syndromes from the Swedish Survey of 681 Cases Born 1959 to 1967

Hemiplegia	
	75% term—most antenatal predisposition/cause
	25% preterm—some antenatal predisposition/cause
Diplegia	
	50% term—antenatal cause
	50% preterm—most very low gestations; periventricular leukomalacia
Tetraplegia	
	100% term—similar to severe term diplegia
Dyskinesia	
	75% term—majority perinatal, severe birth asphyxia; some antenatally predisposed
	25% preterm—some very preterm with perinatal complications

Source: Data from Hagberg & Hagberg (1984).

were more intellectually disabled and had more severe motor handicaps than low birth-weight survivors in earlier epochs.

> Our previous statement that the average preterm CP child is mildly diplegic, with a rather discrete motor disability, normally gifted or only slightly dull, no longer holds. Certainly the main neurologic pattern (i.e., diplegia) still applies to infants born in the period 1979–82, but a shift toward more cases with additional mental retardation, epilepsy, infantile hydrocephalus, and marked motor disability has now taken place (Hagberg et al., 1989a).

Table 17.5 shows the most frequently occurring motor subtypes with their gestational age, birthweight, and gender descriptions for the two most recent time periods in WA. The birthweight and gestational age patterns for spastic hemiplegia have not changed significantly, whereas for the other spastic syndromes those recorded as preterm have increased, and dramatically so for spastic quadriplegia. The mean birthweight has fallen for all spastic categories, and the proportions classified as intrauterine growth retarded and preterm have also risen. The numbers of dyskinetic cases are too small to merit comment. Thus, these changes reflect an increase in growth-retarded (? antenatally damaged) and preterm spastic cerebral palsy. Unfortunately, differences in classification between the Swedish and WA data make other comparisons between Tables 17.4 and 17.5 difficult.

Sex

An excess of males with cerebral palsy has been noted in most studies and is still obvious in WA data, although this pattern does seem to be changing, with more females affected in recent cohorts (Table 17.6). This pattern is interesting and may offer some clues to causation. There are many possible reasons for a male excess, which have been reviewed in earlier reports (Ounsted & Taylor, 1972; Stanley, 1984). We have conducted an epidemiologic study of spastic quadriplegia in WA to investigate genetic and other reasons for the increased

Table 17.5. Summary of Features of Cerebral Palsy Syndromes from Western Austrialian Cerebral Palsy Register Cases Born 1976 to 1980 and 1981 to 1985

Features	1976–80		1981–85	
	Hemiplegia			
	N = 69		N = 86	
% term	60.9		65.1	
% preterm	34.8		34.9	
	Term	Preterm	Term	Preterm
Mean BW(g)	3387	1730	3313	1674
Mean GA (wks)	39.5	31.1	39.6	31.3
% males	64.3	50.0	50.0	56.7
% IUGR	14.0	12.0	14.0	14.0
	Diplegia			
	N = 68		N = 64	
% term	55.9		42.2	
% preterm	42.7		57.8	
	Term	Preterm	Term	Preterm
Mean BW(g)	3188	1828	3168	1473
Mean GA (wks)	39.6	32.5	39.3	30.3
% males	57.9	72.4	48.1	51.4
% IUGR	17.3	17.3	17.2	25.0
	Quadriplegia			
	N = 21		N = 42	
% term	85.7		59.5	
% preterm	14.3		40.5	
	Term	Preterm	Term	Preterm
Mean BW(g)	3203	1770	3196	1598
Mean GA (wks)	39.2	32.2	39.6	30.8
% males	100.0	66.7	56.0	58.8
% IUGR	21.7	4.4	11.9	16.7
	Dyskinesia			
	N = 15		N = 22	
% term	86.7		95.5	
% preterm	13.3		4.5	
	Term	Preterm	Term	Preterm
Mean BW(g)	3018	1400	3288	1715
Mean GA (wks)	39.7	30.5	39.5	32.0
% males	38.5	0 (n=0)	38.1	100.0 (n=1)
% IUGR	23.5	0 (n=0)	13.6	4.6 (n=1)

Abbreviations: BW = birthweight; GA = gestational age; IUGR = intrauterine growth retardation.

male occurrence (Stanley et al., unpublished data). No obvious chromosomal, metabolic, perinatal risk factors, or patterns of structural brain lesions accounted for the male excess. More males than females were severely affected and had dysmorphic features suggestive of an antenatal influence.

Intrauterine Growth Retardation

Several papers have investigated the relationship between poor growth in utero and cerebral palsy. Until recently the literature on the contribution of intra-

Table 17.6. Total Cerebral Palsy and Spastic Syndromes by Gender in Western Australia, 1982 to 1985

		All CP		Hemiplegia		Diplegia		Quadriplegia	
		Male	Female	Male	Female	Male	Female	Male	Female
1982	No.	24	16	9	7	5	5	5	3
	%	60.0	40.0	56.3	43.8	50.0	50.0	62.5	37.5
1983	No.	27	24	9	10	10	6	5	2
	%	52.9	47.1	47.4	52.6	62.5	37.5	71.4	28.6
1984	No.	24	24	8	8	4	5	6	6
	%	50.0	50.0	50.0	50.0	44.4	55.6	50.0	50.0
1985	No.	20	31	3	11	7	11	6	4
	%	39.2	60.8	21.4	78.6	38.9	61.1	60.0	40.0

uterine growth retardation (IUGR) to cerebral palsy suffered from methodologic problems, notably the validity of the measurement itself, with resulting misclassification of the exposure. Population data are needed to accurately classify newborns as growth retarded, and growth charts need to be specific for important nonpathologic factors that affect fetal growth, such as infant gender, maternal parity, height, and race. Including data from preterm births in the creation of growth charts is a problem because infants delivered prematurely are not likely to be a morphologically representative sample of all infants of that gestation. Inaccuracies in gestational estimates are still a problem, although more pregnancies are now being dated by early ultrasound.

The odds ratios (see Chapter 1) for spastic cerebral palsy by percent of expected birthweight (a measure of being small for gestational age) from the WA data are shown in Figure 17.5 (Blair & Stanley, 1990). The percent of expected birthweight was calculated by multiplying birthweight by 100% and dividing by expected birthweight. Expected birthweight was taken as the median birthweight of WA liveborn, white, singleton population of the same gestation, sex, maternal height, and parity. A strong association of spastic cerebral palsy with decreasing expected birthweight is shown. However, the relationship between odds ratios and birthweight percentiles varied with gestation of delivery. In term infants (>37 weeks) there was a significant inverse relationship only below the 10th percentile. In moderately preterm infants (34 to 37 weeks), the relationship was stronger and continued across all percentiles; whereas for more premature infants (≤33 weeks) the weaker inverse relationship observed could have been due to chance.

Table 17.7 shows that 18.5% of term cases and 47.7% of cases born at 34 to 37 weeks could be attributed to some correlate of their being below the 10th percentile for birthweight and that the majority of these attributed cases were below the 3rd percentile birthweight. These data agree with recent studies from Sweden (Uvebrant, 1988) on the importance of growth retardation in cerebral palsy. The mechanism may be a direct effect—the factor causing the growth retardation may also influence the developing brain or interfere with neuronal migration. Or it may be that intrauterine growth retardation makes the infant more vulnerable to the effects of other influences. It could even be that intrauterine growth retardation is the result of a cerebral palsied fetus not moving

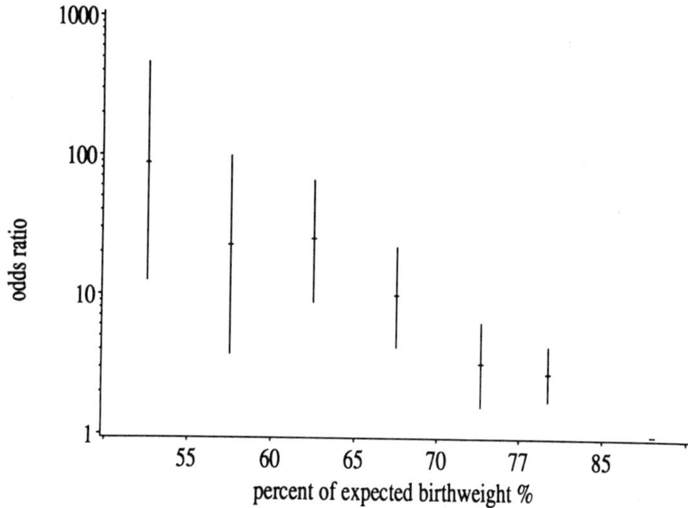

Fig. 17.5. Odds ratios and 95% confidence intervals against small-for-gestational-age cases belonging to the normal birthweight distribution compared with cases >85% of expected birthweight (equivalent to >10th percentile birthweight) (Blair & Stanley, 1990).

or growing well in utero. The association demands further investigation and certainly supports the need to pursue antenatal risk factors.

Birth Asphyxia

The relationship between intrapartum asphyxia and later cerebral palsy has received more attention since 1984 than any other risk factor. It was then still widely assumed that children with cerebral palsy developed their handicap because of birth asphyxia, which may have been prevented by better intrapartum care (Hey, 1985; Paneth et al., 1981). Overestimation of the risk of impairment from intrapartum problems and obstetric mismanagement may have led to the inappropriate use of some obstetric interventions or at least justified their increasing use (Editorial, 1989). In the 1970s proponents of intrapartum electronic fetal monitoring suggested that "early recognition and elimination of fetal distress should reduce, by half, the incidence of handicapping conditions or mental

Table 17.7. Percent of Spastic Cerebral Palsy Attributable to Being Small for Gestational Age

		Percentile Birthweight		
Gestational age (weeks)	No.	<3rd	3–10th	All <10th
>37	101	11.3	7.2%	18.5
34–37	34	35.8	11.9%	47.7
<34	34	2.9	1.7%	4.6

Source: From Blair & Stanley (1990).

retardation" (Quilligan & Paul, 1975). As recently as 1988 parents were still being promised a perfect baby (Amiel-Tison et al., 1988). Courts of law have interpreted those aspects of Little's paper that describe the association of birth problems and later cerebral palsy (Little, 1862) in awarding damages to affected children, even though his observations are now 130 years old and possibly out of date! Such litigation in the United States, and more recently in the United Kingdom and Australia, is having adverse effects on both obstetric care and the obstetric profession (Shearer, 1986).

If major reductions in the occurrence of cerebral palsy were to follow the increased use of obstetric intervention in labor, it would follow that cerebral palsy must be frequently caused by intrapartum events that can be prevented by such interventions (Stanley & Blair, 1991). Evidence is now available from several types of studies that suggests that (1) birth asphyxia may not be as important a cause of cerebral palsy as previously thought; (2) neonatal signs of birth asphyxia, such as difficulty in initiating and maintaining respiration, and abnormal neonatal neurologic signs including seizures may be early manifestations of cerebral palsy from a variety of causes, of which birth asphyxia is only one; (3) infants with birth asphyxia and neurologic damage may not, even with alternative obstetric care, have fared better, and (4) the majority of children with cerebral palsy probably had some antenatal insult or condition that either was the cause of their handicap or made them particularly vulnerable to birth events (Blair & Stanley, 1988; Ellenberg & Nelson, 1988; Freeman & Nelson, 1988; Nelson & Ellenberg, 1981, 1984, 1986; Peters et al., 1984; Stanley & Blair, 1991).

The various sequences that could result in cerebral palsy are illustrated in Figure 17.6. Most researchers believe that it is important to separate term and preterm infants in the study of the relationship between birth asphyxia and cerebral palsy. Many more preterm infants have markers of perinatal asphyxia than term infants, and the association of asphyxia with cerebral palsy is weaker among preterm than term infants (Blair & Stanley, 1988).

The study of birth asphyxia poses problems for epidemiologists specifically because possible confounding factors (gestational age and other morbidity) and the low incidence of outcome (cerebral palsy) demand a large sample size and

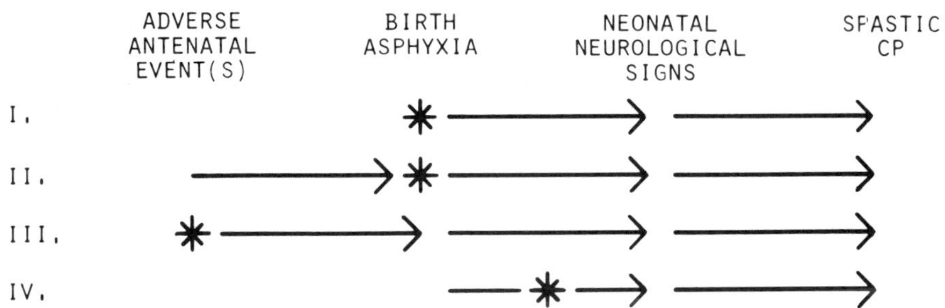

Fig. 17.6. Routes to brain damage.

because there is often selection bias in the populations studied (see Chapter 1). It challenges all researchers because there is no direct measure of oxygenation of cerebral tissue in humans, and thus a variety of secondary measures of questionable accuracy are used. Positron emission tomography measures metabolic changes and neuronal death, but can currently only be used on very small numbers of children (J Wyatt, personal communication).

Cohort studies would provide the best data on the relationship between asphyxia and cerebral palsy, but there are few large enough to examine cerebral palsy alone. Instead, innumerable studies have followed up selected populations of low birthweight infants (Escobar et al., 1991), but few involve heavier infants, with and without asphyxia, to ascertain the respective contributions to cerebral palsy. Table 17.8 shows data from the U.S. Collaborative Perinatal Project, a cohort study of 50,000 births from 1959 to 1963 from a large number of hospitals (Ellenberg and Nelson, 1988). Although the data are now old, they are still the best cohort data available to address the association between birth asphyxia and cerebral palsy. The relationship between low Apgar score (<5 at 5 minutes), neonatal signs (i.e., decreased activity after the first day of life, need for incubator care > 3 days, feeding problems, poor suck, or respiratory difficulties), newborn seizures, and later cerebral palsy is well demonstrated. However, most cases of cerebral palsy (62.7%) occurred in the group of children without any perinatal signs. The highest risk for cerebral palsy (545.5 per 1000) was in the very small proportion of children (0.06%) with all three early characteristics. Neonatal neurologic signs, particularly seizures, were good predictors of cerebral palsy, but even these occurred in only 36% (13.3 + 2.7 + 4.0 + 16.0) of all cases. The most likely explanation for the strong associations is that these neonatal signs are early manifestations of cerebral palsy, rather than being indicative of perinatal damage per se. The majority of the cases with signs suggestive of

Table 17.8. Predicted Risk of Cerebral Palsy (CP), Percent of Population in Each Risk Group, and Percent of CP Contributed by Perinatal Characteristics, 1959 to 1963 Births, United States

Early Characteristics					
Low Apgar Score	Neonatal Signs	Newborn Seizures	Predicted Risk* CP/1000	Children in Risk Group (%)	Cases of CP in Risk Group (%)
–	–	–	1.3	90.1	62.7
+	–	–	2.9	0.9	1.3
–	–	+	1.3	0.06	0.0
+	–	+	2.9	0.01	0.0
–	+	–	3.2	8.1	13.3
+	+	–	7.0	0.7	2.7
–	+	+	96.8	0.08	4.0
+	+	+	545.5	0.06	16.0

*Predicted risk based on multiple logistic model with Apgar score, presence or absence of neonatal signs, or newborn seizures and their interactions as predictor variables. An Apgar score was considered low if <5 at 5 minutes. Neonatal signs were decreased activity after the first day of life, need for incubator care >3 days, feeding problems, poor suck, or respiratory difficulties.

Source: From Ellenberg & Nelson (1988).

newborn encephalopathy were not born after complicated deliveries in which intrapartum asphyxia had been diagnosed, and many had antenatal factors that could have been implicated in their brain damage. Nelson and Ellenberg (1986) suggest that less then 10% of these cases of cerebral palsy were due to birth asphyxia, and asphyxia tended to be severe and prolonged.

Susser et al. (1985) reviewed a large body of data and estimated that 25% of cerebral palsy may be attributable to perinatal asphyxia. However, they acknowledged that this ignored the probable antenatal factors contributing to perinatal problems.

Case-control studies also have been used because of the expense of large cohort studies (see Chapter 1). However, they present challenges to the epidemiologist who must attempt to identify birth asphyxia retrospectively from hospital records, with most cases not having cord blood or other blood gas studies performed and, at best, using markers of asphyxia that are imprecise and can also result from a variety of other perinatal or antenatal problems. These are the same data that litigation lawyers and expert witnesses employ in cases coming to courts of law.

Table 17.9 lists the markers for birth asphyxia usually available to epidemiologists and illustrates their inadequacies in relation to low buffer base levels in the umbilical artery, which is perhaps the best available measure of fetal cerebral tissue oxygenation (Low, 1990). There has been considerable literature suggesting that the best of these markers is the presence of early neonatal seizures (Brann, 1985; Grant, 1987; Minchom et al., 1987). Most of these markers for birth asphyxia are, however, poor predictors of later cerebral palsy (Dijxhoorn et al, 1985; Freeman & Nelson, 1988; Lumley, 1988; Ruth & Raivio, 1988), and the majority of children with cerebral palsy did not have any of these signs in the neonatal period (Blair & Stanley, 1988; Nelson & Ellenberg, 1986). Although neonatal seizures are strongly related to cerebral palsy, it is obvious from Table 17.9 that many infants with seizures did not have low buffer base levels and that many infants with low buffer base levels did not have seizures or other signs of newborn encephalopathy. Thus, many of the measures that describe poor condition at birth may reflect factors other than birth asphyxia.

Table 17.10 shows the WA data (Blair & Stanley, 1988). Of 183 cases of spastic cerebral palsy (all cases from the register over a 6-year period), two thirds (124, or 67.8%) had no perinatal problems. Of the remainder (59), 30 had

Table 17.9. Adequacy of Markers of Fetal/Birth Asphyxia Compared with Umbilical Artery Buffer Base <34 mmol/L

	Sensitivity (%)	False Positive (%)
Late decelerations FHR	50	>50
Moderate/severe meconium	32	95
Apgar score 0–3 at 1 minute	46	84
Apgar score 0–3 at 5 minutes	8	73
NE* severe	23	79

*Defined as seizures and recurrent apnea.

Source: From Low (1990).

Table 17.10. Estimation of Birth Asphyxia or Trauma Having Caused the Brain Damage in Children with Spastic Cerebral Palsy

	Estimation*				
Birth Status	1	2	3	4	All
No birth asphyxia or newborn encephalopathy	92	0	0	0	92
Birth asphyxia but no newborn encephalopathy	32	0	0	0	32
Newborn encephalopathy but no birth asphyxia	22	5	3	0	30
Both birth asphyxia and newborn encephalopathy	10	7	3	9	29
Total	156	12	6	9	183

*1 = definitely not, 2 = most unlikely, 3 = possible, 4 = very likely.

Source: From Blair & Stanley (1988).

abnormal neurologic signs at birth, but no clinical evidence of birth asphyxia (fetal distress, low Apgar scores, prolonged time to breathe) and thus may well have had neurologic signs as the first clinically observed indication of earlier brain damage. And, of the 29 with signs of birth asphyxia and abnormal neonatal neurology, in only 12 was there a definite or possible chance that the cerebral palsy may have resulted from intrapartum factors. Accordingly, a total of 8.2% were assessed (by two independent observers) as having been likely to have had brain damage from birth asphyxia. In cerebral palsy cases who apparently experience asphyxia, it is impossible to assess whether it could have been avoided and thus whether such avoidance would have prevented the cerebral palsy. It is interesting that in one case whose cerebral palsy was ascribed as most likely due to birth asphyxia in the above study (category 4 in Table 10), a later pedigree study showed a dominant genetic disorder (Blair et al., 1992). There are those who argue strongly that Freud's theory may well be the more relevant and that these children show signs of asphyxia because they are already damaged or abnormal (Pharoah et al., 1990). Abnormal neonatal neurologic signs or newborn encephalopathy may also be an early manifestation of (already existing) cerebral palsy, rather than an indicator of birth asphyxia. "Determining the precise role of a specific asphyxia-related variable in the causal sequence leading to cerebral palsy will require more extensive analysis of its relation to antecedent factors" (Paneth, 1986).

Obstetricians should accept that they can only promise perfection at the end of labor if there is perfection at the beginning. Few of the trials of interventions to reduce birth asphyxia, specifically those involving electronic fetal monitoring (Lumley, 1988), have included follow-up to the age when cerebral palsy can be diagnosed confidently. Those that have (Grant et al., 1989), although showing a significant reduction in neonatal seizures, did not demonstrate any difference in cerebral palsy rates. The implication is that monitoring can reduce birth asphyxia as measured by seizures, but not cerebral palsy, and thus few cases of cerebral palsy seem to be related to birth asphyxia.

Antenatal Factors

Determining the relationship between the occurrence of an event in pregnancy and the diagnosis of a cerebral palsy syndrome, which may not be until the child is 4 or 5 years old, presents many epidemiologic challenges. Most authors agree that the majority of full-term cerebral palsy children without obvious intrapartum or postnatal events probably experienced their "brain-damaging" event antenatally. A large number of individually rare occurrences causing cerebral palsy have been documented, including genetic syndromes with obvious monogenic inheritance of motor handicap (Blair et al., 1992), the antenatal death of a co-twin (Melnick, 1977; Szymonowicz et al., 1986), and the presence of intrauterine viral infection (Stanley et al., 1986). Iodine deficiency (Pharoah et al., 1971) and exposure to methyl mercury in pregnancy (Amin-Zaki et al., 1979; Murakami, 1972) suggest that chemical teratogenesis may also be a mechanism in some cases. Monreal (1985) compared 62 families of children with cerebral palsy in his neurology practice with 62 families of children with headaches, 62 with school or behavior problems, and 62 randomly selected normal children. The families of the cerebral palsy children reported more relatives with cerebral palsy, mental retardation, or seizures compared with controls. Problems with such studies include biased family histories because those with problems are better informed of problems in their families than are control families. Some recent research observed that children with cerebral palsy have more non cerebral malformations and dysmorphic features than matched controls, suggesting that antenatal maldevelopment may have occurred more frequently in cases than controls (Miller, 1989). There are excellent reviews of abnormalities of neuronal migration that would fit the pattern seen in cerebral palsy, but the challenge is to be able to study them in human populations (Barth, 1987; Sarnat, 1987). Several papers are now appearing using new and sophisticated forms of cerebral scanning; it will be most interesting to see how these contribute to the determination of timing and etiology of cerebral palsy in the future. The problems of inter- and intraobserver variation in interpretation of these scans is significant, but once they are addressed, it may be that clinicopathologic correlations can be described.

Interventions

Given the above review of the epidemiology of the cerebral palsies, it is clear that little further can be done currently to reduce the incidence of these severe motor handicaps and that present medical care is actually resulting in more survivors than before. Instead of halving the handicap rate and producing perfect babies (Amiel-Tison et al., 1988; Quilligan & Paul, 1975), increased use of electronic fetal monitoring and cesarean section has resulted in more litigation with adverse effects on obstetric care in the United States, United Kingdom, and Australia. We can only hope that as the rate of low birthweight cerebral palsy rises, neonatologists will not be similarly accused. Careful counseling of parents whose children are in neonatal intensive care units and the involvement of these parents in decisions about care, now normal practice in such units, may prevent litigation from becoming the frightening force it currently is in the practice of obstetrics.

Major reductions in cerebral palsy rates will only result from greater knowledge of their antenatal causes. Some causes may be related to preterm birth, but a decline in preterm birth will not necessarily reduce the incidence of cerebral palsy. It is clear that the evidence does not support that premise as yet. Further declines may result from better care of the preterm infant in neonatal intensive care units, particularly if neonatal care can reduce the incidence of intraventricular hemorrhage and serious infections in tiny babies.

The 10% of all cerebral palsy attributed to postneonatal events is the most "preventable" group because these cases are mostly due to infections, such as bacterial meningitis and viral encephalitis, accidental and nonaccidental head injury, and near drowning (Stanley et al., unpublished data). These are all tragedies that health promotion activities should target as priorities. The measures needed include vaccination to prevent maternal rubella infections in pregnancy (see Chapter 9), as well as infections in the first year of life, such as measles, along with measures to prevent injury and drownings.

Management

In the same way that the epidemiology of the cerebral palsies has been dominated by birth asphyxia and low birthweight survival, the management arena has been dominated by conductive education (Cottam & Sutton, 1986) and, more recently, by selective posterior rhizotomy (Cahan, 1988; Cahan et al., 1990). Both these new approaches—the first based on dedicated specialized physical and educational therapists, and the second on specialized and highly technical neurophysiology—seem promising. They have not, however, been put to rigorous evaluation by randomized controlled trials, and thus they remain experimental and are currently being used in an uncontrolled way. Because they are costly and their harmful effects as yet not evaluated, it is imperative that they are appropriately tested as soon as possible to avoid them becoming too far advanced to be evaluated properly, thereby delaying the detection of any adverse effects to the detriment of those with cerebral palsy.

Significant increases in the prevalence of cerebral palsy are now occurring due to both the increased survival of low birthweight infants and the longer lifespan of affected individuals. It is therefore important that more epidemiologic studies be conducted in conjunction with government personnel responsible for disability services to plan for the needs of young and older adults with cerebral palsy and to ensure that the laudable policy of encouraging these people to work and live in the community is supported adequately.

It will be most interesting to keep monitoring the trends in the cerebral palsies over the next decade, to observe progress made in unraveling the etiology of preterm births and their outcomes, and to monitor the levels of interventions in obstetrics, as knowledge about their limitations becomes more widespread.

Acknowledgments

We are grateful for the continued support of the Child Health Research Foundation of Western Australia (formerly the TVW Telethon Foundation for Medical Research), which has funded the WA Cerebral Palsy Register since 1979, and to Linda Watson for maintenance of Register data and assistance with all aspects of our cerebral palsy research.

References

Amiel-Tison C, Sureau C, Shnider SM. Cerebral handicap in full-term neonates related to the mechanical forces of labour. In: Patel N, guest ed. *Bailliere's Clinical Obstetrics and Gynaecology: International Practice and Research. Antenatal and Perinatal Causes of Handicap*. London: Bailliere Tindal; 1988; 2:145–166.

Amin-Zaki L, Majeed MA, Elhassani SB, Clarkson TW, Greenwood MR, Doherty RA. Prenatal methyl mercury poisoning. *Am J Dis Child* 1979; 133:172–177.

Barth PG. Disorders of neuronal migration. *Can J Neurol Sci* 1987; 14:1–16.

Bax M. Terminology and classification of cerebral palsy. *Dev Med Child Neurol* 1964; 6:295–297.

Blair E, Stanley FJ. Interobserver agreement in the classification of cerebral palsy. *Dev Med Child Neurol* 1985; 27:615–622.

Blair EM, Stanley FJ. Intrapartum asphyxia: a rare cause of cerebral palsy. *Pediatrics* 1988; 112:515–519.

Blair E, Stanley FJ. Intrauterine growth and spastic cerebral palsy. I: Association with birth weight for gestational age. *Am J Obstet Gynecol* 1990; 162:229–237.

Blair EM, Stanley FJ, Hockey A. Intrapartum asphyxia and cerebral palsy [letter]. *J Paediatr* 1992; 121:170–171.

Brann A. Factors during neonatal life that influence brain disorders. In: Freeman JM ed. *Prenatal and Perinatal Factors Associated with Brain Disorders*. Bethesda, MD: NIH Publication No. 85-1149; 1985:263–358.

Cahan LD. Selective dorsal rhizotomy for children with cerebral palsy. *Cont Neurosurg* 1988; 10:106.

Cahan LD, Adams JM, Perry J, Beeler LM. Instrumented gait analysis after selected dorsal rhizotomy. *Dev Med Child Neurol* 1990; 32:1037–1043.

Cooke RWI. Trends in preterm survival and incidence of cerebral haemorrhage 1980–9. *Arch Dis Child* 1991; 66:403–407.

Cottam PJ, Sutton A. *Conductive Education: A System for Overcoming Motor Disorder*. London: Croom Helm; 1986.

Dijxhoorn MJ, Visser GHA, Huisjes HJ, Fidler V, Touwen BCL. The relationship between umbilical pH values and neonatal neurological morbidity in full term appropriate-for-dates infants. *Early Hum Dev* 1985; 11:33–42.

Dowding VM, Barry CM. Cerebral palsy: changing patterns of birth weight and gestational age (1976/81). *Irish Med J* 1988; 81:25–29.

Editorial. Cerebral palsy, intrapartum care and a shot in the foot. *Lancet* 1989; 2:1251–52.

Ellenberg JH, Nelson KB. Cluster of perinatal events identifying infants at high risk for death or disability. *J Pediatr* 1988; 113:546–552.

Emond A, Golding J, Peckham C. Cerebral palsy in two national cohort studies. *Arch Dis Child* 1989; 64:848–852.

Escobar GJ, Littenberg B, Pettiti DB. Outcome among surviving very low birth weight infants: a meta-analysis. *Arch Dis Child* 1991; 66:204–211.

Evans P, Elliott M, Alberman E. Evans S. Prevalence and disabilities in 4 to 8 year olds with cerebral palsy. *Arch Dis Child* 1985; 60:940–945.

Evans P, Johnson A, Mutch L, Alberman E. Report of a meeting on the standardisation of the recording and reporting of cerebral palsy [letter]. *Dev Med Child Neurol* 1986; 28:547–548.

Evans P, Johnson A, Mutch L, Alberman E. A standard form for recording clinical findings in children with a motor deficit of central origin. *Dev Med Child Neurol* 1989; 31:119–127.

Freeman JM, Nelson KB. Intrapartum asphyxia and cerebral palsy [special articles]. *Pediatrics* 1988; 82:240–249.

Freud S. *Infantile Cerebral Paralysis*. Coral Gables, FL: University of Miami Press; 1968: 142 (Russiu LA, translator).

Gee V. *Perinatal Statistics in Western Australia*. Seventh Annual Report of the Western Australian Midwives' Notification System 1989. Perth: Health Department of Western Australia; 1990.

Grant A. The relationship between obstetrically preventable intrapartum asphyxia, abnormal neonatal neurological signs and subsequent motor impairment in babies born at or after term. In: Kubli F, Patel N, eds. *International Workshop on Perinatal Events and Cerebral Handicap*. Berlin: Springer-Verlag; 1987:149–159.

Grant A, O'Brien N, Joy M-T, Hennessy E, MacDonald D. Cerebral palsy among children born during the Dublin randomised trial of intrapartum monitoring. *Lancet* 1989; 2:1233–1235.

Grether JK, Cummins SK, Nelson KB. Cerebral palsy in California: a population-based registry. Abstract for American Academy for Cerebral Palsy and Development Medicine, Annual Meeting 1991. *Dev Med Child Neurol* 1991; 33(suppl 64):11.

Haerer AF, Anderson DW, Schoenberg BS. Prevalence of cerebral palsy in the biracial population of Copiah County, Mississippi. *Dev Med Child Neurol* 1984; 26:195–199.

Hagberg B, Hagberg G. Prenatal and perinatal risk factors in a survey of 681 Swedish cases. In: Stanley F, Alberman E, eds. *The Epidemiology of the Cerebral Palsies*. Spastics International Medical Publications, Clinics in Developmental Medicine, No. 87. Oxford: Blackwells Scientific Publications; 1984; 116–134.

Hagberg B, Hagberg G, Olow I. The changing panorama of cerebral palsy in Sweden. IV. Epidemiological trends 1959–78. *Acta Paediatr Scand* 1984; 73:443–440.

Hagberg B, Hagberg G, Olow I, von Wendt L. The changing panorama of cerebral palsy in Sweden. V. The birth year period 1979–82. *Acta Paediatr Scand* 1989a; 78:293–290.

Hagberg B, Hagberg G, Zetterstrom R. Decreasing perinatal mortality—increase in cerebral palsy morbidity? *Acta Paediatr Scand* 1989b; 78:664–670.

Hey E. Fetal hypoxia and subsequent handicap: the problem of establishing a causal link. In: Chamberlain GVP, Orr CJB, Sharp F, eds. *Litigation and Obstetrics and Gynaecology*. London: Royal College of Obstetricians and Gynaecologists; 1985; 233–242.

Holst K, Andersen E, Philip J, Henningsen I. Antenatal and perinatal conditions correlated to handicap among 4-year-old children. *Am J Perinatol* 1989; 6:258–267.

Ingram TTS. A historical review of the definition and classification of the cerebral palsies. In: Stanley F, Alberman E, eds. *The Epidemiology of the Cerebral Palsies*. Spastics International Medical Publications, Clinics in Developmental Medicine, No. 87. Oxford: Blackwells Scientific Publications; 1984; 1–11.

Jarvis SN, Holloway JS, Hey EN. Increase in cerebral palsy in normal birth weight babies. *Arch Dis Child* 1985; 60:1113–1121.

Kitchen WA, Doyle LW, Fox GW, Rickards AL, Lissenden JV, Ryan MM. Cerebral palsy in very low birth weight infants surviving to 2 years with modern perinatal intensive care. *Am J Perinatol* 1987; 4:29–35.

Leviton A, Paneth N. White matter damage in preterm newborns—an epidemiologic perspective. *Early Hum Dev* 1990; 24:1–22.

Little WJ. On the influence of abnormal parturition, difficult labours, premature birth and asphyxia neonatorum, on the mental and physical condition of the child, especially in relation to deformities. *Trans Obstet Soc* 1862; 3:293–344.

Low JA. The significance of fetal asphyxia in regard to motor and cognitive deficits in infancy and childhood. In: Tejani N, ed. *Obstetrical Events and Development Sequelae*. Boca Raton: CRC Press; 1990; 43–58.

Lumley J. Does continuous intrapartum fetal monitoring predict long-term neurological disorders? *Pediatr Perinat Epidemiol* 1988; 2:299–307.

MacDonald AD. *Children of Very Low Birth Weight*. MEIU Monograph No. 1. London: Spastics Society with Heinemann; 1967.

Melnick M. Brain damage in survivor after in-utero death in monozygous co-twin [letter]. *Lancet* 1977; 2:1287.

Miller G. Minor congenital anomalies and ataxic cerebral palsy. *Arch Dis Child* 1989; 64:557–562.

Minchom P, Niswander K, Chalmers I, Dauncey M, Newcombe R, Elbourne D, Mutch L, Andrews J, Williams G. Antecedents and outcome of very early neonatal seizures in infants born at or after term. *Br J Obstet Gynaecol* 1987; 94:431–439.

Monreal FJ. Consideration of genetic factors in cerebral palsy. *Dev Med Child Neurol* 1985; 27:325–330.

Murakami U. Organic mercury problems affecting intrauterine life. In: Klingberg MA, Abromovic A, Clark J, eds. *Drugs and Fetal Development*. Proceedings of an International Symposium on the Effects of Prolonged Drug Usage on Fetal Development. New York: Plenum Press; 1972.

Nelson K, Ellenberg JH. Epidemiology of cerebral palsy. *Adv Neurol* 1978; 19:421–435.

Nelson KB, Ellenberg JH. Apgar scores as predictors of chronic neurologic disability. *Pediatrics* 1981; 68:36–44.

Nelson KB, Ellenberg JH. Obstetric complications as risk factors for cerebral palsy or seizure disorders. *JAMA* 1984; 251:1843–1848.

Nelson KB, Ellenberg JH. Antecedents of cerebral palsy. Multivariate analysis of risk. *N Engl J Med* 1986; 315:81–86.

Notzon FC. International differences in the use of obstetric interventions. *JAMA* 1990; 263:3286–3291.

Ounsted C, Taylor DC (cds). *Gender Differences, Their Ontogeny and Significance*. Edinburgh: Churchill Livingstone; 1972.

Paneth N. Birth and the origins of cerebral palsy [editorial]. *N Engl J Med* 1986; 315:124–126.

Paneth N, Kiely JL. The frequency of cerebral palsy: a review of population studies in industrialised nations since 1950. In: Stanley F, Alberman E, eds. *The Epidemiology of the Cerebral Palsies*. Spastics International Medical Publications, Clinics in Development Medicine, No. 87. Oxford: Blackwells Scientific Publications; 1984; 46–56.

Paneth N, Kiely JL, Stein Z, Susser M. Cerebral palsy and newborn care. II: Estimated prevalence rates of cerebral palsy under differing rates of mortality and impairment of low birth weight infants. *Dev Med Child Neurol* 1981; 23:801–817.

Paneth N, Rudelli R, Monte W, Rodriquez E, Pinto J, Kairam R, Kazam E. White matter necrosis in very low birth weight infants: neuropathologic and ultrasonographic findings in infants surviving six days or longer. *J Pediatr* 1990; 116:975–984.

Peters TJ, Golding J, Lawrence CJ, Fryer JG, Chamberlain GVP, Butler NR. Delayed onset of regular respiration and subsequent development. *Early Hum Dev* 1984; 9:225–239.

Pharoah POD. The epidemiology of chronic disability in childhood. *Int Rehabil Med* 1985; 7:11–17.

Pharoah POD, Buttfield IH, Hetzel BS. Neurological damage to the fetus resulting from severe iodine deficiency during pregnancy. *Lancet* 1971; 1:308–310.

Pharoah POD, Cooke T, Cooke RWI, Rosenbloom I. Birth weight specific trends in cerebral palsy. *Arch Dis Child* 1990; 65:602–606.

Quilligan EJ, Paul RH. Fetal monitoring: is it worth it? *Obstet Gynecol* 1975; 45:96–100.

Rantakallio P, von Wendt L. Prognosis for low birth weight infants up to the age of 14: a population study. *Dev Med Child Neurol* 1985; 27:655–663.

Rantakallio P, von Wendt L. A prospective comparative study of the aetiology of cerebral palsy and epilepsy in a one-year birth cohort from Northern Finland. *Acta Paediatr Scand* 1986; 75:586–592.

Read AW, Waddell VP, Prendiville WJ, Stanley FJ. Trends in Caesarean section in Western Australia, 1980–1987. *Med J Aust* 1990; 153:318–323.

Riikonen R, Raumavirta S, Sinivuori E, Seppala T. Changing pattern of cerebral palsy in Southwest region of Finland. *Acta Paediatr Scand* 1989; 78:581–587.

Robinson R. Cerebral palsy. In: Eyre J, Boyd R, eds. *Paediatric Specialty Practice for the 1990s*. London: Royal College of Physicians; 1991:65–79.

Ruth VJ, Raivio KO. Perinatal brain damage: predictive value of metabolic acidosis and the Apgar score. *Br Med J* 1988; 297:24–27.

Sarnat HB. Disturbances of late neonatal migrations in the perinatal period. *Am J Dis Child* 1987; 141:969–90.

Shearer MH. When perinatal caregivers enter the insurance business. *Birth* 1986; 13:151–154.

Stanley FJ. Social and biological determinants of the cerebral palsies. In: Stanley FJ, Alberman E, eds. *The Epidemiology of the Cerebral Palsies*. Spastics International Medical Publications, Clinics in Developmental Medicine No. 87. Oxford: Blackwells Scientific Publications; 1984:69–86.

Stanley FJ. Survival and cerebral palsy in low birthweight infants: implications for perinatal care. *Paediatr Perinat Epidemiol* 1992; 6:298–310.

Stanley FJ, Alberman E. eds. *The Epidemiology of the Cerebral Palsies*. Spastics International Medical Publications, Clinics in Developmental Medicine, No. 87. Oxford: Blackwells Scientific Publications; 1984.

Stanley FJ, Blair EM. Postnatal risk factors in the cerebral palsies. In: Stanley F, Alberman E, eds. *The Epidemiology of the Cerebral Palsies*. Spastics International Medical Publications, Clinics in Developmental Medicine, No. 87. Oxford: Blackwells Scientific Publications; 1984:135–149.

Stanley FJ, Blair E. Why have we failed to reduce the frequency of cerebral palsy? *Med J Aust* 1991; 154:623–626.

Stanley FJ, Watson L. The cerebral palsies in Western Australia: trends 1968 to 1981. *Am J Obstet Gynecol* 1988; 158:89–93.

Stanley FJ, Sim M, Wilson G, Worthington S. The decline in congenital rubella syndrome in Western Australia: an impact of the school girl vaccination program? *Am J Pub Health* 1986; 76:35–39.

Susser M, Hauser WA, Kiely JL, Paneth N, Stein Z. Quantitative estimates of prenatal and perinatal risk factors for perinatal mortality, cerebral palsy, mental retardation and epilepsy. In: Freeman JM, ed. *Prenatal and Perinatal Factors Associated with Brain Disorders*. Bethesda, MD: NIH Publication No. 85-1149, 1985:359–439.

Szymonowicz W, Preston H, Yu VY. The surviving monozygotic twin. *Arch Dis Child* 1986; 61:454–458.

Takeshita K, Ando Y, Ohtani K, Takashima S. Cerebral palsy in Tottori, Japan. Benefits and risks of progress in perinatal medicine. *Neuroepidemiology* 1989; 8:184–192.

Uvebrant P. Hemiplegic cerebral palsy. Aetiology and outcome. *Acta Paediatr Scand* 1988, Suppl 345.

Wariyar UK, Richmond S. Morbidity and preterm delivery: importance of 100% follow-up [letter]. *Lancet* 1989; 1:387–388.

18

Prediction of Adult Disease

MICHAEL E.J. WADSWORTH

The notion that childhood provides the basis of the adult's intellectual and moral status is extremely old. However, with the exception of studies of height growth, the idea that the foundation of adult health is prepared in the early years of life has been slower to develop. In Britain the findings of the Boer War recruiting medical examinations (MacKenzie & Matthew, 1904) and the Interdepartmental Committee on Physical Deterioration (British Parliamentary Papers, 1904) raised anxieties about the health of the nation's young people. Although the outcome was of great value in terms of the public health care of mothers and infants (Dwork, 1987), the implications for epidemiologic studies of etiology were recognized much more slowly.

Since the early 1960s, however, epidemiologic studies of respiratory and cardiovascular health have begun to find long-term associations between health in childhood and in adult life. The intention of this chapter is to describe the development of questions asking whether there may be associations between early and adult health and to illustrate how the epidemiologic search for such associations has been carried out, commenting on the methods and the progress. Since this kind of epidemiologic work has been most consistent in studies of cardiovascular disease and lower respiratory illness, the chapter concentrates on those topics.

Heart Disease

Large Population Investigations Using Historical Sources

Northern European countries where national mortality records have been kept for long periods offer an opportunity to review long-term trends. English and Welsh data for the period 1845 to 1925, and Swedish data for 1751 to 1925, provide the first substantial evidence of the importance of child health and social circumstances for health in adult life. In their review of this information, Kermack et al. (1934) compared mortality rates throughout life for generations of children born during each specified period. They found that each generation carried a strikingly similar mortality risk profile from childhood into old age, with later-born generations carrying gradually less risk than those born at earlier times. These authors concluded that their findings were "consistent with the hypothesis that the death rates of the adolescent and adult depend on the constitution acquired during the first 15 years or so of life . . . as if the expectation of life was determined by the conditions which existed during the child's earlier years (Kermack et al., 1934).

This early work was developed further in later studies of both cardiovascular mortality and its risk factors. Using comparable sets of mortality data, the findings of Kermack et al. (1934) were further explored using Norwegian information for the period 1964 to 1967 (Forsdahl, 1977), English and Welsh information from 1937 to 1971 and from 1968 to 1978 (Williams et al., 1979), and data on deaths in 17 U.S. States between 1961 and 1971 (Buck & Simpson, 1982). It was surprising that in the years after World War II when standards of living had risen rapidly, these associations should still have been found. This led Forsdahl (1977) to conclude that the observed risk of death in adult life from arteriosclerotic heart disease, in populations born into poor socioeconomic circumstances, might be accounted for by their shift in adult life to relative affluence. He later added that raised cholesterol level caused by affluent living was possibly the process through which the observed association had its effect (Forsdahl, 1978). In the English and Welsh data, Williams et al. (1979) found that regions that had high infant mortality rates in the past, and in which social class differences in living standards persisted, were also those that currently had high mortality rates from ischemic heart disease. They therefore concluded that continuing risk was caused by continuing poverty, but they did not suggest a biologic process that might account for this relationship. The association of poverty with high mortality from heart disease was supported by finding a relationship in 17 U.S. states between high infant mortality from diarrhea and enteritis at ages 0 to 2 years in 1917 to 1921 and high adult mortality from arteriosclerotic heart disease in 1961 (at ages 40 to 44 years), and in 1971 (at ages 50 to 54 years; Buck & Simpson, 1982). These authors speculated that the observed association might be the result of the childhood infections facilitating the production of autoimmune complexes, which in turn promoted the later development of arteriosclerotic lesions. Alternatively, it was suggested that "breast feeding is the common denominator, protecting the infant against diarrhea on the one hand and, on the other, inducing enzymes that promote efficient metabolism of cholesterol not only in infancy but throughout adult life" (Buck & Simpson, 1982).

Barker and Osmond (1986a) extended the findings of Williams et al. (1979), also using national mortality data but in finer detail. They found that despite the general rise in ischemic heart disease mortality as prosperity increased, mortality for this cause remained highest in the least affluent districts. They showed a strong relationship between infant mortality rates in 1921 to 1925 and high adult ischemic heart disease mortality in the same districts in 1968 to 1978, noting that the adult rates were most strongly correlated with neonatal and postneonatal mortality. The areas that had had high infant mortality were also, at the time of the adult deaths, areas of "hard" water, high cigarette smoking, and high dietary fat consumption. Yet, these factors did not account for the observed relationship, which was concluded to be the result of adult susceptibility to the effects of an affluent diet among those poorly fed in childhood. Again, using English and Welsh national mortality data, Barker and Osmond (1987) noted a strong geographic correlation between past high maternal mortality and current death from stroke. In view of the established relationship between maternal mortality and poor maternal health and physique, Barker and Osmond (1987) suggested that the maternal influence on stroke risk might be mediated through maternal health: maternal hypertension, for example, is known to be associated with the risk of hypertension in offspring, which is in turn a risk for stroke.

Data on place of birth recorded for a trial period on English and Welsh death certificates were used to show that place of birth predicted the risk of ischemic heart disease and stroke (Osmond et al., 1990). Significantly increased risk of death from these diseases was found among those born in northern and industrial towns and in Wales, compared with a lower risk of these causes of death in those born in London and the surrounding areas. It was concluded that this study provided "further evidence that the environment in intrauterine life and early childhood has a larger effect on cardiovascular disease than has previously been supposed" (Osmond et al., 1990).

Retrospective Studies

In addition to demographic and vital statistical information, other historical sources have been ingeniously used to investigate the association of child health with adult health through the follow-up of individuals born at earlier times. By moving from the population to the individual level of investigation, considerable progress has been made.

In their study of early life and prenatal effects on adult blood pressure, Barker et al. (1989a) used data from birth records maintained in one English county from 1911 to 1930 to "catch up" in middle and later life with the same population's ischemic heart disease mortality, blood pressure, glucose tolerance, and lipid metabolism. They found that standardized mortality ratios from ischemic heart disease were increasingly reduced in relation to increasing weight at birth and, even more strongly, in relation to weight at 1 year. Heavier babies and those who were heaviest after the first year of life had the lowest risk of death from ischemic heart disease.

Barker et al. (1990) also located birth records from 1935 to 1943 for women admitted to a hospital in the north of England. The records contained information on the babies' birthweight, length, head circumference, and the weight of the placenta. This team again followed up a sample of the babies; 86% of singleton births to married women between 1935 and 1943 were traced, and of those still living in the county of birth, 89% (449) agreed to be visited. They found that the highest blood pressures and risk of hypertension were among people who had been small babies with large placentas. This relationship was independent of information on current alcohol consumption and body mass index and did not differ between birth orders or socioeconomic circumstances at birth or in adult life. It was argued that the intrauterine environment, through maternal nutrition, may have been the key to this association. The investigators suggested that poor maternal nutrition, both in pregnancy and before, could be estimated from their data using the mother's external conjugate diameter—the distance between the symphysis pubis and the fifth lumbar vertebrae. This diameter was lowest in those whose babies were subsequently of lowest birthweight; the greater the external conjugate diameter during pregnancy, the greater the subsequent birthweight. Short maternal stature was already known to be associated with low birthweight (Butler & Alberman, 1969; see Chapter 3). Mothers with poor nutritional status, it was argued, were at risk of greatest discordance of placental and fetal growth, which was found to be associated with a decrease in the ratio of babies' length to head circumference.

> This disproportionate growth is consistent with diversion of blood away from the trunk in favour of the brain. Reduced blood flow to the trunk induced in a fetus that is small in relation to its placenta could have irreversible consequences, perhaps by influencing arterial structure (Butler & Alberman, 1969).

Law et al. (1991) studied a population of 4-year-olds whose birth notes and mothers' obstetric notes were available. They found that low placental and birthweights, small head circumference, reduced length at birth, and possibly also reduced maternal hemoglobin were associated with higher blood pressure in the children. These findings of a relationship between neonatal size and later childhood blood pressure were in accordance with studies of adult blood pressure (Barker et al., 1992).

The two populations obtained from birth records and followed up in middle and later life were investigated further. Those who had grown least in infancy had the greatest adult vulnerability to coronary risk factors (Barker et al., 1992), and the greatest risk of a high adult waist/hip ratio was also associated with reduced growth before birth and during the first year of life (Law et al., 1992). Least growth in the first year of life was associated with relatively high adult mean plasma fibrinogen and factor VII concentrations, and among those whose placental weight was known, fibrinogen concentrations fell as the ratio of placental weight to birthweight decreased (Barker et al., 1992).

Again using a population obtained from birth records and first followed up in middle and later life, Fall et al. (1992) found that both prolonged breast feeding (longer than 1 year) and exclusive bottle feeding were associated with a significantly greater risk of death from ischemic heart disease. These feeding patterns were also significantly associated with higher serum total cholesterol, low-density lipoprotein cholesterol, and apolipoprotein β concentrations, but not with high-density lipoprotein, cholesterol, triglyceride, or apolipoprotein $\alpha 1$ concentrations. Although the authors concluded that a critical period of development may exist during which prolonged breast feeding or exclusive bottle feeding may partly determine the concentration of fibrinogen and factor VII, they offered no specific ideas on possible processes. Instead, they referred to demonstrations of such programming in animal studies. They also noted that exclusively breast-fed babies often develop low iron stores in the latter half of infancy and that breast milk may be vitamin deficient, particularly for vitamin D, if the mother is malnourished. These findings concur with the observation that among the long-term breast-fed group those with higher birthweights but lower weights at 1 year had increased death rates from ischemic heart disease.

A raised risk of impaired glucose tolerance and non-insulin-dependent diabetes was also found in these historically based catch-up study populations, significantly so among those who had low birthweight and relatively poor weight gain in the first year of life. Fetal and infant growth seemed "to protect against the deleterious effects of higher body mass in adult life, and conversely, . . . lower body mass protects against the deleterious effects of reduced early growth" (Hales et al., 1991). The authors proposed this working hypothesis:

> Diabetes is a consequence of poor nutrition during critical periods of fetal life and infancy, with consequent impaired development of β cell function. If poor nutrition continues, the reduced ability to produce insulin is not a disadvantage. It becomes so only if nutrition becomes abundant, when increased demand for insulin outstrips the capacity for production. . . . The long-term effects of poor nutrition during early life may depend on the nature, timing, and intensity of deprivation, which will determine the specific tissues in which development is impaired. This phenomenon may underlie several Western diseases other than diabetes, most importantly ischemic heart disease" (Hales et al., 1991).

Cross-Sectional and Prospective Studies

Several studies have sought evidence for differences in adult risk factors in populations of children; for example, in blood cholesterol concentrations, atherosclerotic plaque, and blood pressure. Labarthe (1992) concludes that such studies suggest that "children in populations with historically high rates of coronary mortality will tend to have higher levels of the risk factors than children in populations with historically low rates." The aspect of such risk most frequently investigated in epidemiologic studies of children has been tracking of blood pressure—that is, individual children who appear consistently in one part of the distribution of blood pressure measures. Findings from the Bogalusa longitudinal study of children reported evidence of tracking, and because they were "based on reliable, basal-like measurements, point to a high degree of persistence, and very likely establish a background for the early diagnosis of primary hypertension" (Levine et al., 1978). In this study Levine et al. (1978) reported that tracking began after age 6 months, but found "no evidence that hypertensive adults may be identified with any degree of certainty solely on the basis of casual blood pressure determinations during infancy or childhood." Similarly, Hofman et al. (1985) found that the predictive value of childhood blood pressure for later hypertension was not useful until after 15 years or later.

Many studies of tracking concentrate on its value as a predictor of the individual's later risk of hypertension, but pay less regard to the question of why tracking occurs. Studies of within-family similarity of blood pressure offer some further evidence.

For example, in the Tecumseh study, Johnson et al. (1965) found consistently positive correlations between parents' and children's (and siblings') blood pressures, and Zinner et al. (1985) also found a familial aggregation of blood pressure in childhood. The Bogalusa study reported a similar finding (Shear et al., 1986), i.e., a relationship between consistently raised blood pressure and a family history of hypertension, diabetes mellitus, or stroke. Likewise, Feinleib et al. (1977) showed that there was a familial aggregation of blood pressure, glucose intolerance, uric acid, triglyceride level, and, possibly, obesity. Law et al. (1991) found that blood pressure in children aged 4 years was more closely associated with their mothers' than their fathers' blood pressure. Furthermore, Margetts et al. (1991) reported from a study in a rural African population that the blood pressure of children under 8 years was related to their mother's weight at 6 months of that pregnancy, but in older children blood pressure was strongly inversely related to mothers' weight gain in the last trimester. These authors offer the tentative explanation "that among younger children blood pressure levels are largely determined by rates of maturation, which are themselves determined by, among other factors, maternal size. Among older children, however, the long-term effects of adverse intrauterine influences become apparent" (Margetts et al., 1991). The Brompton follow-up study of children during the first 10 years of life (de Swiet et al., 1992) found an increasing relationship with age in both tracking and correlation of mother's and child's blood pressure, and a relationship with height (and more strongly with weight) (Clarke et al., 1986; Whincup et al., 1989). In the Brompton study, despite the evidence of tracking, the variability of blood pressure up to age 10 years was not sufficiently strong for the authors to recommend screening of unselected children for later life risk.

Prospective studies (see Chapter 1) of the associations of childhood health and circumstances with later blood pressure confirm many of these relationships. Simpson et al. (1981) in a birth cohort study showed an association of children's blood pressure measured at age 7 with low birthweight. Marmot et al. (1980) found a relationship between breast feeding and lower mean plasma cholesterol in a sample of women selected from a national birth cohort study at age 32 years. In the whole population of the same birth cohort, Wadsworth et al. (1985) noted that low birthweight and systolic blood pressure at age 36 were related. This association held after excluding the effects of several possible confounders, including cigarette smoking (see Chapter 1). Similarly, Barker et al. (1989b), using data from two national birth cohort studies, reaffirmed the low birthweight relationship with adult and childhood blood pressure and also showed that it was independent of gestational age. This investigation found that, although there were no longer large geographic variations in birthweight among children born in Britain in 1970, nevertheless mothers and children who lived in areas of current high cardiovascular mortality were significantly shorter than others, and these mothers had higher mean diastolic blood pressures.

Geographic studies provide evidence both for and against associations among child health, social circumstances, and adult cardiovascular risk. Whincup et al. (1988) measured blood pressure in children aged 5 to 7 in nine British towns and found intertown variation in means corresponding to those of middle-aged men in the same towns and to town-specific risks for stroke mortality. They concluded that "population blood pressure levels in adults may be affected by factors which are of less importance in childhood (particularly alcohol consumption), or which do not differ to the same extent between children as between adults (particularly body build)" (Whincup et al., 1988). However, other studies provide reminders of the importance of the environment by showing the effect on blood pressure of migration (Beaglehole et al., 1978; Marmot, 1984). In Britain, a place-of-birth study showed that regional variation in blood pressure among adult men was strongly associated with the place where the most years of life had been spent, rather than with the place of birth (Elford et al., 1990).

Respiratory Illness

Large Population Investigations Using Historical Sources

In an historical study of childhood respiratory infection and adult chronic bronchitis, Barker and Osmond (1986b) found in the 212 administrative areas of England and Wales a strong correlation between infant mortality from bronchitis and pneumonia in 1921 to 1925, and mortality from chronic bronchitis in the population aged 35 to 74 years in 1968 to 1978. Areas of highest infant mortality from bronchitis and pneumonia in the past were most likely to be those with the highest adult mortality from chronic bronchitis 40 and more years later. These infant-adult correlations prompt the authors to conclude that "high mortality from chronic bronchitis in England and Wales, especially in the towns, is another legacy of poor social conditions which led to high rates of respiratory infection in young children" (Barker & Osmond, 1986b).

In a later analysis, Barker, Osmond, and Law (1989c) found that in the same English and Welsh administrative areas adult mortality from chronic bronchitis between 1968 and 1978 was strongly correlated with postneonatal mortality, but not with neonatal mortality in 1911 to 1925. This is further evidence for the risk of adult chronic bronchitis being established in early childhood, rather than in utero or in very early life.

Large population studies also offer some information about the role played by place of birth. Rosenbaum (1961) found that servicemen carried a risk of experiencing respiratory illness that was significantly related to their place of birth, as did Reid and Fletcher (1971) who showed that British and Norwegian migrants to the United States carried with them their native country's risk of chronic bronchitis. In a national study, Osmond, Barker, and Slattery (1990) analyzed place of birth on English and Welsh death certificates issued between 1969 and 1972 and reported that those born in particular towns and urban areas, which were generally places of high population density and/or concentrations of industry, had a significantly raised risk of death from chronic bronchitis.

Risk Factors

Social and Environmental Factors

Unlike cardiovascular disease, studies of lower respiratory illness have consistently noted that it was much more of a burden on the poor than on other sections of the community. For example, two early postwar studies of London children (Brimblecombe et al., 1958; Payling Wright & Payling Wright, 1945) showed an increased risk of respiratory illness in homes that were below the poverty line, overcrowded, and cold and concluded that these circumstances were conducive to an increased risk of infection.

Findings of greater risk of lower respiratory illness among those in poor socioeconomic circumstances continue to be reported. Holland et al. (1969) found significantly better respiratory function among children in upper social class families, and Mann et al. (1992) showed an increased risk of lower respiratory illness among children in low socioeconomic circumstances.

Naturally, in view of the demographic variation in risk reported above, the environment has been investigated as a source of risk. Before the control of atmospheric pollution from the incomplete combustion of coal, the elevated risk associated with pollution was evident, particularly in the significant increases in urban mortality among the very young and the elderly that occurred during winter fogs in London (Logan, 1956). Although there was a gradual reduction in mortality associated with this source of pollution (Chinn et al., 1981), the expected sharp decline did not follow legislation to control this risk factor (Barker & Osmond, 1986b).

Other environmental risk factors have been investigated inside the home, ranging from poor housing (McCarthy et al., 1985; Ross, et al., 1990), gas cooking (Melia et al., 1982a and b; Ogston et al., 1985), and passive smoking (Colley et al., 1974; Tager et al., 1983) to several more recent comprehensive studies (Taussig et al., 1989, Wright et al., 1989).

A familial similarity in risk for respiratory problems has been a persistent finding (Leeder et al., 1976a and b; Mann et al., 1992), but is not explained by demographic differences or smoking (Speizer et al., 1976). This similarity may possibly have been the result of shared environmental factors, but it may also indicate a familial "constitutional susceptibility" (Fletcher et al., 1976).

An important change in emphasis in social and environmental studies came with Reid's (1969) synthesis of earlier work. He noted the "pessimistic fatalism about the prospects for effective prevention" of chronic bronchitis and suggested that it had been a mistake to concentrate research so much on adults. Reid (1969) concluded it likely that "despite the improvement in adolescence, the bronchitic child is father to the bronchitic man." He also speculated about the clues offered by earlier work:

> Does air pollution or cold aggravate respiratory disease by reducing the resistance of the respiratory tract to secondary invasions? Does the special susceptibility of social classes IV and V lie in some innate poverty of physique, or in the inadequacy of diet or crowded homes? And which comes first, the poor lung function or the repeated attacks of respiratory infection? Or are both poor function and recurrent illness simply different manifestations of an inadequate physical endowment? (Reid, 1969).

This review of evidence based on population-scale investigations indicated the need for long-term studies of individual children using retrospective and prospective data collection methods.

Retrospective Studies

Retrospective research using parents' (or others) reports of early childhood respiratory illness have shown increased risks by measuring contemporary respiratory problems in cases and controls. Lunn et al. (1967) found that 5-year-olds with a reported history of pneumonia or bronchitis had a significantly lower $FEV_{0.75}$ than controls. Burrows et al. (1977) asked adults to report respiratory illness before 16 years and found significantly lower FEV_1 and $VMAX_{25}$ among those with such a history; similarly, Cooreman et al. (1990) noted a significantly increased risk of lower respiratory illness in adults who had such disease in infancy. Fletcher et al. (1976) used the same technique with adult men and found that a reported history of childhood pneumonia, chronic bronchitis, or pleurisy was significantly associated with low FEV values, even after allowing for the effects of age and smoking.

Two studies made use of the catch-up method with populations whose respiratory health had been studied during childhood. An important limitation of this technique arises when the investigator is unable to contact a large proportion of the original population. For example, the findings from Harnett and Mair's (1963) investigation, in which only 46% of patients and 44% of controls could be found 30 years after they had been assessed for recurrent catarrh or bronchitis, are generally discounted because of the small numbers achieved at follow-up. The catch-up approach with hospital patients is, however, usually more complete. After a 10-year period, Pullan and Hey (1982) followed up 72% children seen initially as hospital inpatients with respiratory syncytial virus lower respiratory tract infection during their first year of life. Compared with controls, the index subjects' increased rates of reported wheezing, their threefold increase in bronchial lability (with no excess of atopy), and their reduced maximum expiratory flow rate were concluded to have been the result of damage either to the developing lung through infection or to pre-existing airway differences. This damage might have increased subsequent susceptibility to infection by the virus. Mok and Simpson (1984) also found an increased risk of lower respiratory illnesses, reduced respiratory function, and increased bronchial reactivity 7 years after admission to a hospital for acute lower respiratory disease in infancy. Samet et al. (1983) reviewed such studies and concluded that "injury to the developing lung may introduce permanent changes. Infections by respiratory syncytial virus involved the small airways and clinically severe infections may have lasting effects. Further longitudinal investigations are needed to clarify the complicated interrelationships among atopy, respiratory infection, and airways reactivity."

More recently, Schwartz et al. (1990), in seeking predictors of wheeze and asthma in children up to 11 years in a large national sample in the United States, found an association with low birth weight, after adjustment for confounding variables. Their additional finding of an association of wheeze and asthma with low maternal age offers support for their conclusions that the relationship may be associated with problems in the intrauterine environment. Strope et al. (1991) used early life case notes to establish a relationship of reduced lung function in boys 6 to 18 years after preschool episodes of lower respiratory illness and wheezing. They showed that the episodes of wheezing were necessary for the relationship to retain its significance.

Catch-up studies that begin with medical case notes and find their subjects at later times have also been ingeniously used by Barker et al. (1991). They traced a population of men, born between 1920 and 1930, whose records of birth and health in the first 5 years of life had been preserved. This team traced death certificates of those who had not survived and visited 73% of the survivors who still lived in the same district of birth. Information was collected on current health and past medical and social history. They reported that current mean FEV_1, fell with decreasing birthweight and suggested that this "may be a consequence of an adverse environment in utero which retards the weight gain of the fetus and irrevocably constrains the growth of the airways" (Barker et al., 1991). Among the small number of deaths (55), the death rate from chronic obstructive airways disease fell with increasing birthweight and with weight at age 1 year.

Cross-Sectional and Prospective Studies

The problems of failure of recollection or its distortion, both of which are inherent in retrospective studies, are mostly avoided by prospective studies. The same is true for difficulties experienced in "catching up" with information or with individuals after a few years. Holland et al. (1969) used a mixed design, i.e., by starting a large prospective study of children (aged 5, 11, and 14 years at entry) based on reports of earlier bronchitis or pneumonia. This study found a significant reduction in PEFR at first measurement among those reporting earlier lower respiratory illness. This reduction occurred in children with and without asthma at study entry (Hamman et al., 1975), and at measurements made 5 years later (Bland et al., 1974). The investigators also demonstrated problems of recollection by asking parents on two occasions for their child's history of lower respiratory illness. On the second occasion 17% to 24% did not mention bronchitis or pneumonia (Hamman et al., 1975).

A prospective study, from birth to 5 years, confirmed the findings of a reduced PEFR in those with a history of pneumonia or bronchitis (Leeder et al., 1976a). In a 5-year follow-up study, Kerrebijn et al. (1977) found higher rates of symptoms and increased prevalence of cough in those who had previously reported bronchitis or pneumonia. A 13-year follow-up study, with annual contacts for spirometry and clinical evaluation of children aged 4 to 10 years at entry, found significantly lower FEVs among those who experienced lower respiratory illness before age 2 and also two or more acute lower respiratory illnesses during any 1 year of the study (Gold et al., 1989). Experience of pneumonia or hospital admission for lower respiratory illness before entering the study was associated with low FEV at entry and with a slower increase in FEV at subsequent follow-up. Both this study and that of Taussig (1977) found that at 4 years girls had greater flow rates than boys and suggested that this advantage for girls might offer them greater protection against severe lower respiratory tract illness. This relationship was likely to equalize at around age 5 when boys experience a growth spurt.

The Tucson Children's Respiratory Study followed up 124 children first recruited at age 6 months, before any experience of lower respiratory illness, and with lung function measured at that age (Taussig et al., 1989). After follow-up of this American population during the second and third years of life, Martinez et al. (1991) reported that children who had diminished airway function at entry were at significantly greater risk of subsequent wheezing illness and, if they had also had at least one other respiratory illness episode, were also at significant respiratory disadvantage at the time of this follow-up. In another prospective study of Australian infants selected on the grounds of good respiratory health histories at a mean age of 4½ weeks, Young et al. (1991) found airway responsiveness, which they suggest was present from birth, was associated with either a family history of asthma, parental smoking, or both. These authors concluded that the next task is to find whether this initial level of airway responsiveness is related to "future levels of responsiveness, respiratory problems, and immunological markers after exposure to environmental insults during infancy" (Young et al., 1991). Hanrahan et al. (1992) are following up a population of children whose mothers were selected into the study at registration for antenatal care and whose mothers' smoking during pregnancy was assessed both by reports and by biochemical methods. The babies' pulmonary function tests were undertaken before the end of the 50th postconception week in order to distinguish prenatal from postnatal effects of maternal smoking. This study concluded that prenatal maternal smoking had a considerable deleterious effect on forced expiratory flow levels in very early life; the authors hypothesized that such smoking may contribute to risk of acute and chronic respiratory illness in older children, as other studies have shown, "possibly (by) causing a relative decrease in airway size or altering lung elastic properties (Hanrahan et al., 1992).

Dockery et al. (1983) reported tracking of two indices of lung function in a large community-based sample of children from ages 6 to 11 years. Tracking of a wider range of lung function measures was reported by Hibbert et al. (1990) in a 5-year longitudinal study of healthy children beginning at mean ages 8.8 years and 12.6 years. The authors concluded that "lung growth tracks and that growth of the respiratory system is occurring in an ordered manner relative to the first time point. . . . The high tracking indices continued through adolescence, the period of most rapid growth" Hibbert et al., 1990). It was suggested that growth charts for lung function would permit early detection of deviation from expected lung development.

Attempts to account for apparent associations among childhood respiratory health, social circumstances, and adult respiratory health depend ultimately on studies that follow progress from childhood into adult life. The extended associations from early childhood to adult life hypothesized in the historical, geographic, and environmental studies described above were supported by prospective studies. The three British national birth cohort studies showed that among those who had experienced lower respiratory disease in infancy there was a significantly increased risk of such illness later in childhood (Anderson et al., 1986), in adolescence (Colley et al., 1973), and in adult life (Britten et al., 1987; Kiernan et al., 1976; Mann et al., 1992; Strachan et al., 1988).

The value of these studies lies in their long time span and the opportunity they provide to take account of a wide range of possible confounding factors. For example, the longest of the cohort studies, from birth to 43 years, found that PEFR at 36 years and the experience of lower respiratory illness between ages 20 and 36 years were significantly associated with poor home circumstances and parental bronchitis in early life and with the later life risk factors of smoking, adult asthma/wheeze, and atmospheric pollution. However, the early life factors had the greatest attributable risk (Mann et al., 1992). In this same study, those who had experienced early childhood risk but who were still free from lower respiratory illness at age 36 years had significantly lower PEFR measures at that age.

Discussion

Summary of Methods

This chapter illustrates the range of epidemiologic techniques available for examining evidence of a relationship between health in early life or in utero and health in adulthood. In both the cardiovascular and respiratory studies, the progression of work has often been initiated by large population studies that sought biologically plausible explanations for observed geographic and social variations in infant and adult mortality. Place-of-birth studies have been used to confirm suspected early life long-term effects, whereas migrant studies serve to test for the sensitivity of relationships to environmental and cultural change. The value of existing medical records has been shown repeatedly, both in the follow-up studies of patients and in the catch-up studies of individuals whose early medical records could be traced. These studies and the population investigations have also made extensive use of death certificate data. The prospective studies have searched for associations over long periods, with the benefit of information on possible confounding factors during the intervening years.

Comments on Methods

Most epidemiologic discussion of this kind of work has been concerned with the validity of findings from the large population studies. Commentators point to the problems of interpretation when such portmanteau variables as socioeconomic status are used (Davey Smith & Phillips 1991). These authors note how difficult it is to take account of confounding factors in population studies. Ben Shlomo and Davey Smith (1991), commenting on the Barker and Osmond (1986a) report of correlations between infant mortality and later adult mortality from ischemic heart disease (IHD), showed that after adjustment for the effects of current (1971) social deprivation, there was no longer a significant correlation between infant mortality in 1895 to 1908 and adult death rates from IHD in 1969 to 1973. However, they also caution that this "cannot be taken as showing that early life factors have no role in the aetiology of adult disease. It is essential to remember that neither infant mortality nor the deprivation score is a direct cause of disease; they are crude proxy measures of whatever factors are truly causal" (Ben Shlomo & Davey Smith, 1991). Elford et al. (1992) noted that another problem in the interpretation of these population studies' findings is that "those born into relative disadvantage at the beginning of the century may experience poor health as adults as a result of continuing hardship" (see also Bradley, 1991). However, long-term effects of childhood factors on adult respiratory problems and on adult blood pressure and cardiovascular risk have been found after controlling for social class (Barker & Martyn 1992, Mann et al., 1992).

There has also been some criticism of the hypotheses put forward by researchers who present large population study findings on cardiovascular disease. In the ten studies reviewed by Elford, Shaper, and Whincup (1992) there seemed to be a lack of specificity in several aspects, e.g., in the timing of early life disadvantage and the role of poverty, adversity, and prosperity. They also criticized the concentration on cardiovascular mortality and were concerned with the relative lack of consistency of findings and of hypotheses to account for them. However, as they acknowledge, such investigations are often best viewed as "hypothesis generating" (see Chapter 1), and it should be noted, those reviewed have been carried out over a period of 14 years, during which time ideas have changed. On the other hand, large population studies have generated enthusiasm for moving to the next stage of epidemiologic research. This stage demands ingenuity in devising data collection methods to permit the study of individuals over sufficiently long periods in order to explore possible pathways from early life to adult health.

Studies of individuals are also not without their own problems of method. Elford et al. (1991) reviewed 15 longitudinal and case-control studies of individuals' early life experience and later cardiovascular risk and illness. They noted a lack of specificity in formulating hypotheses, an inconsistency in relationships, and insufficient control of confounding factors. But, as Robinson (1992) noted, the results of only two papers conflicted with the findings of a relationship between early life factors and adult cardiovascular disease and associated risk factors. Studies of individuals that rely on recall (and nearly every method does so to some degree) are subject to the problems of forgetting and memory distortion and are therefore bound by the constraints on what it is reasonable to ask a person to remember. Prospective studies offer the opportunity to explore the sequence and accumulation of risk and the pathways through which risk increases or is reduced. They must, however, decide which information to collect to test hypotheses that may not become testable, or even current, until many years have passed (Wadsworth, 1991). Because beginning a new prospective study on the relationship of early life factors to adult health involves a wait of many years, researchers have made good use of the opportunities offered by the few such studies that exist and by sets of birth records that have survived for 50 years and more. Any single prospective study also has the problems of not knowing whether the same relationships would be found if the study was undertaken at another time or in another culture. The opportunity to use a prospective design to investigate period effect on individuals in cohorts born at different times is rarely available. However, a mixed design, such as that used by Holland et al. (1969), enables that requirement to be achieved in a relatively short period in one study by the simultaneous initiation of studies of groups at different ages. Cross-cultural comparisons are rare, except in cross-sectional studies (e.g., Marmot, 1992; Poulter et al., 1984), and they raise particularly difficult problems in the long-term study of health.

Explanations

The epidemiologic studies of relationships between health in childhood and adult cardiovascular disease offer two kinds of explanations. First, those concerned with the uterine environment involve conclusions based on associations of poor maternal health in pregnancy or poor child health in early life with increased adult risk of heart disease indicators: raised blood pressure, raised plasma fibrinogen and factor VII concentrations, impaired glucose tolerance, or death from ischemic heart disease. Explanations offered involve the "effects on physiology and metabolism imposed by an adverse environment during critical periods of life" (Barker & Martyn, 1992), and such postulated mechanisms are supported by evidence from studies of developing animals (Barker & Martyn, 1992; Bock & Whelan, 1991).

The second group of explanations concerns adversity in childhood. They are largely derived from studies of breast feeding, which has been suggested to be a source of long-term protection from cardiovascular risk (perhaps by protecting against diarrhea and promoting efficient metabolism of cholesterol) and, rather less speculatively, a source of risk. A catch-up study showed increased adult cardiovascular risk and death in individuals who had been breast fed for a year or more or exclusively bottle fed, and explanations included infant programming of lifetime lipid metabolism (Fall et al., 1992; Lucas, 1991). A nutritional programming process has also been proposed to explain the epidemiologic relationship of early fetal and infant growth and its association with the raised risk of cardiovascular disease and non-insulin-dependent diabetes (Hales et al., 1991; Robinson et al., 1991).

Similar explanations have been suggested for the associations between early life factors and adult respiratory health. Barker et al. (1991) suggested that risk is established by poor airway growth in utero, and this hypothesis is supported both by results of animal studies and by the findings of Schwartz et al. (1990), Martinez et al. (1991), Young et al. (1991), and Hanrahan et al. (1992). These last authors also speculated that reduced lung elasticity may be associated with problems experienced in utero. Yet, whereas Barker et al. (1991) suggested malnutrition and poor socioeconomic circumstances as sources of such problems, the work of Young et al. (1991) implicates parental smoking and a family history of asthma. As Barker et al. (1991) noted, mothers in their study were pregnant at a time when maternal smoking was uncommon, and therefore both of these hypothesized sources of fetal insult may be damaging to airway development and perhaps also to lung elasticity. The long-term deleterious effects of lower respiratory illness in the first 2 years of life, as found in many studies, are thought to increase the vulnerability to insult encountered in later life through damage to the developing lung by host factors, air pollutants, or viral infections (Glezen, 1989).

Tracking of blood pressure and lung function in childhood, and of lung function in adolescence, also adds support to the notion that long-term functional capacity is established in early life.

All these postulates have been the subject of controversy, both in relation to method, as already described, and interpretation. Bradley (1991) noted that low birthweight is common in developing countries, but cardiovascular disease is not. However, the processes described by Margetts et al. (1991) as leading to low birthweight in rural African children are also those found to be associated with raised cardiovascular risk on Western countries: therefore it may be that as a longer life-span becomes possible for low birthweight children in developing countries, they will be found to be at correspondingly high risk of cardiovascular problems. It is possible that genetic determinants are responsible for many of the early life problems and their apparent risk to respiratory and cardiovascular health in later life. However, Barker and Martyn (1992) cite Carr-Hill et al. (1987) in support of their claim that "birth weight does not seem to be strongly genetically determined," and they suggest that there is little "evidence that cardiovascular disease has, in the vast majority of people, a major genetic component." Findings of the epidemiologic studies reported in this chapter, particularly those concerned with cardiovascular disease, which are more controversial and currently less widely accepted than those of long-term effects on adult respiratory problems, should not necessarily be seen as being in conflict with those that suggest that risk is largely determined through the adult environment. It is becoming clear that many adult risk factors, such as being overweight (Law et al., 1992), choice of diet (Braddon et al., 1988), and exercise habits (Kuh and Cooper 1992), are themselves associated with early life circumstances.

At present there is evidence for in utero and infant long-term effects on the adult risk of cardiovascular and lower respiratory illness. It remains to be seen how far these effects may be the result of genetic predispositions, of environmentally caused damage to the developing fetus or infant at a critical period of growth, or of continuing adverse environmental effects. Biologic programming established by early life prenatal and/or infant damage seems a likely proposition, and so too does cultural programming through the continuing influence of poor socioeconomic circumstances, low educational attainment, and consequent continuing adverse health behavior. These two concepts of programming are not incompatible.

Conclusions

Epidemiologic studies of long-term associations between childhood and adult life have been innovative. Findings from these studies offer strong evidence of the role of early life in the establishment of risk of adult cardiovascular and lower respiratory problems. They suggest new hypotheses to be explored in clinical and laboratory studies and to be investigated in greater detail in new epidemiologic research.

References

Anderson HR, Bland JM, Patel S, Peckham C. The natural history of asthma in childhood. *J Epidemiol Comm Health* 1986; 40:121–129.

Barker DJP, Martyn CN. The maternal and fetal origins of cardiovascular disease. *J Epidemiol Comm Health* 1992; 46:8–11.

Barker DJP, Osmond C. Infant mortality, childhood nutrition and ischaemic heart disease in England and Wales. *Lancet* 1986a; 1:1077–1081.

Barker DJP, Osmond C. Childhood respiratory infection and adult chronic bronchitis in England and Wales. *Br Med J* 1986b; 293:1271–1275.

Barker DJP, Osmond C. Death rates from stroke in England and Wales predicted from past maternal mortality. *Br Med J* 1987; 295:83–86.

Barker DJP, Winter PD, Osmond C, Margetts B, Simmonds SJ. Weight in infancy and death from ischaemic heart disease. *Lancet* 1989a; 2:577–580.

Barker DJP, Osmond C, Golding J, Kuh D, Wadsworth MEJ. Growth in utero, blood pressure in childhood and adult life, and mortality from cardiovascular disease. *Br Med J* 1989b; 298:564–567.

Barker DJP, Osmond C, Law CM. The intrauterine and early postnatal origins of cardiovascular disease and chronic bronchitis. *J Epidemiol Comm Health* 1989c; 43:237–240.

Barker DJP, Bull AR, Osmond C, Simmonds SJ. Fetal and placental size and risk of hypertension in adult life. *Br Med J* 1990; 301:259–262.

Barker DJP, Godfrey KM, Fall C, Osmond C, Winter PD, Shaheen SO. The relation of birthweight and infant respiratory infection to adult lung function and death from chronic obstructive airways disease. *Br Med J* 1991; 303:671–675.

Barker DJP, Godfrey KM, Osmond C, Bull AR. The relation of fetal length, ponderal index and head circumference to blood pressure and the risk of hypertension in adult life. *Paediatr Perinat Epidemiol* 1992a; 6:35–44.

Barker DJP, Meade TW, Fall CHD, Lee A, Osmond C, Phipps K, Stirling Y. Relation of fetal and infant growth to plasma fibrinogen and factor VII in adult life. *Br Med J* 1992b; 304:148–152.

Beaglehole R, Eyles E, Salmond C, Prior I. Blood pressure in Tokelau children in two contrasting environments. *Am J Epidemiol* 1978; 108:283–288.

Ben-Shlomo Y, Davey Smith G. Deprivation in infancy or adult life: which is more important for mortality risk? *Lancet* 1991; 337:530–534.

Bland JM, Holland WW, Elliott A. The development of respiratory symptoms in a cohort of Kent schoolchildren. *Bull Physiopathol Respir* 1974; 10:699.

Bock GR, Whelan J. *The Childhood Environment and Adult Disease*. Ciba Foundation Symposium 156. Chichester: John Wiley; 1991.

Braddon FEM, Wadsworth MEJ, Davies JMC, Cripps HA. Social and regional differences in food and alcohol consumption and their measurement in a national birth cohort. *J Epidemiol Comm Health* 1988; 17:525–529.

Bradley PJ. Fetal and infant origins of adult disease. *Br Med J* 1991; 302:113.

Brimblecombe FSW, Cruickshank R, Masters PL, Reid DD, Stewart GT, Sanderson D. Family studies of respiratory infections. *Br Med J* 1958; 1:119–128.

Britten N, Davies JMC, Colley JRT. Early respiratory experience and subsequent cough and peak expiratory flow rate in 36 year old men and women. *Br Med J* 1987; 294:1317–1320.

British Parliamentary Papers. *Report of the Interdepartmental Committee on Physical Deterioration*. Cmnd. 2175, 2210, 2186. London: HMSO; 1904.

Buck C, Simpson H. Infant diarrhoea and subsequent mortality from heart disease and cancer. *J Epidemiol Comm Health* 1982; 36:27–30.

Burrows B, Knudson RJ, Lebowitz MD. The relationship of childhood respiratory illness to adult obstructive airway disease. *Am Rev Respir Dis* 1977; 115:751–760.

Butler NR, Alberman ED. *Second Report of the 1958 British Perinatal Morbidity Survey*. Edinburgh: Churchill Livingstone; 1969.

Carr-Hill R, Campbell DM, Hall MH, Meredith A. Is birth weight determined genetically? *Br Med J* 1987; 295:687–689.

Chinn S, Florey Cdu V, Baldwin IG, Gorgol M. The relationship of mortality in England and Wales to measurements of air pollution. *J Epidemiol Comm Health* 1981; 35:174–179.

Clarke WR, Schrott HG, Burns TL, Sing CF, Lauer RM. Aggregation of blood pressure in the families of children with labile high systolic blood pressure. *Am J Epidemiol* 1986; 123:67–80.

Colley JRT, Douglas JWB, Reid DD. Respiratory disease in young adults; Influence of early childhood lower respiratory tract illness, social class, air pollution, and smoking. *Br Med J* 1973; 2:195–198.

Colley JRT, Holland WW, Corkhill RT. Influence of passive smoking and parental phlegm on pneumonia and bronchitis in early childhood. *Lancet* 1974; 2:1031–1034.

Cooreman J, Redon S, Levallois M, Liard R, Perdrizet S. Respiratory history during infancy and childhood, and respiratory conditions in adulthood. *Int J Epidemiol* 1990; 19:621–627.

Davey Smith G, Phillips A. Socioeconomic conditions and ischaemic heart disease. *Br Med J* 1991; 302:113–114.

de Swiet M, Fayers P, Shinebourne EA. Blood pressure in first 10 years of life; the Brompton study. *Br Med J* 1992; 304:23–26.

Dockery DW, Berkey CS, Ware JH, Speizer FE, Ferris BG. Distribution of forced vital capacity and forced expiratory volume in one second in children 6 to 11 years of age. *Am Rev Respir Dis* 1983; 128:405–412.

Dwork D. *War is Good for Babies and Other Young Children. A History of the Infant and Child Welfare Movement in England 1898–1918*. London: Tavistock Publications; 1987.

Elford J, Phillips A, Thomson AG, Shaper AG. Migration and geographic variations in blood pressure in Britain. *Br Med J* 1990; 300:291–295.

Elford J, Whincup P, Shaper AG. Early life experience and adult cardiovascular disease: longitudinal and case control studies. *Int J Epidemiol* 1991; 20:833–844.

Elford J, Shaper AG, Whincup P. Early life experiences and adult cardiovascular disease: ecological studies. *J Epidemiol Comm Health* 1992; 46:1–11.

Fall CHD, Barker DJP, Osmond C, Winter PD, Clark PMS, Hales CN. Relation of infant feeding to adult serum cholesterol concentration and death from ischaemic heart disease. *Br Med J* 1992; 304:801–805.

Feinleib M, Garrison RJ, Fabsitz R, Christian JC, Hrubec Z, Borhani NO, Kannel WB, Rosenman R, Schwartz JT, Wagner JO. The NHLBI twin study of cardiovascular disease risk factors: methodology and summary of results. *Am J Epidemiol* 1977; 106:284–295.

Fletcher CM, Peto R, Tinker C, Speizer FE. *The Natural History of Chronic Bronchitis and Emphysema*. Oxford: Oxford University Press; 1976.

Forsdahl A. Are poor living conditions in childhood and adolescence an important risk factor for arteriosclerotic heart disease? *Br J Prev Soc Med* 1977; 31:91–95.

Forsdahl A. Living conditions in childhood and subsequent development of risk factors for arteriosclerotic heart disease. *J Epidemiol Comm Health* 1978; 32:34–37.

Glezen WP. Antecedents of chronic and recurrent lung disease: childhood respiratory trouble. *Am Rev Respir Dis* 1989; 140:873–874.

Gold DR, Tager IB, Weiss ST, Tosteson TD, Speizer FE. Acute lower respiratory illness in childhood as a predictor of lung function and chronic respiratory symptoms. *Am Rev Respir Dis* 1989; 140:877–884.

Hales CN, Barker DJP, Clark PMS, Cox LJ, Fall C, Osmond C, Winter PD. Fetal and infant growth and impaired glucose tolerance at age 64. *Br Med J* 1991; 303:1019–1022.

Hamman RF, Halil T, Holland WW. Asthma in school children: demographic characteristics and peak expiratory flow rate compared in children with bronchitis. *Br J Prev Soc Med* 29:228–238.

Hanrahan JP, Tager IB, Segal MR, Tosteson TD, Castile RG, VanVunakis H, Weiss ST, Speizer FE. The effect of maternal smoking during pregnancy on early infant lung function. *Am Rev Respir Dis* 1992; 145:1129–1135.

Harnett RWF, Mair A. Chronic bronchitis and the catarrhal child. *Scot Med J* 1963; 8:175–184.

Hibbert ME, Hudson IL, Lanigan A, Landau LI, Phelan PD. Tracking of lung function in healthy children and adolescents. *Pediatr Pulmonol* 1990; 8:172–177.

Hofman A, Valkenburg HA, Maas J, Groustra FN. The natural history of blood pressure in childhood. *Int J Epidemiol* 1985; 14:91–96.

Holland WW, Halil T, Bennett AE, Elliott A. Factors influencing the onset of chronic respiratory disease. *Br Med J* 1969; 2:205–208.

Johnson BC, Epstein FH, Kjelsberg MO. Distributions and familial studies of blood pressure and serum cholesterol levels in a total community. *J Chron Dis* 1965; 18:147–160.

Kermack WO, McKendrick AG, McKinlay PL. Death rates in Great Britain and Sweden: some general regularities and their significance. *Lancet* 1934; 226:698–703.

Kerribijn KF, Hoogeveen S, Schroot HCN, van der Wal MC. Chronic non-specific respiratory disease in children: a five year follow-up study. *Acta Paediatr Scand* 1977; 261(suppl):3–72.

Kiernan KE, Colley JRT, Douglas JWB, Reid DD. Chronic cough in young adults in relation to smoking habits, childhood environment and chest illness. *Respiration* 1976; 33:236–244.

Kuh DJL, Cooper C. Physical activity at 36 years: patterns and childhood predictors in a longitudinal study. *J Epidemiol Comm Health* 1992; 46:114–119.

Labarthe DR. Coronary risk factors in childhood. In: Marmot MG, Elliott P, eds. *Coronary Heart Disease Epidemiology*. Oxford: Oxford University Press; 1992.

Law CM, Barker DJP, Bull AR, Osmond C. Maternal and fetal influences on blood pressure. *Arch Dis Child* 1991; 66:1291–1295.

Law CM, Barker DJP, Osmond C, Fall CHD, Simmonds SJ. Early growth and abdominal fatness in adult life. *J Epidemiol Comm Health* 1992; 46:184–186.

Leeder SR, Corkhill RT, Irwig LM, Holland WW, Colley JRT. Influence of family factors on asthma and wheezing during the first five years of life. *Br J Prev Soc Med* 1976a; 30:213–218.

Leeder SR, Corkhill RT, Wysocki MJ, Holland WW. Influence of personal and family factors on ventilatory function in childhood. *Br J Prev Soc Med* 1976b; 30:219–224.

Levine RS, Henneker CH, Klein B, Gourley B, Briese FW, Hokanson J, Gelband H, Jesse J. Tracking correlates of blood pressure levels in infancy. *Pediatrics* 1978; 61:121–125.

Logan WPD. Mortality from fog in London, January 1956. *Br Med J* 1956; 2:722–725.

Lucas A. Programming by early nutrition in man. In: Bock GR, Whelan J, eds. *The Childhood Environment and Adult Disease*. Ciba Foundation Symposium 156, Chichester: John Wiley; 1991.

Lunn JE, Knowelden J, Handyside AJ. Patterns of respiratory illness in Sheffield infant schoolchildren. *Br J Prev Soc Med* 1967; 21:7–16.

Mackenzie WL, Matthew E. *The Medical Inspection of School Children*. Edinburgh: William Hodge; 1904.

Mann SL, Wadsworth MEJ, Colley JRT. Accumulation of factors influencing respiratory illness in members of a national birth cohort and their offspring. *J Epidemiol Comm Health* 1992; 46:286–292.

Margetts BM, Rowland MGM, Foord FA, Cruddas AM, Cole TJ, Barker DJP. The relation of maternal weight to the blood pressures of Gambian children. *Int J Epidemiol* 1991; 20:938–943.

Marmot MG. Geography of blood pressure and hypertension. *Br Med Bull* 1984; 40:380–386.

Marmot MG. Coronary heart disease: rise and fall of a modern epidemic. In: Marmot MG, Elliott P, eds. *Coronary Heart Disease Epidemiology*. Oxford: Oxford University Press, 1992.

Marmot MG, Page CM, Atkins E, Douglas JWB. Effect of breast-feeding on plasma cholesterol and weight in young adults. *J Epidemiol Comm Health* 1980; 34:164–167.

Martinez FD, Morgan WJ, Wright AL, Holberg C, Taussig LM. Initial airway function is a risk factor for recurrent wheezing respiratory illnesses during the first three years of life. *Am Rev Respir Dis* 1991; 143:312–316.

McCarthy P, Byrne D, Harrison S, Keithley J. Respiratory conditions: effect of housing and other factors. *J Epidemiol Comm Health* 1985; 39:15–19.

Melia RJW, Florey Cdu V, Morris RW, Goldstein BD, Clark D, John HH. Childhood respiratory illness and the home environment. I. Relation between nitrogen dioxide, temperature and relative humidity. *Int J Epidemiol* 1982a; 11:155–163.

Melia RJW, Florey Cdu V, Morris RW, Goldstein BD, Clark D, John HH, Craighead IB, MacKinlay JC. Childhood respiratory illness and the home environment. II. Association between respiratory illness and nitrogen dioxide, temperature and relative humidity. *Int J Epidemiol* 1982b; 11:164–169.

Mok JYQ, Simpson H. Outcome for acute bronchitis, bronchiolitis, and pneumonia in infancy. *Arch Dis Child* 1984; 59:306–309.

Ogston SA, Florey Cdu V, Walker CHM. The Tayside infant morbidity and mortality study: effect on health of using gas for cooking. *Br Med J* 1985; 290:957–960.

Osmond C, Barker DJP, Slattery JM. Risk of death from cardiovascular disease and chronic bronchitis determined by place of birth in England and Wales. *J Epidemiol Comm Health* 1990; 44:139–141.

Payling Wright G, Payling Wright H. Etiological factors in broncho-pneumonia amongst infants in London. *J Hyg* 1945; 44:15–30.

Poulter NR, Khaw KT, Hopwood BEC, Mugambi M, Peart WS, Rose GA, Sever PS. Blood pressure and its correlates in an African tribe in urban and rural environments. *J Epidemiol Comm Health* 1984; 38:181–185.

Pullan CR, Hey EN. Wheezing, asthma, and pulmonary dysfunction 10 years after infection with respiratory syncytial virus. *Br Med J* 1982; 284:1665–1669.

Reid DD. The beginnings of chronic bronchitis. *Proc Roy Soc Med* 1969; 62:311–316.

Reid DD, Fletcher CM. International studies in chronic respiratory disease. *Br Med Bull* 1971; 27:59–64.

Robinson R. Is the child father of the man? Controversy about the early origins of cardiovascular disease. *Br Med J* 1992; 304:789–790.

Robinson SM, Wheeler T, Hayes MC, Barker DJP, Osmond C. Fetal heart rate and intrauterine growth. *Br J Obstet Gynaecol* 1991; 98:1223–1227.

Rosenbaum S. Home localities of national servicemen with respiratory disease. *Br J Prev Soc Med* 1961; 15:61–67.

Ross A, Collins M, Sanders C. Upper respiratory tract infection in children, domestic temperatures and humidity. *J Epidemiol Comm Health* 1990; 44:142–146.

Samet JM, Tager IB, Speizer F. The relationship between respiratory illness in childhood and chronic air-flow obstruction in adulthood. *Am Rev Respir Dis* 1983; 127:508–523.

Schwartz J, Gold D, Dockery DW, Weiss ST, Speizer FE. Predictors of asthma and persistent wheeze in a national sample of children in the United States. *Am Rev Respir Dis* 1990; 142:555–562.

Shear CL, Burke GL, Freedman DS, Berenson GS. Value of childhood blood pressure measurements and family history in predicting future blood pressure status: results from 8 years of follow-up in the Bogalusa heart study. *Pediatrics* 1986; 77:862–869.

Simpson A, Mortimer JG, Silva PA, Spears GF, Williams S. Correlates of blood pressure in a cohort of Dunedin seven year old children. In: Onesti G, Kim K, eds. *Hypertension in the Young and Old.* New York: Grune and Stratton; 1981; 155–163.

Speizer FE, Rosner B, Tager I. Familial aggregation of chronic respiratory disease. *Int J Epidemiol* 1976; 5:167–172.

Strachan DP, Anderson HR, Bland JM, Peckham C. Asthma as a link between chest illness in childhood and chronic cough and phlegm in young adults. *Br Med J* 1988; 296:890–893.

Strope GL, Stewart PL, Henderson FW, Ivins SS, Steadman HC, Henry MM. Lung function in school age children who had mild lower respiratory illness in early childhood. *Am Rev Respir Dis* 1991; 144:655–662.

Tager IB, Weiss ST, Munoz A, Rosner B, Speizer FE. Longitudinal study of the effects of maternal smoking on pulmonary function in children. *N Engl J Med* 1983; 309:699–703.

Taussig LM. Maximal expiratory flow rates at functional residual capacity: a test of lung function in young children. *Am Rev Respir Dis* 1977; 116:1031–1038.

Taussig LM, Wright AL, Morgan WJ, Harrison HR, Ray CG. The Tucson children's respiratory study: I, design and implementation of a prospective study of acute and chronic respiratory illness in children. *Am J Epidemiol* 1989; 129:1219–1231.

Wadsworth MEJ. *The Imprint of Time: Childhood, History, and Adult Life.* Oxford: Oxford University Press; 1991.

Wadsworth MEJ, Cripps HA, Midwinter RA, Colley JRT. Blood pressure at age 36 years and social and familial factors, cigarette smoking and body mass in a national birth cohort. *Br Med J* 1985; 291:1534–1538.

Whincup PH, Cook DG, Shaper AG. Early influences on blood pressure: a study of children age 5–7 years. *Br Med J* 1989; 299:587–591.

Whincup PH, Cook DG, Shaper AG, Macfarlane DJ, Walker M. Blood pressure in British children: associations with adult blood pressure and cardiovascular mortality. *Lancet* 1988; 2:890–893.

Williams DRR, Roberts SJ, Davies TW. Deaths from ischaemic heart disease and infant mortality in England and Wales. *J Epidemiol Comm Health* 1979; 33:199–202.

Wright AL, Taussig LM, Ray GC, Harrison HR, Holberg CJ. The Tucson children's respiratory study. II. Lower respiratory tract illness in the first year of life. *Am J Epidemiol* 1989; 129:1232–1246.

Young S, le Souef P, Geelhoed GC, Stick SM, Turner KJ, Landan LI. The influence of a family history of asthma and parental smoking on airway responsiveness in early infancy. *N Engl J Med* 1991; 324:1168–1173.

Zinner SH, Rosner B, Oh W, Kass EH. Significance of blood pressure in infancy: familial aggregation and predictive effect on later blood pressure. *Hypertension* 1985; 7:411–416.

Index

Note: Page numbers followed by t indicate tables; those followed by f refer to figures.

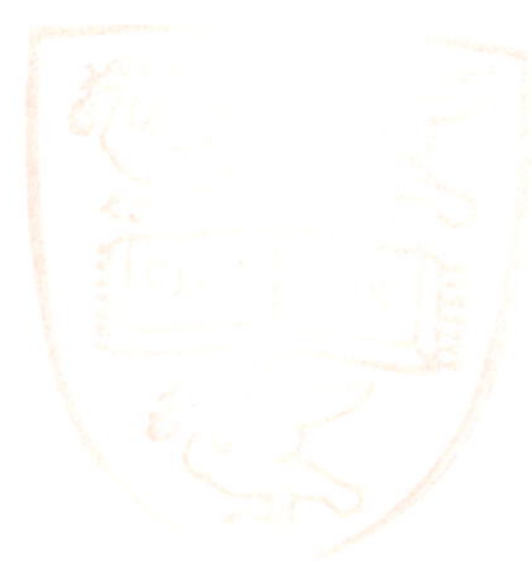